ANNUAL REPORTS IN MEDICINAL CHEMISTRY

Volume 13

CONTRIBUTORS

ANNUAL REPORTS IN MEDICINAL CHEMISTRY

Volume 13

Sponsored by the Division of Medicinal Chemistry of the American Chemical Society

Editor-in-Chief: ***FRANK H. CLARKE***

CIBA-GEIGY CORPORATION
ARDSLEY, NEW YORK

SECTION EDITORS

JOHN KRAPCHO • LESLIE HUMBER • GEORGE WHITFIELD

HANS-JÜRGEN HESS • H. B. RENFROE • CHRISTOPHER WALSH

ACADEMIC PRESS New York San Francisco London 1978

A Subsidiary of Harcourt Brace Jovanovich, Publishers

ACADEMIC PRESS RAPID MANUSCRIPT REPRODUCTION

ACADEMIC PRESS, INC.
111 Fifth Avenue, New York, New York 10003

United Kingdom Edition published by
ACADEMIC PRESS, INC. (LONDON) LTD.
24/28 Oval Road, London NW1 7DX

LIBRARY OF CONGRESS CATALOG CARD NUMBER: 66–26843

ISBN 0–12–040513–X

PRINTED IN THE UNITED STATES OF AMERICA

CONTENTS

I. CNS AGENTS

Section Editor: Leslie G. Humber, Ayerst Laboratories, Montreal, Canada

II. PHARMACODYNAMIC AGENTS

Section Editor: John Krapcho, Squibb Institute for Medical Research, Princeton, New Jersey

CONTENTS

III. CHEMOTHERAPEUTIC AGENTS

Section Editor: George B. Whitfield, The Upjohn Company, Kalamazoo, Michigan

CONTENTS

CONTENTS

CONTENTS

PREFACE

Annual Reports continues to bring together a composite of timely reviews of traditional subjects, appraisals of modern approaches to drug discovery and short summaries of less familiar subjects that may help to broaden the horizons for medicinal chemists. This volume has reviews of potential new drugs acting on the central nervous and cardiovascular systems and of pharmacodynamic and chemotherapeutic agents. These traditional sections have been retained but many of the chapters discuss current research trends. Thus, the CNS section has chapters which consider dopamine agonists, agents affecting GABA and interactions with the opiate receptor. Reflecting the increased importance of enzymes in medicinal research, there are chapters on agents affecting the renin-angiotensin system, on β-lactamases, on enzyme inhibitors and on proteolytic enzymes. Other modern topics include peptide conformation and interactions with DNA. Three chapters discuss drug metabolism from different points of view. Some subjects which normally are reviewed less frequently have been updated. These include diabetes, glucocorticoids and QSAR. Iron chelation and agents for heart failure are considered in this volume and there is a chapter on asymmetric synthesis.

These volumes of Annual Reports are made possible by the cooperative work of dedicated scientists and their secretaries who have taken time from busy schedules to serve as editors, authors and typists. We are all very much indebted to them and I wish to express sincere gratitude.

Frank H Clarke

Ardsley, New York
June 1978

Section I - CNS Agents

Editor: Leslie G. Humber, Ayerst Laboratories, Montreal, Canada

Chapter 1. Antidepressants

Ivo Jirkovsky and Wilbur Lippmann, Ayerst Laboratories, Montreal, Canada

In 1977, interest has continued in the discovery and evaluation of compounds which are relatively selective blockers of serotonin (5-HT) or noradrenalin (NA) uptake in view of the concept of subclasses of depression. Agents that block dopamine (DA) uptake or 5-HT receptors also received attention as potential antidepressants. For the first time, a clinical efficacy of relatively selective 5-HT uptake blockers has been demonstrated. Repeating the pattern noted last year, studies were carried out on the mode of action of antidepressants at the molecular level. New pharmacological methods to identify or to further distinguish between antidepressant agents were reported. Several compounds have remained in the focus of interest for a number of years, and the reader would find value in consulting the past issues of this series[1,2] for background information. Specific reviews on chlorimipramine,[3,4] doxepin,[5] maprotiline,[6] viloxazine,[7] lofepramine,[8] nomifensin,[9] and TRH[10,11] have appeared. Current knowledge on the depressive disorders[12] and serotonin neurons in the CNS[13] have been summarized. Also, clinical use of lithium in psychiatry[14] and antidepressant therapy by sleep deprivation[15] have been reviewed.

Fluvoxamine (1) was demonstrated to exhibit almost exclusive 5-HT uptake inhibiting properties being effective both *in vitro* and *in vivo* in rat brain.[16] The potency of 1 was similar to or greater than that of imipramine. It showed activities related to this action such as decreasing rat brain 5-HT turnover and potentiating the 5-HTP behavioral syndrome in the mouse. NA uptake *in vitro* and *in vivo* in rat brain and related pharmacological activities were unaffected, or only slightly inhibited; also, no inhibition of displacement of DA from rat brain *in vitro* was exhibited. A preliminary clinical trial was carried out with 1 in endogenous depressed patients employing a 5-week treatment (rising dose) with mean daily dosages of approximately 150 mg.[17] A marked improvement of the overall and detailed psychopathology was observed as early as the end of the first week of treatment and leveled off from the third week on. Bipolar patients tended to improve more than the unipolars, retarded depressions more than agitated ones.

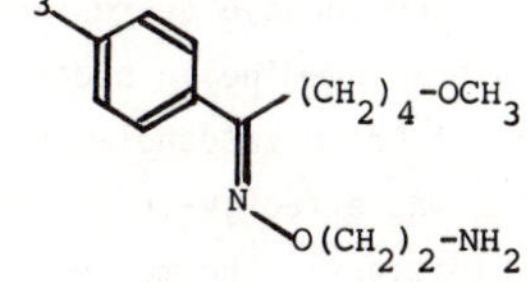

1

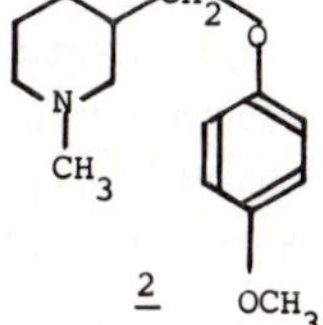

2

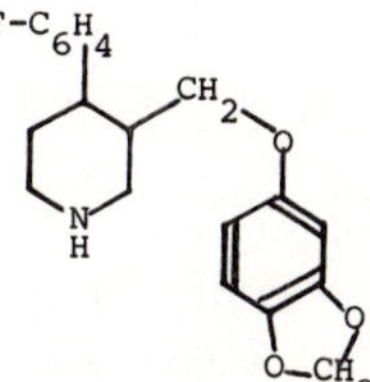

3

Femoxetine (FG-4963, 2) was found to be significantly inferior (at 3x200 mg/day) to amitriptyline (at 3x50 mg/day) in treatment of endogenously depressed patients over a 6-week period.[18] Effects of 2 on tyramine and NA pressor responses were weaker than those of amitriptyline. An analog FG-7051 (3) produced hypermotility and an anticonvulsant effect in combination with 5-HTP when given 1-6 h (0.4-1 mg/kg) or 24 h (5-15 mg/kg) prior to 5-HTP.[19] Chlorimipramine was active only at 20-50 mg/kg and 1-2 h before 5-HTP administration.

ISBN 0-12-040513-X

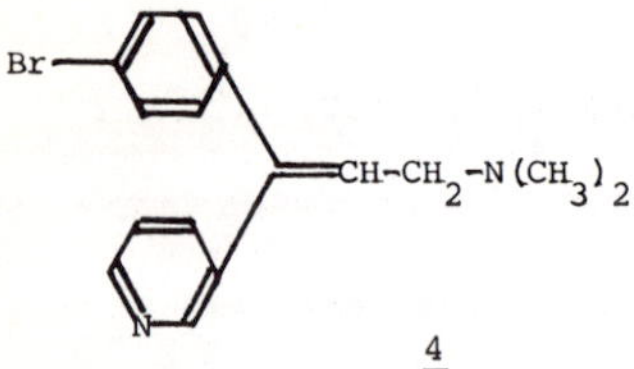

4

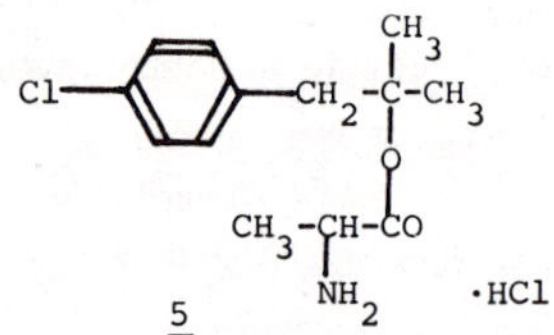

5

Zimelidine (H-102-10, 4) enhanced the spontaneous efflux of 5-HT from rat brain synaptosomes, but significantly inhibited its induced increase.[20] An initial clinical trial[21] with 4 in depressed patients utilized biochemical methodology and indicated potential usefulness of the drug. The 5-HT uptake was markedly inhibited in vitro by the plasma samples drawn from the patients. The study also confirmed that the desmethyl metabolite is approx. 10x as potent as the parent drug in inhibiting 5-HT uptake. Zimelidine was found to be a less potent cardiac depressant (myocardial contractility in dogs) than amitriptyline, although higher doses, by infusion, produced serious circulatory depression.[22] In an open clinical study,[23] 4 was administered for 20 days (150 mg/day) to 10 depressed female patients and good to moderate therapeutic responses were observed in 7 patients between the 4th and 12th day. The treatment had to be discontinued in 3 cases because of agitation symptoms. Alaproclate (A-23189, 5) was 3-30x less effective than chlorimipramine in increasing the induced efflux of 5-HT from rat brain synaptosomes.[20] The kinetics indicated competitive antagonism between 5 and p-chloroamphetamine. In blocking 5-HT uptake, 5 was less potent than chlorimipramine (8x in vitro and 2.5x in vivo).[24] Interestingly, 5 exhibited a 100-fold greater potency in blocking 5-HT than NA uptake. The SAR studies of alaproclate analogs suggested that the presence of the geminal dimethyl moiety was critical for the activity.

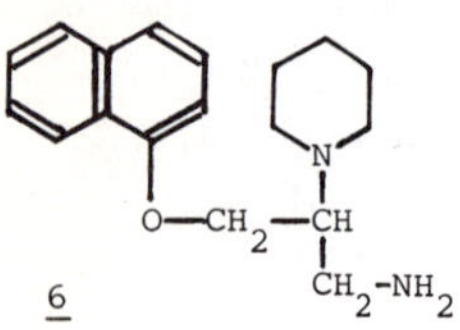

6

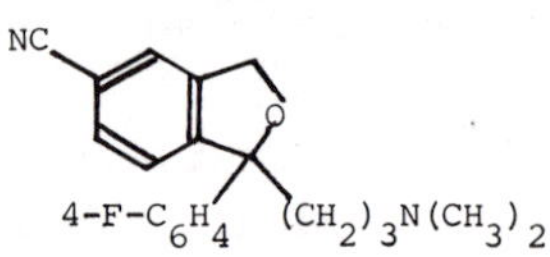

7

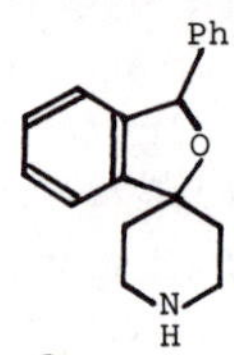

8

Compound 6, a derivative of (naphthalenyloxy)propanediamine, was reported to be a potent and specific inhibitor of the 5-HT neuronal uptake mechanism.[25] Similarly to chlorimipramine, 6 antagonized the depletion of rat brain 5-HT induced by various agents in vivo, potentiated the behavioral effects of 5-HTP and antagonized fenfluramine-induced anorexia. Compound 6 decreased rat brain 5-HT turnover. In vitro 6 was also equivalent in potency to chlorimipramine in blocking 5-HT uptake into rat brain. In vivo 6 and chlorimipramine did not block rat brain catecholamine uptake; 6 did not inhibit NA uptake in mouse heart whereas chlorimipramine was effective. Compound 6 did not exhibit appreciable anticholinergic effects or MAO inhibition in the mouse.

Citalopram (Lu 10-171, 7) is a new phthalane derivative exhibiting selective and potent inhibitory action on 5-HT uptake mechanism.[26] In this regard 7 was 2-10x more active than chlorimipramine in vitro or in vivo in different animal species and preparations. The metabolites of 7, i.e., the desmethyl-, didesmethyl-derivative and the corresponding N-oxide, showed generally weaker inhibitory activities. Compound 7 and its metabolites were devoid of NA uptake inhibiting activity, in contrast to chlorimipramine, and inhibited DA uptake only at extremely high concentrations; chlorimipramine exhibited the latter inhibitory activity at lower concentrations.

Citalopram reduced rat brain 5-hydroxyindoleacetic acid for 1-24 h, maximally at 2-6 h, whereas that of 5-HT was practically unchanged.[27] Thus, 7 decreased the turnover of brain 5-HT and this was confirmed in other models. In pharmacological tests, 7 potentiated the activities of 5-HT, 5-HTP and tryptophan in various species in vivo and in vitro and was 5-10x more active than chlorimipramine; the various metabolites were generally of lower potency.[28] Compound 7 induced or potentiated hyperthermia in animals treated with agents which increased 5-HT. Induced ptosis and immobility were only very weakly antagonized; very weak in vitro anticholinergic and antihistaminic activities were observed. These weak activities are in contrast to those of tricyclic antidepressants.[28] The spiro(isobenzofuran-piperidine) 8 (HP-505) was reported to prevent tetrabenazine ptosis and to inhibit brain NA uptake at lower concentrations than desipramine.[29] Relative to chlorimipramine, 8 was 2.5x less potent in blocking 5-HT uptake. Analogs of 8 containing a heteroatom attached to the nitrogen were prepared, and only the N-hydroxy derivative was equipotent with 8 in preventing tetrabenazine ptosis.[30]

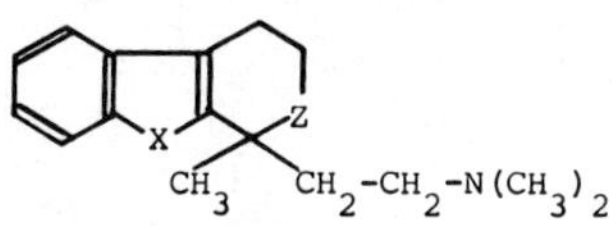

9 X = N-Et Z = S

10 X = N-Et Z = CH_2

11 X = CH_2 Z = O

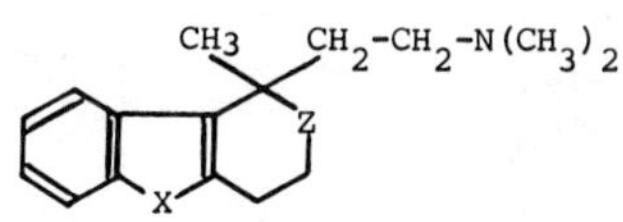

12 X = N-Et Z = S

13 X = CH_2 Z = O

Tandamine (AY-23,946, 9) was shown to inhibit DA uptake into human blood platelets.[31,32] In healthy subjects, 9 exhibited anticholinergic effects, and it was twice as active as desipramine in inhibiting tyramine pressor responses. Pharmacological screening of tandamine and related compounds demonstrated[33] that the desmethyl derivative, a major metabolite of 9, is considerably less potent than 9 in reversing reserpine hypothermia. The reversed annelation of thiopyrano and indole rings (compound 12) modified both chemical and biological properties to a great extent.[33,34] In depressed patients, various studies with 9, i.e. clinical, psychometric and EEG studies, suggested that the drug has no anticholinergic effects, it is well tolerated, and may be of benefit in retarded depressions.[35] An improvement in the depressive symptomatology became statistically significant between the 1st and 2nd week of therapy. The potency of a related tetrahydrocarbazole 10 with respect to the inhibition of NA uptake in vivo was similar to that of desipramine.[36] Several modifications of the pirandamine molecule (11) have been reported,[37] and the biological results indicate that within this series there are no stringent structural requirements in regard to antidepressant-like properties.[37,38] The reversed annelation of pyrano and indene rings (compound 13) caused only moderate changes in activity.

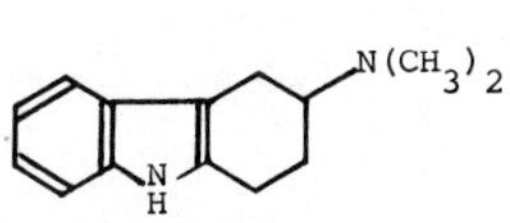

14

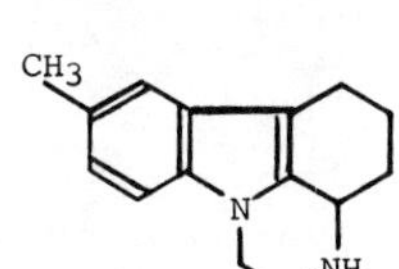

15

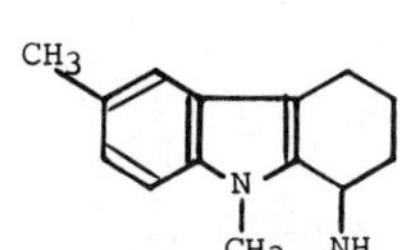

16

Cycloindole (WIN 27147-2, 14),a structurally modified dimethyltryptamine, prevented both the reserpine ptosis and amphetamine stereotyped behavior at 10 mg/kg.[39] Its 6,8-difluoroderivative is a chlorpromazine-like compound. In an uncontrolled clinical study with 14 (200-600 mg/day), all patients showed an improvement and adverse effects were not severe.[40] A placebo controlled trial confirmed that 14 has antidepressant-anxiolytic effects and sedative properties.[41] Recently, studies with 14 were discontinued due to toxicity problems (thrombocytopenia and bleeding). Pyrazidol (15) was 10x less potent than imipramine in inhibiting brain NA uptake; in contrast to imipramine, 15 also inhibited GABA uptake.[42] This compound prevented reserpine ptosis, increased phenamine group toxicity, potentiated 5-HTP head shaking, inhibited pressor response to tyramine, and inhibited NA uptake in isolated rat heart.[43] The seco-analog 16 exhibited a comparable activity only in the potentiation of 5-HTP. The SAR studies within this series have demonstrated the importance of the 8-methyl group.[43] A single injection of pyrazidol had no effect on brain or heart NA, but chronic administration or a higher dose increased heart NA levels.[44]

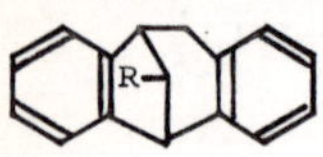

17 R = CH_2-$N(CH_3)_2$

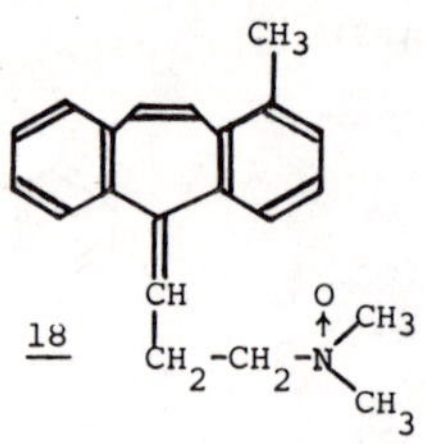

18

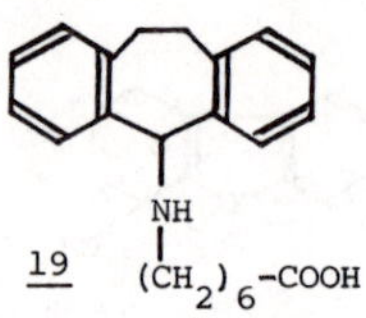

19

The phramacological profile of R-806 (17) was found to be similar to that of imipramine, except that 17 displays less anticholinergic activity.[45] Compound 17 potentiates the pressor response to NA, and in vitro, inhibits the NA uptake into rat brain more effectively than imipramine. In an open clinical trial[46] in endogenously depressed patients, treatment with 17 (10-30 mg/day) proved to be beneficial, and no anxiolytic or sedative effects were observed. The 1-methyl derivative of cyclobenzaprine N-oxide (Ro-8-1998, 18) was compared clinically with imipramine in a double-blind study[47] with a dose relationship of 2:1. The patients markedly improved in both groups and there was no difference in the overall results. The study did not confirm the expectation (based on animal experiments) that 18 might cause less anticholinergic side-effects than imipramine. After 10 days of treatment with 18, a significant decrease of systolic blood pressure and leucocytes was observed. The aminoacid S 1694 (19) produced an increased locomotor activity in mice, competitively inhibited DA uptake, and also caused a significant release of DA at low concentrations.[48] Similar effects on NA and 5-HT uptake and release mechanisms were obtained with higher concentrations of 19.

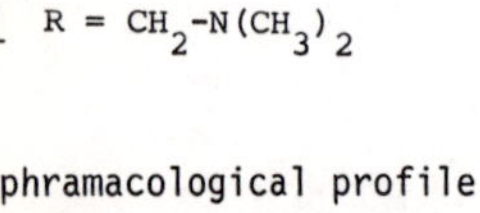

20

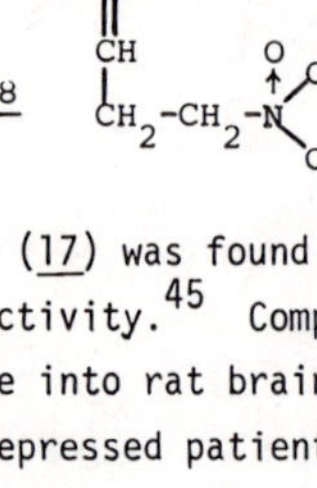

21

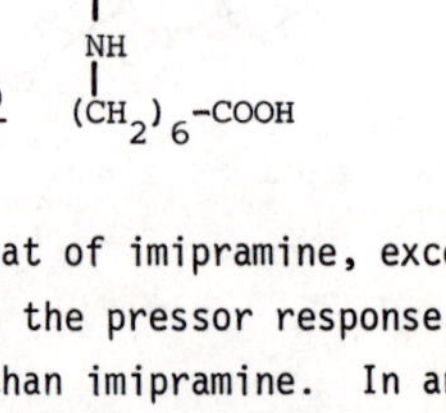

22 R = CH_3

23 R = H

Bupropion (Wellbatrin, 20) was reported to prevent tetrabenazine-induced sedation and ptosis in mice, and to antagonize reserpine hypothermia, although at slightly higher doses than amitriptyline.[49] In contrast to amitriptyline, 20 reduced both the intense motor activity and mortality caused by amphetamine. In in vitro rat brain preparations, bupropion had little effect on 5-HT uptake, and it was 60x less potent than imipramine in inhibition of NA uptake. On the other hand, as an inhibitor of DA uptake, 20 was 6-fold and 20-fold more potent than imipramine and amitriptyline, respectively. When tested clinically in endogenous depression (double-blind, 20 vs placebo), therapeutic responses were noted after 1 week.[50] Danitracen (WA-335, 21), a base structurally related to cyproheptadine and pimethixen, elicited strong binding to 5-HT and histamine receptors.[51] Compared to imipramine, 21 was considerably less potent in reversing the reserpine hypothermia, but its sedative and anticholinergic effects were greater.[52] In healthy subjects, low doses of 21 caused quantitative EEG alterations that were typical for antidepressants.[53] In a double-blind trial with 3x1 mg/day of 21 vs 3x50 mg/day of amitriptyline, two-thirds of the patients showed a 50% improvement (Hamilton score) in both groups after 20 days.[54] Similar results were reported with a low dose of 21 (3 mg/day), however, a dose of 6 mg/day produced marked sedation.[55] Recently, 21 has also been shown to antagonize the action of oxotremorine[56] and the 5-HTP syndrome.[57]

The structure of fluotracene (SKF-28175, 22) bears resemblance to that of melitracene and dimethacrine. Interestingly, 22 exhibited properties of both antidepressant and antipsychotic agents.[58] It was more potent than imipramine in preventing reserpine ptosis and hypothermia, and its neuroleptic profile was comparable to that of thioridazine. Preliminary uncontrolled clinical studies with 22 indicated that this compound might be useful in both depressive and psychotic states. The 10-desmethyl analog (SKF-25971, 23) had a full range of neuroleptic properties in animals, and it was considerably more potent than chlorpromazine in many of the tests.

Melanocyte-stimulating hormone release inhibiting factor I (MIF-I), H-Pro-Leu-Gly-NH_2(L,L), given orally in double-blind studies with a placebo control, caused substantial improvement in endogenously depressed patients and this was observed within a few days.[59,60] The improvement was greater at lower doses (e.g., 60 and 75 mg/day) than at higher doses (e.g., 150 and 750 mg/day). This biphasic pattern of response was similar to that observed clinically with MIF-I in Parkinson's disease[60] and in tardive dyskinesia.[61] Improvement in the mood of parkinsonian patients receiving MIF-I has also been reported.[62,63] Various pharmacological studies in animals suggested the antidepressant activity of MIF-I;[64] the biphasic pattern was also reported. Neurochemically, some studies,[65,66] but not others,[67,68] demonstrated that MIF-I increases DA turnover. Recently, novel synthetic analogs of MIF-I were reported.[69] Some of the analogs exhibited a MIF-I-like behavioral potentiation (DOPA response in the mouse) with the most potent being H-Pro-MeLeu-Gly-NH_2(L,D) although it was less potent than MIF-I (the L-MeLeu analog being inactive).[70] The biphasic pattern of response was observed with the analog. In other pharmacological evaluation it was shown to be active orally.[70] Neurochemically, the analog at a higher dose than MIF-I, increased rat brain DA turnover.[66] Neither the analog nor MIF-I affected rat brain 5-HT turnover or the 5-HTP-induced behavioral syndrome in the mouse. The analog decreased rat brain NA turnover, while in contrast, MIF-I was ineffective even at a higher dose. It is of relevance in this regard[66] that tricyclic antidepressants, such as desimipramine,[71] also decrease NA turnover after a single dose.

Mianserin (Org GB 94, 24), a clinically effective antidepressant,[72-76] does not exhibit an antidepressant-like profile in conventional animal screening tests.[77] Compound 24 possesses 5-HT receptor blocking properties like methysergide and cinanserin.[78] In a determination in rats of the ability of 24 and other drugs to antagonize the incapacitating effect of morphine on the performance of a two-way active avoidance response, 24 caused a significantly greater number of escapes and intertrial responses than in placebo-treated animals.[79] The restoration of activities was also exhibited by methysergide and cinanserin, although not to as great an extent. However, the antidepressants amitriptyline and imipramine were ineffective. This further demonstrates a pharmacological difference between 24 and the tricyclic antidepressants. In vitro, 24 blocked the noradrenergic uptake mechanism being similar in potency to imipramine and amitriptyline.[80] In vivo, 24 was less active than tricyclic antidepressants in preventing the induced-decrease in rat heart and brain NA. Like tricyclic antidepressants, 24 was essentially devoid of the ability to block dopaminergic uptake mechanism in vitro and in vivo. The blockade by 24 of the 5-HT uptake mechanism in vitro was appreciably less than that of the tricyclic antidepressants and the drug was essentially devoid of activity in vivo. The lack of an appreciable effect in vivo on NA uptake would be consistent with an inability to block tyramine-induced effects in human subjects.[81] Compound 24 has been suggested to act by blocking presynaptic noradrenergic α-receptors, similar to phentolamine and phenoxybenzamine.[82] This would result in an increase in concentration of NA in the synaptic cleft. In regard to the latter, 24 blocked the NA uptake mechanism which would also lead to an increase in the NA concentration. Various additional observations[83] also suggest that the increase in the turnover of catecholamines is a specific action of 24 which is not exhibited by other antidepressants. Compound 24 also possessed post-synaptic α-receptor blocking activity under certain conditions; however, the role of such an activity in the overall action of the drug has yet to be defined.[82] Furthermore, the importance of the presynaptic α-blocking activity in the central action of the drug is not yet clear. Compound 25 was found to be a major metabolite of 24 in several animal species and in man.[84] This metabolic path seems to be general for similar compounds possessing a piperazine ring, and the N-oxide and the N-desmethyl derivative of 24 were also precursors of 25. Further studies indicated a role of microsomal enzymes in the formation of 25.[84]

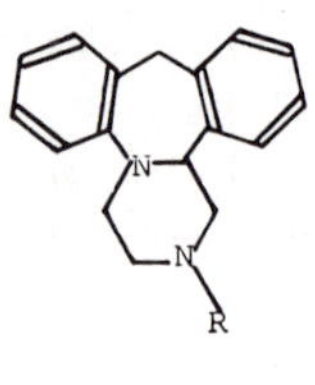

24 R=CH_3

25 R=$(CH_2)_2COCH_3$

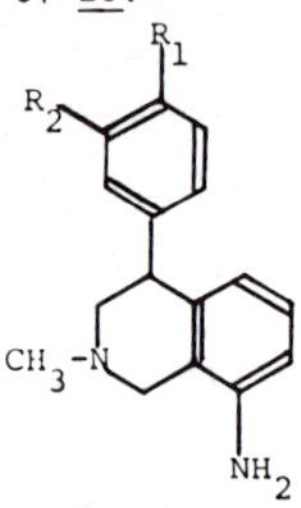

26	R_1=R_2=H	
27	R_1=OH	R_2=H
28	R_1=OH	R_2=OCH_3
29	R_1=OCH_3	R_2=OH

In a single-blind comparative study[85] in elderly depressed patients with physical disability, both nomifensin 26 (75 mg/kg) and viloxazine[1,7] (150 mg/day) exhibited antidepressant activity. From the second week of treatment on, 26 showed more effect than viloxazine. Physical disability evaluation showed no differences for the two drugs at any period of the trials. No side effects were spontaneously reported by the patients.[85] Of 3 metabolites of 26, compound 27 was the most active one, while 28 and 29 exhibited little or no effect in pharmacological tests in mice.[86] In contrast to 26, the metabolite 27 possessed serotoninergic activity comparable to imipramine and chlorimipramine. In in vitro rat brain, 26 was a potent inhibitor of DA uptake[86] (of competitive type[87]) and of NA uptake;[86,87] 27 was similar in activity with regard to DA[86] and twice as active,[86] or slightly less active,[87] with respect to NA. Compounds 28 and 29 exhibited reduced activities.[86,87] All four compounds were more potent than imipramine, desipramine and chlorimipramine in inhibiting DA uptake.[86]

An *in vitro* study employing crude synaptosomal preparations from various rat brain regions was reported in which relevance of the DA uptake in the mechanism of action of various antidepressants was considered.[88] None of the numerous antidepressant drugs and other biogenic amine uptake blocking agents examined exhibited selective DA uptake inhibition. NA uptake inhibition was always greater, and generally much greater, even with the most potent DA uptake blocker 26.[88,89] It was pointed out[88] that it is difficult to ascribe the antidepressant effect to inhibition of uptake of a particular biogenic amine. The clinical doses of the drugs including 26 were cited to be 50-300 mg/day while there was much greater difference in the inhibitory uptake values. The importance of DA uptake was emphasized; it was also recognized that NA, DA and 5-HT might all be of relevance in the antidepressant effects and that their interactions might also be of importance.

Viloxazine possesses unique psychotropic activity in animals[90-92] and clinical results suggested that it might have a rapid antidepressant effect.[93] However, in a recent controlled trial, viloxazine at 3x100 mg/day was not as effective as placebo at the end of 1 week.[94]

Good therapeutic responses were obtained[95] in the treatment of different types of depression (10,000 patients in general practice) with 75 mg/day of maprotiline.[1,6] The results of 3 separate clinical studies[97] with maprotiline were in variance with the "reversed" catecholamine hypothesis of depression,[96] since no biphasic therapeutic response was observed, and the urinary MHPG concentrations were increased.[97]

In a preliminary open trial with salbutamol (3 mg infused twice daily), a drug which exhibits β_2-adrenergic receptor agonist activities, dramatic antidepressant effect was reported in endogenous depression with the effect appearing as early as 3 days; a distinct improvement in mood, retardation and anxiety was also observed by the third day.[98]

In the area of new models for the detection of antidepressant activity of drugs, the potential use of the bulbectomized rat[99] was further studied. Bilateral ablation of the olfactory bulbs of rats resulted in diverse behavioral changes and most of these were reversed by chronic pretreatment with antidepressant drugs.[100] The anxiosoif test is utilized in the assessment of the behavioral changes and the test is essentially a passive avoidance paradigm in which thirsty rats learn to avoid an electrified water spout. Bulbectomized rats showed deficient avoidance behavior. Various antidepressants reversed this effect; in contrast, anxiolytic and neuroleptic drugs aggravated the deficiency. A distinction was made between mianserin and other antidepressant drugs since removal of the olfactory bulbs tended to produce an increase in base-line levels of drinking in most experiments and this effect was reversed by mianserin but not by various other antidepressants.[100] A new behavioral model for detection of antidepressant agents was described based upon behavioral despair in rats[101] and mice.[102] A depressed state was induced by forcing the animals to swim in a narrow cylinder from which they could not escape. After a brief period of vigorous activity the animals adopted a characteristic immobile posture which was readily identifiable. Immobility was reduced by tricyclic antidepressants, MAO inhibitors and atypical antidepressants, such as iprindole, mianserin and viloxazine, as well as by electroconvulsive shock. Psychostimulants also reduced immobility, but in contrast to antidepressants, caused marked motor stimulation. Immobility was not affected by minor or major tranquilizers. The mouse assay was more rapid, and thus, more suitable for the primary screening of potential antidepressant drugs.[102]

In a study of the mechanisms of the seizures induced by antidepressants which antagonize the uptake of biogenic amines, baboons with photosensitive epilepsy were employed.[103] Imipramine, chlorimipramine, and maprotiline, lowered the seizure threshold to a comparable extent. In contrast, nomifensin did not enhance myoclonic responses to photic stimulation, thereby being less epileptogenic. The tricyclic antidepressants, which can block 5-HT uptake, did not exhibit the augmentation of photically-induced epileptic responses after administration of 5-HTP. Thus, it was suggested that enhancement of serotoninergic activity following blockade of 5-HT reuptake within the brain is unlikely to be responsible for enhanced myoclonic responses and epileptogenic seizures observed after tricyclic antidepressants.

Antidepressant drugs such as amitriptyline and imipramine inhibited histamine- and dimaprit (S-[3-(N,N-dimethylamino)propyl]isothiourea, a potent and highly specific histamine$_2$-receptor agonist)-activated adenylate cyclase _in vitro_ (e.g., homogenates of guinea pig hippocamus); dibenzepin and iprindole were 100x less active than amitriptyline.[104] The blockage of the H_2-receptors, in addition to other activities, may be of relevance for some of the pharmacological effects of the antidepressant drugs. Amitriptyline exhibited higher affinity for the H_2-receptor than the H_2-antagonist cimetidine, a clinically effective antiulcer agent.[105,106] Antidepressants also decrease gastric acidity and ulcers in animals and man (see references in 107;108).

The mode of action at the molecular level of the antidepressant drugs continues to be explored with regard to determining the basis for the discrepancy between the time-course of the biochemical and pharmacological responses which are observed within minutes or hours and their clinical antidepressant action which requires administration of the drugs for weeks in order to attain clinical efficacy.[109] Studies have suggested that the therapeutic action of tricyclic antidepressants may be related to postsynaptic adaptive changes in the sensitivity of the noradrenergic adenylate cyclase receptor system rather than to acute presynaptic events.[110] Chronic administration of antidepressants leads to subsensitivity of NA-stimulated adenylate cyclase _in vivo_.[110] This resistant state of the adenyl cyclase appears to be due to a decrease in the number of β-adrenergic receptors present.[109] In this regard it has been suggested that through regulation of the number of β-adrenergic receptors, the β-adrenergic catecholamines can regulate catecholamine sensitivity of tissues _in vivo_.[111] However, other factors appear to be of relevance. Although findings with the antidepressant desimipramine on the number of β-adrenergic receptors present are in accord, iprindole, which also causes β-adrenergic receptor subsensitivity, only exerts minimal effect at presynaptic neurons (see 109 for references) and thus the concentration of the NA at the synaptic cleft is not the only mechanism for the regulation of β-adrenergic receptor concentration.[109]

References

1. P.F. von Voigtlander, in "Annual Reports in Medicinal Chemistry", Vol. 11, p. 3-12, F.H. Clarke ed., Academic Press, 1976
2. R.A. Lahti, in "Annual Reports in Medicinal Chemistry", Vol. 12, p. 1-9, F.H. Clarke ed., Academic Press, 1977
3. Proceedings of a symposium on biological aspects of clomipramine, Postgraduate Med. J. 52, Suppl. 3(1976); _ibid._, 53, Suppl. 4(1977)
4. A symposium on Anafranil in general practice, J. Intern. Med. Res. 5, Suppl. 1(1977)
5. R.M. Pinder, R.N. Brogden, T.M. Speight, and G.S. Avery, Drugs 13, 161-218(1977)
6. _Ibid._, 321-352
7. _Ibid._, 401-421
8. S.R. Baehring-Kuhlmey, Med. Actual. 13, 205-209(1977)
9. Proceedings of a symposium on nomifensin, Brit. J. Clin. Pharmacol. 4, Suppl. 2(1977)

10. J.C. Pecknold and T.A. Ban, Int. Pharmacopsychiat. 12, 166-173(1977)
11. H. Kruse, Arch. Pharmacol. 297, Suppl. 1, 61-62(1977)
12. A symposium on depression held at the Silver Hill Found. (Oct. 10, 1975), Dis. Nerv. Syst. 37, No. 3, Section 2, 1-34(1976)
13. Symposium "Pharmacology of serotonin neurons in the CNS", 60th Ann. Meeting of the Fed. Amer. Soc. Exptl. Biol., Anaheim, Cal., April 14, 1976, Fed. Proc. 36, No. 8, 2133-64(1977)
14. R.R. Fieve, Drugs 13, 458-466(1977)
15. G.A.E. Rudolf, B. Schilgen and R. Toelle, Nervenarzt 48, 1-11(1977)
16. V. Claassen, J.E. Davies, G. Hertting and P. Placheta, Brit. J. Pharmacol., 60, 505(1977)
17. B. Saletu, M. Schjerve, J. Grünberger, H. Schanda and O.H. Arnold, J. Neural Transmission, 41, 17(1977)
18. K. Ghose, R. Gupta, A. Coppen and J. Lund, Eur. J. Pharmacol. 42, 31(1977)
19. J.B. Lassen, Acta Pharmacol. Toxicol. 41, Suppl. 4, 43(1977)
20. S.B. Ross and K. Kelder, Acta Physiol. Scand. 99, 27(1977)
21. B. Siwers, V.A. Ringberger, J.R. Tuck and F. Sjoqvist, Clin. Pharmacol. Ther. 21, 194(1977)
22. L.B. Cobbin and P. Dhumma Upakorn, Clin. Exp. Pharmacol. Physiol. 4, 208(1977)
23. O. Benkert, G. Laakmann, L. Ott, A. Strauss and R. Zimmer, Arzneim.-Forsch. 27, 2421(1977)
24. U.H. Lindberg, S.O. Thorberg, S. Bengtsson, A.L. Renyi, S.B. Ross and S.O. Ogren, Acta Pharm. Suecica (in press)
25. T.A. Pugsley and W. Lippmann, Arch. Int. Pharmacodyn. Ther. 228, 322(1977)
26. J. Hyttel, Psychopharmacology 51, 225(1977)
27. J. Hyttel, Acta Pharmacol. Toxicol. 40, 439(1977)
28. A.V. Christensen, B. Fjalland, V. Pedersen, P. Danneskiold-Samsoe and O. Svendsen, Eur. J. Pharmacol. 41, 153(1977)
29. H.M. Geyer, S.A. Ridlon, U. Schacht and W.J. Novick Jr., Fed. Proc. 35, 784(1976)
30. S.S. Klioze, V.J. Bauer and H.M. Geyer, J. Med. Chem. 20, 610(1977)
31. R.S.B. Ehsanullah, K. Ghose, M.J. Kirby and D. Witts, Brit. J. Clin. Pharmacol. 3, 950P(1976)
32. R.S.B. Ehsanullah, K. Ghose, M.J. Kirby, P. Turner and D. Witts, Psychopharmacol. 52, 73(1977)
33. I. Jirkovsky, L.G. Humber, K. Voith and M.P. Charest, Arzneim.-Forsch. 27, 1642(1977)
34. W. Lippmann and T.A. Pugsley, Biochem. Pharmacol. 25, 1179(1976)
35. B. Saletu, P. Krieger, J. Grunberger, H. Schanda and I. Sletten, Int. Pharmacopsychiat. 12, 137(1977)
36. T.A. Pugsley and W. Lippmann, Experientia 33, 37(1977)
37. I. Jirkovsky, L.G. Humber and R. Noureldin, Eur. J. Med. Chem. 11, 571(1976)
38. W. Lippmann and T.A. Pugsley, Pharmacol. Res. Commun. 8, 387(1976)
39. A. Mooradian, P.E. Dupont, A.G. Hlavac, M.D. Aceto and J. Pearl, J. Med. Chem. 20, 487(1977)
40. J.N. Nestoros, T.A. Ban and H.E. Lehmann, Int. Pharmacopsychiat. 12, 86(1977)
41. E.D. Eckert, R. Zimmermann, L. Dehnel and B.C. Schiele, Curr. Ther. Res. 22, 644(1977)
42. M.D. Mashkovskii, K.S. Raevskii, N.I. Maisov, Yu. G. Sandalov, N.I. Andreeva, Khim.-Farm. Zh. 10, 3(1976)
43. N.I. Andreeva, L.B. Altukhova, V.V. Asnina, L.G. Vasilevikh, V.Z. Gorkin and M.D. Mashkovskii, Khim.-Farm. Zh. 10, 46(1976)
44. V.V. Asnina and N.I. Andreeva, Farmakol. Toksikol. 39, 682(1976)
45. C.L. Mitchell, A.C. Conway, N.J. Tresnak and W.J. Hammar, Fed. Proc. 35, 784(1976)
46. G. Pinard, Curr. Ther. Res. 21, 368(1977)
47. B. Woggon and J. Angst, Int. Pharmacopsychiat. 12, 38(1977)
48. J. Offermeier, B. Potgieter, H.G. Du Preez and P.J. Meiring, South African Med. J. 51, 62(1977)
49. F.E. Soroko, N.B. Mehta, R.A. Maxwell, R.M. Ferris, D.H. Schroeder, J. Pharm. Pharmac. 29, 767(1977)
50. L.F. Fabre Jr., D. McLendon and A. Mallette, Clin. Pharmacol. Ther. 21, 102(1977)
51. G. Engelhardt, Arzneim.-Forsch. 25, 1723(1975)
52. J. Kaehling, H. Ziegler and H. Ballhause, Arzneim.-Forsch. 25, 1737(1975)
53. B. Saletu, J. Grunberger, R. Flener, L. Linzmayer and H. Sieroslawaki, Curr. Ther. Res. 20, 810(1976)
54. N. Matussek, O. Benkert, K. Fidetzis, D. Flach, H.U. Hermann, S. Kaumeier, H. Kindt, E. Kinzler, E. Ruther and W. Watzka, Arzneim.-Forsch. 26, 1160(1976)
55. S. Kaumeier, J. Dohren and D. Flach, Curr. Ther. Res. 21, 108(1977)
56. B. Oderfeld Nowak, A. Wieraszko and B. Heiler, Pol. J. Pharmacol. & Pharm. 29, 215(1977)
57. J. Maj, L. Baran, A. Rawlow and H. Sowinska, Pol. J. Pharmacol. & Pharm. 29, 213(1977)
58. P.J. Fowler, C.L. Zirkle, E. Macko, P.E. Setler, H.M. Sarau, A. Misher and D.H. Tedeschi, Arzneim.-Forsch. 27, 1589(1977)
59. R.H. Ehrensing and A.J. Kastin, Arch. Gen. Psychiatr. 30, 63(1974)
60. A. Barbeau, M. Roy and A.J. Kastin, Can. Med. Assoc. J. 114, 120(1976)
61. R.H. Ehrensing, A.J. Kastin, P.F. Larsons and G.A. Bishop, Dis. Nerv. Sys. 38, 303(1977)
62. P.A. Fischer, E. Schneider, P. Jacobi and H. Maxion, Eur. Neurol. 12, 360(1974)
63. A. Barbeau, Lancet 2, 683(1975)

64. N.P. Plotnikoff, A.J. Kastin, M.S. Anderson and A.V. Schally, Neuroendocrinol. 11, 67(1973)
65. E. Freidman, J. Friedman and S. Gershon, Science 182, 831(1973)
66. T.A. Pugsley and W. Lippmann, Arzneim.-Forsch. 27, 2293(1977)
67. N.P. Plotnikoff, F.N. Minard and A.J. Kastin, Neuroendocrinol. 14, 271(1974)
68. R.M. Kostrzewa, M.A. Spirtes and A.J. Kastin, Pharmacologist 16, 320(1974)
69. A. Failli, K. Sestanj, H.U. Immer and M. Götz, Arzneim.-Forsch. 27, 2286(1977)
70. K. Voith, Arzneim.-Forsch. 27, 2290(1977)
71. J. Schubert, H. Nybäck and G. Sedvall, J. Pharm. Pharmacol. 22, 136(1970)
72. J.E. Murphy, J. Int. Med. Res. 3, 251(1975)
73. D. Wheatley, Curr. Ther. Res. 18, 849(1975)
74. H.P. Vogel, Int. Pharmacopsychiat. 11, 25(1976)
75. M.O. Jaskari, V.G. Ahlfors, L. Ginman, K. Lydekcne and P. Tienari, Pharmakopsychiat. Neuro-Psychopharmakol. 10, 101(1977)
76. A. Coppen, R. Gupta, S. Montgomery, K. Ghose, J. Bailey, B. Burns and J.J. de Ridder, Brit. J. Psychiat. 129, 342(1976)
77. H. Van Riezen, Arch. Int. Pharmacodyn. Ther. 198, 256(1972)
78. B.B. Vergaftig, J.L. Coignet, C.J. De Vos, H. Grijsen and I.L. Bonta, Eur. J. Pharmacol. 16, 336(1971)
79. E. Preston, H. Rigter and C. Strijbos, Brit. J. Pharmacol. 59, 456P(1977)
80. I. Goodlet, S.E. Mireylees and M.F. Sugrue, Brit. J. Pharmacol. 61, 307(1977)
81. K. Ghose, A. Coppen and P. Turner, Psychopharmacology 49, 201(1976)
82. P.A. Baumann and L. Maitre, Naunyn-Schmiedeberg's Arch. Pharmacol. 300, 31(1977)
83. B.E. Leonard and W.F. Kafoe, Biochem. Pharmacol. 25, 1939(1976)
84. F. Van der Veen and G.D. De Jongh, Xenobiotica 7, 99(1977)
85. J. Moizeszowicz and S. Subira, J. Clin. Pharmacol. 17, 81(1977)
86. H. Kruse, I. Hoffmann, H.J. Gerhards, M. Leven and U. Schacht, Psychopharmacology 51, 117(1977)
87. J. Toumisto, Eur. J. Pharmacol. 42, 101(1977)
88. A. Randrup and C. Braestrup, Psychopharmacology 53, 309(1977)
89. B.K. Koe, J. Pharmacol. Exp. Ther. 199, 649(1976)
90. K.B. Maillion, A.H. Todd, R.W. Turner, J.G. Bainbridge, D.T. Greenwood, J. Madinaveitia, A.R. Somerville and B.A. Whittle, Nature (London) 238, 157(1972)
91. D.T. Greenwood, J. Int. Med. Res. 3, Suppl. 3, 18(1975)
92. W. Lippmann and T.A. Pugsley, Can. J. Physiol. Pharmacol. 54, 494(1976)
93. F.J. Bereen, Lancet 1, 379(1973)
94. J. Guy Edwards, Brit. Med. J. 2, 1327(1977)
95. W.A. Forrest, J. Intern. Med. Res. 5, 42(1977)
96. D.S. Segal, R. Kuczenski and A.J. Mandell, Biol. Psychiat. 9, 147(1974)
97. T.A. Ban, M. Amin and H.E. Lehmann, Curr. Ther. Res. 22, 886(1977)
98. D. Widlöcher, Y. Lecrubier, R. Jouvent, A.J. Puech and P. Simon, Lancet 2, 767(1977)
99. H. Rigter, H. Van Riezen and A. Wren, Brit. J. Pharmacol. 59, 451P(1977)
100. H. Van Riezen, H. Schnieden and A. Wren, Brit. J. Pharmacol. 57, 426P(1976)
101. R.D. Porsolt, M. Le Pichon and M. Jalfre, Nature (London) 266, 730(1977)
102. R.D. Porsolt, A. Bertin and M. Jalfre, Arch. Int. Pharmacodyn. Ther. 229, 327(1977)
103. M. Trimble, G. Anlezark and B. Meldrum, Psychopharmacology 51, 159(1977)
104. J.P. Green and S. Maayani, Nature 269, 163(1977)
105. G. Bodemar and A. Walan, Lancet 2, 161(1976)
106. W.S. Blackwood, D.P. Maudgal, P.G. Pickard, D. Lawrence and T.C. Northfield, Lancet 2, 174(1976)
107. W. Lippmann and K. Seethaler, Life Sci. 20, 1393(1977)
108. L. Nitter, Jr., A. Haraldsson, P. Holck, Chr. Hoy, J. Munthe-Kaas, K. Myrhol and W. Paulsen, Scand. J. Gastroenterol. 12, S43, 39(1977)
109. S.P. Banerjee, L.S. Kung, S.J. Riggi and S.K. Chanda, Nature 268, 455(1977)
110. J. Vetulani, R.J. Stawarz, J.V. Dingell and F. Sulser, Naunyn Schmiedeberg's Arch. Pharmacol. 293, 109(1976)
111. C. Mukherjee, M.G. Caron and R.J. Lefkowitz, Proc. Natn. Acad. Sci. 72, 1945(1975)

Chapter 2. Antipsychotic Agents and Dopamine Agonists

by John McDermed
Wellcome Research Laboratories
Research Triangle Park, N.C. 27709
and Richard J. Miller
Department of Physiological and Pharmacological Sciences
University of Chicago, Chicago, Illinois 60637

A large body of indirect but compelling pharmacological data implies the existence of dopaminergic defects in the brains of patients suffering from schizophrenic psychosis. Direct demonstration of a causative biochemical lesion in this disorder is still almost completely lacking, and other neurohumoral systems may be involved.[1,2] However, the dopamine (DA) hypothesis has provided fertile soil from which much of the recent progress in the understanding and treatment of schizophrenia and other diseases of the CNS has grown.

Dopamine Receptors. The use of receptor binding assays, which was reviewed by Creese and Snyder[3] in the previous volume of this series, has accounted for much of the progress of the past year in the characterization of the DA receptor in normal and disease states. The tritiated DA agonists and antagonists which have now been successfully used to label DA receptors *in vitro* include ^{3}H-DA, ^{3}H-apomorphine (APO), ^{3}H-dihydroergotamine, ^{3}H-haloperidol, and ^{3}H-spiroperidol.[3-12] However, it is not clear that all these label the same population of receptors. It has been previously reported that DA agonists are more effective in displacing ^{3}H-DA than ^{3}H-haloperidol from binding sites in rat and calf caudate and that DA antagonists have the opposite effect, although these binding sites are closely associated.[3,13] This has been explained by suggesting that agonists and antagonists selectively interact with different conformations of the same DA receptor.[14] More recently Seeman, *et al*. have examined the abilities of drugs to displace the binding of five different ligands from DA receptors in calf caudate.[7] They obtained biphasic displacement curves in some cases which led them to suggest the existence of two entirely separate receptor populations in brain. Further data from the same group suggest that these distinct receptors may represent pre- and postsynaptic dopaminergic receptors. Thus it has been found that 6-hydroxydopamine lesions in the nigro-striatal pathway of the rat decrease the binding of ^{3}H-APO but increase the binding of ^{3}H-haloperidol.[15] The authors therefore suggested that APO selectively labels presynaptic sites (destroyed by the lesion) and haloperidol selectively labels postsynaptic (supersensitive) receptors. It should also be noted that other groups have also proposed the existence of functionally distinct classes of DA receptors in brain to explain behavioral[16,17] and electrophysiological[18] data.

Several groups have begun to examine the changes in DA receptors in various pathological states or in experimental models of them. For example, rats may be treated chronically with neuroleptic drugs to produce a model of tardive dyskinesia. In such animals, it is found that there is an increase in the total number of DA receptors in the basal

ISBN 0-12-040513-X

ganglia.[19,20] However, similar increases do not occur in the number of opiate or noradrenergic receptors in the same animals.[20] Animal models of Parkinson's disease may also be produced by 6-hydroxydopamine lesions of the nigrostriatal DA pathways or by electrocoagulation of the substantia nigra.[21] Behavioral supersensitivity to DA agonists is seen in such animals, together with an increase in the number of binding sites for ^{3}H-haloperidol.[21] It is highly significant that postmortem samples of caudate nucleus from brains of parkinsonian patients show similar increases over controls.[22] In these same samples ^{3}H-APO binding is reduced, which is entirely consistent with results in rats with 6-hydroxydopamine lesions noted above. Decreases in ^{3}H-spiroperidol binding have also been recorded from brains of patients with Huntington's chorea.[23] In such cases a decrease in the concentration of choline acetylase in the basal ganglia was also seen, leading to the suggestion that some of the haloperidol binding sites may be on cell bodies of cholinergic neurons of the basal ganglia. In support of this suggestion it has also been found that injection of kainic acid into the basal ganglia, which selectively destroys cell bodies of cholinergic and GABAergic neurons, also leads to a decrease of haloperidol binding in this area.[24] It also leads to a decrease in DA-sensitive adenylate cyclase activity.

A very important observation has been made with respect to the state of DA receptors in the basal ganglia and elsewhere in the brains of patients with schizophrenia.[25] Lee and Seeman found that in the postmortem samples of brains from such patients there was an increased number of receptors for haloperidol binding in the putamen, caudate nucleus, and nucleus accumbens, but not in the frontal cortex. This provocative observation suggests that an increased number of DA receptors could be the biochemical defect responsible for the symptoms of schizophrenia. However, more work is required in this system, particularly to determine if this result was from a primary lesion characteristic of the disease or a secondary one resulting from long term treatment with neuroleptic drugs.

Another novel use of binding assays has been reported by Creese and Snyder, who have used this technique to assay for neuroleptic drugs in the sera of schizophrenic patients undergoing drug therapy. In this system the amount of circulating drug is monitored by observing the ability of the patient's plasma to inhibit the binding of ^{3}H-spiroperidol to calf caudate membranes.[26] This single procedure is simultaneously applicable to all the commonly used antipsychotic drugs and even any active metabolites, and should be a considerable aid to psychiatrists trying to establish optimal drug regimens for their patients.

One other DA-linked system has been increasingly investigated over the past year. That is the ability of DA agonists to decrease, and of DA antagonists to increase, the secretion of prolactin from the anterior pituitary.[27] This is believed to be a direct effect of dopaminergic agents on the prolactin-secreting cells of the anterior lobe. In fact, binding of tritiated ligands to such cells has been observed.[28,29] It is quite clear that the ability of DA antagonists to act as antipsychotic drugs correlates well with their ability to increase prolactin secretion in the rat. It may therefore be that this is another important and useful system for monitoring DA antagonists both in vitro and in the clinic.[30] In addition, one paper has reported very interesting dopaminergic effects in cells of the bovine parathyroid gland.[31] However, the pharmacology of this system has not as yet been extensively elucidated.

Antipsychotic Agents. Considerable interest in recent years has been focused on the mode of action of sulpiride (1), because this antipsychotic is generally believed to be largely free from the liabilities of extrapyramidal side effects and tardive dyskinesia encountered with the classical neuroleptics. Recent clinical studies have confirmed the antischizophrenic efficacy of sulpiride,[32-4] though it should be noted that in the largest of these[33] (76 inpatients, double-blind vs. haloperidol) sulpiride did produce a significant number of "extrapyramidal disturbances" (8 cases vs. 12 for haloperidol). Several pharmacological studies have provided evidence that sulpiride exhibits many, although not all, of the effects of classical neuroleptics. In common with other neuroleptics sulpiride inhibits APO-induced behavior in animals,[35] increases dopamine turnover and accumulation of metabolites,[35-36] increases prolactin secretion,[34,37] and inhibits binding of ^{3}H-haloperidol to dopamine receptors in homogenates of rat caudate.[38] Rather high doses are required in some of these systems as well as for antischizophrenic activity in man. On the other hand, sulpiride is apparently atypical in other regards. It does not produce catalepsy and does not block the DA-sensitive adenylate cyclase in striatum and nucleus accumbens.[39] In the periphery it has been shown to have an unusually high specificity for DA receptors vs. α-adrenergic receptors,[40] in comparison to other neuroleptics. There are particularly interesting reports that sulpiride is atypical in producing selective effects on DA metabolism in the limbic system,[41] entorhinal cortex,[42] and retina,[43] rather than in the striatum. It should also be noted that sulpiride may be acting at the presynaptic level to an unusual degree.[44]

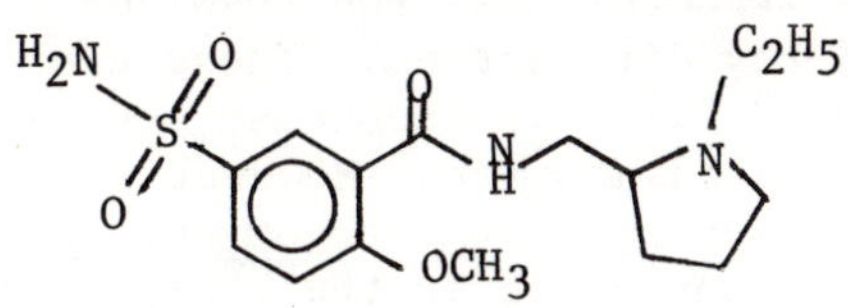

1

Perhaps the most intensively studied subject of neurobiology during very recent years has been the endogenous opioids, the endorphins and enkephalins.[45,46] The profound behavioral effects of endorphins injected into the brain have led some authors to speculate that endogenous opiate peptide systems may be involved in the pathogenesis of schizophrenia.[47] Consequently, it has also been suggested that opiate peptides may be effective antipsychotic agents in certain cases. Several studies have pointed to interaction of enkephalinergic systems with central dopaminergic pathways. For example, β-endorphin and analogs of enkephalin, as well as classical narcotics, have been shown to produce typically "dopaminergic" responses such as hypermotility and catalepsy.[48] Moreover, high concentrations of these peptides have been found in the regions of the basal ganglia which are also densely innervated by dopaminergic neurons.[49] At the biochemical level, it has been shown that β-endorphin and enkephalins increase the turnover of DA and accumulation of metabolites in the basal ganglia and decrease the turnover of DA in the hypothalamus.[50] It is well known that opiates and opiate peptides are effective in increasing the release of prolactin from the pituitary.[51] In spite of the evidence above, it should be stressed that antipsychotic efficacy has not yet been demonstrated in any opioids.

Some information has recently appeared on chiral neuroleptics which may ultimately provide new insights into receptor topography. Although numerous neuroleptics have been resolved into optical isomers and many of these show a high degree of stereoselectivity, the absolute configurations of very few of these are yet known. The best studied of these is butaclamol, whose DA receptor blocking activity is exclusively a property of the dextro enantiomer.[52] Recently the structures of two resolved dibenzothiepins have been determined by X-ray diffraction. These are octoclothepin (2)[53] and the related compound 3.[54] In each case neuroleptic activity is found only in the (+)-10S enantiomer. However, it might be noted that some controversy exists over whether or not some related dibenzothiepins are completely stereospecific in their biological activities.[55-57]

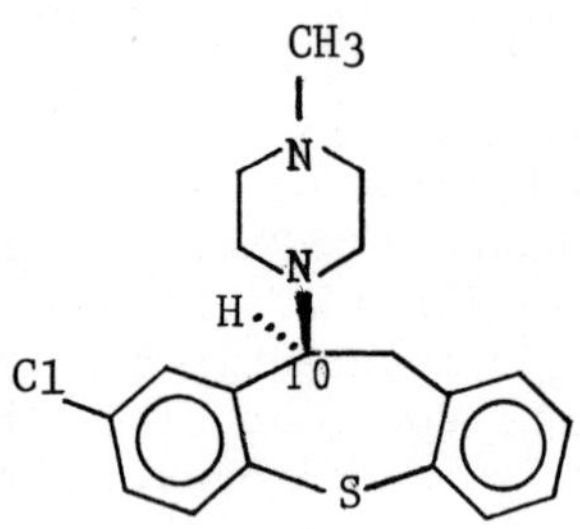

(+)-2

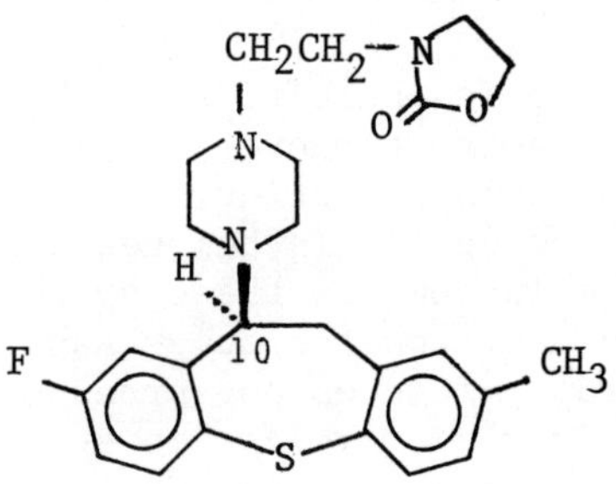

(+)-3

The absolute configuration of SU 23397 (4), a stereospecifically active neuroleptic of a very different structural type, has been determined by chiral synthesis.[58] Comparison of the structures and configurations of these chiral antagonists with each other and with chiral DA agonists should offer an improved understanding of the mode of interaction of these drugs with their receptors.[52]

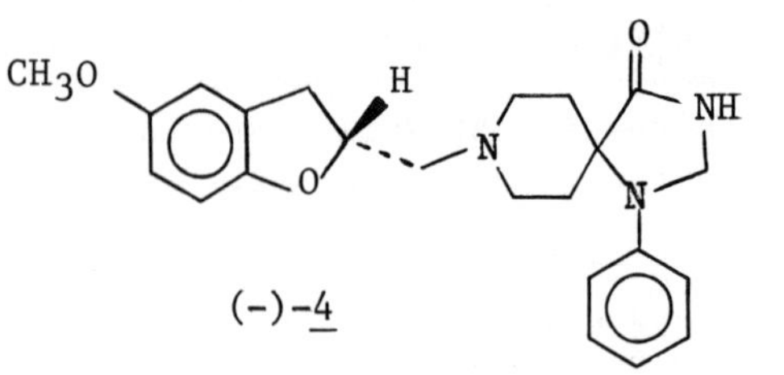

(-)-4

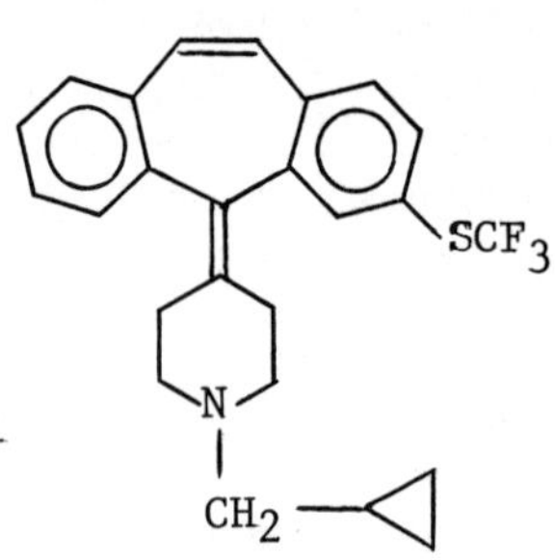

5

From the standpoint of chirality, the novel compound 5 is interesting.[59] This drug, which was made as an analog of cyproheptadine, is optically active. Although it lacks a chiral carbon atom, severely hindered inversion of the non-planar 7-membered ring renders it permanently asymmetric. (-)-5 blocks the conditioned avoidance response (CAR) in squirrel monkeys (0.6 X haloperidol) and APO-induced stereotypy in rats (0.1 X haloperidol). Its enantiomer, (+)-5, blocks neither the CAR nor the stereotypy, but it appears to possess central anticholinergic activity.

Protiva's group has reported[60] that the compound VUFB-10699 (6) is an orally-active cataleptic and blocks APO-induced emesis. Although it is obviously a derivative of octoclothepin (2), those workers noted that it also bears some structural resemblance to drugs of the pimozide type.

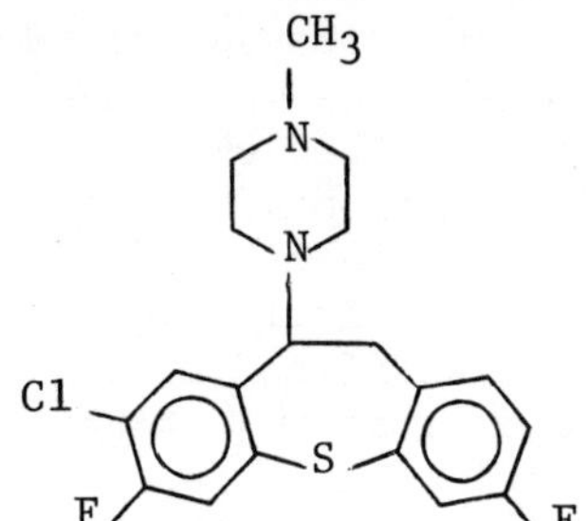

6

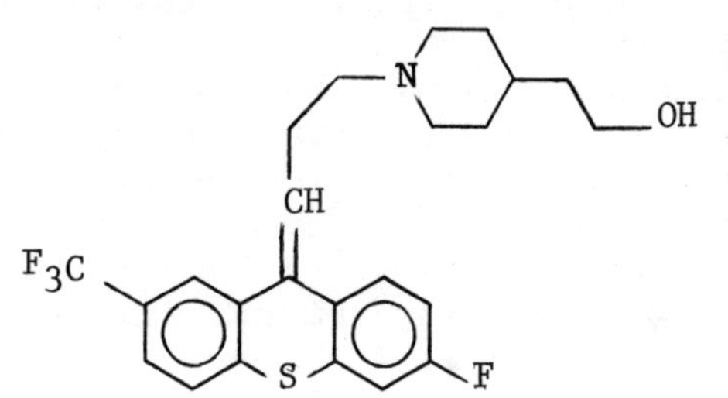

7

A Lundbeck group has reported that piflutixol (7), the 6-fluoro derivative of flupenthixol, is even more potent that its distinguished parent as a neuroleptic in animal models.[61] This compound, whose geometrical isomerism is unstated, is more potent (4-10x) than cis-flupenthixol in blocking APO- and amphetamine-induced stereotypy and in inducing catalepsy. It is the most potent blocker known for the DA-sensitive adenylate cyclase of striatum ($IC_{50}=9.7 \times 10^{-10}$M). It is a potent and long-acting sedative. Typical of neuroleptic drugs, 7 increases DA turnover and elevates the metabolites HVA and DOPAC in rodent brain.[62]

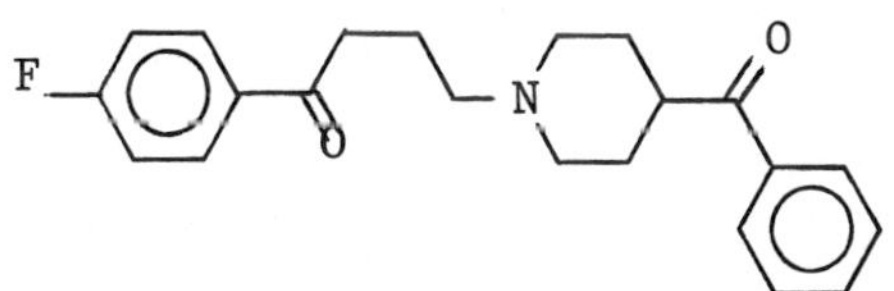

8

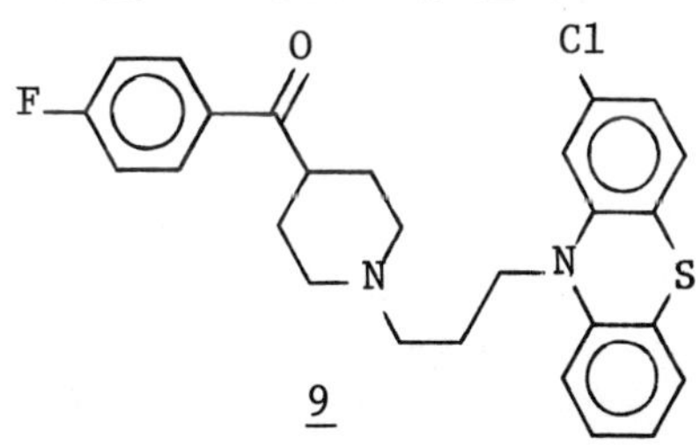

9

An approach to drug design which is often attempted but rarely rewarded is the incorporation of two separate pharmacophores into the same molecule. This approach appears to have succeeded twice in the case of neuroleptics. Lenperone (AHR 2277; 8) may be viewed as containing two butyrophenone moieties in the same molecule. It is an effective antipsychotic drug in man and has a rapid onset of action with minimal extrapyramidal and autonomic side effects.[63] It appears to show greater selectivity than haloperidol in blocking APO-induced behavior in animals.[64] Using this as a model, Boswell, et al.,[65] have combined butyrophenone and phenothiazine groups to produce compound 9, which is the most interesting of a series of five. It is long-acting in suppression of CAR in mice and in protection against amphetamine toxicity in aggregated mice.

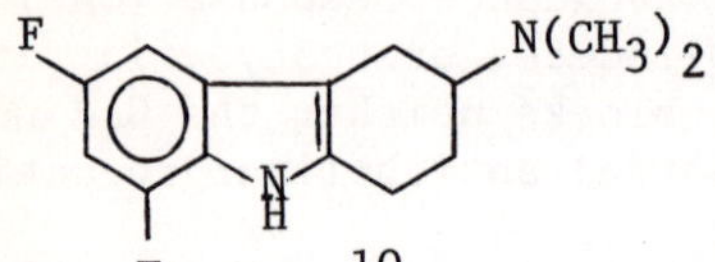

10

One of the more novel structures reported this year to have neuroleptic potential is 10, which was the only active analog in a large series.[66] It was active (6x chlorpromazine) in blocking amphetamine-induced stereotypy, but no further indications of neuroleptic activity were reported. Removal of the fluorine groups gave a compound with imipramine-like activity.

Dopamine Agonists. APO (11) is easily the most thoroughly investigated DA agonist and is the basis for a large number of widely used pharmacological models. It is the subject of a valuable recent review by Colpaert, *et al.*[67] Subsequent to this review, some papers have appeared which are pertinent to the use of APO in pharmacological models. Ljundberg and Ungerstedt[68] reported that APO elicits two distinguishable patterns of behavior in rats (gnawing *vs.* locomotion, sniffing, *etc.*), depending on apparently trivial change in the point of s.c. injection, and that such behavioral changes are not merely dose-dependent intensity changes as is commonly assumed. Cools, *et al.*, have made similar observations and have noted rapid conditioning with APO.[69] Additional evidence has accumulated that various behavioral and neurochemical effects of APO are mediated at presynaptic sites,[70] whose existence is supported by binding studies.[21] Corsini, *et al.*, have demonstrated that low (non-emetic) doses of APO have a paradoxical antipsychotic effect in schizophrenics.[71] This could be explained by selective action of APO at low doses at the presynaptic level which inhibits release of DA into the synapse and thus decreases the activity of the neuron. This may be an attractive target for future drug design.

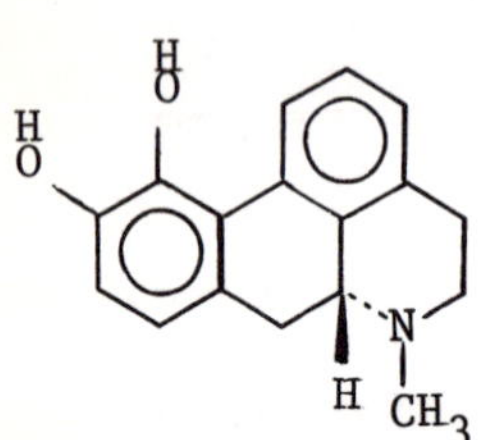

(-)-11

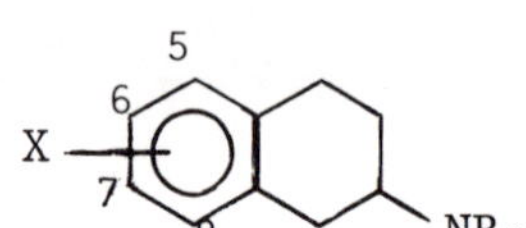

12

a. X=5,6-$(OH)_2$
b. X=6,7-$(OH)_2$
c. X=5-OH

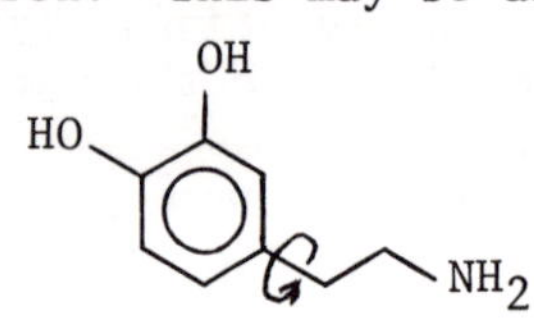

DA, α-rotamer

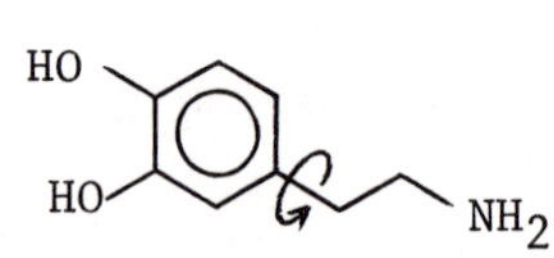

DA, β-rotamer

In recent years 2-aminotetralins (12) have received considerable attention as DA agonists. They were envisioned to be the principal pharmacophore of APO and have lately been used to infer conformational preferences of DA at its receptors. Cannon, *et al.*,[72] have now reported that the pattern of stereotypy-hyperactivity induced by numerous compounds of types 12a and 12b depends on the mode of administration (see also refs. 68, 69) and on the substitution pattern. Compound 12a, R=Pr,[73,74] was the most potent of all. They suggest that compounds of type 12a (α-rotamer of DA) may act via a mechanism different from that of 12b (β-rotamer of DA), and that the α-rotamer represents the preferred conformation of DA in the caudate. This latter suggestion stands in interesting contrast to the effects of these compounds in stimulation of DA-sensitive adenylate cyclase from striatum,[75] in dilation of the canine renal artery,[76] and in binding studies,[77] in which models the β-rotamer is preferred. Of course, the possibility of different receptors in different models must be considered.[40] The earlier report[78] that in vivo activity of compound 12c, R=Pr, is an exclusive property of the levo enantiomer has been subsequently found to have biochemical correlates in stimulation of DA-sensitive adenylate cyclase from retina[79] and in binding to striatal membranes.[77] A compound possibly related to 12c which has been reported to have dopaminergic agonist activity in mice is 3-[2-(dipropylamino)ethyl]phenol,[80] a homolog of m-tyramine.

Ergot alkaloids, which bear little structural resemblance to the dopaminergic aporphines and tetralins, continue to be a rich source of therapeutically useful DA agonists. Parkinson's disease is a condition in which a functional deficit of DA has been clearly established.[81] Reports demonstrating the benefit of bromocriptine (CB 154; 13) in this condition have been rapidly accumulating.[82-87] Of particular interest are the observations in these reports that patients who fail or cease to respond to L-Dopa may respond well to 13. More limited clinical experience with lergotrile (14) in Parkinson's disease[88] appears to parallel that with 13. It would appear that the efficacy of 13 is indeed due to a

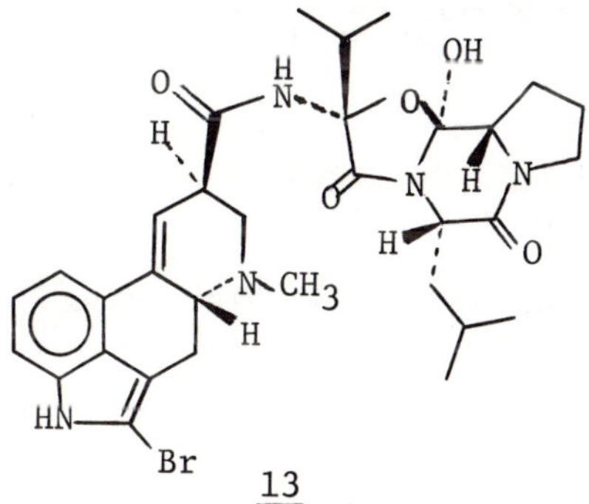

13

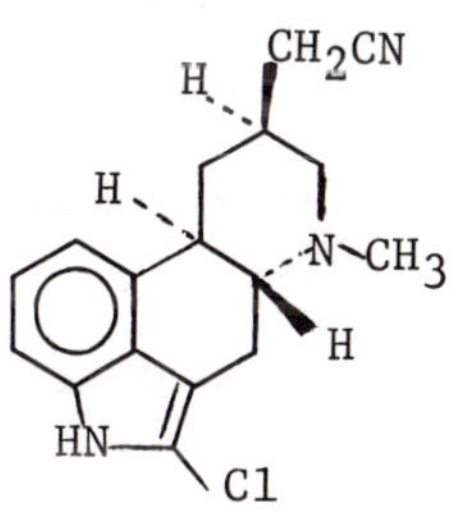

14

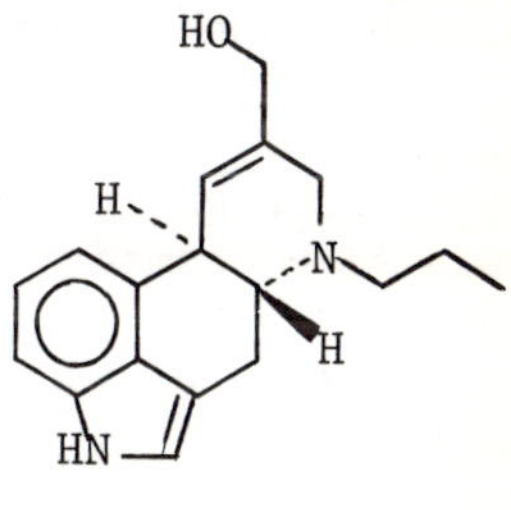

15

DA agonist effect. For example, 13 inhibits release of prolactin.[89] Like APO, it raises secretion of growth hormone from normal pituitary, but paradoxically, 13 lowers it in the condition of benign pituitary adenoma. This last property has made it the drug of choice for treatment of acromegaly.[90,91] The pharmacology of 13 and 14 is complex and appears to include both post- and presynaptic activity[92-96] and possible metabolic activation.[92] Interestingly, while both inhibit binding of agonists in vitro,[94] 14 is an antagonist in the DA-sensitive adenylate cyclase preparation.[97]

Two reports describing synthetic analogs of ergot alkaloids have appeared using inhibition of prolactin secretion in rats to assess activity. Compound 15 was found to be very active in this model.[98] Simpler fragments of the ergoline structure were generally inactive.[99]

L-Dopa, of course, remains the classic treatment of Parkinson's disease. Two groups have reported attempts to improve the bioavailability of L-Dopa, itself a prodrug of DA, by a prodrug approach. Bodor, et al.,[100] systematically prepared derivatives of L-Dopa with one or more of the functional groups blocked, and dipeptides of L-Dopa with multiple protecting groups. Plasma levels of L-Dopa and DA in dogs given such prodrugs orally were found to be significantly higher than after oral L-Dopa. A different approach was taken by Maeda, et al.[101-102] They showed that 3,4-dihydroxyphenylpyruvic acid was rapidly metabolized to L-Dopa by transamination in homogenates of liver and kidney. However, this particular prodrug appears to be hampered by poor absorption *in vivo*.

L-Dopa has been reported to reverse DA receptor supersensitivity,[103,104] and this finding may have implications for the treatment of tardive dyskinesia[104,106]. L-Dopa has also been found to induce recovery from septal lesion-induced rage.[105]

There is a very provocative report by Cotzias, et al.,[107] that chronic L-Dopa treatment produces a dose-dependent increase in longevity of normal mice. This is particularly interesting in view of recent epidemiological studies which indicate that L-Dopa treatment may increase longevity of parkinsonian patients.[108]

Virtually all of the preceeding discussion has pertained to DA agonists and antagonists in the CNS, but more recently the importance of DA mechanisms in the periphery has been noted and reviewed.[40,109] Hypertension is a particular focus of attention.[110] There is an interesting report that prolactin levels in 19 young men with essential hypertension were consistently and significantly higher than in 8 normotensive controls.[111] Bromocriptine was effective in reducing both prolactin levels and blood pressure in these hypertensives. The involvement and possible therapeutic relevance of DA control of cerebral blood flow is also being examined.[112-114]

REFERENCES

1. D.P. Van Kammen, Am. J. Psychiatry, *134*, 138 (1977).
2. R. Freedman, Biol. Psychiatry, *12*, 181 (1977).
3. I. Creese and S.H. Snyder, in "Ann. Rpt. Med. Chem.," Vol. 12, F.H. Clarke, Ed., Academic Press, N.Y., 1977, p. 249.
4. J.E. Leysen, W. Gommeren and P. Laduron, Biochem. Pharmacol., *27*, 307 (1977).
5. P. Laduron, P.F.M. Janssen and J.E. Leysen, Biochem. Pharmacol., *27*, 317 (1977.)
6. P. Laduron, P.F.M. Janssen and J.E. Leysen, Biochem. Pharmacol., *27*, 323 (1977).
7. M. Titeler, P. Weinreich, D. Sinclair and P. Seeman, Proc. Nat. Acad. Sci. USA, *75*, in press (1978).
8. M. Titeler, P. Weinreich and P. Seeman, Proc. Nat. Acad. Sci. USA, *74*, 3750 (1977).
9. P. Seeman, T. Lee, M. Chau-Wong, J. Tedesco and K. Wong, Proc. Nat. Acad. Sci. USA, *73*, 4354 (1976).
10. P. Seeman, M. Chau-Wong, J. Tedesco and K. Wong, Proc. Nat. Acad. Sci. USA, *72*, 4376 (1975).
11. P. Seeman, J.L. Tedesco, T. Lee, M. Chau-Wong, P. Muller, J. Bowles, P.M. Whitaker, C. McManus, M. Titeler, P. Weinreich, W.C. Friend and G.M. Brown, Fed. Proc., *37*, in press (1978).
12. P. Seeman, Biochem. Pharmacol., *26*, 1741 (1977).
13. I. Creese, D. Burt and S. Snyder, Science, *192*, 481 (1976).
14. D. Burt, I. Creese and S. Snyder, Mol. Pharmacol., *12*, 800 (1976).
15. T. Nagy, T. Lee, P. Seeman and C. Fibiger, Nature, in press (1978).
16. A.R. Cools in "Adv. Biochem. Psychopharmacol.," Vol. 16, E. Costa and G.L. Gessa, Eds., Raven Press, N.Y., 1977, p215.
17. N.C. Tye, L. Horsman, F.C. Wright, B.T. Large and I.A. Pullar, Eur. J. Pharmacol., *45*, 87 (1977).
18. G.K. Aghajanian and B.S. Bunney in "Adv. Biochem. Psychopharmacol.," Vol. 16, E. Costa and G.L. Gessa, Eds., Raven Press, N.Y., 1977, p 433.

19. D.R. Burt, I. Creese and S.H. Snyder, Science, *196*, 326 (1977).
20. P. Muller and P. Seeman, Life Sci., *21*, 1751 (1977).
21. I. Creese, D.R. Burt and S.H. Snyder, Science, *197*, 596 (1977).
22. T. Lee, P. Seeman, A. Rajput, I. Farley and O. Hornykiewicz, Nature, in press (1978).
23. T.D. Reisine, J.Z. Fields, L.Z. Stern, P.C. Johnson, E.D. Bird and H.I. Yamamura, Life Sci., *21*, 1123 (1977).
24. I. Creese, R. Schwarcz, J.T. Coyle and S.H. Snyder, 7th Ann. Mtg. Soc. Neurosci., Anaheim, Cal., Nov. 6, 1977, Abstr., Vol. 3, no. 1448.
25. T. Lee and P. Seeman, 7th Ann. Mtg. Soc. Neurosci., Anaheim, Cal., Nov. 6, 1977, Abstr., Vol. 3, no. 1414.
26. I. Creese and S. Snyder, Nature, *270*, 180 (1977).
27. H.Y. Meltzer, R.G. Fessler, M. Simonovic, J. Doherty and V.S. Fang, Psychopharmacol., 54, *39* (1977).
28. G. Brown, P. Seeman and T. Lee, Endocrin., *99*, 1407 (1976).
29. I. Creese and S. Snyder, Eur. J. Pharmacol., *46*, 377 (1977).
30. G. Nikitopoulou, M. Thorner, J. Crammer and M. Lader, Clin. Pharmacol. Ther., *21*, 422 (1977).
31. E.M. Brown, R.J. Carroll and G.D. Aurbach, Proc. Nat. Acad. Sci. USA, *74*, 4210 (1977).
32. G.B. Cassano, P. Castrogiovanni, L. Conti and L. Bonollo, Psychopharmacol. Bull., *13*, 41 (1977).
33. D.H. Mielke, D.M. Gallant, J.J. Roniger, C. Kessler and L.R. Kessler, Dis. Nerv. Syst., *38*, 569 (1977).
34. D.H. Mielke, D.M. Gallant and C. Kessler, Am. J. Psychiatry, *134*, 1371 (1977).
35. P.N.C. Elliott, P. Jenner, G. Huizing, C.D. Marsden and R. Miller, Neuropharmacol., *16*, 333 (1977).
36. B. Scatton, J. Dedek and J. Korf, Brain Res., *135*, 374 (1977).
37. R.M. MacLeod and C. Robyn, J. Endocrin., *72*, 273 (1977).
38. P. Seeman, Biochem. Pharmacol., *26*, 1741 (1977).
39. M. Trabucchi, R. Longoni, P. Fresia and P.F. Spano, Life Sci., *17*, 1551 (1975).
40. L.I. Goldberg, P.H. Volkman and J.D. Kohli, Ann. Rev. Pharmacol. Toxicol., in press (1978).
41. B.H. Westerink, B. Lejeune, J. Korf and H.M. Van Praag, Eur. J. Pharmacol., *42*, 179 (1977).
42. L.F. Agnati and C. Gentili, Drugs Exptl. Clin. Res., *1*, 229 (1977).
43. B. Scatton, J. Dedek and J. Korf, Brain Res., *135*, 374 (1977).
44. K. Fuxe, L. Agnati, B.G. Everitt, T. Hökfelt, A. Ljungdahl and M. Perez de la Mora, in "Adv. Biochem. Psychopharmacol.," Vol. 16, E. Costa and G.L. Gessa, Eds., Raven Press, N.Y., 1977, p 489.
45. J. Hughes, T. Smith, H. Kosterlitz, L. Fothergill, B. Morgan and H. Morris, Nature, *255*, 577 (1975).
46. C. Li, Archiv. Biochem. Biophys., *183* 592 (1977).
47. F.E. Bloom, D. Segal, N. Ling and R. Guillemin, Science, *194*, 629 (1977).
48. E. Wei, L.F. Tseng, H.H. Loh and C.H. Li, Life Sci., *21*, 733 (1977).
49. R.J. Miller, K.J. Chang, B. Cooper and P. Cuatrecasas, J. Biol. Chem., *253*, 531 (1978).
50. L. Ferland, K. Fuxe, P. Feroch, J. Gustafsson and P. Skelt, Eur. J. Pharmacol., *63*, 89 (1977).
51. C.J. Shaar, R.C.D. Frederickson, N. Dininger and L. Jackson, Life Sci., *21*, 853 (1977).
52. L.G. Humber, F.T. Bruderlein and K. Voith, Mol. Pharmacol., *11*, 833 (1975).
53. A. Jaunin, T.J. Petcher and H.P. Weber, J. Chem. Soc., Perkin II, 186 (1977).
54. W. Aschwanden, E. Kyburz and P. Schonholzer, Helv. Chim. Acta, *59*, 1245 (1976).
55. T.G. White and J. Schmutz, Experientia, *33*, 1399 (1977).
56. T.K. Gupta, B.R. Vishnuvajjala, D.T. Witiak and M.C. Gerald, Experientia, *33*, 65 (1977).
57. M. Protiva, Drugs of the Future, *11*, 250 (1977).
58. N.K. Chaudhuri, T.J. Ball and N. Finch, Experientia, *33*, 575 (1977).
59. D.C. Remy, K. Rittle, C. Hunt, P. Anderson, B. Arison, E. Engelhardt, R. Hirschmann, B. Clineschmidt, V. Liotti, P. Bunting, R. Ballentine, N. Papp, L. Flataker, J. Witoslawski and C. Stone, J. Med, Chem., *20*, 1013 (1977).
60. K. Sindelar, J. Metysova, J. Holubek, Z. Sedivy and M. Protiva, Coll. Czech. Chem. Commun., *42*, 1179 (1977).
61. I. Moller Nielsen, V. Boeck, A. V. Christensen, P. Danneskiold-Samsoe, J. Hyttel, J. Langeland, V. Pedersen and O. Svendsen, Acta Pharmacol. Toxicol., *41*, 369 (1977).
62. J. Hyttel, Acta Pharmacol. Toxicol., *41*, 449 (1977).
63. B. Woggon, A. Franke, H. Hucker, E. Ruether, D. Athen, J. Angst and H. Hippius, Int. Pharmacopsychiat., *12*, 113 (1977).
64. R.M. Quock and R.A. Louie, 7th Ann. Mtg. Soc. Neurosci., Anaheim, Cal., Nov. 6, 1977, Abstr., Vol. 3, no. 813.
65. R.F. Boswell, Jr., W.J. Welstead, Jr., R.L. Duncan, Jr., D.N. Johnson and W.H. Funderburk, J. Med. Chem., *21*, 136 (1978).
66. A. Mooradian, P.E. Dupont, A.G. Hlavac, M.D. Aceto and J. Pearl, J. Med. Chem., *20*, 487 (1977).
67. F.C. Colpaert, W.F.M. Van Bever and J.E. Leysen in "Intl. Rev. Neurobiol.," Vol. 19, C.C. Pfeiffer, Ed., Academic Press, N.Y., 1976, p 225.
68. T. Ljungberg and U. Ungerstedt, Eur. J. Pharmacol., *46*, 41 (1977).
69. A.R. Cools, C.L.E. Broekkamp and J.M. Van Rossum, Pharmacol. Biochem. Behav., *6*, 705 (1977).
70. A. Carlsson in "Pre- and Postsynaptic Receptors," E. Usdin and W. Bunney, Eds., Marcel Dekker, N.Y., 1975, p 49.
71. G.U. Corsini, M. Del Zompo, S. Manconi, C. Cianchetti, A. Mangoni, and G.L. Gessa in "Adv. Biochem. Psychopharmacol.," Vol. 16, E. Costa and G.L. Gessa, Eds., Raven Press, N.Y., 1977, p 645.
72. J.G. Cannon, T. Lee, H.D. Goldman, B. Costall and R.J. Naylor, J. Med. Chem., *20*, 1111 (1977).
73. J.D. McDermed, G.M. McKenzie and A.P. Phillips, J. Med. Chem., *18*, 362 (1975).
74. B. Costall, R.J. Naylor and R.T. Owen, Eur. J. Pharmacol., *45*, 357 (1977).

75. G.N. Woodruff, K.J. Watling, C.D. Andrews, J.A. Poat and J.D. McDermed, J. Pharm. Pharmacol., *29*, 422 (1977).
76. P.H. Volkman, J.D. Kohli, L.I. Goldberg, J.G. Cannon and T. Lee, Proc. Nat. Acad. Sci. USA, *74*, 3602 (1977).
77. J.L. Tedesco, J. Bowles, J.D. McDermed and P. Seeman, 7th Ann. Mtg. Soc. Neurosci., Anaheim, Cal., Nov. 6, 1977, Abstr., Vol. 3, no. 1476.
78. J.D. McDermed, G.M. McKenzie and H.S. Freeman, J. Med. Chem., *19*, 547 (1976).
79. M. Schorderet, J. McDermed and P. Magistretti, J. Physiol. (Paris), in press (1978).
80. H.E. Geissler, Arch. Pharm., *310*, 749 (1977).
81. K.G. Lloyd, L. Davidson and O. Hornykiewicz, J. Pharmacol. Exp. Ther., *195*, 453 (1975).
82. D.B. Calne, P.F. Teychenne, L.F. Claveria, R. Eastman, J.F. Greenacre and A. Petrie, Br. Med. J., *4*, 442 (1974).
83. U. Gron, Acta Neurol. Scand., *56*, 269 (1977).
84. O. Kristensen and E. Hansen, Acta Neurol. Scand., *56*, 274 (1977).
85. J.D. Parkes, A.G. Debono and C.D. Marsden, J. Neurol. Neurosurg. Psychiat., *39*, 1101 (1976).
86. R. Kartzinel, M. Perlow, P. Teychenne, A.C. Gielen, M.M. Gillespie, D.A. Sadowsky and D.B. Calne, Lancet 2, 272 (1976).
87. A. Lieberman, M. Kupersmith, E. Estey and M. Goldstein, New Eng. J. Med., *295*, 1400 (1976).
88. A. Lieberman, M. Kupersmith, E. Estey and M. Goldstein, Lancet 2, 515 (1976).
89. K. Mashiter, E. Adams, M. Beard and A. Holley, Lancet 2, 197 (1977).
90. J.A.H. Wass, M.O. Thorner, D.V. Morris, L.H. Rees, A.S. Mason, A.E. Jones and G.M. Besser, Brit. Med. J., 875 (1977).
91. J. Cassar, K. Mashiter and G.F. Joplin, Metabolism, *26*, 539 (1977).
92. E.K. Silbergeld, H. Adler, S. Kennedy, and D.B. Calne, J. Pharm. Pharmacol., *29*, 632 (1977).
93. E.K. Silbergeld and R.F. Pfeiffer, J. Neurochem., *28*, 1323 (1977).
94. J.Y. Lew, F. Hata, T. Ohashi and M. Goldstein, J. Neural Trans., *41*, 109 (1977).
95. G. Di Chiara, L. Vargiu, M.L. Porceddu and G.L. Gessa in "Adv. Biochem. Psychopharmacol.," Vol. 16, E. Costa and G.L. Gessa, Eds., Raven Press, N.Y., 1977, p 443.
96. M. Trabucchi, V.M. Andreoli, L. Frattola and P.F. Spano in "Adv. Biochem. Psychopharmacol.," Vol. 16, E. Costa and G.L. Gessa, Eds., Raven Press, N.Y., 1977, p 661.
97. J.W. Kebabian, D.B. Calne and P.R. Kebabian, Commun. Psychopharmacol., *1*, 311 (1977).
98. A.M. Crider, J.M. Robinson, H.G. Floss, J.M. Cassady and J.A. Clemens, J. Med. Chem., *20*, 1473 (1977).
99. D.B. Rusterholz, C.F. Barfknecht and J.A. Clemens, J. Med. Chem., *20*, 85 (1977).
100. N. Bodor, K.B. Sloan, T. Higuchi and K. Sasahara, J. Med. Chem., *20*, 1435 (1977).
101. T. Maeda and H. Shindo, Chem. Pharm. Bull., *25*, 1992 (1977).
102. T. Maeda, N. Miyakoshi and H. Shindo, Chem. Pharm. Bull., *25*, 2001 (1977).
103. A.J. Friedhoff, H. Rosengarten, K. Bonnet and M. Alpert, 7th Ann. Mtg. Soc. Neurosci., Anaheim, Cal., Nov. 6, 1977, Abstr., Vol. 3, no. 1453.
104. C. Ezrin-Waters and P. Seeman, Life Sci., in press (1978).
105. R.F. Marotta, N. Logan, M. Potegal, M. Glusman and E. L. Gardner, Nature, *269*, 513 (1977).
106. B.J. Carroll, G.C. Curtis and E. Kokmen, Am. J. Psychiatry, *134*, 785 (1977).
107. G.C. Cotzias, S.T. Miller, L.C. Tang and P.S. Papavasiliou, Science, *196*, 549 (1977).
108. R.J. Marttila, U.K. Rinne, T. Siirtola and V. Sonninen, J. Neurol., *216*, 147 (1977).
109. R.G. Pendleton and P.E. Setler, Gen. Pharmacol, *8*, 1 (1977).
110. B.J. Clark, Acta Med. Scand., Suppl. 606, 95 (1977).
111. K.O. Stumpe, R. Kolloch, M. Higuchi, F. Kruck and H. Vetter, Lancet 2, 211 (1977).
112. J. McCulloch and A.M. Harper, Acta Neurol. Scand., (Suppl.) 56 (64), 100 (1977).
113. A. Nilsson, J. Risberg, M. Johanson and L. Gustafson, Acta Neurol. Scand. (Suppl.) 56 (64), 478 (1977).
114. M.H. Lavyne, W.A. Koltun, J.A. Clement, D.L. Rosene, K.S. Pickren, N.T. Zervas and R.J. Wurtman, Brain Res., *135*, 76 (1977).

Chapter 3 Anti-Anxiety Agents, Anticonvulsants and Sedative-Hypnotics

William J. Houlihan and Gregory B. Bennett
Pharmaceuticals Div., Sandoz, Inc., East Hanover, New Jersey

Benzodiazepines and Related Compounds

General — A specific benzodiazepine receptor has been found in rat and human brain cells that may mediate their pharmacological activities.[1, 2a] Binding sites in the rat are unevenly distributed throughout the brain and a loose parallel between the pharmacological potency and receptor affinity was found. The cerebral and cerebellar cortical regions of the human brain contain the highest density of binding sites and the receptors are very similar to those of rat brain.[1,2a] The proposal that benzodiazepines act on the glycine or GABA receptor now seems unlikely since neither glycine or its antagonist strychnine displaced ^{3}H-diazepam binding on the benzodiazepine receptor[1] and chronic administration of diazepam (1a) to mice led to tolerance of anti-strychnine and anti-bicuculline, but not anti-pentylenetetrazole activity.[2b]

Animal studies indicate that the pharmacological actions of benzodiazepines are derived at least in part from activating effects on the 5-HT receptor in the brain[3,4,5] and are probably mediated by several neurotransmitters.[6] The CNS pharmacological activities of benzodiazepines were correlated with some calculated physical parameters[7, 8] and the quantitative SAR in the minor tranquilizer series of benzodiazepinooxazoles (2) was studied.[9]

Changes in the plasma binding of benzodiazepines can be correlated with the lipophilic nature of the ring substituents[10] and diazepam (1a) binding to human serum albumin has been reported.[11]

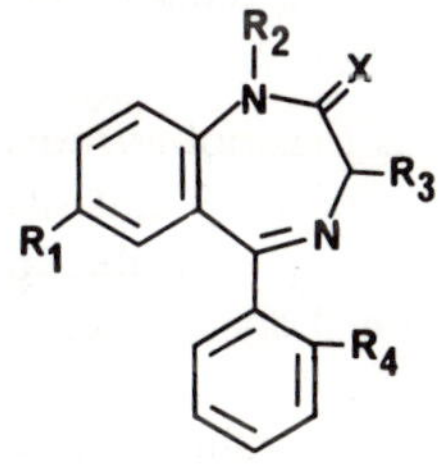

1

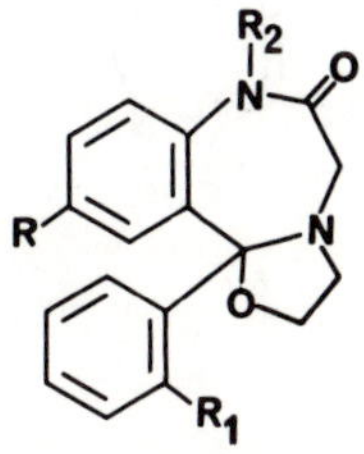

2

2a, R = Cl, R_1 = F, R_2 = CH_2CH_2OH

	R_1	R_2	R_3	R_4	X
1a	Cl	CH_3	H	H	O
1b	Cl	CH_2POMe_2	H	H	O
1c	Cl	CH_3	OH	H	O
1d	Cl	H	OH	H	O
1e	Cl	$CH_2CH_2NEt_2$	H	F	O
1f	Cl	$CH_2C{\equiv}CH$	H	H	O
1g	Cl	H	OH	Cl	O
1h	NO_2	CH_3	H	H	O
1i	NO_2	H	H	Cl	O
1j	Cl	CH_2-cyclopropyl	H	H	O
1k	Cl	CH_3	$OCONMe_2$	H	O
1l	Cl	CH_3	H	F	O
1m	Cl	CH_2CF_3	H	H	O
1n	Cl	CH_3	H	H	H_2
1o	Cl	H	H	Cl	O
1p	Cl	CH_3	H	H	S
1q	NO_2	CH_3	H	F	O
1r	Cl	CH_2CF_3	H	F	S

The behavioral[12] and neural[13] mechanisms of benzodiazepines were reviewed and the monkey behavioral studies of fosazepam[14] (1b), diazepam, temazepam (1c) and oxazepam (1d) were reported.[15]

ISBN 0-12-040513-X

Metabolic studies of diazepam in patients with liver diseases[16], flurazepam (1e) in human portal and hepatic systems[17] and the in vitro liver microsomal metabolism of diazepam and pinazepam (1f) in rat, dog and guinea pig[18] and several desmethyldiazepines[19] in rats are reported.

The clinical pharmacokinetics of a number of benzodiazepines has been reviewed.[20,21,22] Additional pharmacokinetic studies of lorazepam (1g) intramuscular in humans,[23] oral triazolam (3a) in humans,[24] oxazepam (1d) in man and dog[25] and diazepam, temazepam (1c) and oxazepam (1d) in macca ·mulatto monkeys[15] have appeared. Hydrolysis kinetics of diazepam, oxazepam,[26] nitrazepam[27] (1h), ripazepam (4) and other pyrazoloazepinones[28] are reported. A specific radioimmunoassay for determining clonazepam (1i) in human plasma[29] and gas liquid chromatography procedures for separating a variety of benzodiazepines are given.[30]

Acute overdosages with benzodiazepines,[31] toxicity of high dose flurazepam (1e) in hospitalized elderly patients[32] and the use of benzodiazepines in nonpsychiatric medical practice[33] are reviewed.

Dietary administration of diazepam (1a), flurazepam (1e), nitrazepam (1h), oxazepam (1d), and prazepam (1j) at subneurotoxic doses to Swiss-Webster mice led to reduced postnatal survival of off-spring.[34]

Three cases of acute psychotic illness following sudden withdrawal[35] and disorganization of thought as manifested in speech[36] are reported with benzodiazepine therapy.

Anti-Anxiety Agents — Alprazolam (U31, 889, 3b) at 1.5-3.0 mg daily gave moderate to marked improvement in patients suffering from anxiety and tension after alcohol withdrawal.[37] Camazepam[38] (SB 5883, 1k) at 30 mg, fludiazepam[39] (1l) at 7 mg, halazepam[40] (1m) at 120 mg, lorazepam[41,42] (1g) at 3-6 mg, medazepam[43] (1n) at 16 mg and clobazam[44,45] (HR 376, 5) at 20-40 mg daily doses were useful for relieving anxiety in adult patients. Chlordesmethyldiazepam (1o) at 6 mg daily was effective in female neurotic patients.[46] Chlordiazepoxide at 30 mg daily in anxious patients induced increases in verbal interpersonal hostility following frustration.[47]

The imidazobenzodiazepine[48] 6, ethoxy benzodiazepine[49] 7 and the as-triazinobenzodiazepine[50] 8 all have potent minor tranquillizer activity in mice. Triazobenzodiazepine[51] 9 and RGH-3331[52] (10) gave anxiolytic activity in rats. The pyrolobenzodiazepine 11 was more potent than diazepam in reducing anxiety in rats and is used in veterinary medicine as an animal anesthetic.[53] Agressive behavior in untamed cats was markedly inhibited by MS 4101[54] (2a).

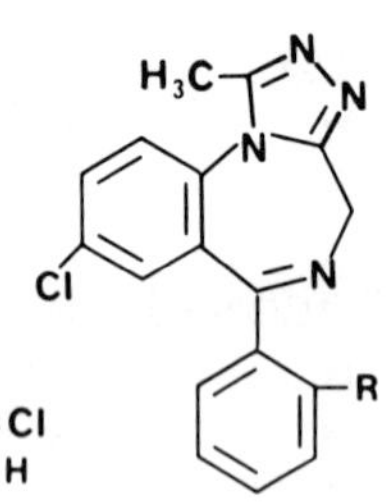

3a R=Cl
3b R=H

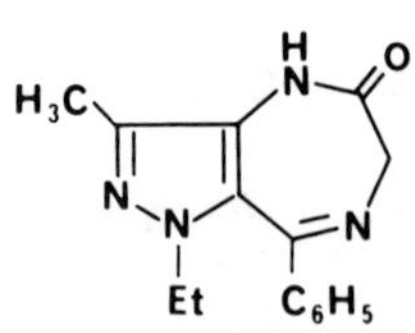

4

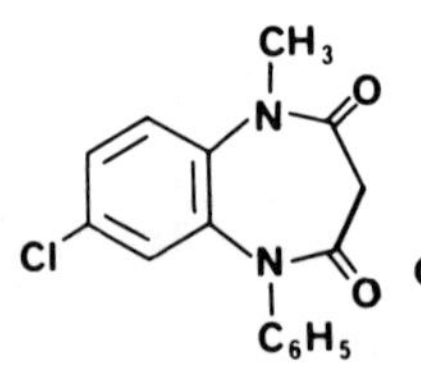

5

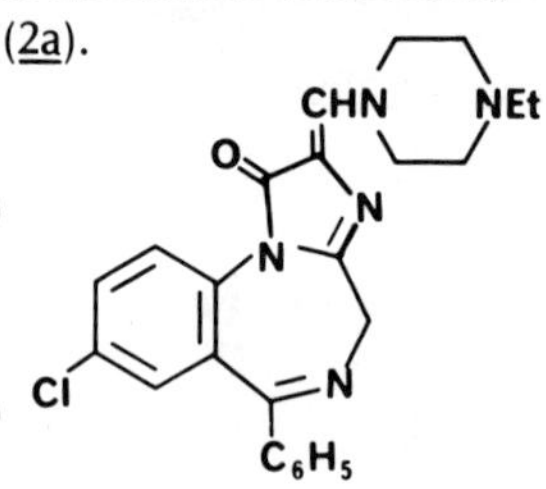

6

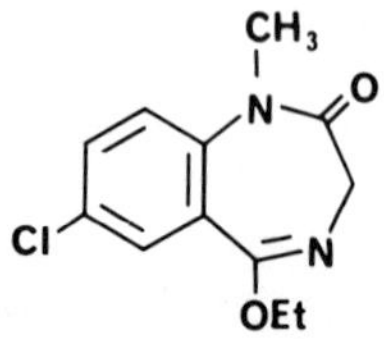

7

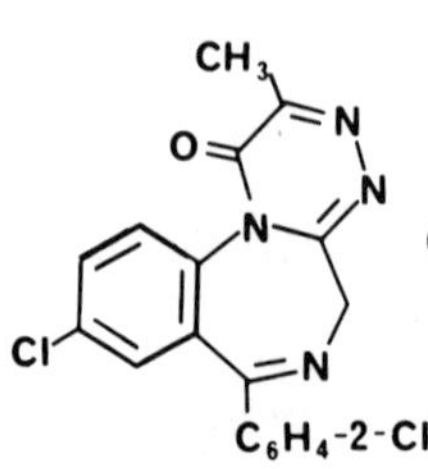

8

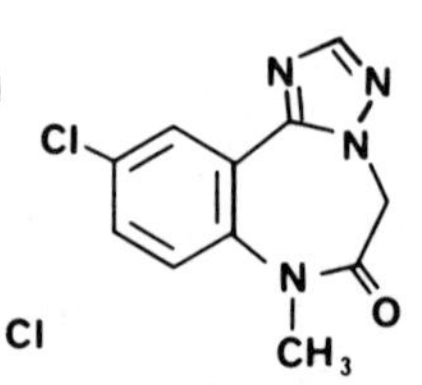

9

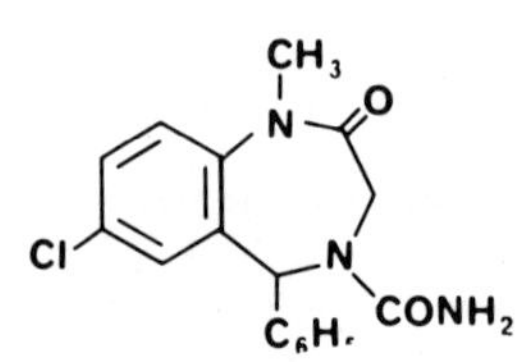

10

Anticonvulsant Agents — Clonazepam (1i) was clinically useful in the treatment of tonic-clonic convulsions,[55] photosensitive epilepsy,[55] focal epilepsy,[55,56] and the stiff-man syndrome[57] caused by diazepam. Studies in dogs, mice and rats indicate that the anticonvulsant activity of clonazepam is partially due to the inhibition of synaptic recovery and the enhancement of presynaptic inhibition.[58]

The benzodiazepine 12 showed anticonvulsant activity greater than diazepam in mice.[59] Sulazepam (1p) was active against corazol induced convulsions,[60] the benzodiazepine 13 against metrazole convulsions[61] and the pyrolodiazepine 14 against pentylenetetrazole convulsions.[62]

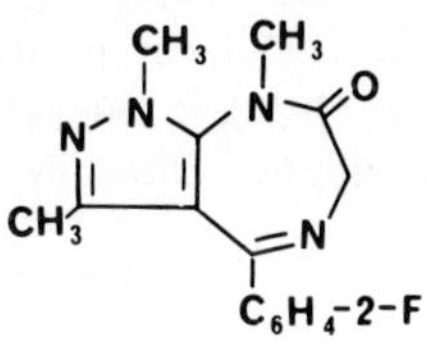

11

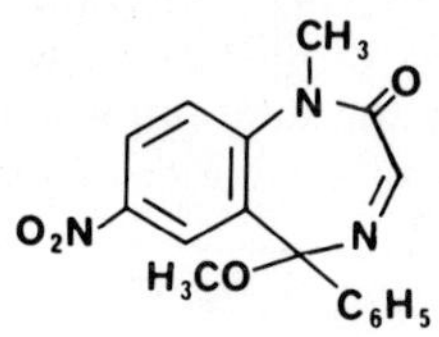

12

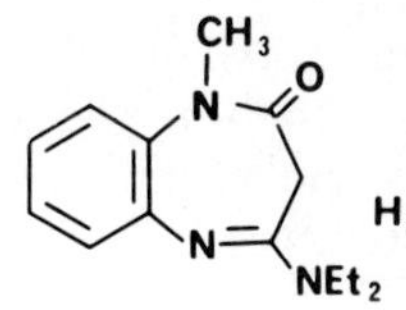

13

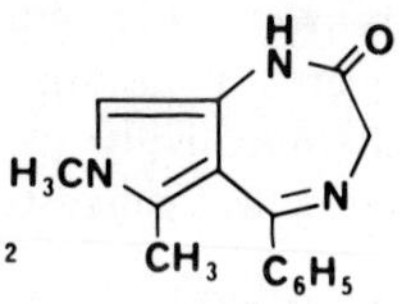

14

Sedative-Hypnotics — Triazolam (3a) at 0.25-0.5 mg was an effective sleep inducer devoid of significant side effects,[63] showed no evidence of toleration,[64,66] but caused increased thought disorders, and congnitive-intellectual impairment.[67]

Flunitrazepam (1q) at 1 mg in normal subjects[68] and at 2 mg in sleep disorder[69,70] or minor gynecological surgery patients[71] was effective in inducing sleep. Hangover and rebound phenomena was found with flurazepam (1e), flunitrazepam (1q) and nitrazepam (1h) in healthy subjects.[72]

Temazepam (1c) at 10-30 mg is a useful hypnotic in general practice with no hangover effects.[73] Chlordesmethyldiazepam (1o) at 2 mg induced sleep in long lasting severe insomniacs[74] but caused behavioral performance impairment at the same dose.[75] Useful sleep induction was given by Sch 16134 (1r) at 50 mg.[76]

Non-Benzodiazepine Compounds

Anti-Anxiety Agents — Several clinical strategies,[41,77] a new anxiolytic rating scale[78] and an intensive design analysis[79] for evaluating anxiolytic agents were reported. The joint use of antidepressant and anxiolytic therapy for the alleviation of anxiety was indicated.[80] A social isolation syndrome in monkeys was proposed as a model for human psychoses.[81]

The tranquilizer phenigam (15) potentiates sedation.[82] Compound 16 was active in monkeys and rodents [83] as an anti-anxiety agent, and 17 appears similar in mice i.p. to chlordiazepoxide.[04]

Based on an increased NE turnover in rats and no effect on DA turnover, it was anticipated that pyrroxan (18) would display anti-anxiety action together with sedation and tranquilizing effects.[85]

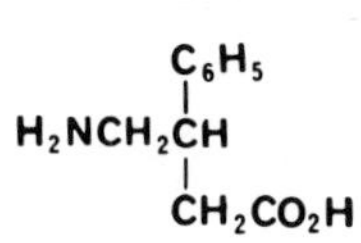

15

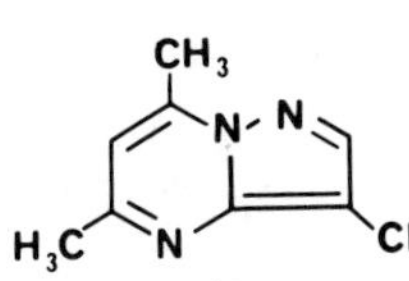

16

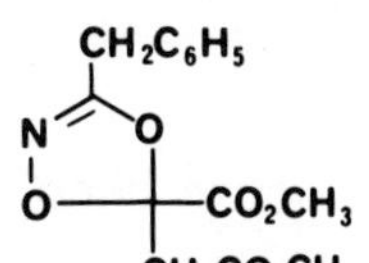

17

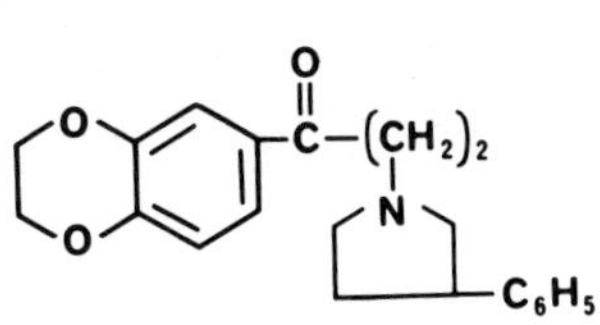

18

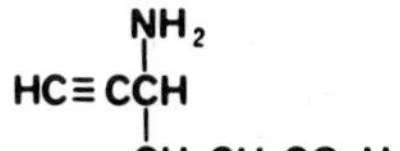

19

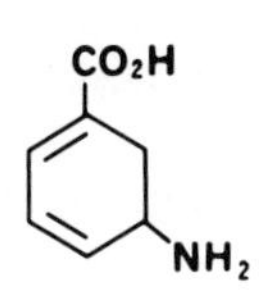

20

Anticonvulsants — The drug interaction of antiepileptic agents,[86] drugs in common use to control clinical seizures,[87] indications for determining serum levels of antiepileptic agents[88] and the metabolic correlation between epilepsy and transmitters[89] are reviewed. A theory was postulated which might explain the relationship between psychosis and epilepsy that occurs in a subgroup of schizophrenic patients.[90] New rodent models for status epilepticus[91] and petit mal epilepsy[92] were reported. The teratogenic activity of several antiepileptic drugs in mice is compared[93] and the teratogenesis of phenytoin is postulated to result from the covalent binding of phenytoin epoxide to constituents of the gestational tissues.[94]

Intracerebroventricular administration of GABA to mice inhibited electrically or pentylenetetrazole induced convulsions.[95] The role played by the transmitter pool of GABA in the convulsant action of chemoconvulsants and in the anticonvulsant effect of antiepileptics clinically used in petit mal epilesy was suggested.[96]

GAG (RMI 71675, 19) produces a sustained elevation of brain GABA concentration, protected against electroshock, thiosemicarbazide and strychnine seizures.[97] Gabaculine (20), a potent inhibitor of GABA transaminase, given i.v. or i.p., elevated brain GABA content and prevented picrotoxin and thiosemicarbazide, but not electroshock induced convulsions.[98]

Carbamazepine (21) produced qualitative control of focal seizures and reduced intracortical spike propagation,[99] and caused less side effects than phenytoin,[100] with no hematotoxic complications. It is less likely to interfere with mental functions in children than equivalent doses of sedative anticonvulsants.[101]

Mephenytoin (22a) was effective against seizures of focal origin, but was of little value in other seizures.[102] The binding of pentobarbital (23a) and diphenylhydantoin (22b) to blood cells was found to be independent of total drug concentration within therapeutic levels.[103]

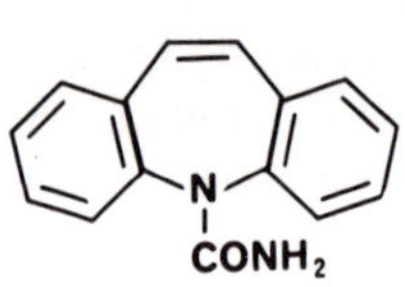

21

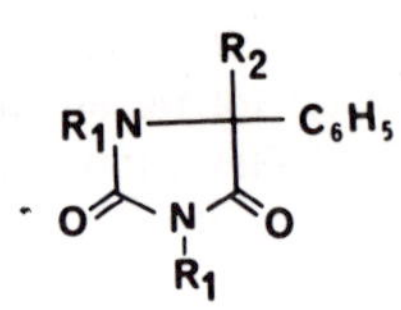

22a, R_1=Me, R_2=Et

22b, R_1=H, R_2=C_6H_5

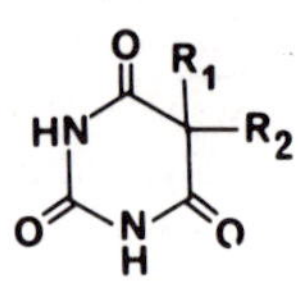

	R_1	R_2
23a	CHMeEt	Et
23b	Ph	Et
23c	CHMeEt	allyl

$(C_3H_7)_2CHCO_2Na$

24

$C_3H_7C(CO_2H){=}CHC_2H_5$

25

Sodium valproate (24) at 600-1200 mg daily was useful in the treatment of grand mal seizures and atonic attacks.[104,105] The bioavalibility,[106] therapeutic efficacy in epilepsy and the mechanism of action[107] of sodium valproate are reviewed. The related pentenoic acid 25 exhibited anxiolytic action by inhibiting 2-oxoglutarate transaminase in animals.[108]

The structure activity correlation between inhibition of tetrazole seizures and partition coefficients of various thiobarbiturates[109] and hydantoins[110] were studied. GS 223 (26a) was the most active member of a series protecting rodents against MES and pentylenetetrazole seizures.[111a] The related succinimide PB 385 (26b) has been proposed for clinical studies as an anticonvulsant agent.[111b]

Glutarimides, (R)-27,[112] 28,[113] and 29[114] protected against MES and tetrazole induced seizures in mice. X-ray studies of phenacetamide (30) support the concept that the stereochemical features confer anticonvulsant action against grand mal epilepsy.[115]

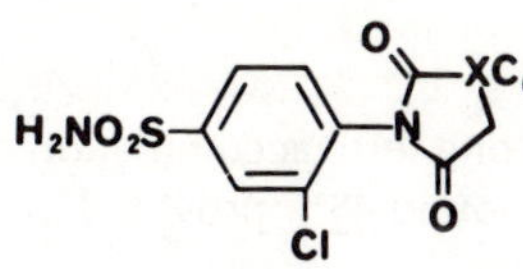

26a X=N
26b X=CH

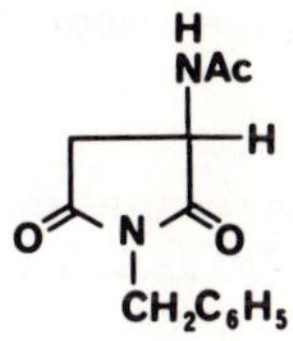

27

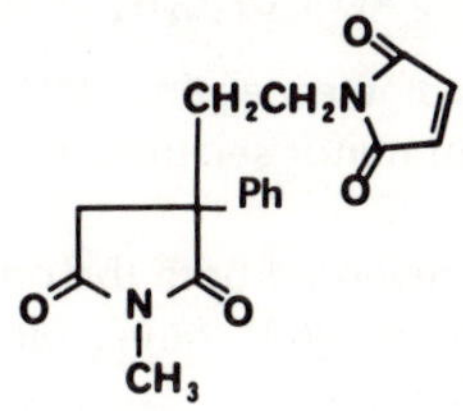

28

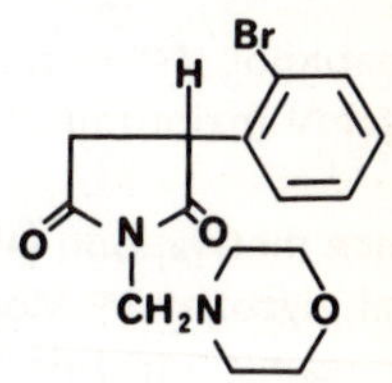

29

Thiocarbamate 31[116] and mercaptotriazole 32[117] protected mice against pentylenetetrazole induced convulsions. Other ureas providing protection in mice against MES or pentylenetetrazole induced convulsions include 33,[118] 34,[119] 35,[120] 36,[121] and 37.[122]

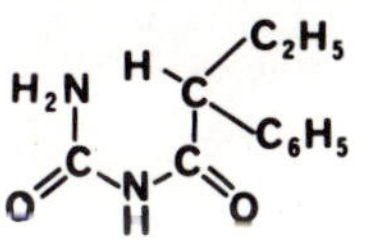

30

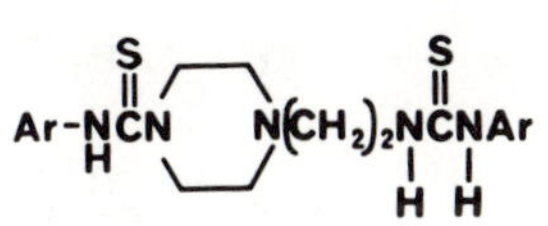

31

Ar=4$C_2H_5OC_6H_4$

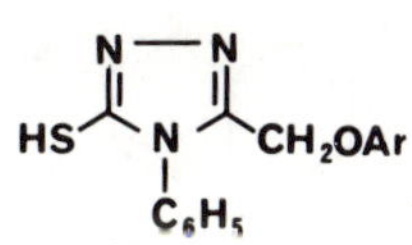

32

Ar= 2, 6-$(CH_3)_2C_6H_4$

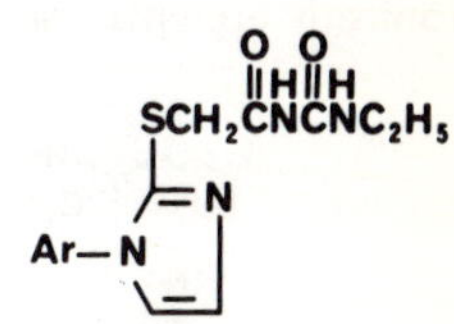

33

Ar=4-$CH_3C_6H_4$

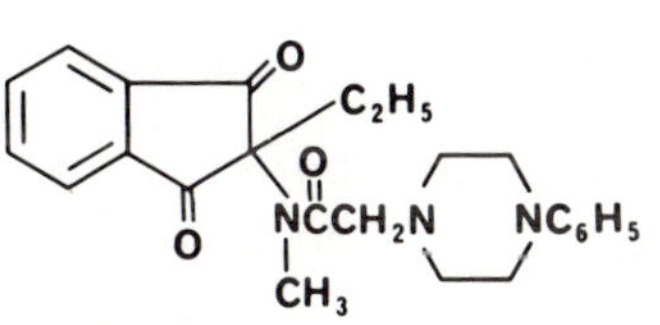

34

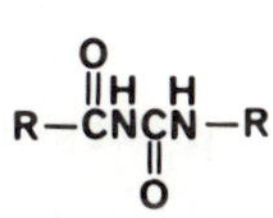

35

R=$CH(C_6H_5)_2$

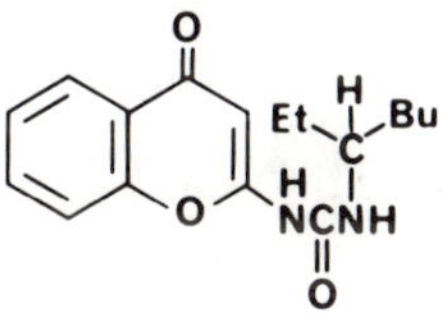

36

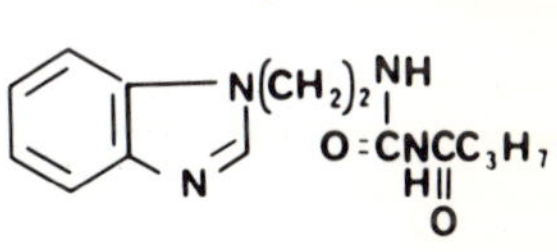

37

Piperazinimine SC 13504 (38) was shown to be a very selective anticonvulsant when fixed interval operant responses were used to compare behavioral toxicities.[123] Benzylideneaminoxypropionic acid 39 prevented convulsions induced by aminoxyacetic acid.[124]

p-Chlorophenylalanine (40) caused a marked reduction in the susceptibility of inbred mice to audiogenic seizures.[125] Compounds 41a,[126] 42,[127] and 43[128] were active against MES induced convulsions in mice.

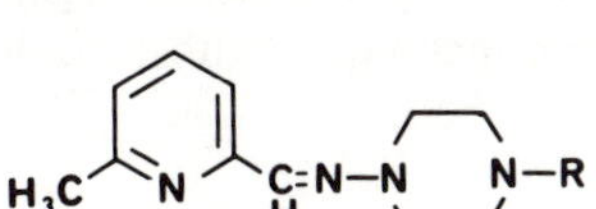

38
R=$CH(C_6H_5)_2$

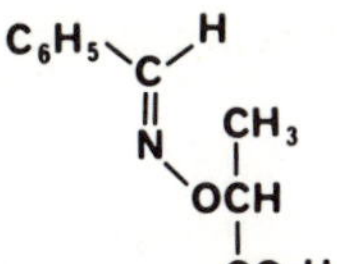

39

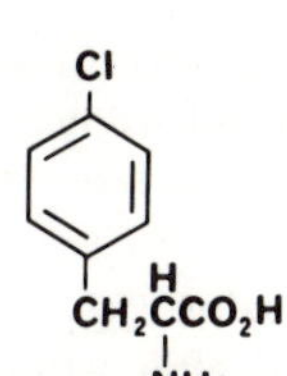

40

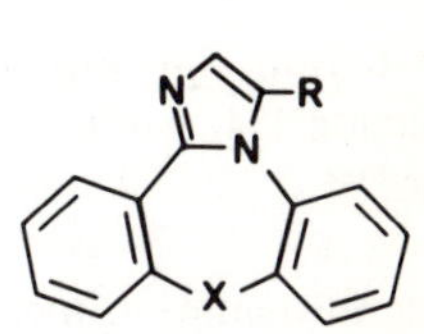

41a R=H, X=NH
41b R=CH_3, X=O

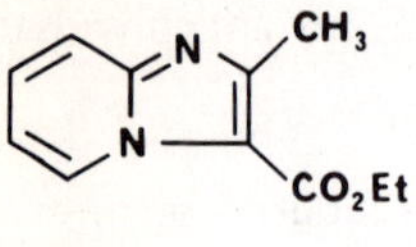

42

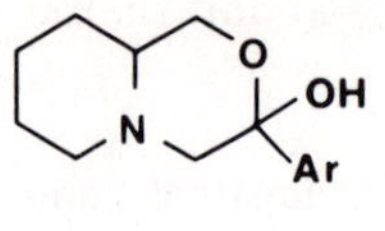

43

Ar = 3-$CF_3C_6H_4$

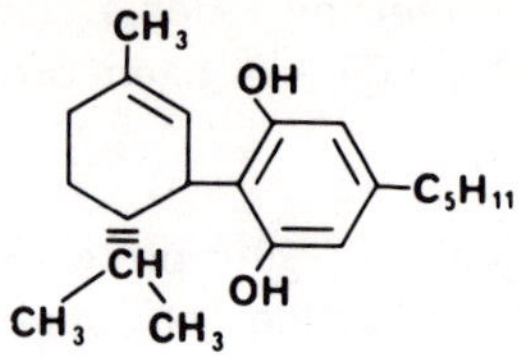

44

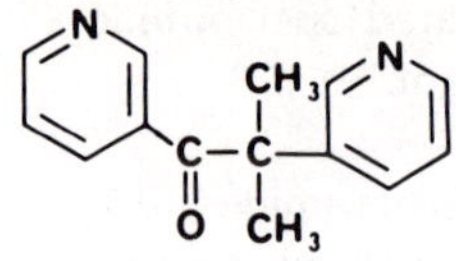

45

Cannabidiol (44) in rats protected against MES and audiogenic seizures indicating its effectiveness against major rather than minor seizures.[129]

In mice metyrapone (45) prevented both the onset of seizures and the long term accumulation of cerebral glycogen.[130] Morpholine 46,[131] quinazolone 47[132] as well as compound 48[133] provided protection against tetrazole convulsions.

Diphenylsilanediol (49) was shown to be orally active in the mouse electroshock model and idiopathic epileptic dogs refractory to seizure control by several anticonvulsants.[134] Swertiamarin (50) was effective against MES and pentylenetetrazole.[135] Glycine choline ester 51[136] was effective in mice and taurine[137] (52) caused a disappearance of the chemical manifestation of seizures in the chronically epileptic cat.

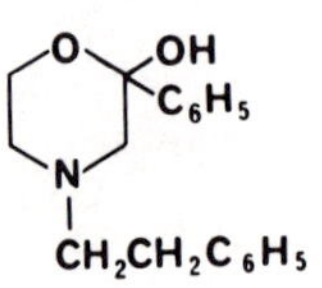

46

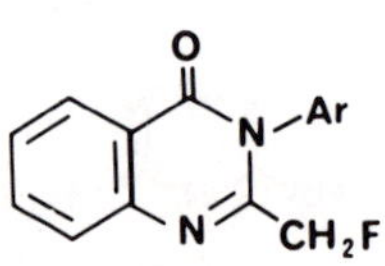

47

Ar = 2-$CH_3C_6H_4$

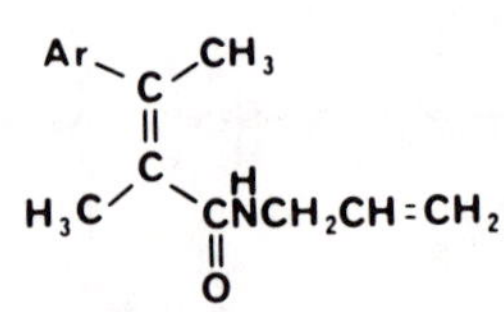

48

Ar = 4-FC_6H_4

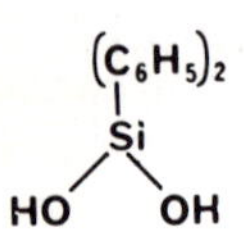

49

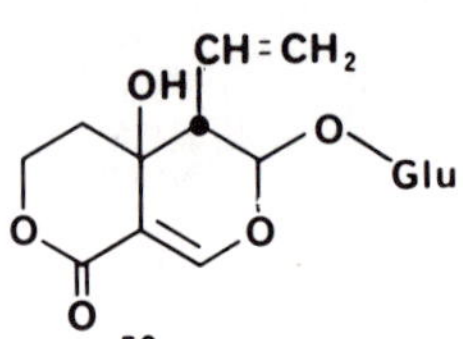

50

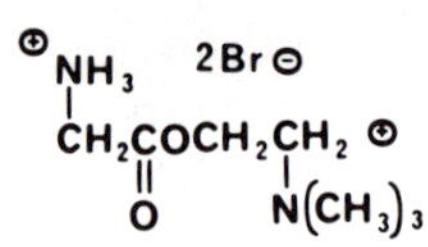

51

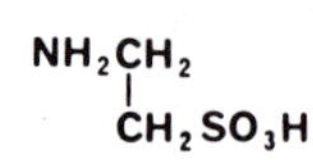

52

Sedative-Hypnotics — A standard protocol was reported to study hypnotic drugs in separate sleep laboratories.[138] Stress induced insomnia in rats was reported to be a reliable model for screening potential hypnotic agents[139] and several laboratory screens for detecting thalidomide-like hypnotic activity were described.[140] The metabolism of phenobarbital[141] (23b) and secobarbital[142] (23c) and the pharmacokinetics of glutethimide[143] (54) were reported.

Methyprylon (53) was found more frequently superior to placebo than pentobarbital (22a) and glutethimide (54) when assessed using both subjective and objective techniques with chronic insomniacs.[144]

The antihistamine trimeprazine (55) acts as a sleep inducer, increasing both REM and slow wave sleep with no REM rebound after withdrawal.[145] It was shown that large doses of nicotinamide (56) result in an increased brain 5-HT level and consequently an increase in REM sleep.[146]

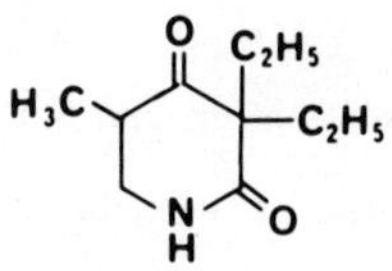
53

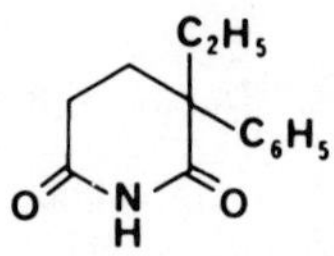
54

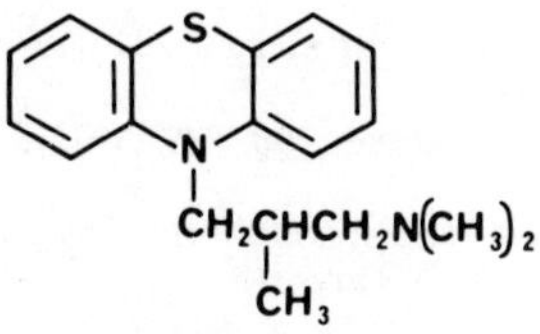
55

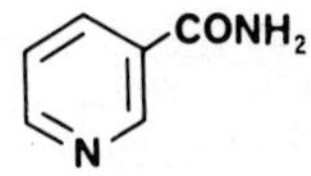
56

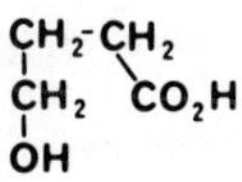
57

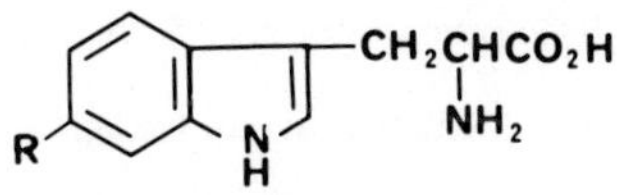
58a, R=H
58b, R=F

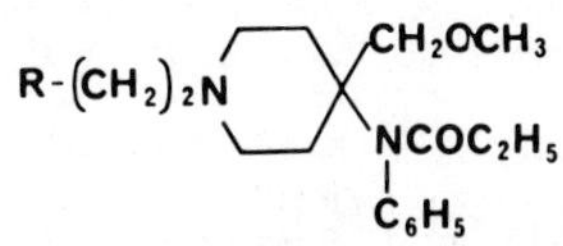
59
R=2-thienyl

While only lasting 2-3 hrs., γ-hydroxybutyric acid (57) induced a sleep indistinguishable from natural sleep by subjective, behavioral and EEG criteria.[147] In humans, ℓ-tryptophan (58a) reduced sleep latency without distorting sleep physiology, both on long term administration and after drug withdrawal[148] and sufentanil (59) had greater hypnotic activity than ten fold higher doses of fentanyl.[149]

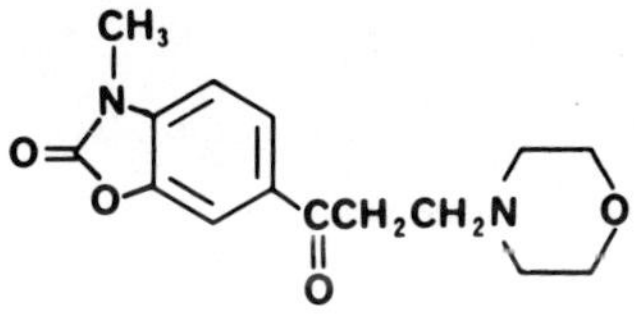
60

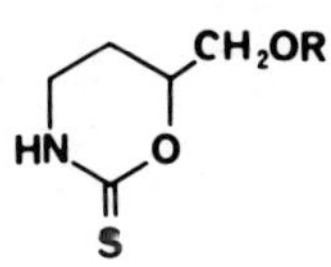
61
R=4-FC$_6$H$_4$

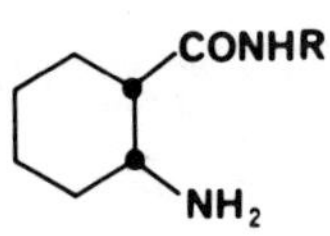
62

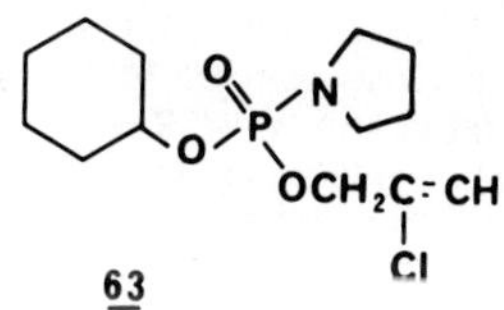
63

Several peptide fragments related to bradykinin injected intracerebrally in mice prolonged pentobarbital sleeping times[150] and the isolation and pharmacology of the controversial rabbit δ-EEG enhancing nonapeptide were reported.[151] Compound 41b[126] caused sedation in rats while 60,[152] 61,[153] 62,[154] and 63[155] were active in mice. In rats, ip., 6-flurotryptophan (58b) produce a significant reduction is sleep latency, but an increase in the number of awakenings.[156] In mice, compound 64[157] and 65[158] potentiated the effects of barbiturates. Pyrazole 66[159] and oxime 67[160] were the most active sedative-hypnotics of their respective series.

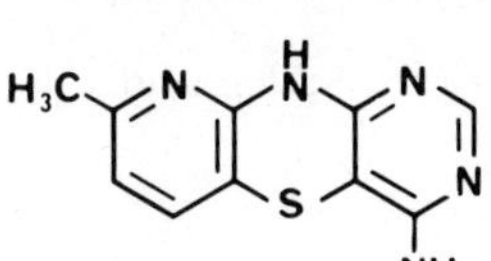
64

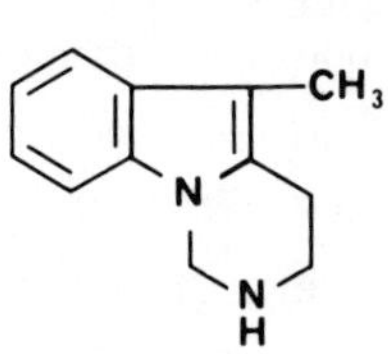
65

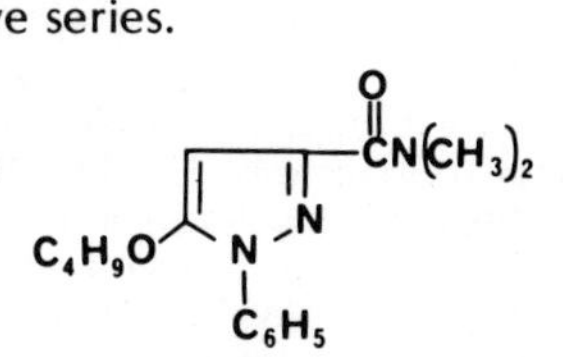
66

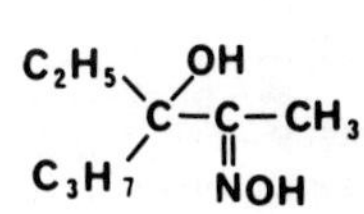
67

References

1. R.F. Squires and C. Braestrup, Nature, 266, 731 (1977); C. Braestrup, R. Albrechtsen and R.F. Squires, ibid., 269, 702 (1977).
2. a. H. Mohler and T. Okada, Science, 198, 849 (1977); b. A. S. Lippa and B. Regan, Life Sciences, 21, 1779 (1977).
3. M. Nakamura and H. Fukushima, Psychopharmacology, 53, 121 (1977).
4. R. B. Rastogi, R. A. Agarwal, Y. D. Lapierre and R. L. Singhal, Eur. J. Pharmacol., 43, 91 (1977).
5. W. J. Weiner, C. Goetz, P. N. Nausieda and H. L. Klawans, ibid., 46, 21 (1977).
6. S. H. Synder, S. J. Enna and A. B. Young, Am. J. Psychiatry, 134, 662 (1977).
7. T. Blair and G. A. Webb, J. Med. Chem., 20, 1206 (1977).
8. N. Y. Golovenko, A. V. Bogatkii, G. Y. Kolomeichenko and S. A. Andronati, Khim. Farm. Zh., 10, 14 (1976).
9. M. Yoshimoto, T. Kamioka, T. Miyadera, S. Kobayashi, H. Takagi and R. Tachikawa, Chem. Pharm. Bull. (Tokyo) 25, 1378 (1977).
10. R. W. Lucek and C. B. Contினho, Mol. Pharmacol., 12, 612 (1976).
11. N. Roosdorp, B. Wann and I. Sjoholm, J. Biol. Chem., 252, 3876 (1977).
12. F. E. Bloom, Am. J. Psychiatry, 134, 669 (1977).
13. L. Stein, J. D. Belluzzi and D. Wise, ibid., 134, 665 (1977).
14. A. N. Nicholson and C. M. Wright, Br. J. Clin. Pharmacol., 4, 494 (1977).
15. S. H. Curry, R. Whelpton, A. N. Nicholson and C. M. Wright, ibid., 61, 325 (1977).
16. U. Klotz, K. M. Antonin, H. Brugel and P. R. Bieck, Clin. Pharmacol. Ther., 21, 430 (1977).
17. W. A. Mahon, T. Inaba and R. M. Stone, ibid., 22, 228 (1977).
18. V. Comi, A. Fossati and G. B. Gervasi, Farmaco Ed. Sci., 32, 278 (1977).
19. E. Mussini, F. Marcucci, L. Airoldi, T. Facehinetti and S. Garattini, J. Pharm. Sci., 66, 1482 (1977).
20. R. I. Shader and D. J. Greenblatt, Am. J. Psychiatry, 134, 652 (1977).
21. E. Van der Kleijn, R. B. Vree and P. J. M. Guelen, Psychopharmacology, 52, 997 (1977).
22. R. I. Shader and D. J. Greenblatt, Am. J. Psychiatry, 134, 652 (1977).
23. D. J. Greenblatt, T. H. Joyce, W. H. Comer, J. A. Knowles, R. I. Shader, A. A. Kyriakopoulos, D. S. Mac Laughin and H. W. Ruelius, Clin. Pharmacol. Ther., 21, 222 (1977).
24. C. M. Metzler, H. Ko, M. E. Royer, W. Veldkamp and O. I. Linet, ibid., 21, 111 (1977).
25. F. Sjoqvist and A. Sundwall, Acta Pharmacol. Toxicol., 40, 5 (1977).
26. W. W. Han, G. J. Yakatan and D. D. Maness, J. Pharm. Sci., 66, 573 (1977).
27. W. W. Han, G. J. Yakatan and D. D. Maness, ibid., 66, 795 (1977).
28. W. H. Hong, C. Johnston and D. Szulczewski, ibid., 66, 1703 (1977).
29. W. R. Dixon, R. L. Young, R. Ning and A. Liebman, ibid., 66, 235 (1977).
30. J. P. Cano, J. Guintrand, C. Aubert and A. Viala, Arzneim.-Forsch., 27, 338 (1977).
31. D. J. Greenblatt, M. D. Allen, B. J. Noel and R. I. Shader, Clin. Pharmacol. Ther., 21, 497 (1977).
32. D. J. Greenblatt, M. D. Allen and R. I. Shader, ibid., 21, 355 (1977).
33. L. Lasagna, Am. J. Psychiatry, 134, 656 (1977).
34. F. J. Guerriero and K. A. Fox, Pharmacol. Res. Comm., 9, 187 (1977).
35. S. H. Preskorn and L. J. Denner, J. Am. Med. Assoc., 237, 36 (1977).
36. L. A. Gottschalk, Curr. Ther. Res., 21, 192 (1977).
37. L. F. Fabre, Jr., A. Gainey and S. Kemple, J. Int. Med. Res., 5, 26 (1977).
38. A. Tammaro, M. T. Picceo, P. Gemmellaro and O. Bonaccorso, Arzneim.-Forsch., 27, 2177 (1977).
39. M. Tanaka, H. Isozaki and K. Inanago Japan J. Pharmacol., 27, 517 (1977).
40. K. Rickels, J. Pereira-Ogan, I. Csanalosi, R. J. Morris, H. Rosenfeld, L. Sobolsky, A. Schless and J. H. Werblowsky, Psychopharmalacology, 52, 129 (1972).
41. R. I. H. Wang, R. L. Wiesen, S. Stockdale and E. Hieb, J. Clin. Pharmacol., 17, 269 (1977).
42. K. Schapira, H. A. McClelland and D. J. Newell, Am. J. Psychiatry, 134, 25 (1977).
43. N. C. Moore, Psychopharmacology, 52, 103 (1977).
44. S. Deventhan and S. Channabasavanna, Curr. Ther. Res., 21, 361 (1977).
45. O. Landano, M. Peralta, L. Lujan, N. Aparicio and J. Moizeszowicz, J. Clin. Pharmacol., 17, 441 (1977).
46. V. Andreoli, F. Maffei, N. Montanaro and G. Morandini, Arzneim.-Forsch., 27, 436 (1977).
47. G. E. Kochansky, C. Salzman, R. I. Shader, J. S. Harmatz and A. M. Ogletree, Arch. Gen. Psychiatry, 34, 1457 (1977).
48. I. R. Ager, G. W. Danswan, D. R. Harrison, D. P. kay, P. D. Kennewell and J. B. Taylor, J. Med. Chem., 20, 1035 (1977).
49. J. H. Gogerty, R. G. Griot, D. Habeck, L. I. Iorio and W. J. Houlihan, ibid., 20, 952 (1977).
50. R. B. Moffett, G. N. Evenson and P. F. Vonvoigtlander, J. Heterocycl. Chem., 14, 3956 (1977).
51. H. Breuer, Tetrahedron Lett., 1935 (1976).
52. J. Rohricht, L. Kisfaludy, F. Darvas, E. Palosi and L. Szporny, Gyogyszereszet, 21, 50 (1977).
53. H. A. DeWald, S. Lobbestael and D. E. Butler, J. Med. Chem., 20, 1562 (1977).

54. K. Anezaki, S. Sakurada, R. Ando, K. Kisara and H. Nakahama, Nippon Yakurigaku Zasshi, 72, 725 (1976).
55. R. N. Nanda, R. H. Johnson, H. J. Keogh, D. G. Lambie and I. D. Melville, J. Neurol. Neurosurg. Psychiatry, 40, 538 (1977).
56. J. W. Lance and M. Anthony, Arch. Neurology, 34, 14 (1977).
57. U. Westblom, J. Am. Med. Assoc., 237, 1930 (1977).
58. T. Yajima, K. Uritani, R. Aoki, T. Suzuki and K. Nakamura, Nippon Yakurigaku Zasshi, 72, 763 (1977).
59. M. Ogata, H. Matsumoto and K. Hirose, J. Med. Chem., 20, 776 (1977).
60. N. Y. Golovenko and V. G. Zimkovsky, Byul. Eksp. Biol. Med., 82, 1078 (1976).
61. G. Roma, A. Balbi and A. Ermili, Farmaco, Ed. Sci., 32, 393 (1977).
62. L. Fantanella, L. Mariani, G. Tarzia and N. Corsico, Eur. J. Med. Chem., 11, 217 (1976).
63. J. C. Chatwin and W. L. Johns, Curr. Ther. Res., 21, 207 (1977).
64. R. L. Reeves, J. Clin. Pharmacol., 17, 319 (1977).
65. R. I. H. Wang, J. Int. Med. Res., 5, 184 (1977).
66. L. F. Fabre, L. Gross, V. Pasigajen and C. Metzler, J. Clin. Pharmacol., 17, 402 (1977).
67. L. A. Gottschalk and H. W. Elliott, Res. Commun. Psychol. Psychiatry Behav., 1, 575 (1976).
68. I. Hindmarch, A. C. Parrott and L. Arenillas, Br. J. Clin, Pharmacol., 4, 229 (1977).
69. U. J. Jovanovic, J. Int. Med. Res., 5, 77 (1977).
70. E. O. Bixler, A. Kales, C. R. Soldatos and J. D. Kales, J. Clin. Pharmacol., 17, 569 (1977).
71. I. Freuchen, J. Ostergaard and O. Mikkelsen, Curr. Ther. Res., 20, 36 (1976).
72. I. Hindmarch, Act. Psychiat. Scand., 56, 373 (1977).
73. L. K. Fowler, J. Int. Med. Res., 5, 295 (1977); L. K. Fowler, ibid., 5, 297 (1977).
74. G. Cesco, S. Giannico, I. Fabbrucci, L. Scaggiante and N. Montanaro, Arzneim.-Forsch., 27, 146 (1977).
75. C. Z. Tansella, M. Tansella and M. Lader, J. Clin. Pharmacol., 16, 481 (1977).
76. F. R. Freemon, M. S. H. Al-Marashi and J. C. M. Lee, ibid., 17, 398 (1977).
77. E. H. Uhlenhuth, Am. J. Psychiatry, 134, 659 (1977).
78. S. M. Free and J. E. Overall, Psychopharmacol. Bull., 13, 8 (1977); R. I. Wang and C. Larson, ibid., 13, 6 (1977).
79. E. H. Uhlenhuth, D. A. Turner, G. Purchatzke, T. Gift and J. Chassan, Psychopharmacology, 52, 79 (1977).
80. R. L. McGhie, H. O'Hara, J. O'Hara, N. H. Brodie, H. G. Dunckley and A. A. Schiff, J. Int. Med. Res., 5, 354 (1977).
81. A. B. Noble, W. T. McKinney, C. Mohr and E. Moran, Am. J. Psychiatry, 133, 1165 (1976).
82. R. A. Khaunina and I. P. Lapin, Khim. Farm. Zh., 10, 125 (1976).
83. W. E. Kirkpatrick, T. Okabe, I. W. Hillyard, R. K. Robins, A. T. Dren and T. Novinson, J. Med. Chem., 20, 386 (1977).
84. N. D. Heindel, W. P. Fives and R. A. Carrano, J. Pharm. Sci., 66, 772 (1977).
85. T. A. Pugsley and W. Lippmann, Psychopharmacology, 52, 113 (1977).
86. A. Richens, Drugs, 13, 266 (1977).
87. D. K. Ziegler, Drugs of Choice, 267 (1976-7).
88. W. Froscher, Arzneim.-Forsch., 27, 1729 (1977).
89. G. A. Buscaino and S. Striano, Acta Neurology, 31, 413 (1976).
90. M. Trimble, Biol. Psychiatry, 12, 299 (1977).
91. K. M. Taber, J. J. McNamara and S. F. Zornetzer, Electroenceph. Clin. Neurophysiol., 43, 707 (1977).
92. D. E. Shearer, D. E. Fleming and E. D. Begler, Epilepsia, 17, 429 (1976).
93. F. M. Sullivan and P. R. McElhatton, Toxicol. Appl. Pharmacol., 40, 365 (1977); P. R. McElhatton and F. M. Sullivan, Brit. J. Pharmacol., 59, 494P (1977).
94. F. Martz, C. Failinger III and D. A. Blake, J. Pharmacol. Exp. Ther., 203, 231 (1977).
95. K. Rusinov, M. Lazarova and S. A. Shopova, Acta. Physiol. Pharmacol. Bulg., 2, 69 (1976).
96. W. Loscher and H. H. Frey, Arch. Pharmacol., 296, 263 (1977).
97. P. J. Schechter, Y. Tranier, M. J. Jung and A. Sjoerdsma, J. Pharmacol. Exp. Ther., 201, 606 (1977).
98. Y. Matsui and T. Deguchi, Life Sciences, 20, 1291 (1977).
99. J. David and R. S. Grewd, Epilepsia, 17, 415 (1976).
100. A. Troupin, L. M. Ojemann, L. Halpern, C. Dodrill, R. Wilkens, P. Friel and P. Freigl, Neurology, 27, 511 (1977).
101. R. J. Schain, J. W. Ward, and D. Guthrie, ibid., 27, 476 (1977).
102. A. Troupin, L. M. Ojemann and C. A. Dodrill, Epilepsia, 17, 403 (1976).
103. M. Ehrnebo and I. Oder Cederlof, Eur. J. Clin. Pharmacol., 11, 37 (1977).
104. R. M. Pinder, R. N. Brogden, T. M. Spreight and G. S. Avery, Drugs, 13, 81 (1977); W. R. Cuabe and R. J. Gumnet, Epilepsia, 18, 117 (1977).
105. J. S. Lockard, R. H. Levy, ibid., 17, 477 (1976).
106. W. Oelkers, G. Stoffels, H. Schafer and H. Reith, Arzneim.-Forsch., 27, 1088 (1977).
107. Issue No. 2, Epilepsia, 18, (1977).

108. R. Misslin, A. Hinschberger, M. Maitre and L. Ciesielski, Pschopharmacology, 50, 53 (1977).
109. B. R. Pandey, K. Raman, J. P. Barthwal, K. Kishor and K. P. Bhargava, Curr. Sci., 46, 366 (1977).
110. M. J. Kowhda, Z. Kleinrok and E. Przegalinski, Pol. J. Pharmacol. Pharm., 28, 329 (1976).
111. a. P. G. Waser, A. J. Ganz and R. W. Pfirrmann, Arzneim.-Forsch., 27, 2125 (1977); b. P. G. Waser, A. J. Ganz and R. W. Pfirrmann, ibid., 27, 1942 (1977).
112. D. T. Witiak, B. R. Vishnuvajjala, W. L. Cook and J. A. Minatelli, J. Med. Chem., 20, 801 (1977).
113. M. J. Kornet, A. M. Crider and E.O. Magarian, ibid., 20, 405 (1977).
114. J. Lange, S. Rump, E. Galecka and I. Ilczak, Pharmazie, 32, 82 (1977).
115. A. Camerman and N. Camerman, Proc. Natl. Acad. Sci, 74, 1264 (1977).
116. S. S. Parmar, M. Chaudhary, S. Chaudhary and H. R. Spiro, Pharmacology, 15, 112 (1977).
117. S. S. Parmar, M. Chaudhary, S. K. Chaudhary, S. Kumar and H. P. Spiro, J. Pharm. Sci., 66, 971 (1977).
118. S. K. Chaudhary, S. S. Parmar, M. Chaudhary and J. P. Barthwal, ibid., 65, 1010 (1976).
119. Y. Y. Ozol, Pharm. Ind., 38, 942 (1976).
120. A. G. Pechenkin, V. K. Groshkova and L. G. Tignibidina, Khim. Farm. Zh., 10, 63 (1976).
121. M. Payard, J. Paris, J. Couquelet and J. Bastide, Eur. J. Med. Chem., 11, 13 (1976).
122. L. V. Skrabova, Khim. Farm. Zh., 10, 49 (1976).
123. S. Peterson, L. Stark, J. Carlisle and D. Barmby, Proc. West Pharmacol. Soc., 20, 159 (1977).
124. G. D. Lahan, G. Osuide and F. Stansfield, West Afr. J. Pharmalcol. Drug Res., 3, 77 (1976).
125. G. J. Alexander and L. M. Kopeloff, Neuropharmacology, 16, 405 (1977).
126. J. P. Maffrand, J. M. Pereillo, F. Eloy and D. Aubert, Eur. J. Med. Chem., 11, 467 (1976).
127. H. Boehme and K. H. Weisel, Arch. Pharm., 309, 959 (1976).
128. G. O. N. Rankin, Diss. Abstr. Int. B, 37, 3906 (1977).
129. P. Consroe and A. Wolkin, J. Pharmacol. Exp. Ther., 201, 26 (1977).
130. A. Berel, P. R. Lehr and J. Gayet, Brain Res., 128, 193 (1977).
131. A. H. Beckett and P. Kourounakis, Arzneim.-Forsch., 26, 1810 (1976).
132. I. R. Ager, D. R. Harrison, P. D. Kennewell and J. B. Taylor, J. Med. Chem., 20, 379 (1977).
133. A. Balsamo, P. L. Barilli, P. Crotti and B. Macchia, ibid., 20, 48 (1977).
134. M. L. Chandler and R. R. LeVier, Pharmacologist, 19, 214 (Abstr. 495) (1977).
135. S. K. Bhattacharya, P. K. S. P. Reddy, S. Ghosal and A. K. Singh, J. Pharm. Sci., 65, 1547 (1977).
136. V. P. Shamshin, O. S. Anisimova, T. Y. Filipenko and V. G. Voronin, Khim. Farm. Zh., 11, 47 (1977).
137. N. M. vanGelder, I. Koyama and H. H. Jasper, Epilepsia, 18, 1 (1977).
138. A. Kales, E. O. Bixler, J. D. Kales and M. B. Scharf, J. Clin. Pharmacol., 17, 207 (1977).
139. D. C. Piper, Br. J. Pharmacol., 59, 509P (1977).
140. R. C. A. Frederickson, I. H. Slater, W. E. Dusenberry, C. R. Hewes, G. T. Jones, and R. A. Moore, J. Pharmacol. Exp. Ther., 203, 240 (1977).
141. B. K. Tang, T. Inaba and W. Kalow, Fed. Proc., 36, 996, (1977).
142. B. G. Hammond and E. W. Maynert, ibid., 36, 996 (1977).
143. J. W. Crow, P. Lain, F. Bochner, D. W. Shoeman and D. L. Azarnoff, Clin. Pharmacol. Ther., 22, 458 (1977).
144. R. I. H. Wang and S. L. Stockdale, J. Clin. Pharmacol., 17, 728 (1977).
145. K. Kayed, T. Hansen and O. B. Godtlibsen, Tidsskr. Nor. Laegenforen, 96, 1722 (1976.
146. C. R. Robinson, G. V. Pegrain, P. R. Hyde, J. M. Beaton and J. R. Symthies, Biol. Psychiatry, 12, 139 (1977).
147. M. Mamelak, J. M. Escrin and O. Stokan, ibid., 12, 273 (1977).
148. E. Hardtmann, Am. J. Psychiatry, 134, 366 (1977).
149. J. Kugler, B. Grote, M. Laub, A. Doenicke and E. Dick, Anaesthesist, 26, 343 (1977).
150. Y. Okada, Y. Tuchiya, M. Yagyu, S. Kozawa and K. Karija, Neuropharmacology, 16, 381 (1977).
151. a. G. A. Schoenberger, P. F. Maier, H. J. Touler and M. Monnier, Eur. J. Physiol., 369, 99 (1977); b. G. A. Schoenberger and M. Monnier, Proc. Nat. Acad. Sci., 74, 1282 (1977).
152. J. C. Cazin, D. Lesieur, C. Lespagnol and M. Cazin, Eur. J. Med. Chem., 11, 33 (1977).
153. G. Raynand, C. Gouret, M. J. Bouniol and M. Mazadier, ibid., 11, 75 (1977).
154. Z. Ecsery, Acta. Chim. Acad. Sci. Hung., 89, 61 (1976).
155. N. P. Grechkin, L. N. Grishina, I. D. Neklesova, M. A. Kudrena and N. N. Anisimova, Khim. Farm. Zh., 11, 43 (1977).
156. A. Fletcher and D. Sugden, Br. J. Pharmacol., 61, 485 p (1977).
157. C. O. Okafor, M. L. Steenberg and J. P. Buckley, Eur. J. Med. Chem., 12, 249 (1977).
158. G. N. Artemenko, Y. I. Vikhlyaev, N. F. Kucherova and L. N. Boresova, Farmakol. Toksikol., 39, 651 (1976).
159. S. Sugiura, S. Ohno, O. Ohtani, K. Izumi, T. Kitamikado, H. Asai, K. Kato, M. Hori, and H. Fujimura, J. Med. Chem., 20, 80 (1977).
160. G. Taillandier, J. L. Benoit-Guyod, A. Boucherle, M. Broll and P. Eymard, Eur. J. Med. Chem., 11, 365 (1976).

Chapter 4. Agents Affecting GABA in the CNS

Jeffrey K. Saelens and Fredric J. Vinick
Research Department, Pharmaceuticals Division
CIBA-GEIGY Corporation, Summit, New Jersey

A considerable body of evidence points to the fact that γ-aminobutyric acid (GABA, 1) is a major inhibitory transmitter in the central nervous system of animals and man. A comprehensive review of GABA function and the importance of the GABA system in certain neurologic and psychiatric disorders has recently been published.[1]

It is well established that GABA itself, GABA-mimetics and certain other agents such as baclofen (2) and γ-butyrolactone (3) will slow the

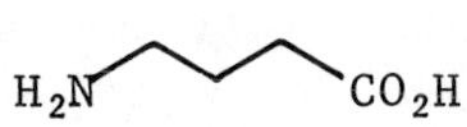

1

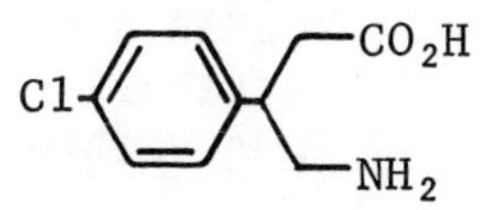

2

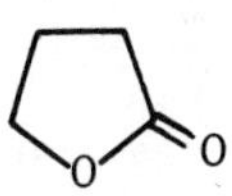

3

firing rate of dopaminergic neurons in two areas of the brain: those in the substantia nigra which project to the striatum[2] and those in the ventral tegmentum which project to the mesolimbic areas and cortex.[3] Since antipsychotic agents are known to block dopamine receptors in these brain areas, the use of GABA-mimetics which also attenuate dopaminergic functions alone or as an adjunct to neuroleptic therapy has received increased attention.[4]

There are several other disease states in which a disruption of a GABA neuronal system has been implicated. In Huntington's chorea a clear loss of GABA function occurs, presumably due to the destruction of the striatal-nigral GABAergic pathway.[5-10] The fact that there is no loss of GABA receptors in the striatum[11] further illustrates that the GABA pathway is not intrinsic to this extra-pyramidal area. Recently, the similarity between the cellular destruction caused by intrastriatal administration of kainic acid (4) and the observed cellular losses in Huntington's chorea has been noted.[12-14] Kainic acid is a structurally rigid

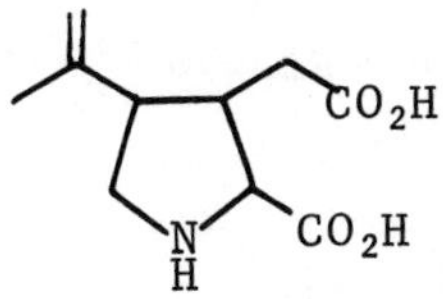

4

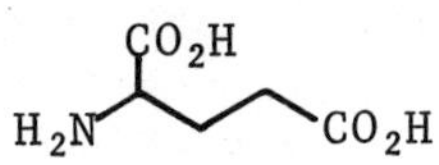

5

analogue of glutamic acid (5). It is a potent neuroexcitatory agent which destroys cells containing glutamic acid receptors.

ISBN 0-12-040513-X

Due to its function as a major inhibitory transmitter in the central nervous system, GABA, or more specifically, the lack thereof, has long been suspected to play a role in epilepsy.[15] Studies have been carried out showing that agents which elevate or mimic GABA prevent seizure activity in animal models[16-18] and that agents which deplete GABA or block its actions cause seizures.[16,19-22] Surprisingly, only one anti-epileptic agent, sodium valproate (6), has been found to have a direct influence on GABA metabolism, and that effect is not the same as those mentioned above.[23,24]

$$(C_3H_7)_2CHCO_2H$$

6

Sodium valproate evidently inhibits succinic semialdehyde dehydrogenase (SSAD), the enzyme necessary to metabolize the product of GABA-transaminase (GABA-T) activity (see Fig. 1 for GABA synthesis/metabolism and section on GABA-T inhibition). Without SSAD activity, GABA-T activity is presumably hampered by end-product inhibition.

The synthesis and metabolism of GABA within a presynaptic neuron is outlined in Fig. 1.

Fig. 1

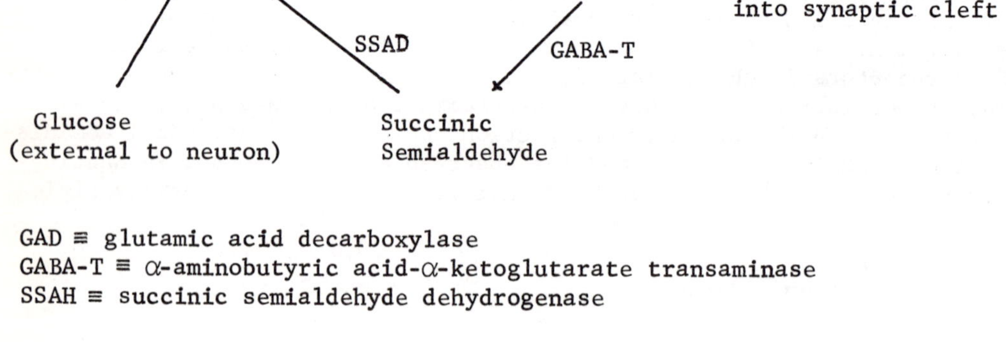

GAD ≡ glutamic acid decarboxylase
GABA-T ≡ α-aminobutyric acid-α-ketoglutarate transaminase
SSAH ≡ succinic semialdehyde dehydrogenase

As can be seen from Fig. 1, glucose from outside the neuron is the fundamental precursor of GABA. GABA itself cannot cross the blood-brain barrier and hence must be synthesized within the neuron.

A depiction of GABA-mediated neurotransmission is presented in Fig. 2.

Fig. 2

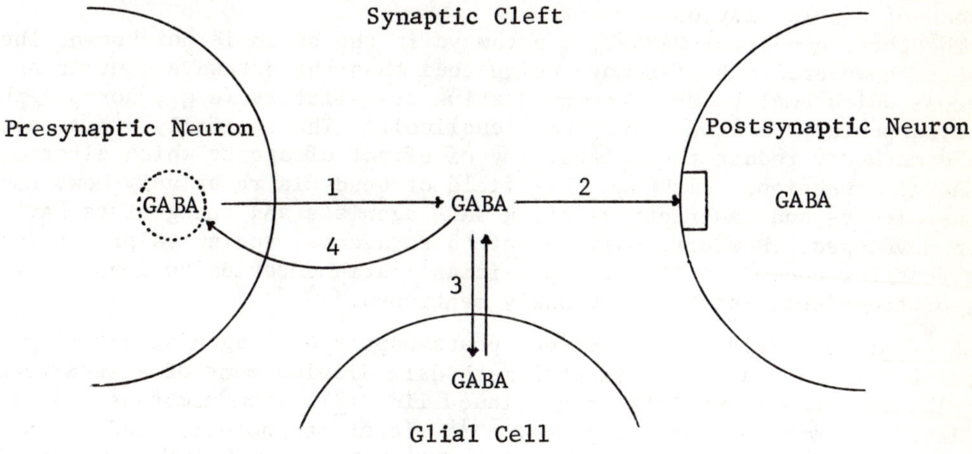

1. Release of stored GABA into synaptic cleft.
2. Receptor interaction.
3. Uptake into perisynaptic glia, or release from glia.
4. Uptake into presynaptic neurons.

In principle, GABA-mediated function could be modified by a drug which would interact with the GABA system at one or more of the locations shown in Fig. 2 and/or with GABA synthesis/metabolism (Fig. 1).

As previously mentioned, GABA is considered to be a major inhibitory transmitter. In most cases, GABA inhibits neurotransmission by increasing cell membrane permeability to chloride ions. Two types of inhibition have been identified.[25] In the first type the release of GABA from a neuron terminal partially depolarizes the terminal of an excitatory neuron. The partial depolarization causes a reduction in the release of the excitatory transmitter. This mode of inhibition between GABA interneurons and sensory neurons in the spinal cord is called presynaptic inhibition. The second, more classical mechanism of inhibition occurs at synapses between GABA neuron terminals and cell bodies. GABA hyperpolarizes the soma and/or dendrites of the next cell in line, giving rise to a higher than normal potential gradient. Since this excessive charge differential cannot be compensated for, the neuron is unable to fire.

GABA is also found in glial cells in the central nervous system.[1] Glial cells, like GABA neurons, have the capacity for high affinity uptake of GABA, and can release GABA when exposed to a sufficiently high external concentration of potassium ions (see Fig. 2). Glial GABA accounts for approximately 50% of the GABA in the brain. The exact role of glial GABA is not known, but is thought to represent a "second line of defense" against localized excessive depolarization. If such a depolarization were to occur, the resultant rise in extracellular potassium ion concentration would induce the release of glial GABA which would, in turn, reduce the spread of depolarization.

The total number of GABAergic pathways in the brain is not known. They appear, however, to be far more ubiquitous than the pathways containing neurons which employ other known putative transmitters (e.g., norepinephrine, dopamine, serotonin and acetylcholine).[1] Theoretically, this fact could markedly reduce the selectivity of effect of agents which alter GABAergic function. Although this field of study is relatively new, numerous direct- and indirecting-acting GABA agonists and antagonists have been developed. However, only one of these agents, sodium valproate (6) has thus far become part of the physician's armamentarium to counteract any of the disease states previously mentioned.

GABA Agonists Evidence for direct postsynaptic GABA agonist activity is obtained via two main experimental methods: displacement of a GABA receptor ligand, such as H^3-GABA or H^3-bicuculline (7), from membrane fragments believed to contain GABA receptors;[27-30] microiontophoretic studies in which the suspected agonist mimics the action of GABA and where the suspected agonist's actions are blocked by a GABA antagonist such as bicuculline[31-32] (microiontophoresis is an electrophoretic technique in which the agent in question is applied very near to the neuronal receptor site). Specific binding to the GABA receptor can be distinguished from binding by the uptake carrier mechanism by omitting sodium ions from the medium. Receptor binding is sodium independent, whereas the neuronal uptake carrier mechanism requires the presence of a physiological concentration of sodium ions.[1] Some of the more potent agents capable of displacing GABA receptor ligands are muscimol (8),[29] 3-aminopropane sulphonic acid (9),[29,30] imidazole-4-acetic acid (10),[29,30] and GABA itself (1).[28-30]

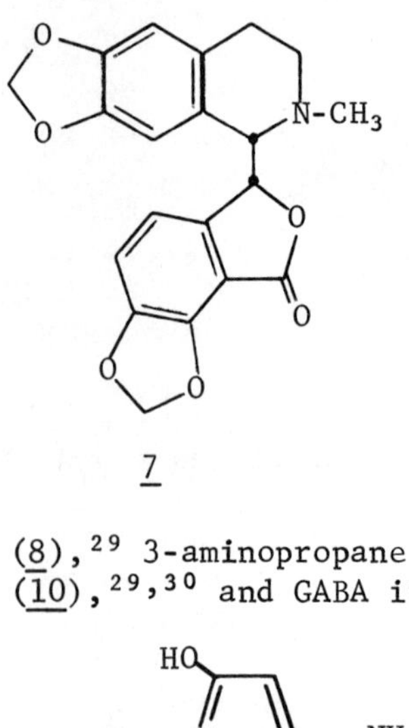

7

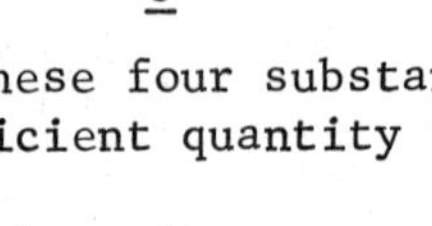

8

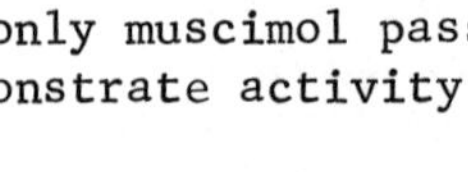

9

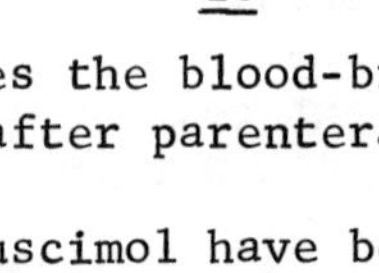

10

Of these four substances, only muscimol passes the blood-brain barrier in sufficient quantity to demonstrate activity after parenteral administration.[33]

A number of agents structurally related to muscimol have been synthesized but not exhaustively tested.[32] The most effective of these compounds, in terms of microiontophoretic potency relative to GABA, were 3-hydroxy-5-(1-aminoethyl)isoxazole (11) and 3-hydroxy-5-(2-aminoethyl)isoxazole (12); however, neither agent was as potent as muscimol itself.

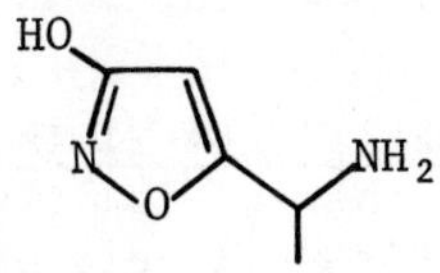

11

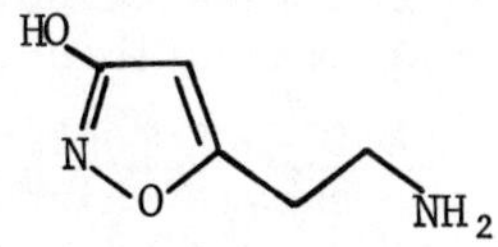

12

Trans-4-aminocrotonic acid (13) has also been claimed to have GABA agonist activity,[34] whereas the cis isomer (14) does not, based on microiontophoretic studies. This observation leads to the hypothesis that in order to be effective as a GABA agonist, a substance must exist in an extended (cf. 13) rather than a folded (cf. 14) conformation. The interpretation of the experimental data is confounded by the fact that trans-4-aminocrotonic acid is also a potent inhibitor of GABA uptake.[35]

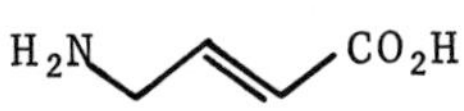

13

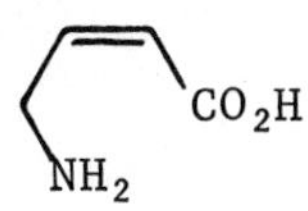

14

GABA Uptake Inhibitors In contrast to GABA receptor binding which is sodium independent, GABA uptake into both neuronal and glial elements is sodium dependent. The uptake mechanisms are not identical, however, since various agents differentially inhibit uptake of GABA in neurons and glial cells. Selective GABA uptake inhibitors in glial cells are α-aminoisobutyric acid (15)[36] and β-alanine (16).[27,37-39]

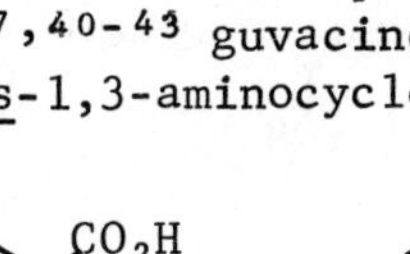

15

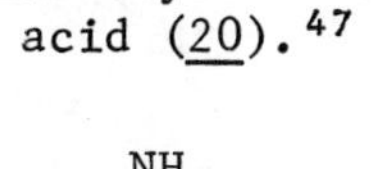

16

Selective GABA uptake inhibitors in neuronal elements are nipecotic acid (17),[27,40-43] guvacine (18),[43] 2,4-diaminobutyric acid (19),[30,35,44-46] and (±)-cis-1,3-aminocyclohexane carboxylic acid (20).[47]

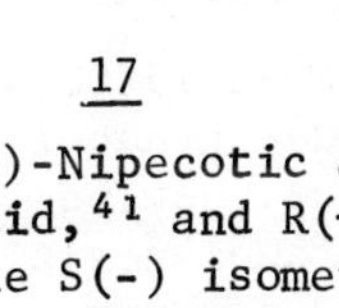

17

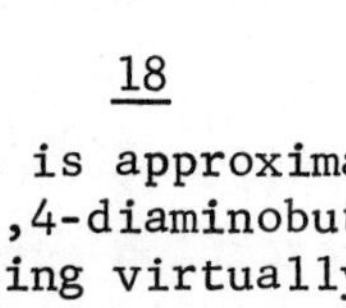

18

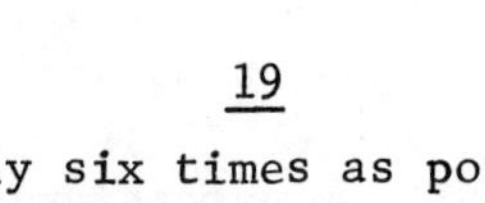

19

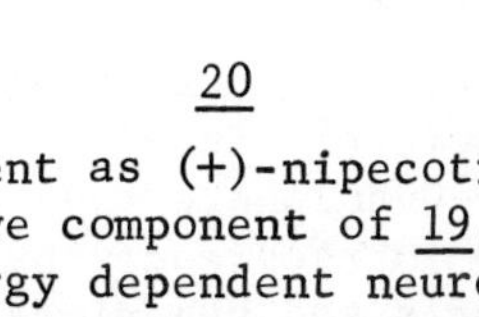

20

(-)-Nipecotic acid is approximately six times as potent as (+)-nipecotic acid,[41] and R(+)-2,4-diaminobutyric acid is the active component of 19, the S(-) isomer being virtually inactive.[44] The energy dependent neuronal uptake process can also be poisoned with p-chloromercuribenzenesulphonic acid[48] and p-aminomercuribenzoic acid.[30]

γ-Aminobutyric Acid-α-Ketoglutarate Transaminase (GABA-T) Inhibitors

GABA-T is the enzyme which metabolizes and thereby inactivates GABA (see Fig. 1). GABA-T inhibitors raise brain tissue levels of GABA and presumably prolong the duration of action of presynaptically released GABA by reducing the extracellular to intracellular concentration gradient. GABA-T is a pyridoxal phosphate-dependent enzyme.[1] The most common and probably the least interesting agents which are claimed to inhibit GABA-T actually do not interfere with the function of GABA-T itself, but rather complex with its coenzyme, pyridoxal phosphate. Examples are aminooxyacetic acid (21),[49] hydrazine,[50] hydrazinopropionic acid (22),[51] isoniazid (23),[52] hydroxylamine,[53] and cycloserine (24).[54]

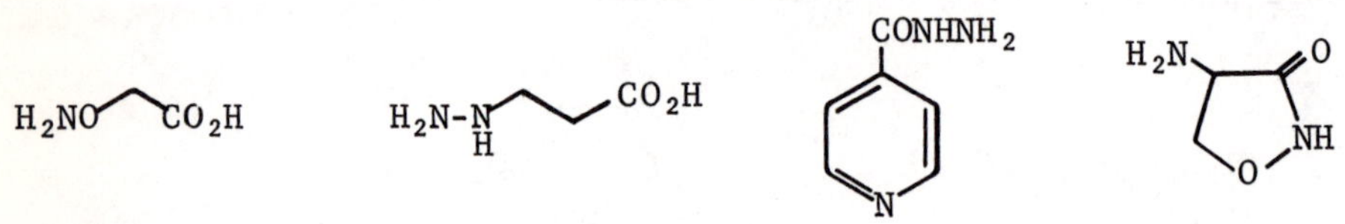

21 22 23 24

A number of irreversible inhibitors have exhibited activity in vitro and in vivo. L-α-Amino-β-chloropropionic hydroxamic acid (25), although related to the carbonyl trapping agents, is specific for GABA-T and causes an increase in mouse brain GABA levels and an increase in the onset time of isoniazid-induced seizures.[16] 4-Amino-hex-5-ynoic acid (26) increased mouse brain GABA levels,[17] decreased GABA-T activity in vitro and in vivo,[55,56] and blocked audiogenic seizures in susceptible mice, as well as electroshock in normal mice.[17] More recently, 4-amino-hex-5-enoic acid (27) was studied in mice and found to enter the brain rapidly and irreversibly inhibit GABA-T.[57,58] A sustained increase in brain GABA concentration was observed. Furthermore, this agent is more selective (GAD is only slightly affected) and longer acting than 26.

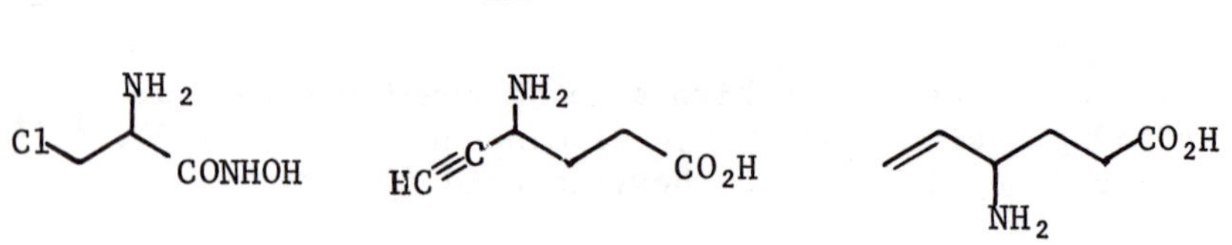

25 26 27

Gabaculine (28) is probably the most potent of the GABA-T inhibitors,[59] active at concentrations at least two orders of magnitude smaller than 26. Specifically, in the equation $E + I \overset{K_I}{\rightleftarrows} EI$ (where E is the enzyme, GABA-T, and I is the inhibitor, gabaculine), K_I is 5.8×10^{-7}M at 15°C. However, the in vivo activity of 28 is not as well established. Ethanolamine-O-sulphate (29) has been extensively studied,[23,60-62] but must be given intracerebroventricularly to observe protection against audiogenic seizures and behavioral changes (piloerection, ptosis, hunched posture, sedation and lack of spontaneous locomotor activity).

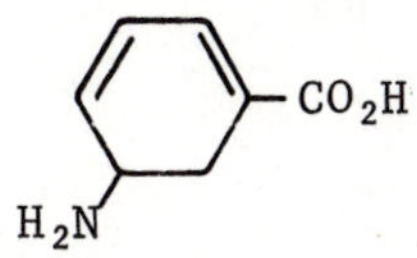

28

29

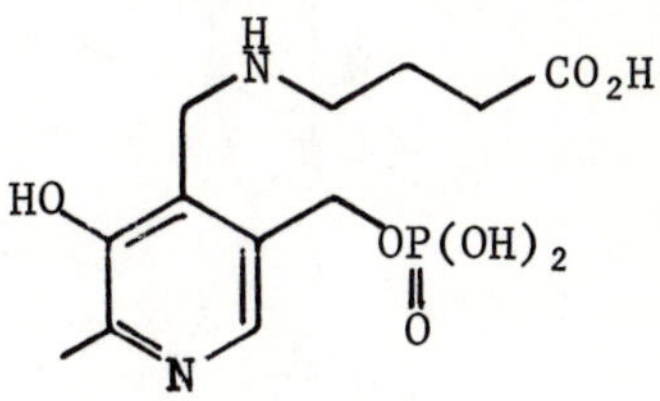

30

N-(5'-Phosphopyridoxyl)-4-aminobutyric acid (30), synthesized from pyridoxal-5'-phosphate and GABA, is a powerful inhibitor of rat brain GABA-T, competitive with GABA itself.[63] It is not known whether this agent can cross the blood-brain barrier.

L-Glutamic Acid Decarboxylase (GAD) Inhibitors

GAD is the neuronal and glial cytoplasmic enzyme which converts glutamic acid to GABA (cf. Fig. 1). Inhibition of GAD *in vivo* leads to seizures and convulsions which have no known or potential medical use. Many of the inhibitors of GABA-T also inhibit GAD, particularly the carbonyl trapping agents (e.g. 21-24).[19] In addition, somewhat more selective inhibitors such as allylglycine (31)[64] have been described.

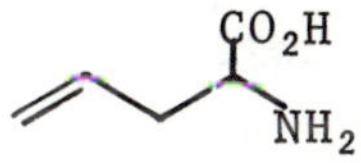

31

GABA Antagonists Like GAD inhibitors, GABA antagonists induce seizures and convulsions in animals and have no known or potential therapeutic value. Picrotoxin (32) was long thought to be a GABA receptor antagonist. However, more recent definitive studies have shown that picrotoxin does not bind to the GABA receptor but most likely "jams" the chloride ion channel.[28]

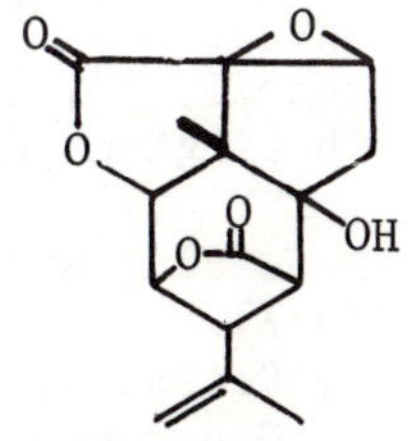

32

Bicuculline (7) and bicuculline methochloride are the best known, true GABA receptor antagonists[28,29,65] and have been extensively used to identify GABA receptors[28,29] and characterize GABA agonists in microiontophoretic studies.[31,32,65,66] Interestingly, (+)-bicuculline methochloride is 400 times more potent a convulsant than the (-)-isomer. In addition, the (+)-isomer is approximately 100 times more potent than the (-)-isomer in inhibiting GABA receptor binding: the IC_{50} (μM) for (+)-bicuculline methochloride is 7.0, whereas the IC_{50} for (-)-bicuculline methochloride is 500.[28] Other GABA antagonists are tetramethylenedisulphotetramine (33)[20,21] and t-butylbicyclophosphate (34).[67-68]

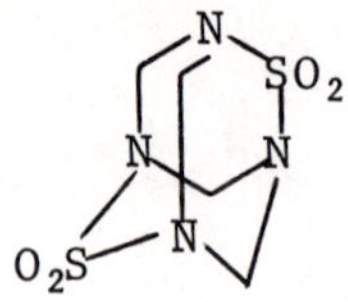

33

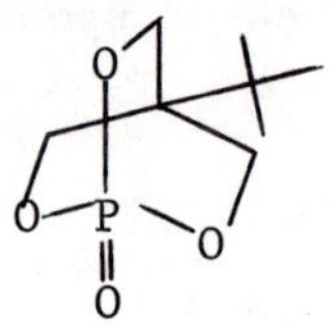

34

References

1. "GABA in Nervous System Function", Kroc Foundation Series, vol. 5, E. Roberts, T.N. Chase and D.B. Tower, Eds., Raven Press, New York (1976).
2. A. Dray and D.W. Straughan, J. Pharm. Pharmacol., 28, 400 (1976).
3. S. Huot, B. Lippert, M.G. Palfreyman and P.J. Schechter, Proc. Brit. Pharmacol. Soc., 264P$_o$(1977).
4. K. Fuxe, T. Hökfelt, Å. Ljungdahl, L. Agnati, O. Johansson and M.P. de la Mora, Med. Biol., 53, 177 (1975).
5. P.L. McGeer and E.G. McGeer, J. Neurochem., 26, 65 (1976).
6. N. Urquhart, T.L. Perry, S. Hansen and J. Kennedy, ibid., 24, 1071 (1975).
7. S.J. Enna, L.Z. Stern, G.J. Wastek and H.I. Yamamura, Life Sciences, 20, 205 (1977).
8. E.D. Bird and L.L. Iversen, Brain, 97, 457 (1974).
9. B.S. Glaeser, W.H. Vogel, D.B. Oleweiler and T.A. Have, Biochem. Med., 12, 380 (1975).
10. B. Mattsson, Acta Psychiat. Scand., Suppl. 255, 211 (1974).
11. S.J. Enna, J.P. Bennett, Jr., D.B. Bylund, S.H. Snyder, E.D. Bird and L.L. Iversen, Brain Res., 116, 531 (1976).
12. R. Schwarcz and J.T. Coyle, Invest. Ophthalmol. Visual Sci., 16, 141 (1977).
13. E.G. McGeer and P.L. McGeer, Nature, 263, 517 (1976).
14. J.T. Coyle and R. Schwarcz, ibid., 263, 244 (1976).
15. B.S. Meldrum, Int. Rev. Neurobiol., 17, 1 (1975).
16. D. Tsui, D.K. Govecki, C.B. Charington and J.D. Wood, Eur. J. Pharmacol. 38, 189 (1976).
17. P.J. Schechter, Y. Tranier, M.J. Jung and A. Sjoerdsma, J. Pharmacol. and Exp. Therap., 201, 606 (1977).
18. Y. Matsui and T. Deguchi, Life Sciences, 20, 1291 (1977).
19. J.D. Wood and S.J. Peesker, J. Neurochem., 23, 703 (1974).
20. J.F. Collins, R.G. Hill and F. Roberts, Proc. Brit. Pharmacol. Soc., 239P (1975).
21. N.G. Bowery, D.A. Brown and J.F. Collins, Brit. J. Pharmacol., 53, 422 (1975).
22. J.D. Wood and S.K. Peesker, J. Neurochem., 25, 277 (1975).
23. R.W. Horton, G.M. Anlezark, M.C.B. Sawaya and B.S. Meldrum, Eur. J. Pharmacol., 41, 387 (1977).
24. S. Simler, L. Ciesielski, M. Maitre, H. Randrianarisoa and P. Mandel, Biochem. Pharmacol., 22, 1701 (1973).
25. S.J. Enna and S.H. Snyder, J. Neurochem., 28, 857 (1977).

26. Y. Miyata and M. Otsuka, J. Neurochem., 25, 239 (1975).
27 E.J. Peck, Jr., A.L. Miller and B.R. Lester, Brain Res. Bull., 1, 595 (1976).
28. S.J. Enna, J.F. Collins and S.H. Snyder, Brain Res., 124, 185 (1977).
29. H. Möhler and T. Okada, Nature, 267, 65 (1977).
30. S.J. Enna and S.H. Snyder, Brain Res., 100, 81 (1975).
31. A. Dray and D.W. Straughan, J. Pharm. Pharmac., 28, 314 (1976).
32. P. Krogsgaard-Larsen, G.A.R. Johnston, D.R. Curtis, C.J.A. Game and R.M. McCulloch, J. Neurochem., 25, 803 (1975).
33. W. Theobald, O. Buch, H.A. Kunz, P. Krupp, E.G. Stenger and H. Heimann, Arzneim. Forsch. 18, 311 (1968).
34. G.A.R. Johnston, D.R. Curtis, P.M. Beart, C.J.A. Game, R.M. McCulloch, and B. Twitchin, J. Neurochem., 24, 157 (1975).
35. R.W. Olsen, J.D. Bayless and M. Ban, Molec. Pharmacol., 11, 558 (1975).
36. G. Ronquist, G. Ågren, J. Ponten and B. Westermark, J. Cell. Physiol., 89, 433 (1976).
37. N.G. Bowery, D.A. Brown, G.G.S. Collins, M. Galvan, S. Marsh, G. Yamini and L. Saunders, Brit. J. Pharmacol., 57, 73 (1976).
38. F. Schon and J.S. Kelly, Brain Res., 86, 243 (1975).
39. G.A.R. Johnston and A.L. Stephanson, ibid., 102, 374 (1976).
40. D. Lodge, G.A.R. Johnston and A.L. Stephanson, J. Neurochem., 27, 1569 (1976).
41. G.A.R. Johnston, P. Krogsgaard-Larsen, A.L. Stephanson and B. Twitchin, ibid., 26, 1029 (1976).
42. P. Krogsgaard-Larsen and G.A.R. Johnston, ibid., 25, 797 (1975).
43. G.A.R. Johnston, P. Krogsgaard-Larsen and A. Stephanson, Nature, 258, 627 (1975).
44. G.A.R. Johnston and B. Twitchin, Brit. J. Pharmacol., 59, 218 (1977).
45. D.P. van Kammen, Am. J. Psychiatry, 134, 138 (1977).
46. D.R. Curtis, C.J.A. Game and D. Lodge, Exp. Brain Res., 25, 413 (1976).
47. N.G. Bowery, G.P. Jones and M.J. Neal, Nature, 264, 281 (1976).
48. D.I.W. Phillips and J.S. Kelly, J. Neurochem., 25, 359 (1975).
49. G.G.S. Collins, Biochem. Pharmacol., 22, 101 (1973).
50. M.A. Medina, J. Pharmacol. and Exp. Therap., 140, 133 (1971).
51. N.M. van Gelder, J. Neurochem., 15, 747 (1968).
52. J.D. Wood and S.J. Peesker, Can. J. Physiol. Pharmacol., 51, 959 (1973).
53. C.F. Baxter and E. Roberts, J. Biol. Chem., 236, 3287 (1961).
54. P. Scotto, P. Monaco, V. Scardi and V. Bonavita, J. Neurochem., 10, 831 (1963).
55. M.J. Jung and B.W. Metcalf, Biochem. Biophys. Res. Comm., 67, 301 (1975).
56. M.J. Jung, B. Lippert, B.W. Metcalf, P.J. Schechter, P. Böhlen and A. Sjoerdsma, J. Neurochem., 28, 717 (1977).
57. M.J. Jung, B. Lippert, B.W. Metcalf, P. Böhlen and P.J. Schechter, ibid., 29, 797 (1977).
58. B. Lippert, B.W. Metcalf, M.J. Jung and P. Casara, Eur. J. Biochem., 74, 441 (1977).
59. R.R. Rando and F.W. Bangerter, J. Amer. Chem. Soc., 98, 6762 (1976).
60. L.J. Fowler, J. Neurochem., 21, 437 (1973).

61. A. Dray, L.J. Fowler, N.R. Oakley, M.A. Simmonds and T. Tanner, Proc. Brit. Pharmacol. Soc., 288P (1975).
62. A. Dray, N.R. Oakley and M.A. Simmonds, J. Pharm. Pharmacol., 27, 627 (1975).
63. G. Tunnicliff, T.T. Ngo and A. Barbeau, Experientia, 33, 20 (1977).
64. R.W. Horton and B.S. Meldrum, Brit. J. Pharmacol., 49, 52 (1973).
65. A.M. Sillito, J. Physiol., 250, 287 (1975).
66. R.W. Olsen, M. Ban and T. Miller, Brain Res., 102, 283 (1976).
67. N.G. Bowery, J.F. Collins and R.G. Hill, Nature, 261, 601 (1976).
68. N.G. Bowery, J.F. Collins, R.G. Hill and S. Pearson, Proc. Brit. Pharmacol. Soc., 275P (1977).

Chapter 5. *Narcotic Analgetics, Endorphins and the Opiate Receptor*

David S. Fries, University of the Pacific, Stockton, CA 95211

Reviews on the endorphins[1-4] and other aspects of opiate research[5-7] have appeared. Research on the opiates has centered on 1) the elucidation of the physiological locations and the functions of endorphins; 2) the discovery of peptide or classical narcotic structural analogs which are clinically effective for the relief of pain but lack addiction liability;[8] 3) the determination of the nature of the opiate-receptor(s). The major advancements in each of these areas are reviewed in this chapter.

Endogenous Opiates

Biosynthesis and Catabolism - Evidence continues to mount that endorphins in the pituitary gland are derived from a larger precursor by the pathway[9-11]: 31K peptidal precursor → β-Lipotropin → β-Endorphin → γ-Endorphin → α-Endorphin. ACTH is also derived from the 31K peptide. Met-enkephalin can be derived from the degradation of larger endorphins; however, the importance of this pathway remains uncertain.[12] The origin of leu-enkephalin remains unknown. The activities of the enkephalins are terminated by the rapid cleavage of the Tyr-Gly peptide bond.[13-15] This cleavage limits the duration of action of these agents and makes quantitative measurements of their activity difficult in all in vivo, and some in vitro, tests.

Distribution - Immunohistochemical,[16-20] radioimmunoassay,[21-24] stereospecific receptor binding,[25-26] and electrically stimulated mouse vas deferens[27] assays were used to map endorphin distribution in several animal species. These studies agree that the larger peptidal endorphins have higher concentration in the pituitary than in other regions of the brain or other tissues. Conversely, the enkephalins predominate in nonpituitary tissues. Within the rat pituitary the endorphins are located in cells of the pars intermedia and pars distalis but are excluded from the neurophypophysis. In rats the enkephalins are distributed in regions of the spinal cord, regions of the brain including the periaqueductal grey matter, thalamus, hypothalamus, and basal ganglia, and in the gut. Studies using either decapitation or microwaves to kill rats have produced equivalent results;[26] however, these results apparently depend on the procedures used to kill the rats.[24] Radioimmunoassays using met-enkephalin specific[18] or met- and leu-enkephalin nonspecific antibodies[21] show equivalent enkephalin distribution patterns indicating that there is little anatomical separation between the two peptides. The distribution of the enkephalins parallels the distribution of opiate receptors in many, but not all, brain regions.

Physiological Actions and Functions - The exact physiological function of endogenous opiates remains unknown.[28] Evidence continues to mount that exogenously administered endorphins and enkephalins produce morphine-like actions in animals.[29] Studies show that met-enkephalin inhibits the morphine abstinence syndrome in mice.[30] β-Endorphin administration to animals

ISBN 0-12-040513-X

causes analgesia and development of tolerance to its analgetic effects.[31-35] Analgesia is produced by injection of enkephalins into areas of the spinal cord.[34-35] The self-administration of the enkephalins by mice suggests that, like morphine, the enkephalins cause euphoria and drive-reduction reward.[36] Rats self-administer leu-enkephalin to a greater extent than met-enkephalin, indicating that leu-enkephalin may play a predominant role in euphoria and behavioral aspects of opiate activity.[36] Leu-enkephalin produced a morphine-like analgetic effect when injected intracerebroventricularly (i.c.v.) into rats (45°C hot-plate); however, when tested in a similar manner, met-enkephalin caused an increased sensitivity to pain and induced reponses resembling those seen in narcotic withdrawal. Injection (i.c.v.) of β-endorphin into cats caused behavioral responses at 12.5 μg and both behavioral and antinociceptive responses at 25.0 and 50.0 μg doses; however, no effect from met-enkephalin was observed.[38] Analgesia, antagonized by naloxone, was produced by met-enkephalin injected into the periaqueductal grey matter of rats.[39] Amnesia produced in rats by enkephalins is not reversed by naloxone.[40] β-Endorphin also inhibits fixed ratio operant behavior in rats.[41] Large doses (1-2 mg) of met-enkephalin injected (i.c.v.) into cats caused emetic and hyperthermic effects similar to those caused by morphine.[42] Hypermotility in rats, which is blocked by naloxone but not haloperidol, is produced by injection of morphine or D-ala-met-enkephalin amide into the nucleus accumbens of rats.[43]

The putative role of enkephalins as neurotransmitters is enhanced by studies which show that electrical stimulation (10 Hz) of guinea pig ileum strips causes release of enkephalins.[44,45] This preparation may provide a valuable model for the study of the synthesis, storage and release of endorphins.[44] The inhibitory effects of met- and leu-enkephalins have been shown on acetylcholine release in myenteric plexus neurons.[46] Inhibition of acetylcholine release and turnover by the enkephalins has been shown in brain tissues.[47-49] The enkephalins have similar inhibitory effects on some dopamine[49,50] and substance P mediated neurons.[51] Microiontophoretic application of endogenous opiates into rat brains showed an inhibitory response on all responsive cells[52,53] except those in the hypothalamus where these compounds caused an excitatory response.[54]

The endorphins cause an opiate-like inhibition of c-AMP formation in neuroblastoma X glioma hybrid cells.[55-57] The effects of endorphins on the release or physiological blood levels of prolactin, luteinizing hormone, follicle stimulating hormone, thyroid stimulating hormone, growth hormone and arginine vasopressin have been studied.[58-62]

The hypothesis that endogenous opiates function in modulating severe stressful or painful stimuli is supported by the elevated endorphin levels found in dehydrated[63] and foot-shock stressed[64] rats. This effect has not been shown in man.[65] Treatment of depressed patients with naloxone failed to give noticeable improvement although the naloxone treatment did cause a decrease in CSF endorphin levels.[66] Naloxone also failed to produce significant effects when tested in a double-blind experiment on schizophrenic patients.[67] Naltrexone, in high doses, does not have beneficial effects on schizophrenic patients.[68] Naloxone causes a dose related antianxiety effect in man.[65] Injection (i.v.) of 1.5 mg of β-endorphin into three schizophrenic patients exacerbated their clinical condition; however, a similar dose of β-endorphin to two depressed patients resulted in marked improvement of their condition.[69] A subsequent treatment of these same patients with β-endorphin obtained from a different synthetic preparation failed to produce the results of the first studies.[69]

Conformation of Enkephalins - Studies continue to show a great deal of conformation mobility for enkephalins and there is disagreement as to the most probable conformation in solution.[70-74] Some of the discrepancies in NMR conformational studies can be explained from the fact that spectral changes occur on dilution with dimeric structures existing at high concentrations,[70] and that the enkephalins can exist in zwitterionic and cationic forms which differ in spectral features.[71] Theoretical studies indicate a number of possible low energy conformations.[75,76] Conformations with a type βII-bend at or a type βI-bend at position 3 and 4 have been proposed. Either of these enkephalin conformations have some structural parameters in common with synthetic opiates.[70,71] A study has been made with a series of enkephalin analogs in which mouse vas deferens activity and receptor binding in brain homogenates were correlated with allowable conformations of the peptide chain. By this procedure a conformational map showing enkephalin conformations allowable for activity was constructed.[77]

Enkephalin Analogs - Selected enkephalin analogs which have been prepared in an attempt to discover analgetic agents with improved pharmacological profiles are reported in Table I. Compound 9 (FK 33-824) is 1000X more potent than morphine (mouse hot-plate, i.c.v.).[85] This compound retains one-fifth the activity of morphine when given orally. A D-amino acid in place of Gly^2 facilitates oral or i.v. activity by decreasing metabolic inactivation of the peptides. Studies have shown that 1 and 9 retain the addicting properties of morphine.[79,85] No peptide with analgetic activity has been reported to be nonaddicting. The enkephalin analogs do have decreased respiratory effects compared to morphine; however, they produce a catatonic state which is unlike morphine's action.[84,85] The danger of depending on in vitro tests to measure analgetic potency is demonstrated by the high in vitro activities seen for hexapeptides 12[84] 13[86] which were poorly active or inactive in vivo.

Reports on the agonist-antagonist activity of several N-allyltyrosyl analogs of enkephalins have appeared. N-Allyl-[D-ala]^2- met-enkephalin[87], and N-allyl-met-enkephalin[87,88] were found not to have appreciable antagonist properties. N-Allyl-leu-enkephalin does have antagonist activity on the guinea pig ileum.[88]

Miscellaneous Endogenous Opiates - Two compounds having opiate-like activity have been detected in the blood of several animal species. These two compounds, called slow moving material (SMM) and fast moving material (FMM) on the basis of their tlc behavior, are not degraded by pronase and show different activities on guinea pig ileum than β-endorphin or met-enkephalin.[89] A nonpeptide morphine like substance (MLS) has been isolated from beef brains and human urine.[90] MLS binds with a specific anti-

Table I. Selected Enkephalin Analogs.

No.	Identification Number	Structural Variations at a.a. Position					Ref.
		1	2	3	4	5	
1	BW180c	H-Tyr	D-Ala	Gly	Phe	D-Leu-OH	78,79
2	ICI120,518	H-Tyr	D-Ala	Gly	Phe	Pro-NHEt	80
3	ICI121,444	H-Tyr	D-Ala	Gly	Phe-NH-	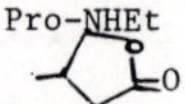	80
4		H-Tyr	D-Met	Gly	Phe	Pro-NH_2	81
5		H-Tyr	D-Met	Gly	Phe	Pro-NHEt	81,82
6		H-Tyr	D-Ala	Gly	Phe	Met-OH	83
7		H-Tyr	D-Nle	Gly	Phe	Pro-NHEt	82
8		H-Tyr	Gly	Gly	Phe	Leu-NH-CH_2-CH_2-$NHCH_3$	84
9	FK33-824	HTyr	D-Ala	Gly	N-Me-Phe	Met(O)-ol	85
10		HTyr	D-Ala	Gly	Phe	Met-ol	85
11		HTyr	D-Ala	Gly	Phe	Met-(O)-ol	85
12		H-Lys-Tyr	D-Ser	Gly	Phe	Met-OMe	84
13		H-Arg-Tyr	Gly	Gly	Phe	Met-OH	86

body to morphine which does not cross react with peptide opiates. MLC binds to opiate receptors in neuroblastma X glioma hybrid cells in a similar fashion to, but 20-40X greater than, naloxone.

Nonpeptide Opiate Agonists and Antagonists

Oripavines - Detailed animal pharmacology of buprenorphine has been reported.[91,92] Buprenorphine is more potent and longer acting as an analgetic, shows less addiction liability, and causes less respiratory depression at high doses, when compared to morphine sulfate.

Morphines and Morphinans - Double-blind[93,94] and placebo-controlled[95] studies with butorphanol show it to be an effective analgetic agent in man. An evaluation of heroin in terminal cancer patients will be made.[96] Formyl and propionyl homologs of 6-acetyl- and 3,6-diacetylmorphine were shown to have 4X longer duration than morphine in monkeys.[97] The (+)-isomer of morphine was synthesized and shown not to be an analgetic, but to retain some of the pharmacological effects of opiates.[98] Multiple receptors were proposed on the basis of the activity of (+)-morphine.

The N-(2'R)-tetrahydrofurfuryl derivative 14a (Mr 2096 CL) was reported to be a mixed agonist-antagonist with 25X the potency of morphine in the mouse writhing test and to partially suppress morphine abstinence in monkeys.[99,100] The epimeric 2'S-analog 14b is a pure antagonist with 0.2 the activity of nalorphine.

Homo- and homoisomorphinan derivatives 15a,b, and 16a,b were reported.[101] Both 15a and 15b are equipotent with morphine in the hot-plate test; however, 15b supports physical dependence while 15a neither sup-

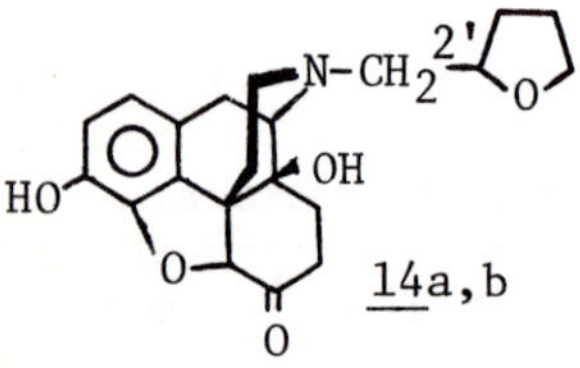

14a,b

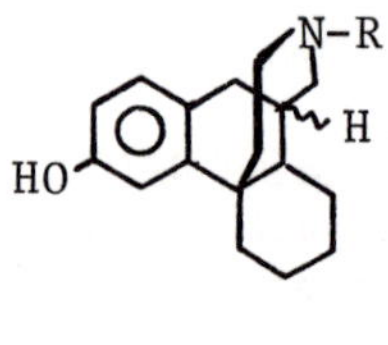

cis B/C	tran B/C	R
15a	15b	Me
16a	16b	CH_2- 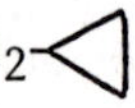

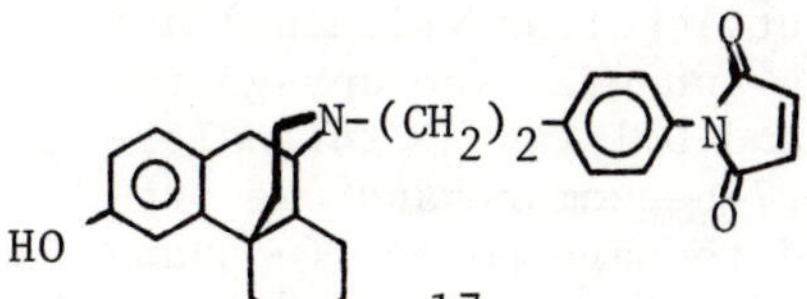

17

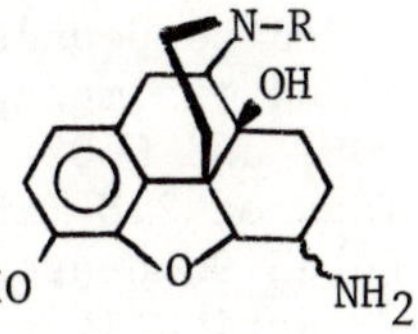

18a,b R = allyl

19a,b R = CH_2-c-C_3H_5

presses nor precipitates withdrawal in monkeys. The cyclopropylmethy derivatives (16a,b) have 0.12 and 0.05 the analgetic activity of morphine, lack antagonist activity and do not substitute for morphine in addicted monkeys. Compound 17, a representative example of a series of N-aralkylmorphinans prepared as potential opiate receptor-site-directed alkylating agents, was 4X as potent as morphine sulfate in the hot-plate test and caused some inhibition of morphine activity in this same test. Receptor binding studies failed to show irreversible binding of 17.[102] Epimeric 6-amino derivatives 18a,b and 19a,b, were found to be less potent, but longer acting antagonists than their keto precursors, naloxone and naltrexone.[103]

Benzomorphans - An excellent review on synthetic and chemical aspects of the benzomorphans was published.[104] A controlled treatment study confirmed that naltrexone produced fewer side effects than cyclazocine in man.[105] A "twin crossover relative potency analgesic assay" in man comparing morphine and 8-methoxycyclazocine (Win 20,836) revealed that doses of 8-methoxycyclazocine equianalgetic with a morphine standard caused unacceptable levels of psychotomimetic side effects.[106]

Compounds 20 and 21 gave respectively 0.20 and 1.0 the analgesia of morphine in the hot-plate test.[107] Antagonist activity greater than that of nalorphine was seen for 21, but 20 is not an antagonist in the tail-flick screen. Neither 20 nor 21 suppressed abstinence signs in morphine dependent monkeys. Benzomorphan analogs 22 and 23 incorporate the 9β-OH in the position equivalent to the 14-position of the morphinan ring nucleus.[108] Compound (-)-22 is equipotent as an agonist (mouse writhing) and 2X more potent than butorphanol as an antagonist (straub tail test). Compound 23 is virtually devoid of agonist activity but slightly more active than naloxone as an antagonist.

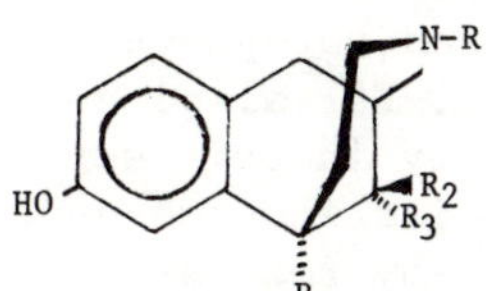

	R	R_1	R_2	R_3
20	n-C_6H_{13}	Me	Et	H
21	CH_2-c-C_4H_7	Me	Et	H
22	CH_2-c-C_3H_5	allyl	OH	H
23	CH_2-c-C_4H_7	allyl	OH	H
24	Me	Me	$(CH_2)_2$-C(OH)(CH_3)-$(CH_2)_3$-H	H
25	CH_2-c-C_3H_5	Me	$(CH_2)_2$-C(OH)$(CH_3)_2$	Me
26	CH_2-c-C_3H_5	Me	$(CH_2)_2$-C(OH)(CH_3)-C$(CH_3)_3$	Me
27	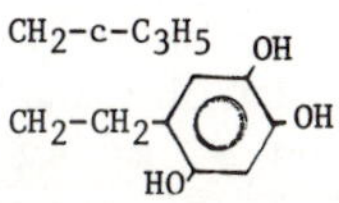	Me	H	Me

A series of eighteen benzomorphans with 9-propanol substituents, as in oripavine structures, included compounds 24,25 and 26.[109] These compounds had agonist ED_{50}'s of 2.6,4.5 and >25 mg/kg (acetylcholine writhing) and antagonist AD_{50}'s of >80, 0.006, and 0.022 mg/kg (phenazocine antagonism) respectively, compared to values of 2.8 (ED_{50}) and 0.1 (AD_{50}) for nalorphine. A series of N-substituted 9α-n-propyl-6,7-benzomorphans was prepared and the N-CH_3 to N-C_6H_{13} derivatives found to have potent (unquantified) and long lasting (to 10 hr) antagonist effects in single dose suppression studies in monkeys.[110] The N-(2,4,5-trihydroxyphenylethyl)normetazocine derivative 27 was prepared in an attempt to deliver a 6-hydroxydopamine-like alkylating moiety to the analgetic receptor; however, this compound has only weak affinity for the opiate receptor (neuroblastoma X glioma cells).[111] The C-ring-N-positional analog of the benzomorphans possesses activity equivalent to codeine (mouse tail pressure).[112] The B,C-methano-bridged analog gave nalorphine level antagonism (rat tail-flick) but only weak agonist effects.[113]

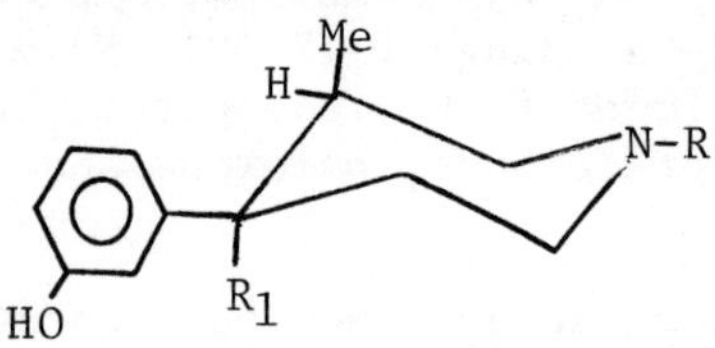

	R	R1
28a	Me	Me
28b	phenethyl	Me
28c	Me	propiophenone
28d	Me	propionoxy

4-Phenylpiperidines - The most exciting report in this area was the potent and pure antagonist activities seen for the 4-(3-hydroxyphenyl)-3-methylpiperidine derivatives of structure 28.[114] Thus 28a, 28b and 28c had AD_{50} values of 0.24, 0.11 and 0.056 mg/kg, s.c. ("rat tail heat" against morphine), respectively, compared to a value of 0.022 mg/kg for naloxone. The (+)-isomer of 28a (AD_{50}=0.029) is more active than the (-)-isomer (AD_{50}=0.22). The cis-3,4-Me compounds are 50-100X less active. The 3-methyl group is believed to confer antagonist properties to this compound since the β-prodine analog 28d is a pure antagonist 2-3X more potent than pentazocine. N-Allyl derivatives of 28 are less potent as antagonists than their N-methyl counterparts.

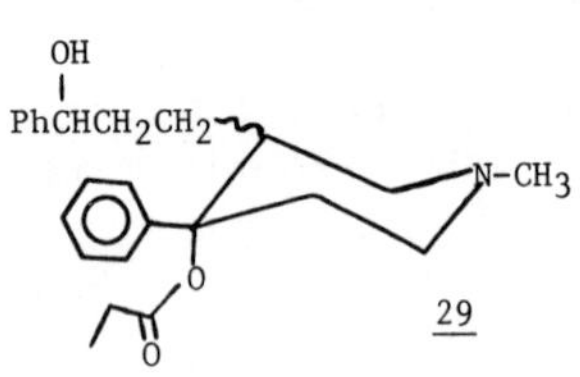

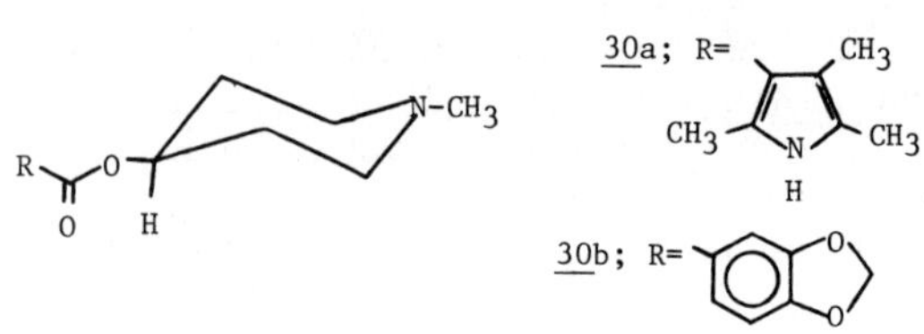

The correlation observed between receptor binding and hot-plate analgesia of α- and β-prodine analogs substituted with Me, Et, allyl and hexyl at the 3-position led to the conclusion that activity in this series is determined by relative receptor affinity rather than distribution and/or metabolism of the compounds.[115] The ester 29, of 3-(3-hydroxy-3-phenylpropyl)piperidine was inactive in the tail-flick test but was a weak agonist in the writhing test (80.5 and 32 mg/kg respectively).[116] 1-Methyl-4-piperidinol esters with bulky aromatic substituents gave codeine level analgetic activity (4.9, 7.3 mg/kg for 30a and 30b, respectively) in the mouse hot-plate test. These compounds showed only weak binding (300-30,000X less than morphine) to opiate receptors in mouse brain homogenates and 30b had no dependence liability in monkeys.[117]

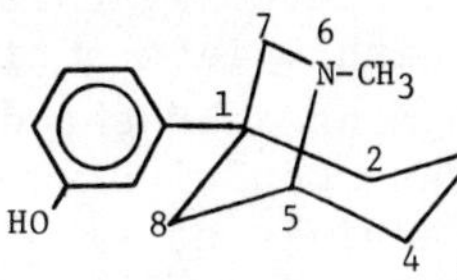
31

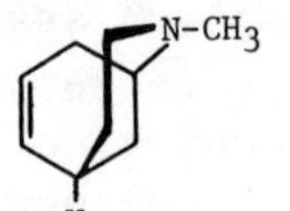
32

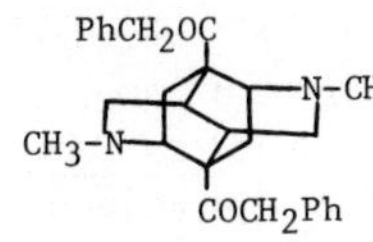
33

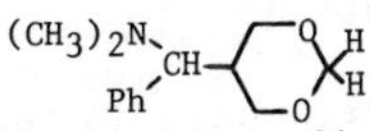
34

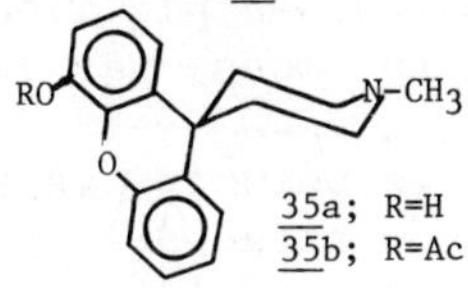
35a; R=H
35b; R=Ac

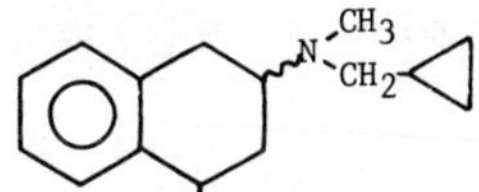
36

Miscellaneous - Extensive SAR on the 6-azabicyclo[3.2.1]octanes (31) were published.[118] Methyl substitution at C-7 enhances agonist activity (7-Me-N-Me, ED_{50}=2.9; hot-plate test) while a methyl at C-8 gives compounds which are inactive as agonists but retain antagonist activity (8-Me-N-Me, AD_{50}=0.18 vs. 0.16 for nalorphine; morphine respiratory depression, rabbits). 7,8-Dimethyl substitution results in inactive compounds. SAR of N-substituted analogs somewhat parallel that observed for other analgetic series with exception of the N-phenethyl substituent which is inactive in the nonmethylated ring system but in combination with a 7-Me substituent produced the most potent agonist of the series (ED_{50}=0.3 mg/kg vs. 1.2 mg/kg for morphine; hot-plate test). None of the compounds displayed appreciable physical dependence capacity. The N-Me-7,8-unsubstituted and the N-Me-7-exo-methyl compounds were resolved and only the (+)-isomers found to be active as agonists; however, the (-)-isomers maintained antagonist activity. Members of other bicycloalkane series such as the 3-hydroxyphenyl derivatives of 2-azabicyclo[2.2.2]octane,[119] 2-azabicyclo[3.2.1]octane[120] and 3-azabicyclo[3.3.1]nonane[121] were inactive as agonists but produced pentazocine level antagonism in the rabbit respiratory depression assay.

The B,C-ring analog (32) of morphine was synthesized but failed to show analgetic activity.[122] The (-)-isomer of the novel 5,11-diazaditwistane derivative 33 had analgetic activity 2X greater than morphine (rat hind paw pressure) while the (+)-isomer was inactive.[123] The (+)-isomer of the 1,3-dioxane 34 gave analgetic activity comparable to codeine (ED_{50}'s 6.2 vs. 6.7 mg/kg, AcOH writhing)[124] which was blocked by naloxone. Replacement of the phenyl with 3-pyridyl or a 2-Me substituent on the dioxane ring gave a 2-3 fold increase in agonist activity. The spiropiperidine analogs 35a (ICI 86,458) and 35b (ICI 91,356) are reported to have 0.5 and 1.0 the potency of morphine in the AcOH writhing assay.[125] Both the cis- and trans-aminotetralin diastereomers of 36 were reported to have codeine level agonist activity (mouse hot-plate) and, at 3 mg/kg, to give a 100% inhibition of an ED_{80} dose of morphine (mouse tail flick).[126]

Opiate Receptors

The differential competitive displacement by narcotic agents of various ^{3}H-labeled peptide and nonpeptide opiates from receptors (stereospecific binding sites) in brain tissue has led a number of investigators to conclude that there are multiple receptors associated with opiate activity.[127-131] The contention of multiple receptors is augmented by the differential in vitro and in vivo pharmacological responses seen with various opiates.[131-135] An example of this is the equipotent activities seen for morphine and met-enkephalin on the guinea pig ileum compared to 30X greater activity of met-enkephalin on the mouse vas deferens.[131]

A quantitative relationship between opiate receptor binding and activity in vivo could be made for ten structurally diverse opiates when lipophilicity was also taken into account.[136] Cases have been reported in which binding ratios in the presence and absence of Na^{+} failed to predict the narcotic antagonist activity which undoubtedly existed in the compounds. Also, some pure agonists have been found to have low sodium binding ratios.[137] Two proposals on the nature of the opiate receptor appeared. One of these is similar to the Beckett model but proposes an extended aromatic (lipophilic) binding region.[138] The other pictures the receptor site as a cup shaped area formed by four pentapeptide segments in antiparallel β-pleated sheets.[139] As with all previous opiate receptor models, both of these proposals are based on SAR correlations of some, but not all agents having opiate activity and neither are supported by experimental evidence.

References

1. S.H. Snyder, Sci. Amer., 236, No.3, 44(1977), Chem. Eng. N., Nov. 28, 1977, p.26, N. Engl. J. Med., 296, 266(1977).
2. R.C.A. Frederickson, Life Sci., 21, 23(1977).
3. W.A. Klee, in "Peptides in Neurobiology," H. Gainer, Ed., Plenum Press, New York, 1977, p.375.
4. Psychoneuroendocrinology, 2, #1, 1977, Entire issue devoted to endogenous opiates.
5. H.L. Borison, Pharmacol. Ther. B., 3, 227(1977).
6. H.J. Sanders, Chem. Eng. N., Mar. 28, 1977, p.30.
7. E.L. May, in "Psychopharmacological Agents," Vol.4, Academic Press, New York, N.Y., 1976, p.35.
8. H. Isbell, Clin. Pharmacol. Ther., 22, 377(1977).
9. J.L. Robers & E. Herbert, Proc. Natl. Acad. Sci., 74, 5300(1977).
10. R.E. Mains, B.A. Eipper, & N. Ling, Proc. Natl. Acad. Sci., 74, 3014(1977).
11. G. Giagnoni, S. Sabol, & M. Nirenberg, Proc. Natl. Acad. Sci., 74, 2259(1977).
12. B.M. Austen, D.G. Smyth, C.R. Snell, Nature, 269, 619(1977).
13. J.L. Meek, H.Y.T. Yang, & E. Costa, Neuropharmacol., 16, 151(1977).
14. W. Fratta, H.Y.T. Yang, J. Hong, & E. Costa, Nature, 268, 452(1977).
15. A. Dupont, L. Cusan, M. Garon, & G. Alvarado-Urbina, Life Sci., 21, 907(1977).
16. R. Simantov, M.J. Kuhar, G.R. Uhl, & S.H. Snyder, Proc. Natl. Acad. Sci., 74, 2167(1977).
17. T. Hokfelt, A. Ljungdahl, L. Terenius, R. Elde & G. Nilsson, Proc. Natl. Acad. Sci., 74,3081(1977).
18. S.J. Watson, H. Akil, S. Sullivan, & J.D. Barchas, Life Sci., 21, 733(1977).
19. F. Bloom, E. Battenberg, J. Rossier, N. Ling, J. Leppaluoto, T.M. Vargo, & R. Guillemin, Life Sci., 20, 43(1977).
20. S.J. Watson, J.D. Barchas, & C.H. Li, Proc. Natl. Acad. Sci., 74, 5155(1977).
21. S.R. Childers, R. Simantov, & S.H. Snyder, Eur. J. Pharmacol., 46, 289(1977).
22. J. Rossier, A. Bayon, T.M. Vargo, N. Long, R. Guillemin, & F. Bloom, Life Sci., 21, 847(1977).
23. J. Rossier, T.M. Vargo, S. Minick, N. Long, F.E. Bloom, & R. Guillemin, Proc. Natl. Acad. Sci., 74, 5162(1977).
24. H.Y. Yang, J.S. Hong, & E. Costa, Neuropharmacology, 16, 303(1977).
25. H. Pollard, C. Llorens-Cortes, J.C. Schwartz, Nature, 268, 747(1977).
26. A.L. Cheung, W.B. Stavinoha, & A. Goldstein, Life Sci., 20, 1285(1977).
27. J. Hughes, H.W. Kosterlitz, & T.W. Smith, Brit. J. Pharmacol., 61, 639(1977).

28. L. Terenius, Acta Pharmacol. Toxicol., 41, 26(1977).
29. W. Feldberg & D.G. Smyth, Brit. J. Pharmacol., 60, 445(1977).
30. H.N. Bhargava, J. Pharmacol., 41, 81(1977).
31. J.M. Van-Ree, D. De Wied, A.F. Bradbury, E.C. Hulme, D.G. Smyth & C.R. Snell, Nature, 264, 792 (1976).
32. J.I. Szekely, A.Z. Ronai, Z. Dunai-Kovacs, E. Miglecz, S. Bajusz & L. Graf, Life Sci., 20, 1259 (1977).
33. M.M. Puig,P. Gascon & J.M. Musacchio, J. Pharmacol., 45, 205(1977).
34. A.W. Duggan, J.G. Hall & P.M. Headley, Brit. J. Pharmacol., 61, 399(1977).
35. T.L. Yaksh, S.P.Huang & T.A. Rudy, Neuroscience, 2, 593(1977).
36. J.D. Belluzzi & L. Stein, Nature, 266, 556(1977).
37. L. Leybin, C. Pinsky, F.S. LaBella, V. Havlicek, M. Rezek, Nature, 264, 458(1977).
38. M. Meglio, Y. Hosobuchi, H.H. Loh, J.E. Adams & C.H. Li, Proc. Natl. Acad. Sci.,74,774(1977).
39. J.B. Malick & J.M. Goldstein, Life Sci., 20, 827(1977).
40. H. Rigter, H. Greven & H. Van Riezen, Neuropharmacology, 16, 545(1977).
41. L. Lichtblau, L.H. Fossom & S.B. Sparber, Life Sci., 21, 927(1977).
42. W.G. Clark, Pro. Soc. Exp. Biol. Med., 154, 540(1977).
43. A. Pert & C. Sivit, Nature, 265, 645(1977).
44. M. Wuster, Arch. Pharmacol., 297, R53(1977).
45. M.M. Puig, P. Gascon, G.L. Craviso & J.M. Musacchio, Science 195, 419(1977).
46. R.A. North & M. Tonini, Brit. J. Pharmacol., 61, 541(1977).
47. F. Moroni, D.L. Cheney & E. Costa, Nature, 267, 267(1977).
48. K. Jhamandas, J. Sawynok, M. Sutak, Nature, 269, 433(1977).
49. N. Subramanian, P. Mitznegg, W. Sprugel, W. Domschke, S. Domschke, E. Wunsch & L. Demling, Arch. Pharmacol., 299, 163(1977).
50. H. Pollard, C. Llorens-Cortes, J.C. Schwartz, Nature, 268, 745(1977).
51. T.M. Jessell, L.L. Iversen, Nature, 268, 549(1977).
52. P.B. Bradley, R.J. Gayton & L.A. Lambert, Brit. J. Pharmacol., 61, 147P(1977).
53. M. Segal, Neuropharmacology, 16, 587(1977).
54. R.A. Nicoll, G.R. Siggins, N. Ling, F.E. Bloom & R. Guillemin, Proc. Natl. Acad. Sci., 74, 2584(1977).
55. S.K. Sharma, W.A. Klee & M. Nirenberg, Proc. Natl. Acad. Sci., 74, 3365(1977).
56. M. Brandt, C. Buchen & B. Hamprecht, FEBS Letters, 80, 251(1977).
57. A. Goldstein, B.M. Cox, W.A. Klee & M. Nirenberg, Nature, 265, 363(1977).
58. J.F. Bruni, D. Van Vugt, S. Marshall & J. Meites, Life Sci., 21, 461(1977).
59. D. Cocchi, A. Santagostino, I. Gil-Ad, S. Ferri & E.E. Muller, Life Sci., 20, 2041(1977).
60. W.F. White, J.V. Nadler, A. Hamberger, C.W. Cotman, Nature, 270, 357(1977).
61. A. Dupont, L. Cusan, M. Garon, F. Labrie & C.H. Li, Proc. Natl. Acad. Sci., 74, 358(1977).
62. R.E. Weitzman, D.A. Fisher, S. Minick, N. Ling & R. Guillemin, Endocrinology, 101, 1643(1977).
63. M.M. Mata, H. Gainer & W.A. Klee, Life Sci., 21, 1159(1977).
64. J. Madden, IV, H. Akil, R.L. Patrick & J.D. Barchas, Nature, 265, 359(1977).
65. P. Grevert & A. Goldstein, Proc. Natl. Acad. Sci., 74, 1291(1977).
66. L. Terenius, A. Wahlstrom & H. Agren, Psychopharmacol., 54, 31(1977).
67. G.C. Davis, W.E. Bunney, Jr. & E.G. Defraites, Science, 197, 74(1977).
68. D.H. Mielke & D.M. Gallant, Amer. J. Psychiat., 134, 1430(1977).
69. N.S. Kline, C.H. Li, H.E. Lehmann, A. Lajtha, E. Laski & T. Cooper, Arch. Gen. Psychiat., 34, 1111(1977).
70. M.A. Khaled, M.M. Long, W.D. Thompson, R.J. Bradley, G.B. Brown & D.W. Urry, Biochem. Biophys. Res., 76, 224(1977).
71. C.R. Jones, V. Garsky & W.A. Gibbons, Biochem. Biophys. Res. Commun., 76, 619(1977).
72. H.E. Bleich, A.R. Day, R.J. Freer & J.A. Glasel, Biochem. Biophys. Res. Commun.,74,592(1977).
73. P.W. Schiller, C.F. Yam & M. Lis, Biochemistry-USA, 16, 1831(1977).
74. M. Anteunis, A.K. Lala, C. Garbay-Jaureguiberry & B.P. Roques, Biochemistry-USA, 16, 1462(1977).
75. C. Humblet, J.L. De Coen & M.H.J. Koch, Arch. Int. Physiol. Biochem., 85, 415(1977).
76. J.L. De Coen, C. Humblet & M.H.J. Koch, FEBS Lett., 73, 38(1977).
77. C.R. Beddell, R.B. Clark, L.A. Lowe, S. Wilkinson, K.J. Chang, P. Cuatrecasas & R. Miller, Brit. J. Pharmacol., 61, 351(1977).
78. M.G. Baxter, R.L. Follenfant, A.A. Miller & D.M. Sethna, Brit. J. Pharmacol., 59, 523P(1977).
79. M.G. Baxter, D. Goff, A.A. Miller & I.A. Saunders, Brit. J. Pharmacol., 59, 455P(1977).
80. A.S. Dutta, J.J. Gormley, C.F. Hayward, J.S. Morley, J.S. Shaw, G.J. Stacey & M.J. Turnbull, Brit. J. Pharmacol., 61, 481P(1977).
81. S. Bajusz, A.Z. Ronai, J.I. Szekely, L. Graf, Z. Dunai-Kovacs & I. Berzetei, FEBS Lett., 76, 91(1977).
82. S. Bajusz, A.Z. Ronai, J.I. Szekely, Z. Dunai-Kovacs, I. Berzetei & L. Graf, Acta Biochem. Biophys. Acad. Sci. Hung., 11, 305(1976).
83. J.M. Walker, G.G. Berntson, C.A. Sandman, D.H. Coy, A.V. Schally & A.J. Kastin, Science, 196, 85(1977).

84. A.S. Dutta, J.J. Gormley, C.F. Hayward, J.S. Morley, J.S. Shaw, G.J. Stacey & M.T. Turnbull, Life Sci., 21, 559(1977).
85. D. Roemer, H.H. Buescher, R.C. Hill, J. Pless, W. Bauer, F. Cardinaux, A. Closse, D. Hauser & R. Huguenin, Nature, 268, 547(1977).
86. P.Y. Law, E.T. Wei, L.F. Tseng, H.H. Loh & E.L. Way, Life Sci., 20, 251(1977).
87. S.N. Kozhechkin, R.U. Ostrovskaya, Nature, 269, 73(1977).
88. E.F. Hahn, J. Fishman, Y. Shiwaku, F.F. Foldes, H. Nagashima & D. Duncalf, Res. Commun. Chem. Pathol. Pharm., 18, 1(1977).
89. R. Schulz, M. Wuster & A. Herz, Life Sci., 21, 105(1977).
90. A.J. Blume, J. Shorr, J.P.M. Finberg & S. Spector, Proc. Natl. Acad. Sci., 74, 4927(1977).
91. A. Cowan, J.C. Doxey & E.J.R. Harry, Brit. J. Pharmacol., 60, 547(1977).
92. A. Cowan, J.W. Lewis & I.R. Macfarlane, Brit. J. Pharmacol., 60, 537(1977).
93. A. Delpizzo, Curr. Ther. Res., 20, 763(1976).
94. I.C. Andrews, Curr. Ther. Res., 22, 697(1977).
95. M. Lippmann, M.S. Mok, S.N. Steen, A.Z. Lane & F.S. Caruso, Curr. Ther. Res., 22, 276(1977).
96. C. Holden, Science, 198, 807(1977).
97. E.L. May & A.E. Jacobson, J. Pharm. Sci., 66, 285(1977).
98. Y.F. Jacquet, W.A. Klee, K.C. Rice, I. Iijima, J. Minawikawa, Science, 198, 842(1977).
99. H. Merz, K. Stockhaus & H. Wick, J. Med. Chem., 20, 844(1977).
100. M.D. Aceto, L.S. Harris, W.L. Dewey & R.L. Balster, Committee on Problems of Drug Dependence, Nat. Acad. Sci., 1976.
101. S. Shiotani & T. Kometani, J. Med. Chem., 20, 976(1977).
102. P.S. Portoghese, R.N. Hanson, V.G. Telang, J.L. Winger & A.E. Takemori, J. Med. Chem., 20, 1020(1977).
103. J.B. Jiang, R.N. Hanson, P.S. Portoghese & A.E. Takemori, J. Med. Chem., 20, 1100(1977).
104. D.C. Palmer & M.J. Strauss, Chem. Rev., 77, 1(1977).
105. L.S. Brahen, T. Capone, V. Wiechert, D. Desiderio, Arch. Gen. Psychiat., 34, 1181(1977).
106. W.T. Beaver & G.A. Feise, J. Clin. Pharmacol., 17, 480(1977).
107. I.M. Uwaydah, E.L. May & L.S. Harris, J. Med. Chem., 20, 1374(1977).
108. M. Saucier, J.P. Daris, Y. Lambert I. Monkovic & A.W. Pircio, J. Med. Chem., 20, 676(1977).
109. W.F. Michne, R.L. Salsbury & S.J. Michalec, J. Med. Chem., 20, 682(1977).
110. K.C. Rice, W.A. Klee, M.D. Aceto, H.H. Swain & A.E. Jacobson, J. Pharm. Sci., 66, 193(1977).
111. K.C. Rice, S. Shiotani, C.R. Creveling, A.E. Jacobson & W.A. Klee, J. Med. Chem., 20, 673(1977).
112. S. Shiotani, T. Kometani & K. Mitsuhashi, J. Med. Chem., 20, 310(1977).
113. T.A. Montzka & J.D. Matiskella, J. Med. Chem., 20, 453(1977).
114. D.M. Zimmerman & R. Nickander, "reported to the Committee on Problems of Drug Dependence," Cambridge, MA, 1977. Reports available through Nat. Acad. Sci. (reported with permission of authors.)
115. M.A. Iorio & W.A. Klee, J. Med. Chem., 20, 309(1977).
116. R. Abbas, R.E. Willette & J.M. Edwards, J. Pharm. Sci., 66, 1583(1977).
117. J.A. Waters, J. Med. Chem., 20, 1094(1977).
118. M. Takeda, H. Inoue, K. Noguchi, Y. Honma, M. Kawamori, G. Tsukamoto, Y. Yamawaki, S. Saito, K. Aoe, T. Date, S. Nurimoto & G. Hayashi, J. Med. Chem., 20, 221(1977).
119. M. Takeda, M. Kawamori, H. Inoue, K. Noguchi & S. Nurimoto, Chem. Pharm. Bull., 25, 775(1977).
120. K. Noguchi, M. Takeda & S. Nurimoto, Chem. Pharm. Bull., 25, 890(1977).
121. M. Takeda, M. Kawamori, K. Noguchi & S. Nurimoto, Chem. Pharm. Bull., 25, 1777(1977).
122. R.C. Cavestri & M. Mokotoff, J. Med. Chem., 20, 1493(1977).
123. M.H. Fisher, E.J.J. Grabowaki, A.A. Patchett, J. ten Broeke, L.M. Flataker, V.J. Lotti & F.M. Robinson, J. Med. Chem., 20, 63(1977).
124. R.N. Booher, S.E. Smits, W.W. Turner, Jr., & A. Pohland, J. Med. Chem., 20, 885(1977).
125. W.R. Buckett, M.J. Crossland, R.H.B. Galt, Z. Matusiak, R.J. Pearce, J.S. Shaw & M.J. Turnbull, Brit. J. Pharmacol., 61, 146P(1977).
126. D.S. Fries & D.J. Bertelli, 174th Nat. ACS Mtg. Chicago, p. MEDI 24, August (1977).
127. L. Terenius, Psychoneuroendocrinology, 2, 53(1977).
128. Y. Audigier, B. Malfroy-Camine & J.C. Schwartz, Eur. J. Pharmacolo., 41, 247(1977).
129. D.T. Wong & J.S. Horng, Res. Commun. Chem. Pathol. Pharm., 16, 749(1977).
130. T.T. Chau-Pham. & W.L. Dewey, Life Sci., 21, 1337(1977).
131. J.A.H. Lord, A.A. Waterfield, H. Hughes & H.W. Kosterlitz, Nature 267, 495(1977).
132. E.T. Wei, L.F. Tseng, H.H. Loh & C.H. Li, Life Sci., 21, 321(1977).
133. J. Knoll, Pol. J. Pharmacol. Pharm., 29, 165(1977).
134. A.A. Waterfield, R.W.J. Smokcum, J. Hughes, H.W. Kosterlitz & G. Henderson, J. Pharmacol., 43, 107(1977).
135. W.R. Martin, P.E. Gilbert, J.A. Thompson & C.A. Jessee, Drug Alc. Depend., 3, 23(1978).
136. A.E. Jacobson, W.A. Klee & W.J. Dunn, Eur. J. Med. Chem., 12, 49(1977).
137. H.W. Kosterlitz & F.M. Leslie, Brit. J. Pharmacol., 59, 478P(1977).
138. R.H.B. Galt, J. Pharm. Pharmacol., 29, 711(1977).
139. J.R. Smythies, Psychoneuroendocrinology, 2, 71(1977).

Section II - PHARMACODYNAMIC AGENTS

Editor: John Krapcho, Squibb Institute for Medical Research, Princeton, N.J. 08540

Chapter 6. Pulmonary and Anti-Allergy Drugs

Stanley C. Bell, Wyeth Laboratories, Inc. Radnor, PA 19087.
Robert J. Capetola, Ortho Pharmaceutical Corp. Raritan, NJ 08869.

Introduction - The main pathophysiological changes underlying asthma are narrowing of the airway due to constriction of the bronchial muscles, edema of the bronchial mucosa, leucocytic infiltration, and hypersecretion of a tenacious sputum, leading to mechanical obstruction of parts of the bronchial tree.[1] The allergic reaction is classified as a Type I inflammatory reaction. The union of sensitizing antigen or hapten with receptive IgE immunoglobulins bound to host mast cells and basophils triggers a series of intracellular events that culminate in the release of various pharmacological mediators. These mediators include histamine, slow reacting substance of anaphylaxis (SRS-A), eosinophil chemotactic factor of anaphylaxis (ECF-A), serotonin, platelet activating factor (PAF), kinins and prostaglandins. More recently, a neutrophil chemotactic factor of anaphylaxis (NCF-A) was described during IgE-mediated asthma in humans.[2]

Several papers have appeared that review the autoregulatory mechanisms and pharmacological control of mediator release.[3-5] It is becoming clearer that both positive and negative feedback mechanisms controlled by these chemical mediators through intermediary cyclic nucleotides provide important means for the intrinsic modulation of Type I inflammatory reactions. For example, the modulation process may be divided into two distinct phases, inhibition and enhancement.[3] Autonomic inhibition of mediator release is achieved principally by β-agonists and is specifically inhibited by β-antagonists such as propranolol. Inhibition of mediator release is also accomplished by histamine stimulation of H_2 receptors (on mast cells and basophils) and by E-series prostaglandins, through negative feedback mechanisms. These inhibitory substances act by increasing cyclic AMP levels which, through mechanisms not completely understood, in turn inhibit mediator release. Enhancement of mediator release is achieved by α-agonists and prostaglandins such as $F_{2}\alpha$ which probably act by antagonizing the action of cyclic AMP.

Cyclic AMP and cyclic GMP have opposing actions in regulating IgE dependent mediator release. The pathophysiology of asthma may depend therefore on the sum of the effects of the endogenous mediators which alter the ratio of cyclic nucleotides.[3]

Histamine has long been regarded as one of the prime mediators of asthma in humans. However the inability to consistently block the action of histamine with classical antihistamines suggests that SRS-A may be the

ISBN 0-12-040513-X

major bronchoconstrictor in human asthma. Recently a report appeared that provides clear evidence that both are involved.[6] Therefore pharmacological control of human airways in vivo may require a drug with polypharmacology, i.e. one that inhibits the release of many mediators or a combination of specific antagonists.

Inhibitors of Mediator Release - The pharmacologic actions of mediators of anaphylaxis and immune and biochemical mechanisms in asthma have been reviewed.[4,5] Disodium cromoglycate (DSCG) continues to be the subject of a number of papers. A study on histamine induced reflex bronchoconstriction in the dog suggests that DSCG may reduce the activity of lung irritant receptors.[7] Two new chromone derivatives FPL52757 (1) and (FPL57787 2) were reported to be active by inhalation or the oral route in experimental and clinical asthma.[8] The administration of 1, given either by inhalation as an aqueous aerosol up to 10 min. before antigen challenge, or in single or multiple oral doses of 50 to 100 mg from 2 to 12 hours before challenge, afforded protection from anaphylactic bronchoconstriction. In a limited study of the tricyclic chromone 2 in experimental asthma good activity was obtained with single or multiple oral doses of 4 to 10 mg.

Benzosubstituted analogs 2-5 of DSCG have been assigned generic names.[9] Terbucromil 3 was also found to have dose related uricosuric properties in man.[10] A series of analogs of the tetracyclic chromone 6 (PR-D-92-EA) were tested for antiallergic activity in the rat PCA.[11] 6 had an ED_{50} of .11 mg/kg. A series of chromonone-2-carboxylic acids with anti-SRS-A activity was reported.[12] The deshydroxy analog (7) of FPL55712 (8) was more potent than 8 (IC_{50}=0.001 μg/ml) but offered no in vivo advantage. Neither 6 nor 8 was reported to be active against bovine SRS-A.[13] The chromone 3-tetrazole 9 and related compounds were reported to be slightly more potent than DSCG.[14]

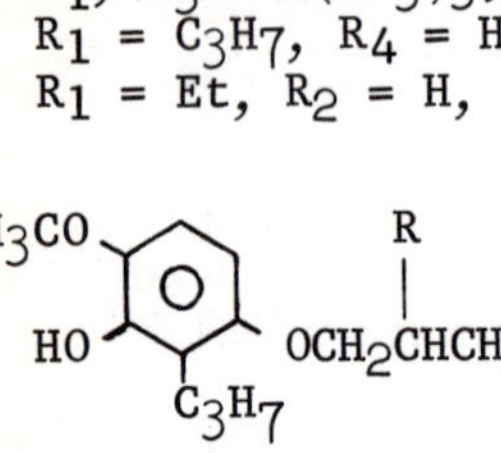

1 R_1, R_3 = Et, R_4 = OH, R_2 = H
2 R_1 = C_3H_7, R_4 = OH, R_2, R_3 = $(CH_2)_4$ Proxicromil
3 R_1, R_3 = $C(CH_3)_3$, R_2, R_4 = H Terbucromil
4 R_1 = C_3H_7, R_4 = H, R_2, R_3 = $(CH_2)_4$ Procromil
5 R_1 = Et, R_2 = H, R_3 = $CH{=}CH_2$, R_4 = OH Evicromil

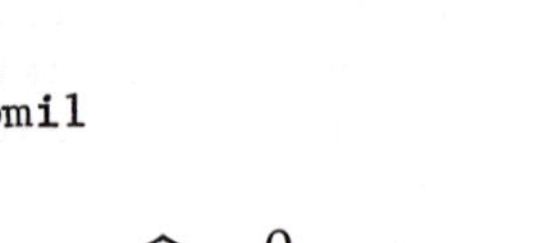

6

7 R = H

8 R = OH

9

A fused bisquinoline carboxylic acid derivative 10 was reported to be 500 x more potent (ID_{50}=.005 mg/kg) than DSCG in the rat PCA[15] administered iv at the time of antigen challenge or ip 30 min. before antigen challenge. The quinoline 11 containing an oxamate group on the fused benzo ring was active *in vivo* (25 x DSCG) in the rat PCA.[16] Pyrimidoquinolin-2-carboxylates were described as being 10-100 x more potent than DSCG with the ester being orally active.[17a] Pirolate 12 the dimethoxy analog appears to be the compound of choice.[17b]

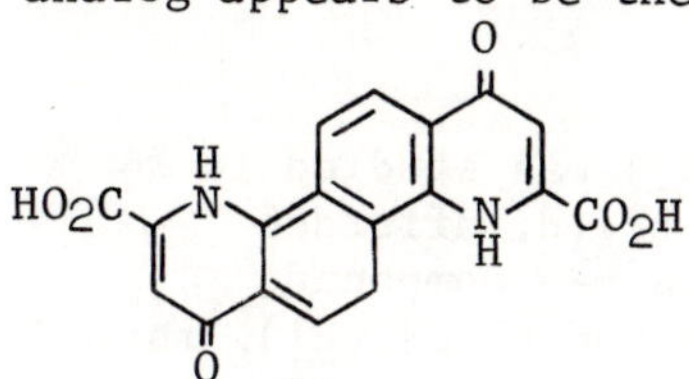

10

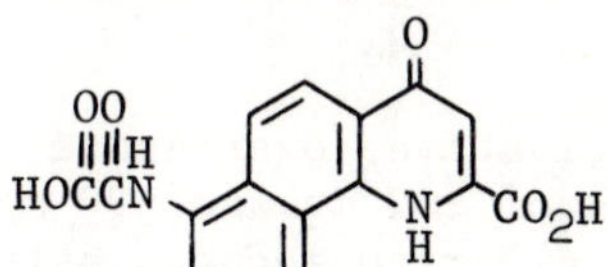

11

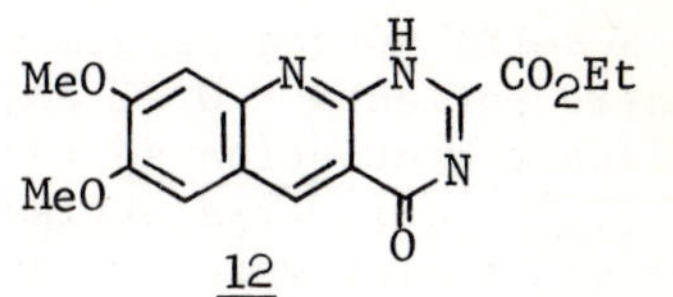

12

A clinical study of lodoxamide 13 tromethamine on asthmatic patients has shown it to be an effective and potent antiallergy compound. Inhalation doses of 0.01, 0.1 and 1.0 mg increased the amount of allergen necessary to cause a $\geq$ 20% fall in forced expiratory volume.[18]

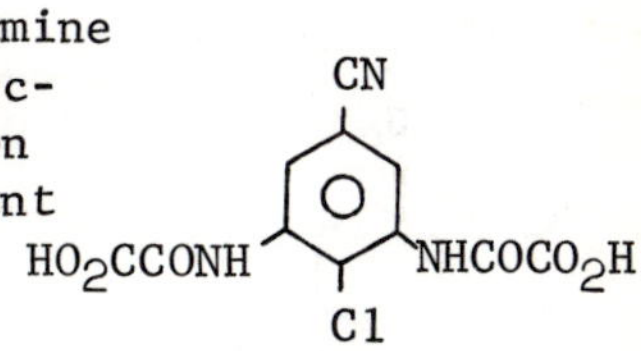

13 Lodoxamide

A variety of diones were found to be potent inhibitors of mediator release. Nivimedone (BRL10833) (14) was studied in seven asthmatic patients both by aerosol (40 mg) and by the oral route (2-10 mg/kg) and was without significant effect.[19]

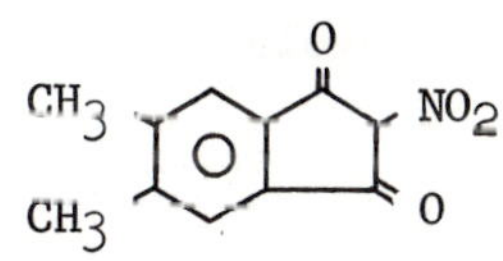

14 Nivimedone

Xanthones and related tricyclics continue to be of considerable interest. Clinical studies of tixanox (R57337) (15), given as an aerosol, report it to be significantly better than placebo in exercise-induced-bronchospasm[20] while studies with doxantrazole 16 (up to 400 mg orally) show it to be ineffective in exercise-induced asthma.[21] Conversion of orally inactive xanthone acids to amides 17 produced compounds with some oral activity (rat PCA).[22]

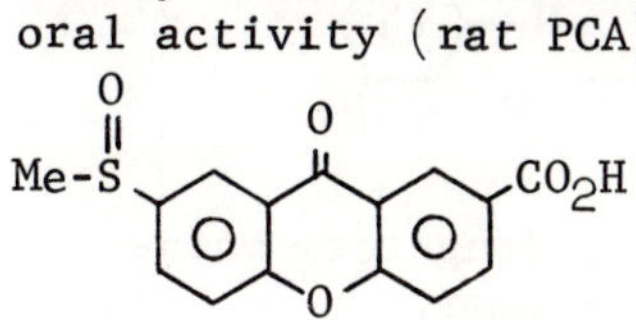

15 Tixanox

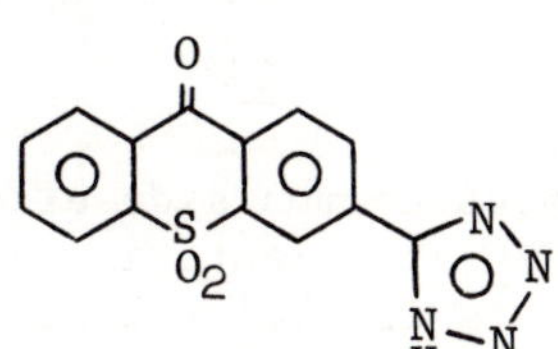

16 Doxantrazole

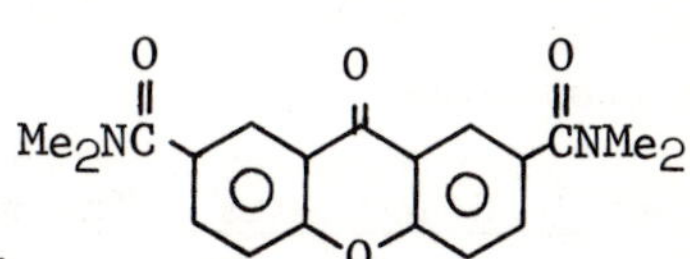

17

The cycloheptathiophene HC20-511 (18) was shown to be effective in the clinic against allergen bronchoprovocation for up to 6 hours with a dose of 1 mg po.[23] The drug was reportedly well tolerated. A review of the pharmacology of ketotifen 18 has appeared.[24]

18 Ketotifen (Zatiden®)

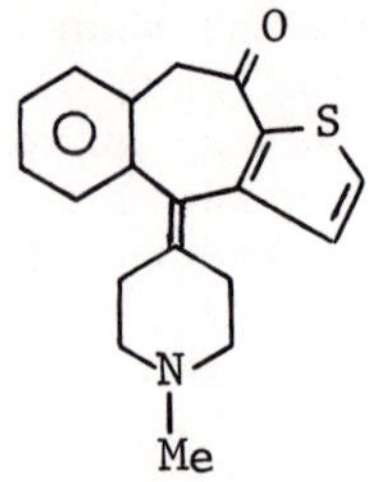

A tetrahydrocarbazole derivative, oxarbazole (19) was studied in 24 asthmatic patients. Oral doses of 200 mg and 300 mg b.i.d. afforded significant protection against allergen-induced asthma.[25] Compound AB-50 (20), a bis (2-acetylsalicylamido) benzoic acid and AB-23 (21), the desacetoxy analog were compared to DSCG in the rat PCA and *in vitro* histamine release (antigen + 48/80).[26] 21 was reported to be more active than DSCG *in vitro*.

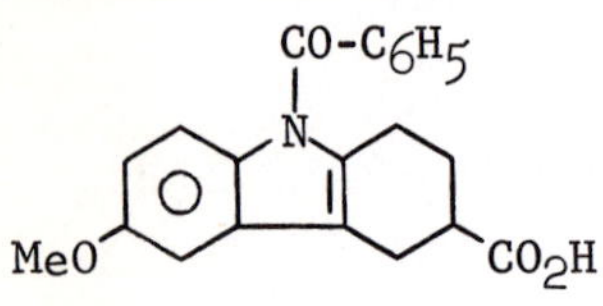

19 Oxarbazole

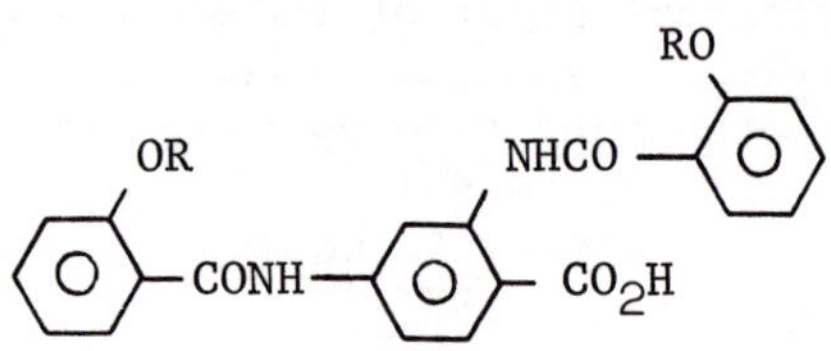

20 R = Ac
21 R = H

The piperazinopropylbenzimidazole (oxatomide R35443) 22 demonstrated clinical effectiveness in a large sample of patients with allergic rhinitis.[27] Oxatomide prevents mediator release and is also a potent H_1 antagonist as well as being orally active.[28] 23 is an orally active piperazinopropyladenine derivative capable of preventing ascaris-induced bronchospasm in dogs.[29]

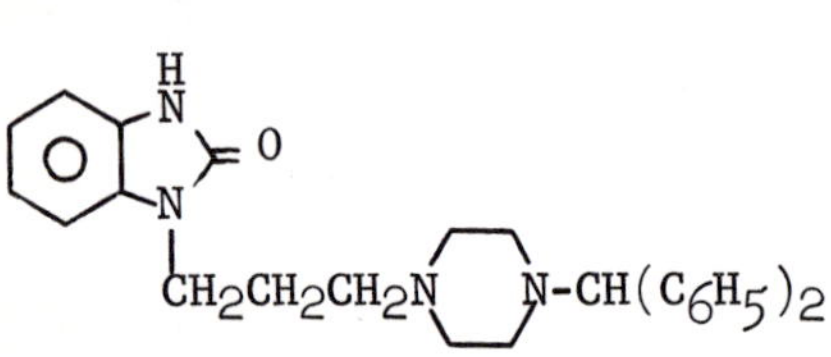

22 Oxatomide

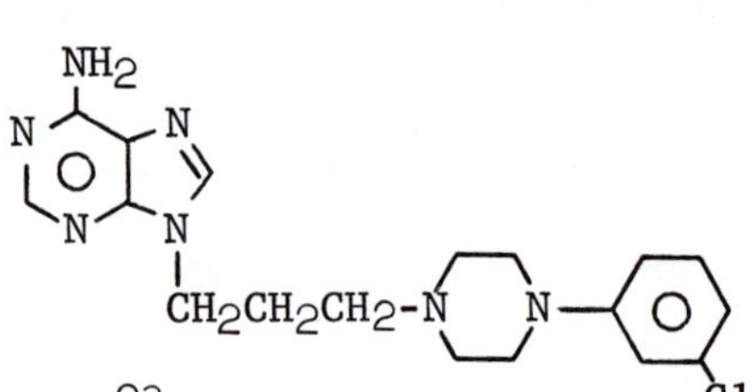

23

β-Adrenergic Stimulants - The most common side effect of long-term maintenance therapy with the newer β_2-stimulants is muscle tremor.[30,31] This effect is mediated by β_2 receptors in skeletal muscle.[32] The search for new agents with greater selectivity for bronchial versus skeletal muscle should continue.

Most new β-stimulants and those undergoing clinical investigation continue to be substituted β-hydroxy-α-phenethylamines. The effects of these substitutuions on β-adrenergic cyclases have been reviewed.[33] The interaction of the receptor and the aromatic moiety of several adrenergic drugs was studied by the SCF-MO-LCAO method.[34] These authors conclude that the "affinity" of the drugs is due to the ethanolamine side chain and the regions of electrophilicity of the phenyl ring and the substituents, while the "intrinsic activity" can be explained by the regions of nucleophilicity of the aromatic ring and the substituents.

Clinical studies in the U.S. continue with fenoterol 24, a potent bronchodilator used for years in Europe.[35,36] It has a rapid onset of action with a duration superior to isoproterenol.[36] In patients with reversible airway obstruction, clenbuterol (NAB365) 25 was found to be about 100 x more potent that salbutamol 26 po.[37] Side effects were similar and included moderate to moderately severe tremors. Orally 25 reaches maximum plasma concentration in 2 hours and has a half-life of 35 hours.[37] In another study 25 was shown to be equiactive with 24 but more potent (24 μg vs. 5 mg given by inhalation).[38a] The bronchodilating effect of salbutamol 26 was significantly superior and of longer duration than that of isoproterenol in another clinical study.[38b] No significant changes in heart rate or blood pressure were noted with 26.

Modification of the aromatic hydroxymethyl group of salbutamol 26 produced compounds 27 of slightly less activity[39] while substitutions of the β-hydroxy group with hydroxymethyl[40] 28 greatly decreases potency. The formamido derivative BD-40-A (29) was 43 x more potent as a bronchodilator than 26 given orally in guinea pigs.[41]

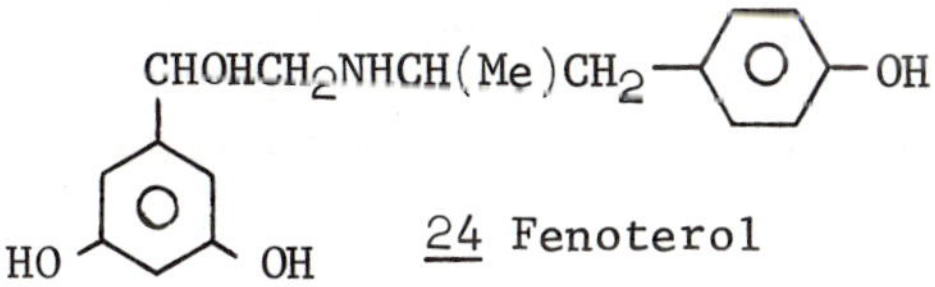

24 Fenoterol

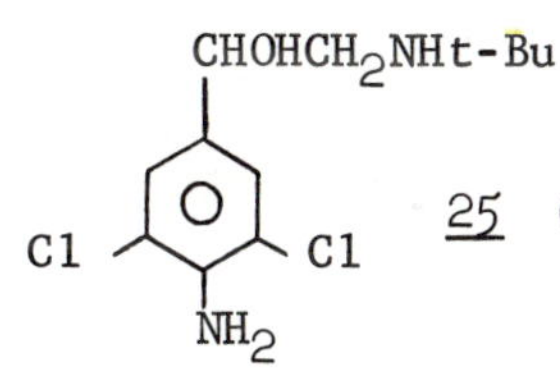

25 Clenbuterol

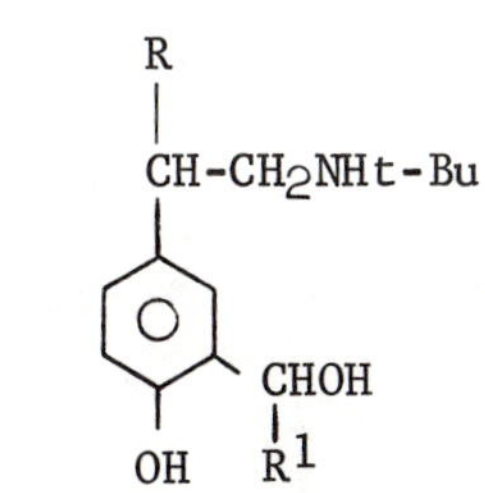

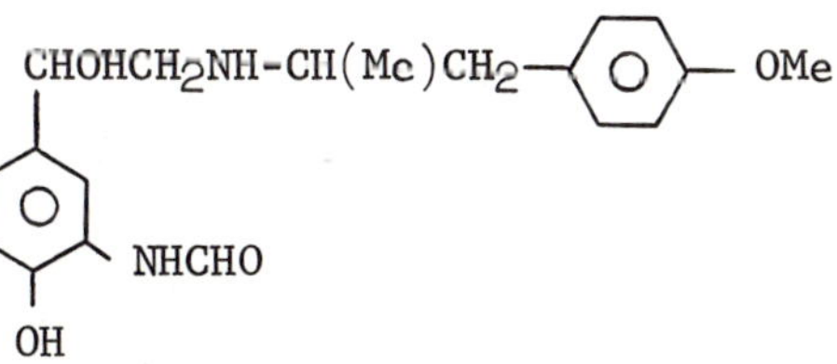

26 R = OH, R^1 = H, Salbutamol
27 R^1 = Me, R = OH
28 R^1 = H, R = CH_2OH

29

Animal data suggest that QH25 (30) is a more selective bronchodilator than both isoproterenol and salbutamol.[42] A study of Sm 220 Cl (31) demonstrates species differences and suggests there would be no tracheobronchial vs. cardiac selectivity in man.[43] Ibuterol 32 (KWD2058), the di-isobutyric ester of terbutaline 33 caused significantly less increase in heart rate, tremor ratio, and pulse amplitude in man when doses causing equal bronchodilation were infused.[44]

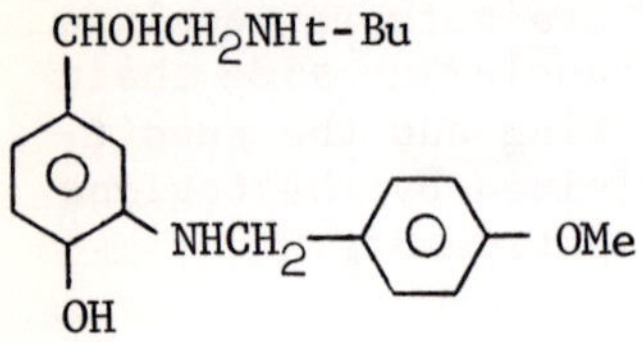

30

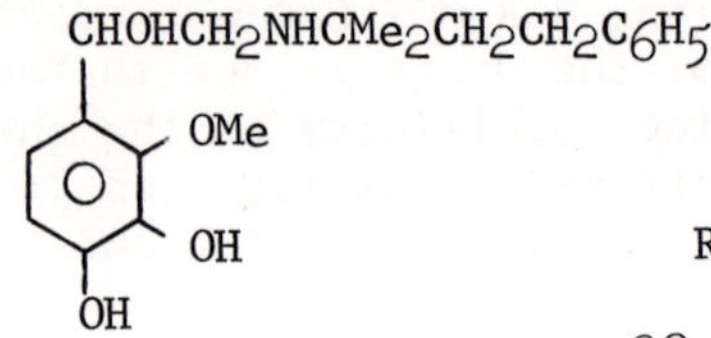

31

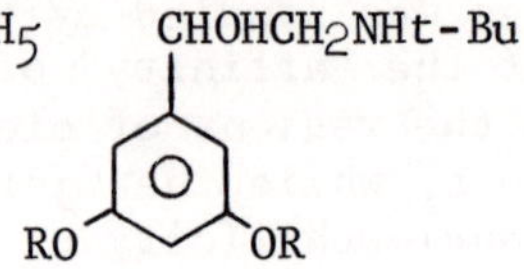

32 R=COCHMe$_2$ Ibuterol
33 R=H Terbutaline

Replacement of the phenyl ring of sulfonterol with pyridyl yielded a compound 34 of equal potency but, more β_2-selective.[45] Carbostyryl derivatives 35a (OPC-2009), and 35b (OPC-2030) [(-) erythro] show high β_2-selectivity in dogs[46] and data suggest their action is mediated through increasing cAMP concentration.[47]

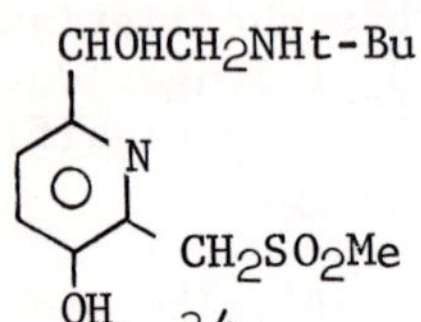

34

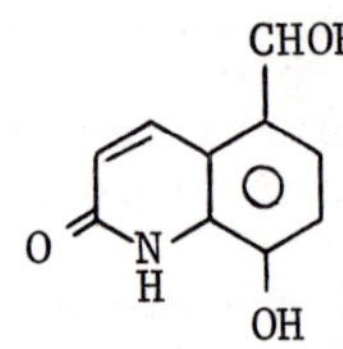

35a R=CH(CH$_3$)$_2$
35b R=Et

The bronchodilating effect of β-agonists such as isoproterenol, salbutamol and chlorprenaline was shown to be markedly enhanced when combined with the α-blocker, dihydroergotoxin.[48] The isoquinoline, trimetoquinol(AQ-110), 36 was compared with a series of analogs[49,50] and the isomer 37 was found to be more β_2 selective although not as potent.[97] Detailed pharmacological and therapeutic reviews have appeared for rimiterol 38[51] and hexoprenaline 39.[52]

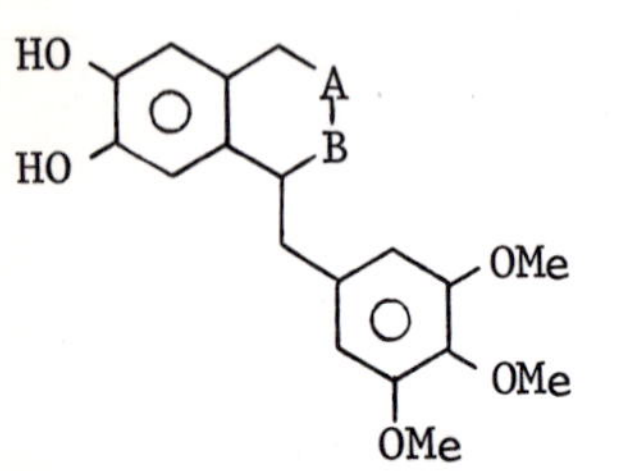

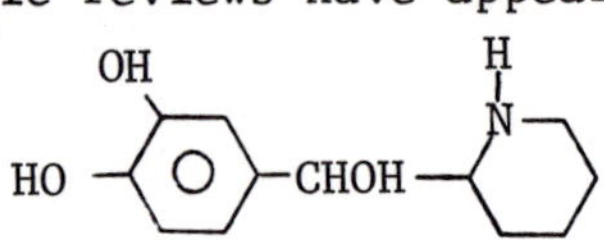

38 Rimiterol

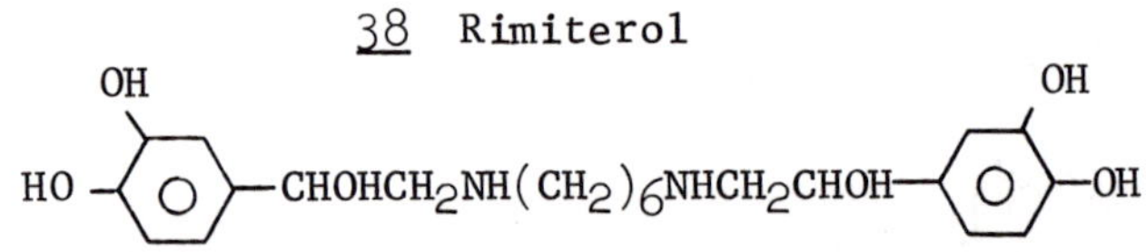

36 Trimetoquinol A = CH$_2$, B = NH
37 A = NH, B = CH$_2$

39 Hexoprenaline

The pharmacology of W10,294A (40) has been outlined. The bronchodilator activity was compared to that of aminophylline and shown to be more potent. The mechanism of action is apparently unrelated to beta stimulation or phosphodiesterase inhibition. 40 reached peak plasma levels in 1.7 hr. with a half-life of 1-2 hours.[53,54]

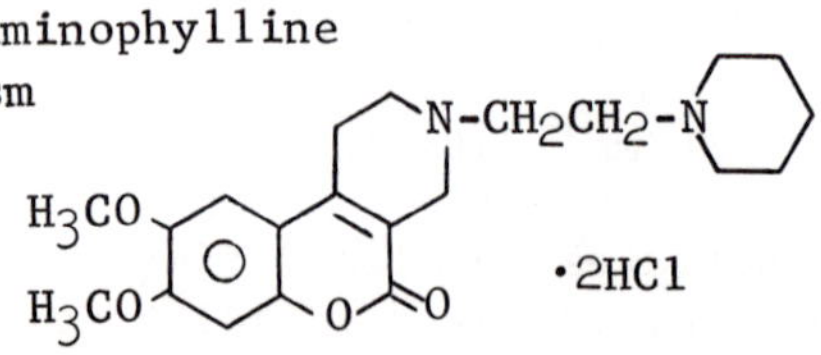

40

Phosphodiesterase Inhibitors - A basically substituted derivative of theophylline 41 was shown to inhibit edema formation or delayed contact allergy (DNCB) in guinea pigs.[55] Interestingly this derivative is a potent competitive antagonist of histamine (H_1).[55] A series of thienoquinoline-1,1-dioxides 42, prepared as potential antiinflammatory agents, was found to possess phosphodiesterase inhibiting activity in the range of theophylline.[56]

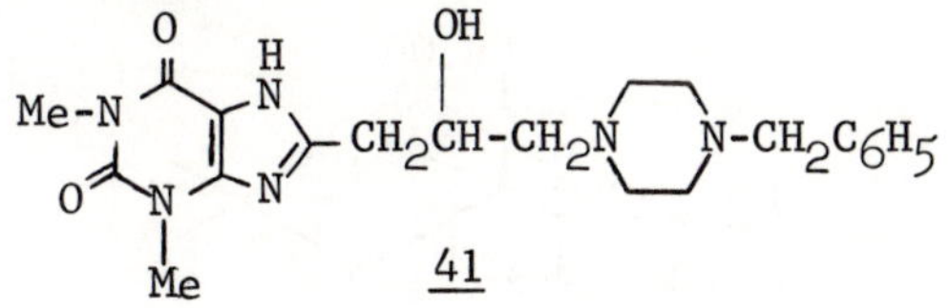

41

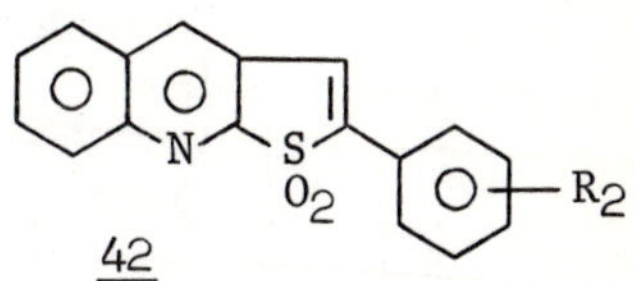

42

A study characterizing the phosphodiesterases in human lung tissue has appeared.[57]

Prostaglandins - The use of prostaglandins as bronchodilators continues to be of considerable interest. Historically, their use has been limited due to pharyngeal irritation and cough when administered by inhalation. 16 (S)-Methyl-20-methoxy PGE_2 (YPG-209) 43, given intraduodenally, was a potent inhibitor (ED_{50} of 19 μg/kg) of increased airway resistance induced by histamine in anesthetized guinea pigs.[58] Intravenously it was 230 x more potent than PGE_2. The substitution of alkoxy groups in the 16 position of PGE_2 generally produces bronchodilators of less potency 44[59] while substitution of 16,16-trimethylene derivatives of PGE_1 and PGE_2 (45)[60] yields compounds with comparable potency but produces a short-lived pulmonary hypertension.

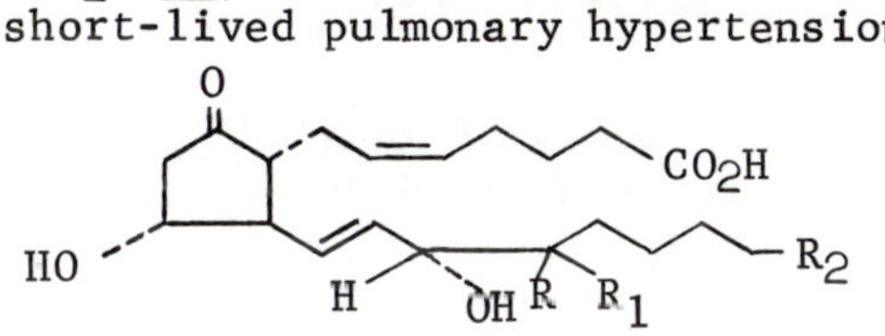

43 R = Me, R_1 = H, R_2 = OMe

44 R = OMe, R_1, R_2 = H

45 R, R_1 = $(CH_2)_3$, R_2 = H

11-Deoxy-15-hydroxy-2,13-diene prostaglandin (46) showed bronchodilating activity comparable to PGA_2 while the isomeric 16-hydroxy-2,14-diene analogs were bronchoconstricting.[61] Prostacyclin, 47 an interesting substance that may be a naturally occurring inhibitor of platelet aggregation was also reported to have significant bronchodilating activity.[62]

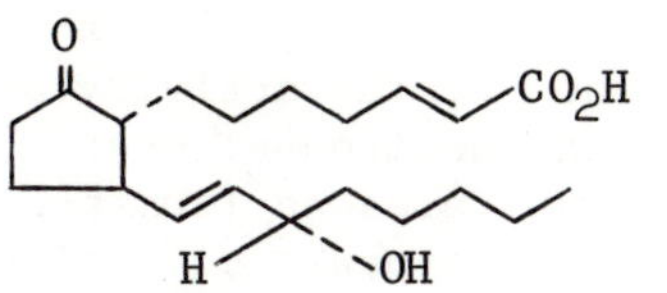

46

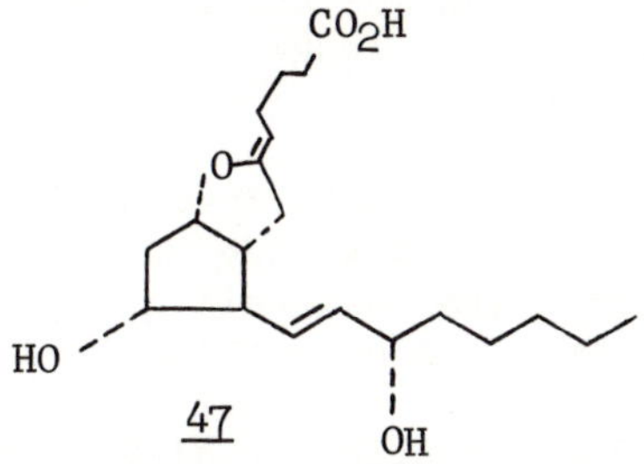

47

Steroids - Clinical testing of beclomethasone dipropionate 48 has been extensive. Its use is intended for the prophylactic treatment of steroid-dependent asthmatics. Therapy with topical steroids yields maximal local and minimal systemic effects with oropharyngeal fungal infections being an important complication. Beclomethasone dipropionate 48 was tested in an 18 month study of steroid-dependent asthmatics and demonstrated a significant improvement with no Candida infections.[63] Flunisolide 49 was tested as a nasal spray in adult hay fever patients and shown to be safe and efficacious in the treatment of seasonal allergic rhinitis.[64]

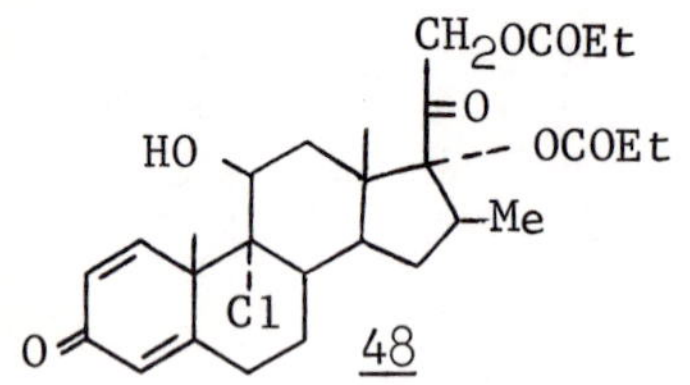

48

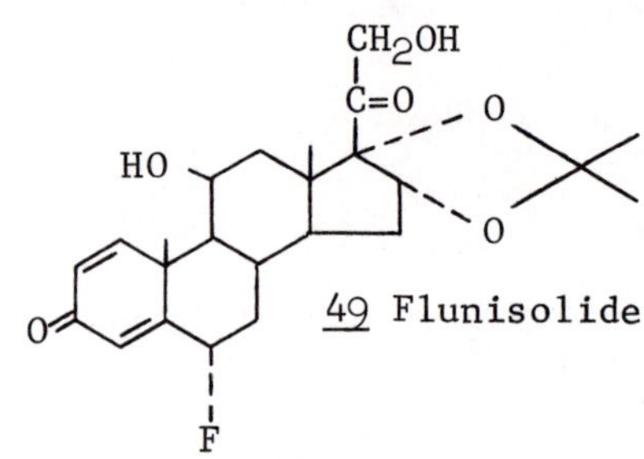

49 Flunisolide

Anticholinergics - The quaternary anticholinergic Sch1000 (ipratropium bromide) (50) has been studied extensively in the clinic and demonstrated to be an effective bronchodilator in asthma. In a recent study 50

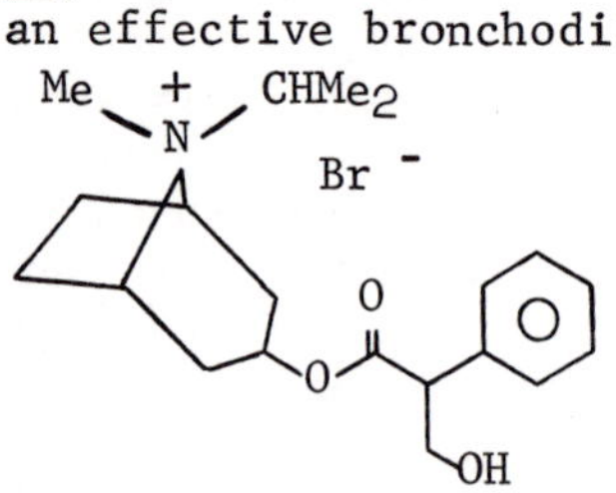

50 Ipratropium Bromide (Atrovent®)

was tested in patients with chronic bronchitis.[65] Doses of inhaled 50 ranged from 10 μg to 80 μg and these doses were superior in duration of action to isoproterenol (75 μg and 150 μg). Bronchodilatory response to 50 lasted up to 4 hours. No significant alterations of pulse or blood pressure were noted. Dryness of the mouth and scratching in the trachea were reported absent. 50 was also assessed alongside DSCG and shown to be effective in exercise-induced asthma.[66] Salbutamol (200 μg), administered as an aerosol, was found to produce a greater degree of bronchodilation during the initial 3 hours following drug administration than the quaternary anticholinergic Sch1000 (40 μg) in asthmatic patients.[67] Comparable bronchodilation was achieved after 4 hours and a combination of the two drugs produced a longer duration of bronchodilation than either drug alone.

Peptides - Previously uncharacterized eosinophil chemotactic activity of apparent M.W. 1500 to 2500 was found preformed in rat peritoneal mast cells, was associated with mast cell granules and was released from sensitized mast cells.[68] Further purification revealed two peaks of eosinophil chemotactic activity. In other experiments, data suggest that histamine and the ECF-A peptides (Val-Gly-Ser-Glu and Ala-Gly-Ser-Glu) not only attract eosinophils selectively in chemotaxis but also increase the number of complement receptors on the eosinophil membrane.[69] The significance of this finding is not known at present.

References

1. H. Formgren, Scand. J. Resp. Dis.(Suppl), 97, 1 (1977).
2. P.C. Atkins, M. Norman, H. Weiner, and B. Zweiman, Ann. Intern. Med., 86, 415 (1977).
3. M.C. Holroyde, J.F. Burka, P. Eyre, Agents and Actions, 7, 421 (1977).
4. P.J. Piper, Pharmac. Ther. B, 3, 75 (1977).
5. T.T. Hubscher, Ann. Allergy, 38, 83 (1977).
6. G.K. Adams III, L.M. Lichtenstein, Nature, 270, 255 (1977).
7. D. M. Jackson, I.M. Richards, Br. J. Pharmac., 61, 257 (1977).
8. J. Augstein, H. Cairns, D. Hunter, T.B. Lee, J. Suschitzky, R.E.C. Altounyan, D.M. Jackson, J. Mann, T.S.C. Orr, and P. Sheard, Agents and Actions, 7, 443 (1977).
9. Brit. Pharmacop. Comm. Approved Names (Suppl. 1), 6, Oct. 1, 1977.
10. J. Augstein, H. Cairns, A. Chambers, J.W. Burns, and H. Radziwonik, J. Pharm. Pharmac., 28, 919 (1976).
11. J.P. Devlin, K. Freter and P.B. Stewart, J. Med. Chem., 20, 205, (1977).
12. R.A. Appleton, J.R. Bantick, T.R. Chamberlain, D.N. Hardern, T.B. Lee, and A.D. Pratt, ibid., 20, 371 (1977).
13. J.F. Burka and P. Eyre, Eur. J. Pharmacol., 44, 169 (1977).
14. A. Nohara, H. Kuriki, T. Saijo, H. Sugihara, M. Kanno and Y. Sanno, J. Med. Chem., 20, 141 (1977).
15. C.M. Hall, J.B. Wright, H.G. Johnson, and A.J. Taylor, J. Med. Chem., 20, 1337 (1977).
16. J.B. Wright and H.G. Johnson, ibid., 20, 166 (1977).
17. a) J.H. Althuis, P.F. Moore, and H.J. Hess, A.C.S. 174 Nat'l Mtg., Chicago, Aug., 1977 Abstr. MEDI - 44. b) J.A.M.A., 238, 1407 (1977).
18. T. Bui, K, Burke, G. Watt, A. Bewtra, R. Townley, 34th Ann. Meeting Am. Acad. of Allergy, Abstr. No. 201 (1978).
19. S. Zwi, S. Hurwitz, H. Kallenbach and H. Goldman, Am. Rev. Resp. Dis., 115, 184 (1977).
20. a) R. R. Rosenthal, J. Oren, J.D. Johnson, and P.S. Norman, Congress Abstracts, Ann. Allergy, 38 #63 (1977). b) J.A.M.A., 236, 1992 (1977).
21. H. Poppius, and B. Stenius, Europ. J. Clin. Pharmacol., 11, 107 (1977).
22. W.J. Jones, Jr., W.L. Albrecht, N.L. Munro and K.T. Stewart, J. Med. Chem., 20, 594 (1977).
23. a) J. P. Girard and M. Cuevas, Acta. Allergol., 32, 27 (1977). b) E. Waldvogel, C. Schwarb, J. M. Bastian, and J.-P. Bourquiss, Helv. Chim. Acta., 59, 866 (1977).
24. U. Martin and D. Roemer, Monogr. Allergy, 12 145 (1977).
25. C.J. Falliers, T.S. Mingo, 34th Ann. Meeting Am. Acad. Allergy, Abst. No. 199 (1978).
26. Y. Ohsugi, T. Matsuno, and Y. Takagaki, Chem. Pharm. Bull., 25, 2437 (1977).
27. R. De Beule, E. Vannieuwenhuyse, J. Callier, W. Verstraete, F. Degreef, M. Gregoire, Y. Robience, W. Stevens and P. Libert, Acta. Allergol., 32, 278 (1977).
28. F. Awouter, C.J.E. Niemegeers, J. Vanden Bark, J.M. Van Nueten, F.M. Leneerts, M. Borgers, K.H.L. Schellekins, A. Broekaert, J. De Cree, and P.A.J. Janssen, Experientia, 33, 1657 (1977).
29. O.I. Zimmermann, W.T. Ulmer and A. Roesch., Arzneim-Forsch., 27 (II) 1999 (1977).
30. D.P. Tashkin, Chest., 71, 125 (1977).
31. M. Weinberger and L. Hendeles, Ration. Drug. Ther., 11, (6) (1977).
32. S. Larsson, Acta. Med. Scand. Suppl., 608 5 (1977).
33. H. Sheppard in "Annual Reports in Medicinal Chemistry", Vol. 12, F.H. Clark, Ed. Academic Press, New York, NY, 1977, P. 173.
34. C. Petrongolo, B. Macchia, F. Macchia, and A. Martinelli, J. Med. Chem., 20, 1645 (1977).
35. W.W. Simi and W.C. Miller, J. Allergy. Clin. Immunol., 59, 178 (1977).
36. C. Emirgil, K. Palmer, L. VanVoorhies, C. Wesson, B.J. Sobol, Ann. Allergy, 39, 415 (1977).
37. P. L. Kamburoff, F.J. Prime, and O.-P. Schmidt, Br. J. Clin. Pharmacol., 4, 67 (1977).
38. a) V.A. Dorow, Arzneim-Forsch., 27 (II) 2020 (1977). b) V.K. Mahajan, J.F. Tomashefski, G.L. Huber, Ann. Allergy, 39, 319 (1977).
39. J. Ven, J.S. Frazee, C. Kaiser, D.F. Colella and J.R. Wardell Jr., J. Med. Chem., 20 1029 (1977)
40. T. Jen, J.S. Frazee, M.S. Schwartz, K.F. Erhard, C. Kaiser, D.F. Colella, and J.R. Wardell Jr., J. Med. Chem., 20, 1263 (1977).
41. K. Murase, T. Mase, H. Ida, K. Takahashi and M. Murakami, Chem. Pharm. Bull., 25, 1368 (1977).
42. J.-J. Larsen and K. Hermansen, Acta. Pharmacol. et. Toxicol., 40, 42 (1977).
43. K. Bohmer and C. Raper, Clin. Exp. Pharmacol. Physiol., 4, 349 (1977).
44. S. Larsson, N. Svedymr, Europ. J. Clin. Pharmacol., 11, 429 (1977).
45. T. Jen, J.S. Frazee, M.S. Schwartz, C. Kaiser, D.F. Colella, and J.R. Wardell, Jr., J. Med. Chem., 20, 1258 (1977).
46. S. Yoshizaki, Y. Manabe, S. Tamada, K. Nakagawa, and S. Tei, J. Med. Chem., 20, 1103 (1977).
47. I. Takayanagi, N. Kondo, H. Yamashita, T. Hongo and K. Takagi, J. Pharm. Pharmac., 29, 187 (1977).

48. S. Kitamura, Y. Ishihara, K. Sasaki, T. Shimizu, and M. Harasawa, Arzneim-Forsch., 27 (II) 1959 (1977).
49. K. Ikezawa, H. Takenaga, M. Sato, H. Nakajima, and A. Kiyomoto, Japan J. Pharmacol., 27 537 (1977).
50. P.F. Kador, R. Venkatraman, D.F. Feller, and D.D. Miller, J. Med. Chem., 20 891 (1977).
51. R.M. Pinder, R.N. Brogden, T.M. Speight, G.S. Avery, Drugs 14, 81 (1977).
52. R.M. Pinder, R.N. Brogden, T.M. Speight, G.S. Avery, Drugs, 14, 1 (1977).
53. F.-J. Leinweber and F.J. DeCarlo, Fed. Proc., 36, 3514 Abs., 1 Mar. 77.
54. R.E. Giles, J.C. Williams, M.P. Finkel, J.P.E.T., 203, 701 (1977).
55. R. Czarnecki, Pol. J. Pharmacol. Pharm., 29, 123 (1977).
56. E.A. Harrison, Jr., K.C. Rice and M.E. Rogers, J. Heterocyclic Chem., 14, 909 (1977).
57. D. Green, G. Guy, J.B. Moore, Jr. and H. Lopezb, Life Sciences 20, 1157 (1977).
58. K. Tomioka, M. Terai, and H. Maeno, Arch. Int. Pharmacodyn., 226, 224 (1977).
59. W.A. Hallett, A. Wissner, C.V. Grudzinskas, R. Partridge, J.E. Birnbaum, M.J. Wriss, and F. Dessy, Prostaglandins, 13, 409 (1977).
60. J.S. Skotnicki, R.E. Schaub, M.J. Weiss, and F. Dessy, J. Med. Chem., 20, 1042 (1977).
61. W. Bartmann, G. Beck, R. Kunstmann, U. Lerch, and H. Teufel, Tetrahedron Lett. 2563 (1977).
62. M.A. Wasserman, D.W. DuCharme, R.L. Griffen, M.G. Wendling and G.L. DeGraaf, The Pharmacologist, 19 ASPET Abstract No. 098 (1977).
63. I. Kass, S.V. Nair, K.D. Patil, Chest, 71, 703 (1977).
64. J.K. Kammermeyer, D.W. Rajtora, J. Anuras, and H.B. Richarson, J. Allergy. Clin. Immunol., 59 287 (1977).
65. W. Baigelman, S. Chodosh, Chest, 71, 324 (1977).
66. M. Chan-Yeung, Chest, 71, 320 (1977).
67. R.E. Ruffin, J.D. Fitzgerald and A.S. Rebuck, J. Allergy Clin. Immunol., 59, 136 (1977).
68. R.N. Boswell, K.F. Austen, E.J. Goetzl, J. Immunol., 120, 15, (1978).
69. A.R.E. Anwar and A.B. Kay, Nature, 269, 522 (1977).

Chapter 7. Diuretics

Robert L. Smith, Otto W. Woltersdorf, Jr. and Edward J. Cragoe, Jr.
Merck Sharp & Dohme Research Laboratories, West Point, Pa. 19486

The medical use of diuretics for edema and hypertension continues to grow more rapidly than the pharmaceutical industry in general. The most promising agents being generated in research are those with novel structures, unique modes of action and increased safety. Some valuable reviews of the field,[1-3] symposia[4] and medical perspectives[5-9] have been published. New insights have developed regarding the role of prostaglandins and related systems in kidney function and in the control of blood pressure.

1-Aralkyl-2-pyrazolin-5-ones (1) - In a search for a new chemical type of salidiuretic with high ceiling and long duration of action, a series of compounds of type 1 was discovered by Horstmann and colleagues.[10,11] Elucidation of the structure-activity (S/A) requirements[11,12] led to the

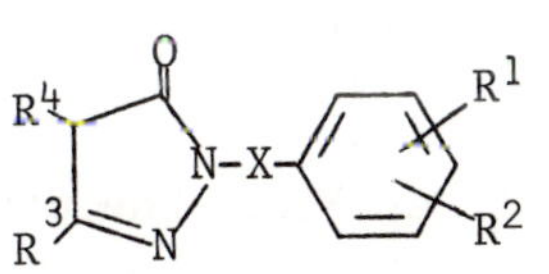

1

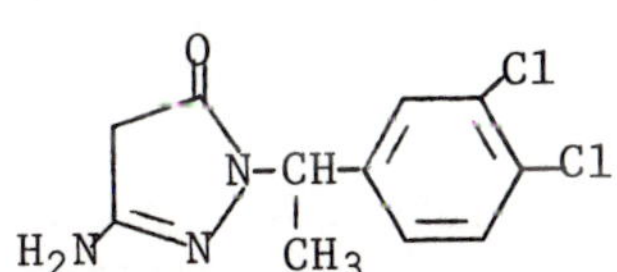

2

selection of 2 (Muzolimine, BAY g 2821) for detailed pharmacological and clinical study.[13,14] Compound 2 is amphoteric, forming soluble salts in acids and bases, and it is more lipophilic than furosemide. The tautomeric form and conformation of 2 were determined by X-ray analysis and quantum-chemical M.O. calculations. Electron density distribution was estimated with the aid of CNDO/2 calculations.[15] In dogs, 2 combines a high ceiling salidiuretic effect similar to furosemide with a somewhat longer duration of action. It was more potent than furosemide; p.o. doses of 0.1 to 3 mg/kg induced a linear increase in saliuresis, while glomular filtration rate (GFR) was unchanged and p-aminohippurate (PAH) clearance was increased.[16] The Na^+/K^+ ratio was somewhat higher than that of furosemide. In rats, 2 was less effective than furosemide, whereas, the duration of action was longer. Compound 2 reduced blood pressure in renal hypertensive dogs and in renal hypertensive and SH rats.[17] The drug appeared to work via inhibition of tubular reabsorption and not by increased filtration. Similar to furosemide, 2 inhibited sodium transport at the medullary portion of the ascending limb of Henle's loop;[18] however, unlike furosemide it acted only from the peritubular side. Apparently, 2 does not work by inhibition of renal Na^+-K^+-ATPase.[19] Studies using isolated frog skins showed that, on the serosal side, 2 increases the Na^+ permeability of the serosal membrane and decreases the active Na^+ transport capacity at the mucosal cell membrane.[20] In normal volunteers, the threshold dose of 2

ISBN 0-12-040513-X

was 10 mg p.o. and responses to doses up to 80 mg were log-linear. Excretion of Na^+ and Cl^- were as high with 30 mg of 2 as seen with 40 mg of furosemide; K^+ excretion was considerably lower.[21] Compound 2 was effective in chronic heart failure patients[22,23] and in those with varying degrees of renal insufficiency.[23-25] The primary site of action appeared to be the thick ascending limb of Henle's loop with possibly some proximal action.[22,26] Single p.o. doses of 40 mg of 2 produced little change in plasma renin, angiotensin II and aldosterone levels; Na^+ levels did not change but a marked decrease in K^+ levels occurred.[27] In patients with hepatogenic ascites, a combination of 2 with spironolactone was more effective than furosemide with spironolactone.[28]

Ticrynafen (3) - Numerous clinical studies[29-35] with 3 revealed its unique characteristics. Doses of 250 to 500 mg produced natriuresis and kaliuresis comparable to 50 mg hydrochlorothiazide. However, in contradistinction to hydrochlorothiazide, 3 induced a plasma urate decrease and bicarbonate increase. Although the drug bears a structural similarity to ethacrynic acid, it appears to act at a different site in the nephron. Instead of inhibiting Na^+ and Cl^- reabsorption in the thick ascending limb of the loop of Henle, it apparently acts primarily within the cortical distal nephron with some action in the proximal nephron.[31,37]

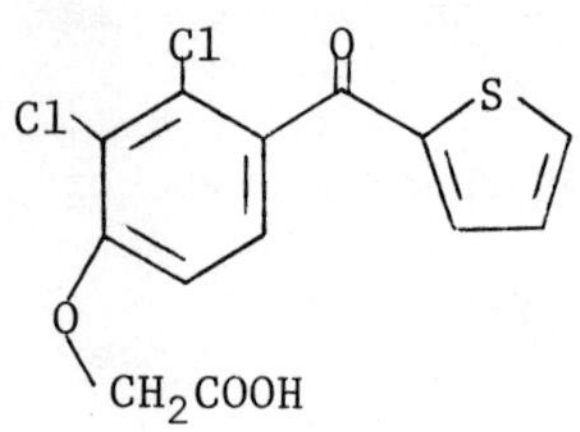

3

Compound 3 also exhibited a significant kaliuretic effect. The drug markedly affected either the reabsorptive or the secretory flux of urate in the proximal tubule; profound uricosuria was produced. This effect is independent of any proximal natriuretic effect of the agent.[31,36,38] Studies in hypertensive patients over periods up to six weeks showed that single daily doses of 250 mg of 3 were less antihypertensive than 50 mg of hydrochlorothiazide. However, when this dose was given twice daily, the antihypertensive effects of the two drugs were similar except that the onset of action of 3 was later than that of hydrochlorothiazide.[39-41]

It is interesting to note that some analogs of 3 wherein the 2-thienyl moiety is replaced by an aryl group have been reported recently. Biological data on the p-fluorophenyl analog in animals closely paralleled that of 3.[42]

Indanones - The S/A relationships of the indanyloxyacetic acid diuretics have been further elucidated.[43,44] MK-196 (4) exhibits potent salidiuretic effects in rats, dogs and chimpanzees[43 45] and is uricosuric in chimpanzees[45-47] and rats.[48] It is antihypertensive in SH rats and in renal hypertensive African green monkeys.[45] Micropuncture studies in rats indicated that the drug acts primarily in the loop of Henle and collecting duct.[49,50] Single and multiple p.o. doses (14 days) of 10 and 20 mg of 4 were compared with

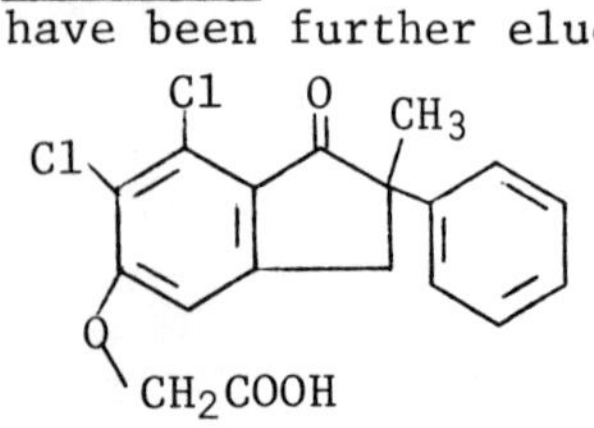

4

40 mg of furosemide in normal volunteers.[51–53] The 10 mg dose of 4 produced slightly less salidiuresis and the 20 mg dose more than 40 mg of furosemide over a 24 hr. period. Neither dose of 4 caused any increase in plasma urate levels, while furosemide caused urate retention. The high dose of 4 produced a temporary uricosuria. In mildly hypertensive patients, a 10 mg or 15 mg p.o. daily dose of 4 for one month produced a hypotensive effect as great or greater than that of 50 mg of hydrochlorothiazide.[54]

Quincarbate (5) - A novel class of 1,4-dioxino[2,3-g]quinolines was discovered and shown to possess potent salidiuretic properties.[55] Detailed S/A studies revealed 5 to be the most active member of the series.[56,57] In the Lipschitz rat assay, the p.o. salidiuretic potency of 5 was much greater than that of furosemide or hydrochlorothiazide. The Na^+/K^+ ratio and high ceiling effects of 5 were similar to furosemide, but the dose-response curve was flatter. 5 was highly effective in dogs and man, weakly effective in rhesus monkeys and inactive in mice and hamsters. The site of action is unknown; mechanisms involving carbonic anhydrase inhibition and aldosterone antagonism have been excluded. Preliminary clinical data indicate p.o. doses as low as 5 mg are effective.[56,57]

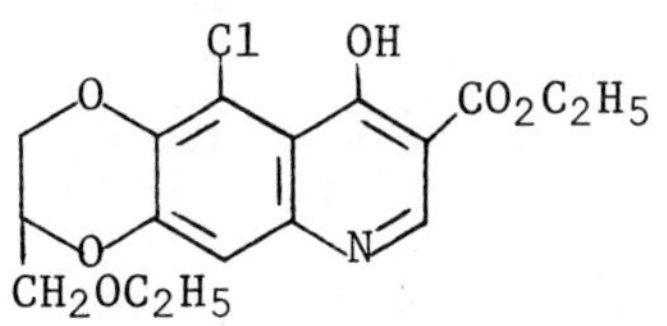

5

Sulfonamide Diuretics - This class continues to be the most widely used of all the diuretics; therefore, the medicinal chemical investigation of this chemical type has continued. The S/A relationships developed by Feit and Nielson in the 3-sulfamoylbenzoic acid series (6) have been both extensive and provocative. After studying the structural requirements of R and R^1

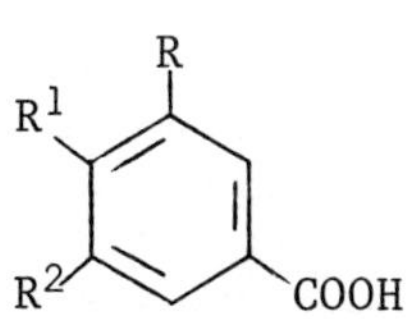

6

R	R^1	R^2	6
$n\text{-}C_4H_9NH$-	C_6H_5O-	H_2NO_2S-	a
$C_6H_5CH_2NH$-	C_6H_5O-	CH_3O_2S-	b
$C_6H_5CH_2NH$-	C_6H_5CO-	CH_3O_2S-	c
$C_6H_5CH_2O$-	C_6H_5CO-	HCONH	d
$(CH_2)_4N$-	C_6H_5O-	H_2NO_2S-	e

which led to the highly potent loop diuretic bumetanide (6a), their current work has focused on R^2. Compounds in which R^2 is mesyl[58] (such as 6b and 6c) or even formamido[59] (6d) are about 1/10 as potent as 6a in standard dog assays. More recently, this study has been extended to include replacements for carboxy, including alkoxymethyl, alkylthiomethyl, aminomethyl and substituted-aminomethyl. Some of these compounds were equipotent with 6a.[60]

Merkel and co-workers have found an analog of 6 (6e, piretanide) that is more potent in rats than 6a. The dose-related effects of 6e, furosemide and 6a on urine and electrolyte were similar; however, the slope of the dose-response excretion pattern of 6 was flatter than those of furosemide and 6a.[61]

Compound 7 (tizolemide, HOE 740) represents an outstanding example of a series of basic sulfonamide diuretics. P.O. studies in rats at 50 mg/kg showed tizolemide to have salidiuretic effects superior to those of hydrochlorothiazide and chlorthalidone and to have the long duration of action characteristic of chlorthalidone.[62,63]

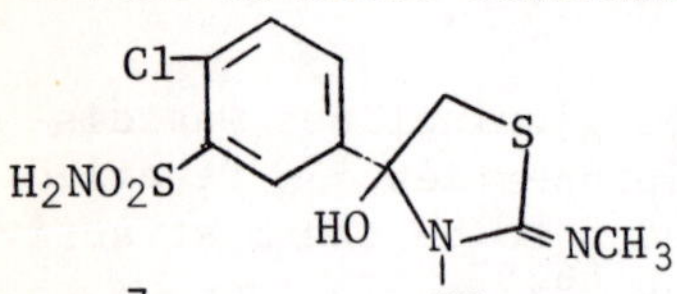

7

A report on the pharmacology of indapamide (8) indicates that it has a salidiuretic potency in normal, acidotic, alkalotic and SH rats equal to trichlormethiazide.[64] Clinical studies have confirmed the antihypertensive activity of this drug.[65,66]

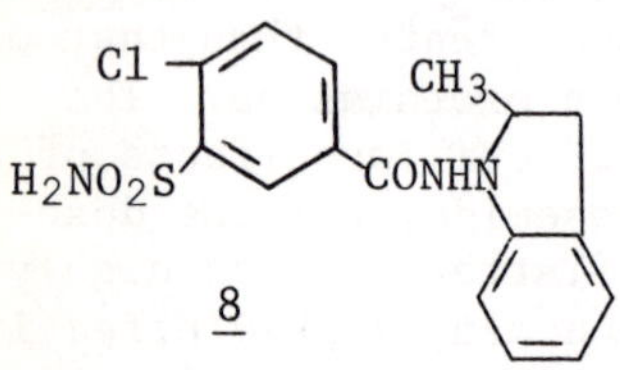

8

Salicylamines - This novel class of diuretics has been disclosed[67,68] and an extensive study of the structural requirements for salidiuretic activity reported.[69] MK-447 (9) was selected for intensive pharmacological evaluation. It was more effective than furosemide in producing saluresis and diuresis in rats, dogs and chimpanzees. In subdiuretic doses, 9 was antihypertensive in SH rats. The antihypertensive effect was reduced by indomethacin which suggests that it is prostaglandin-mediated. Compound 9 was antihypertensive in diuretic doses in renal hypertensive dogs.[70] The drug stimulated the biosynthesis of PGE_2 from arachidonate in ram seminal vesicular microsomes, in intact mouse ovaries and in rat kidney slices. The antiinflammatory properties of 9 were demonstrated by its effect in reducing carrageenan-induced foot edema in rats and the croton oil-induced swelling in mouse ears. Depression of PGG_2 levels was suggested as contributing to the antiinflammatory effect of 9.[71,72] A study in human volunteers at 6.25, 25 and 100 mg p.o. revealed a dose-related diuresis and saliuresis with minimal kaliuresis indicating that 9 is a potent high ceiling diuretic.[73]

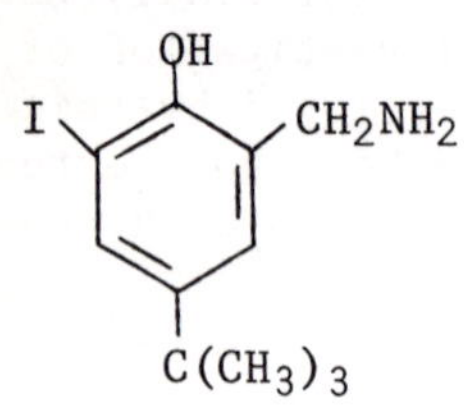

9

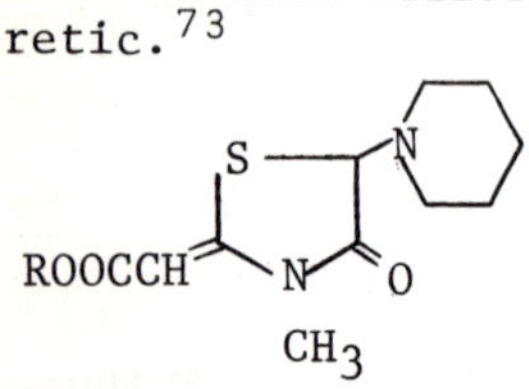

No.	R
10	C_2H_5
11	H

Etozolin (10) was reported a number of years ago;[74] however, only recently has a disclosure of the salidiuretic and choleretic S/A relationships of the chemical series appeared. In addition, its pharmacology, site of action, toxicity and metabolism in laboratory animals and man have been published.[75]

The corresponding carboxylic acid (11,

etozolinic acid), which is a major metabolite of 10, is reported to be somewhat more active and less toxic than 10.[76]

Prostaglandins (PGs) - A comprehensive review[77] examining the actions postulated for the major renal prostaglandins (PGE_2, $PGF_{2\alpha}$, PGD_2 and PGA_2) in the regulation of blood pressure, renal blood flow (RBF) and renal sodium and water excretion was published in mid-1976. This brief review focuses on the highlights gleaned from recent investigations of the intrarenal transport, the sites and modes of metabolism and the pharmacological and physiological functions of renal PGs. Their interrelationships with other regulators of kidney function including diuretic agents are also considered.

Demonstration that endogenous renomedullary PGs most likely enter the tubular fluid at a site in the loop of Henle has been achieved by Oates and colleagues[78] using the stop-flow technique in anesthetized dogs. Neither the influx mechanism nor a determination as to whether PG influx and efflux occur at the same loop site could be made from the experimental data. However, the latter served to substantiate the proposed intrarenal origin of urinary PGs.[79] Furthermore, the identified PG entry site provided support for the hypothesis[79] that PGs elaborated in the medulla, the renal site of maximal PG synthetic capacity,[80] can enter the lumen. They are subsequently transported via the tubular fluid to possible sites of action in the cortex, the renal tissue richest in degradative enzymes[80] but limited in ability to form PGs.[80,81] Whether PGs in tubular fluid influence kidney function remains to be established.

Recent studies[82] on 9-keto PG reductase (9-KPGR) preparations isolated from rabbit and human kidneys have shown that the loop diuretics, ethacrynic acid and furosemide, and the potent PG synthetase inhibitor, indomethacin, inhibit 9-KPGR. At drug concentrations of $5x10^{-4}M$, ethacyrnic acid, indomethacin and furosemide reduced rabbit renal 9-KPGR activity by 79%, 76% and 30%, respectively. Human renocortical 9-KPGR, although found to be less sensitive to inhibition than the rabbit enzyme, was inhibited similarly by ethacrynic acid, indomethacin and furosemide. In both species, ethacrynic acid was markedly more inhibitory than furosemide; interestingly, thiazide diuretics were without significant effect. These observations, coupled with the known ability of ethacrynic acid and furosemide to inhibit 15-hydroxy-PG dehydrogenase (15-HPGDH),[83] the major renocortical deactivating enzyme, led Stone and Hart[82] to suggest that blockade of 9-KPGR and 15-HPGDH may contribute to the therapeutic effects elicited by ethacrynic acid and furosemide in man since modulation of the PGE_2 to $PGF_{2\alpha}$ ratio is thought to exert an important influence on renal function.[84]

Weber et al[85] recently obtained the first definitive evidence that renal 9-KPGR is under the control of NaCl intake by examining the effects of low and high sodium diets on urinary sodium ($U_{Na}V$), urine volume (UV), PGE_2 and $PGF_{2\alpha}$ excretion, plasma renin activity (PRA) and renal 9-KPGR activity in cross-bred rabbits. At high NaCl (2.5 g/100 g diet) intake, $U_{Na}V$ was nine times but UV, only twice, that at low NaCl (0.25 g/100 g diet) intake. PRA decreased from 12.9 to 1.8 $ngml^{-1}h^{-1}$ in going from the low to high NaCl diet. At low NaCl intake, daily urinary excretions of PGE_2 and $PGF_{2\alpha}$ were 1.9 and 2.1 μg, respectively, giving a 1:1.1 ratio of PGE_2 to $PGF_{2\alpha}$; 9-KPGR activity was found to be 0.61 ± 0.07 and 0.1 ± 0.01 nM $PGF_{2\alpha}$ formed $min^{-1}mg^{-1}$ in the cortex and medulla, respectively. At high NaCl intake, 9-KPGR activity increased three-fold in the cortex and two-fold in the medulla; daily urinary excretion of PGE_2 decreased to 0.53 μg, whereas, that of $PGF_{2\alpha}$ (2.43 μg) remained essentially unchanged, giving a 1:4.6 ratio of PGE_2 to $PGF_{2\alpha}$. Based on these results, Weber and co-workers proposed the intriguing concept that renal 9-KPGR is intimately involved in adjusting the activity of the renin-angiotensin system and distal nephron function in response to NaCl ingestion and, accordingly, may play a pivotal role in the regulation of NaCl and water balance. Indeed, such a mechanism may be operative in man, particularly in disease states such as Bartter's syndrome in which changes in the PGE_2 to $PGF_{2\alpha}$ ratio have been observed[86] to accompany variations in sodium and volume homeostasis.

A recent comparative investigation[87] of the renal responses to intrarenal infusions of PGE_2 (0.4 μg $Kg^{-1}min^{-1}$) and PGD_2 (0.4-0.8 μg $Kg^{-1}min^{-1}$) in the anesthetized dog revealed that, whereas, both PGs produced substantial and comparable increases in total RBF and renal venous PRA, only PGE_2 caused a marked diuresis and natriuresis. Further, GFR was not affected by PGE_2 but was reduced significantly by PGD_2 except when the latter was administered at a lower dose (0.04 μg $Kg^{-1}min^{-1}$). The failure of PGD_2 to alter electrolyte and fluid excretion rates concomitantly with the observed, induced renal vasodilation is counter to the results reported in a recent abstract.[89] Furthermore, this behavior is rather surprising since most renal vasodilators, with the exception of secretin,[88] produce a salidiuresis which accompanies elevation of RBF.[90,91] Nonetheless, Bolger et al[87] conclude that PGD_2 of intrarenal origin is likely to be involved primarily in the control of kidney hemodynamics and not in fluid and electrolyte regulation.

While investigating the unilateral ureteral-obstructed rabbit model of hydronephrosis, Needleman and colleagues[92] succeeded in unmasking the presence of TXA_2 synthetase and its potent constrictile product, thromboxane A_2 (TXA_2), in the ureteral-obstructed kidney but not in the contralateral normal kidney. This discovery marks the entry of TXA_2 into the realm of renal PGs. Both arachidonic acid (AA) and the endoperoxide PGH_2 were readily metabolized to TXA_2 by microsomal fractions of homogenates derived from the hydronephrotic kidney. Employing [^{14}C]-AA in this preparation, the percentages of radioactivity converted to PGE_2, $PGF_{2\alpha}$, PGD_2 and TXA_2 (measured as TXB_2) were 15%, 10%, 5% and 2.5-3%, respectively. These workers believe that the potential role of TXA_2 in ureteral obstruction, if TXA_2 is produced in other species, may be in altering regional blood flow to non-functioning kidney locales or in decreasing total RBF to a non-functioning kidney in a pathological situation.

The effect of decreased release of endogenous renal PGs on $U_{Na}V$ has been examined by Kirschenbaum and Stein[93] in conscious dogs undergoing a water diuresis. Intravenous administration of either of two PG synthetase inhibitors, meclofenamate (2 mg Kg^{-1}) and RO 20-5720 (1 mg Kg^{-1}), failed to alter GFR, UV, U_KV, mean arterial pressure or renal plasma flow but elicited a four-fold increase in $U_{Na}V$ resulting primarily from a rise in U_{Na}. These data suggest that inhibition of intrarenal PG synthesis in the conscious dog is associated with a natriuresis without a change in UV or U_KV during water diuresis and, therefore, may indicate that the observed $U_{Na}V$ increase resulted from diminished sodium reabsorption at a site(s) beyond the distal tubule. These investigators were tempted to suggest that a decrease in local PGE release is associated with a commensurate diminution in collecting-duct sodium reabsorption. The tenability of this suggestion is suspect in view of recent studies by Stokes and Kokko[94] in rabbits and Ganguli et al[95] in rats which strongly suggest that endogenous PGE_2 inhibits sodium reabsorption in the collecting tubule.

In conclusion, although notable strides have been achieved in this challenging area of research since the initial discovery of medullin, the full consequences of renal PG involvement in kidney function are yet to be fully delineated and understood.

References

1. P. Y. D. Wong, Pharm. J., 215, 433 (1975).
2. W. Rupp, Arzneim.-Forsch., 27 (1), 289 (1977).
3. A. Lant, Practitioner, 219, 519 (1977).
4. Symposium on the Pharmacology of Diuretics, J. Clin. Pharmacol., 17, 618-680 (10 part 2), (1977).
5. D. G. Vidt, Postgrad. Med., 59 (5), 143 (1976).
6. R. H. Maffly, J. Am. Med. Assoc., 235, 2526 (1976).
7. R. W. Gifford, Jr., J. Am. Med. Assoc., 235, 1890 (1976).
8. W. Modell in Drugs of Choice, 1976-1977, W. Modell, Ed., C. V. Mosby Co., St. Louis, Mo., 1976, p. 92.
9. A. B. Schwartz, Nephrology for the Practicing Physician, Grune & Stratton, New York, N.Y., 1975.
10. E. Möller, K. Meng, E. Wehinger and H. Horstmann, U.D. Patents 3,949,083, April 6, 1976; 3,952,008, April 20, 1976; 3,957,814, May 18, 1977; 3,978,077, August 31, 1976; 4,002,641, January 11, 1977; 4,032,646, June 28, 1977.
11. J. Castañer, Drugs of the Future, 2, 387 (1977).
12. H. Horstmann, E. Moller, E. Wehinger and K. Meng, Abstr. Pap., Am. Chem. Soc., 174th Meet. MEDI 19 (1977).
13. Brit. Pharmacop. Comm. Appr. Names (Suppl. 7) 2 (1977).
14. E. Möller, H. Horstmann, K. Meng and D. Loew, Experientia, 33, 382 (1977).
15. E. Möller, H. Horstmann and K. Meng, Pharmatherapeutica, 1, 540 (1977).
16. D. Loew and K. Meng, Naunyn-Schmedeberg's Arch. Pharmacol., 297 (Suppl. 2), R38 (1977).
17. K. Meng, D. Loew, K. Stoepel and F. Hoffmeister, Curr. Med. Res. Opin., 4, 555 (1977).
18. D. Loew and K. Meng, Pharmatherapeutica, 1, 333 (1977).

19. H. J. Kramer, Pharmatherapeutica, 1, 353 (1977).
20. A. Dorge, R. Rick and E. V. Arnim, Pharmatherapeutica, 1, 341 (1977).
21. D. Lowe, Curr. Med. Res. Opin., 4, 455 (1977).
22. K. J. Berg, S. Jorstad and A. Tromsdal, Pharmatherapeutica, 1, 319 (1977).
23. P. Fauchald and E. Lind, Pharmatherapeutica, 1, 409 (1977).
24. G. Hoppeseyler, A. Heissler, M. Coppencastrop, M. Schindler, P. Schollmeyer and W. Ritter, Pharmatherapeutica, 1, 422 (1977).
25. A. Röckel, Curr. Med. Res. Opin., 4, 574 (1977).
26. M. Mussche and N. Lameire, Curr. Med. Res. Opin., 4, 462 (1977).
27. E. Schnurr, H. Kuppers, K. Wiesen and B. Grabensee, Pharmatherapeutica, 1, 415 (1977).
28. F. Heinrich, D. Loew and J. Dycka, Curr. Med. Res. Opin., 4, 706 (1977).
29. G. Lemieux, A. Kiss, A. Gougoux and P. Vinay, J. Clin. Chem. Clin. Biochem., 14, 306 (1976).
30. K. Lau, R. M. Stote, M. Goldberg and Z. S. Agus, Clin. Sci. Mol. Med., 53, 379 (1977).
31. T. H. Steele, D. R. Prasad and O. G. Reese, Wis. Med. J., 76, S54 (1977).
32. A. K. Jain, F. G. McMahon, R. Vargas and J. R. Ryan, Clin. Pharmacol. Ther., 21, 107 (1977).
33. P. Bessin, J. Bonnet, M. F. Malin, Abstr. Pap., Am. Chem. Soc., 174th Meet. MEDI 5 (1977).
34. A. R. Maass, R. M. Stote, I. B. Snow, R. Erickson, Abstr. Pap., Am. Chem. Soc., 174th Meet. MEDI 6 (1977).
35. O. G. Reese, Jr. and T. H. Steele, Am. J. Med., 60, 973 (1976).
36. D. R. Prasad, I. M. Weiner and T. H. Steele, J. Pharmacol. Exp. Ther., 200, 58 (1977).
37. K. Lau, R. Stote, M. Goldberg and Z. S. Agus, Clin. Res., 24, 405A (1976).
38. G. Lemieux, A. Kiss, P. Vinay and A. Gougoux, Kidney Int., 12, 104 (1977).
39. M. Nemati, M. C. Kyle, E. D. Freis, J. Amer. Med. Assoc., 237, 652 (1977).
40. A. Gillies, G. Morgan and T. Morgan, Aust. N. Z. Med. Med., 7, 443 (1977).
41. R. Vargas, A. Jain, J. Ryan, F. G. McMahon, Clin. Pharmacol. Ther., 21, 119 (1977).
42. P. H. Jones, D. S. Bariana, A. K. L. Fung, Y. C. Martin, J. Kynel and A. Lall, Ger. Offen. 2,642,879, April 7, 1977.
43. O. W. Woltersdorf, Jr., S. J. deSolms, E. M. Schultz and E. J. Cragoe, Jr., J. Med. Chem., 20, 1400 (1977).
44. S. J. deSolms, O. W. Woltersdorf, Jr., E. J. Cragoe, Jr., L. S. Watson and G. M. Fanelli, Jr., J. Med. Chem., 21, in press (1978).
45. L. S. Watson, G. M. Fanelli, H. F. Russo, C. S. Sweet, C. T. Ludden and A. Scriabine, in New Antihypertensive Drugs, A. Scriabine and C. S. Sweet, Eds., Spectrum Publications, Inc., Holliswood, N. Y., 1976, p. 307.
46. G. M. Fanelli, Jr., D. L. Bohn, A. Scriabine and K. H. Beyer, Jr., J. Pharmacol. Exp. Ther., 200, 402 (1977).

47. G. M. Fanelli, Jr., D. L. Bohn and A. G. Zacchei, J. Pharmacol. Exp. Ther., 200, 413 (1977).
48. R. McKenzie, T. Knight and E. J. Weinman, Proc. Soc. Exp. Biol. Med., 153, 202 (1976).
49. M. L. Kauker, Fed. Proc., 35, 224 (1976).
50. M. L. Kauker, J. Pharmacol. Exp. Ther., 200, 81 (1977).
51. B. T. Emmerson, L. Thompson and K. Mitchell, J. Clin. Chem. Biochem., 14, 286 (1976).
52. K. F. Tempero, G. Hitzenberger, Z. E. Dziewanowska, H. Halkin and G. H. Besselaar, Clin. Pharmacol. Ther., 19, 116 (1976).
53. Z. E. Dziewanowska, K. F. Tempero, F. Perret, G. Hitzenberger and G. H. Besselaar, Clin. Res., 24, 253A (1976).
54. K. F. Tempero, J. A. Vedin, C. E. Wilhelmsson, P. Lund-Johansen, C. Vorburger, C. Moerlin, H. Aaberg, W. Enenkel, J. Bolognese and Z. E. Dziewanowska, Clin. Pharmacol. Ther., 21, 119 (1977).
55. T. A. C. Boschman and J. G. Korsloot, U.S. Patent 3,865,832, February, 1975.
56. J. van Dijk and J. Hartog and T. A. C. Boschman, J. Med. Chem., 19, 982 (1976).
57. T. A. C. Borschman, J. van Dijk and J. Hartog, 5th Intern. Symp. Med. Chem., Paris, July (1976).
58. P. W. Feit and O. B. T. Nielson, J. Med. Chem., 19, 402 (1976).
59. P. W. Feit and O. B. T. Nielson, J. Med. Chem., 20, 1687 (1977).
60. P. W. Feit and O. B. T. Nielson, Abstr. Pap., Am. Chem. Soc. 174th Meet. MEDI 2 (1977).
61. W. Merkel, D. Bormann, D. Mania, R. Muschaweck and M. Hropot, Eur. J. Med. Chem., 11, 399 (1976).
62. H-J. Lang, B. Knabe and R. Muschaweck, Abstr. Pap., Am. Chem. Soc. 174th Meet. MEDI 3 (1977).
63. Hoechst A.G. Belg. Pat. 850,451, January, 1976.
64. Y. Suzuki, Y. Hamaguchi and I. Yamagami, Nippon Yakurigaku Zasshi, 73, 321 (1977).
65. G. Gragnoli, F. Puccetti, R. Nami, I. Tanganelli, F. Favilli and E. Betti, Minerva Med., 68, 749 (1977).
66. P. Turner, G. N. Volans and H. J. Rogers, Curr. Med. Res. Opin., 4, 596 (1977).
67. E. J. Cragoe, Jr. and E. M. Schultz, U.S. Patents 3,794,734, February, 1974; 3,928,624, December, 1975 and 4,029,816, June, 1977.
68. E. M. Schultz and E. J. Cragoe, Jr., U.S. Patents 3,809,721, May, 1974; 3,864,401, February, 1975; 3,979,361, September, 1976 and 4,044,153, August, 1977.
69. R. L. Smith, G. E. Stokker and E. J. Cragoe, Jr., Abstr. Pap., Am. Chem. Soc. 174th Meet. MEDI 7 (1977).
70. A. Scriabine, L. S. Watson, H. R. Russo, C. T. Ludden, C. S. Sweet, G. M. Fanelli, Jr., N. Bohidar and C. A. Stone, Fed. Proc., 37, 921 (1978).
71. F. A. Kuehl, Jr., J. L. Humes, R. W. Egan, E. A. Ham, G. C. Beveridge and C. G. Van Arman, Nature, 265, 170 (1977).
72. F. A. Kuehl, Jr., R. W. Egan, J. L. Humes, G. C. Beveridge and G. C. Van Arman, New Biochemical Aspects of Prostaglandins and Thromboxans, Academic Press, N. Y., (1978).

73. M. B. Affrime, D. T. Lowenthal, G. Onesti, P. Busby, C. Swartz and B. Lei, Clin. Pharmacol. Ther., 21, 97 (1977).
74. G. Satzinger, Justus Liebig's Ann. Chem., 665, 150 (1963).
75. Elkapin[R] (Etozolin, GO 687), Arzneim.-Forsch., 27 (II), 1741 (1977).
76. G. Satzinger, M. Herrmann and K-O. Vollmer, U.S. Patent 3,971,794, July, 1976.
77. R. J. Anderson, T. Berl, K. M. McDonald and R. W. Schrier, Kidney Int., 10, 205 (1976).
78. W. M. Williams, J. C. Frölich, A. S. Nies and J. A. Oates, ibid, 11, 256 (1977).
79. J. C. Frölich, T. W. Wilson, B. J. Sweetman, M. Smigel, A. S. Nies, K. Carr, J. T. Watson and J. A. Oates, J. Clin. Invest., 55, 763 (1975).
80. K. Crowshaw and J. Z. Szlyk, Biochem. J., 116, 421 (1970).
81. C. Larsson and E. Änggard, Eur. J. Pharmacol., 21, 30 (1973).
82. K. J. Stone and M. Hart, Prostaglandins, 12, 197 (1976).
83. R. V. Patak, B. K. Mookerjee, C. J. Bentzel, P. E. Hysert, M. Babej and J. B. Lee, ibid, 10, 649 (1975).
84. K. U. Malik and J. C. McGiff, Circ. Res., 36, 599 (1975).
85. P. C. Weber, C. Larsson and B. Scherer, Nature, 266, 65 (1977).
86. J. R. Gill, J. C. Frölich, R. E. Bowden, A. A. Taylor, H. R. Keiser, H. W. Seyberth, J. A. Oates and F. C. Bartter, Am. J. Med., 61, 43 (1976).
87. P. M. Bolger, G. M. Eisner, P. T. Shea, P. W. Ramwell and L. M. Slotkoff, Nature, 267, 628 (1977).
88. G. R. Marchand, K. A. Hubel and H. E. Williamson, Proc. Soc. Exp. Biol. Med., 139, 1356 (1972).
89. O. Oelz, B. J. Sweetman, J. A. Oates, A. S. Nies and J. L. Data, Pharmacologist, 18, 163 (1976).
90. P. G. Baer and L. G. Navar, Kidney Int., 4, 12 (1973).
91. T. M. Daugharty, L. J. Belleau, J. A. Martino and L. E. Earley, Am. J. Physiol., 215, 1442 (1968).
92. A. R. Morrison, K. Nishikawa and P. Needleman, Nature, 267, 259 (1977).
93. M. A. Kirschenbaum and J. H. Stein, J. Clin. Invest., 57, 517 (1976).
94. J. B. Stokes and J. P. Kokko, ibid, 59, 1099 (1977).
95. M. Ganguli, L. Tobian, S. Azar and M. O'Donnell, Circ. Res., 40, I-135 (1977).

Chapter 8. Antihypertensive Agents

W. Lesley Matier and William T. Comer, Mead Johnson & Company
Evansville, Indiana

Introduction - This review covers advances in the understanding and drug treatment of hypertension during the past year. Diuretics remain the most widely used class of antihypertensives, and the first agent selected for mild hypertensives is usually a diuretic; these agents are discussed in Chapter 7. A new mechanistic approach to treating hypertension with angiotensin converting enzyme inhibitors is covered separately in Chapter 9. The structures of drugs discussed in this chapter are shown or may be found in recent volumes of "Annual Reports in Medicinal Chemistry."

General - The clinical pharmacology[1] of antihypertensive drugs, their use in hypertensive emergencies,[2] and in rational combinations,[3] have been reviewed. In the U.S.A., the Joint National Committee on Detection, Evaluation and Treatment of High Blood Pressure recommends a stepwise approach to treating hypertension starting with a diuretic.[4] The causes of hemodynamic changes in essential hypertension and their normalization by drug treatment was the topic of a symposium,[5] as was the important role of the sympathetic nervous system in the etiology and maintenance of hypertension.[6] As with renin levels, subgroups of patients with elevated plasma catecholamine levels have now been identified.[7] The vascular damage associated with hypertension may be due to increased synthesis and deposition of collagen in arteries resulting in fibrosis.[8] Vascular damage in hypertensives may also be related to blood velocity;[9] propranolol and clonidine decrease blood velocity and may therefore be preferred over methyldopa and hydralazine which increase blood velocity.

Centrally Acting Antihypertensives - The centrally acting drugs, α-methyldopa and clonidine, continue to be widely used. The action of methyldopa or clonidine is not dependent on patients' renin states although these drugs do lower renin levels.[10,11] A decarboxylase inhibitor failed to block methyldopa's hypotensive action,[12] and its active metabolite, α-methylnorepinephrine, was found more potent than norepinephrine in impairing sympathetic transmission by presynaptic α-receptor stimulation.[13] Methyldopa,[14] but not clonidine,[15] allowed stable blood pressure control when given once daily in high dose.

Clonidine causes physiological changes in patients similar to propranolol, but by an entirely different mechanism. It has been used in place of a β-blocker[16] and in combination with the vasodilator minoxidil.[17] Clonidine has been reported to induce diuresis in hypertensive patients being treated with minoxidil and propranolol.[17]

Studies on the action of clonidine in cats support inhibition of

ISBN 0-12-040513-X

central sympathetic outflow as its major hypotensive mechanism.[18] Similarly, in tetraplegic patients with cervical spinal cord transection, clonidine did not lower blood pressure, indicating that in man, as in animals, intact bulbospinal pathways are needed.[19] Stimulation of peripheral presynaptic α-receptors may contribute to the reduction of catecholamines and blood pressure caused by clonidine,[20] whereas stimulation of postsynaptic α-receptors may account for decreased hypotensive actions of clonidine at higher doses in cats[18] and patients.[21] It has been proposed that these presynaptic α-receptors be classified as α_2 based on the response to various α-agonists. Alpha receptors in the brain mediating hypotensive effects, in the kidney mediating renin release and receptors inhibitory to melanocyte-stimulating hormone, also appear to be α_2; postsynaptic vascular α-receptors, involved in vasoconstrictor responses, are α_1.[22]

The involvement of central histamine receptors in the hypotensive action of clonidine remains uncertain. The action of this drug is antagonized by *i.c.v.* administered metiamide, a specific histamine H_2-antagonist, but the selective histamine H_2-stimulant, dimaprit (4-methylhistamine), raises blood pressure.[23] A histamine metabolite, imidazole acetic acid, exerts a strong, central, hypotensive action antagonized by metiamide and may possibly be an inhibitory neurotransmitter.[24]

Sedation and dry mouth remain the most bothersome side effects associated with clonidine therapy, whereas rebound hypertension is potentially the most dangerous. Reports of hypertensive crises associated with withdrawal of this drug continue to appear.[25,26] The hypertensive response appears to be due to a sudden reversal of the central inhibitory action of clonidine resulting in increased plasma norepinephrine levels.[27] Sedation[28] and paradoxical sleep[29] appear to be mediated by central α_2-receptors and not by histamine H_2-receptors,[30] so separation of sedation from clonidine's antihypertensive effects may not be possible. Both clonidine and methyldopa inhibit conditioned salivation in conscious dogs which is a useful animal model that correlates with the effect in man.[31]

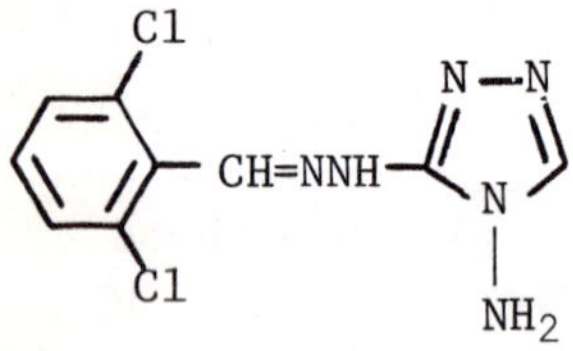

1

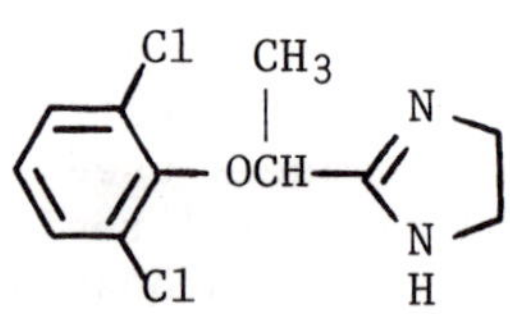

2 lofexidine

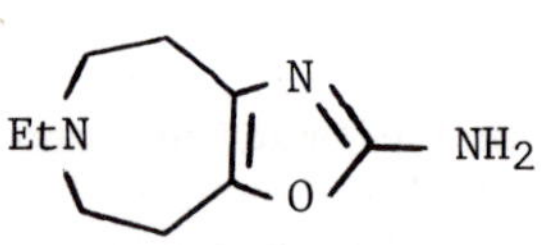

3

Several groups have reported QSAR studies of aromatic substituted analogs of clonidine.[32,33] Clonidine-like agents continue to be investigated clinically. Flutonidine,[34] guanabenz,[35] and guanfacine[36] (BS 100-141) are clinically effective agents but are not free of clonidine-type side effects. Tiamenidine, presently in clinical trials in Europe and the U.S., is reported to not cause spontaneous rebound hypertension.[37] Guanabenz[38] and the structurally similar FLA-136[39] (1) reduce norepinephrine turnover in the rat brain. The latter appears to selectively stimulate presynaptic α-receptors without affecting central or peripheral postsynaptic receptors.[40] Lofexidine (2) is a new centrally acting antihypertensive in animals and man.[41] Rebound hypertension may not be a problem with this drug since urinary catecholamine excretion changed very little after its withdrawal. B-HT933 (3) is an interesting new structure showing typical clonidine-like effects in animals.[42] It has been suggested that the centrally acting antihypertensive agent, R28935, inhibits central noradrenergic neurotransmission by blocking central postsynaptic α-receptors in contrast to the stimulation of presynaptic α-receptors by clonidine and related drugs.[39]

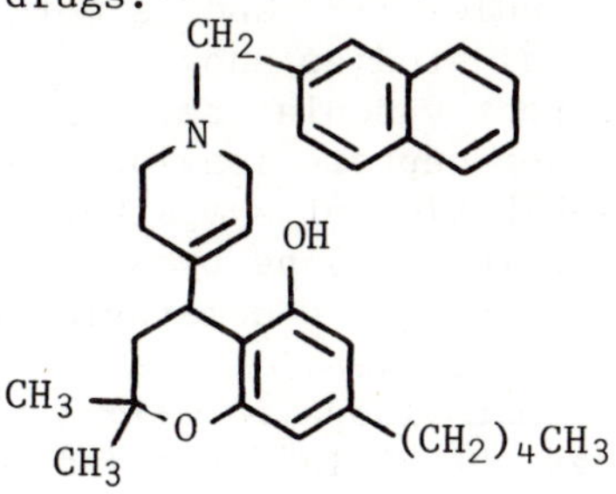

4

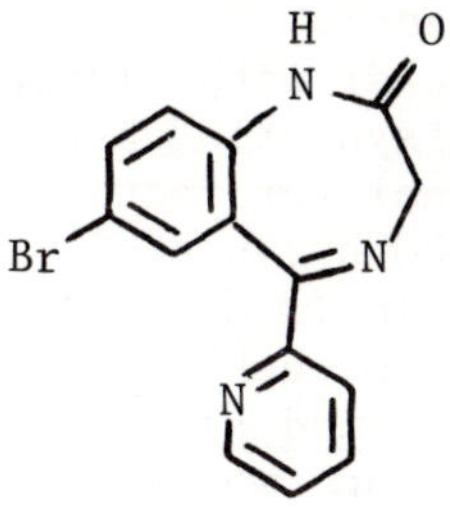

5 bromazepam

The hypotensive and bradycardic effects of Δ^9-tetrahydrocannabinol, a psychoactive constituent of marihuana, is at least partly mediated via activation of central α-receptors.[43] BRL-13776 (4), resulting from structural modification of tetrahydrocannabinols, is antihypertensive in animals, probably as a consequence of central catecholamine depletion.[44] The new benzodiazepine antianxiety agent, bromazepam (5), lowered the blood pressure of a large group of hypertensives without affecting heart rate.[45]

Antihypertensive Vasodilators - The clinical use of hydralazine has been reviewed.[46] It is a valuable drug when combined with β-blockers and diuretics. Its cardiac stimulating actions may be due to direct effect on the myocardium in addition to reflex activation of cardiac sympathetic nerves secondary to a decrease in blood pressure.[47] Alpha blockade enhances hydralazine's hypotensive effect by blocking the vasoconstrictor actions of reflexly released catecholamines whereas propranolol did not cause a synergistic effect.[48] Hydralazine is extensively metabolized in man mainly by N-acetylation and cyclization to triazolo derivatives and by hydrazone formation.[49] Several of these hydrazone metabolites are potent vasodilators but the triazoles are inactive.[50-52] Acetylator phenotype determines the response to hydralazine and other drugs that are extensively acetylated in man.[53] Most of the metabolites from the antihypertensive hydrazone, budralazine (DJ1461, 6), in rats arise from initial formation of hydralazine.[54] Initial clinical experiences with propyldazine[55] (ISF2123, 7) and BQ22-708[56] (8) show them to be effective hypotensives at much lower doses than hydralazine and with the expected side effects of potent vasodilators. Hydralazine, (7) and analogs with free hydrazine groups inhibit diamine oxidases at hypotensive doses.[57]

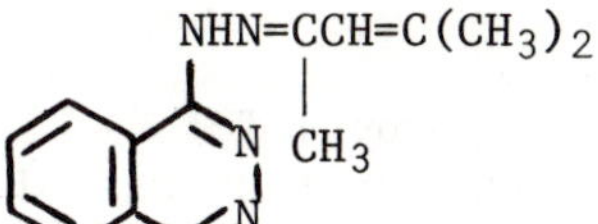

6 budralazine

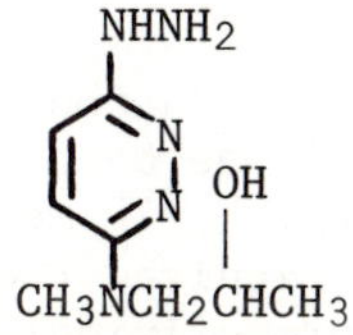

7 propyldazine

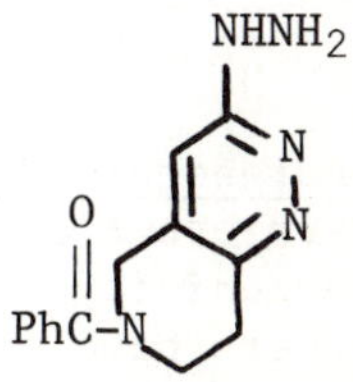

8

The pharmacology and clinical use of prazosin has been thoroughly reviewed[58-60] and discussed in symposia.[61,62] Many clinical studies confirm its hypotensive actions. As the sole therapy, it was found as effective as methyldopa[63] but less than hydrochlorothiazide.[64] It does not alter renal function, cardiac output, or plasma renin, but it may cause fluid retention[65] and has shown better efficacy in combination with thiazide diuretics.[66,67] The major use for this drug may be in combination with a diuretic and β-blocker in place of hydralazine. The incidence of first-dose fainting and dizziness is quite high in some studies[68,69] and is more pronounced in patients on a low sodium diet.[70] Animal studies show prazosin to be a selective α-blocker with little direct vascular relaxant action.[71,72] It blocks only postsynaptic vascular α-receptors leaving presynaptic α-receptors operational for feedback inhibition of sympathetic neurotransmitter release.[73,74] Both types of α-receptors may be present in postsynaptic tissue.[75] Prazosin is metabolized mainly by O-demethylation and glucuronide formation[76] to weakly active derivatives.[77] The prazosin analog, trimazosin, was found as active as methyldopa in mild hypertensives[78] and first reports on two new analogs, BL-5111A[79] (9) and E 643[80] (10), have appeared.

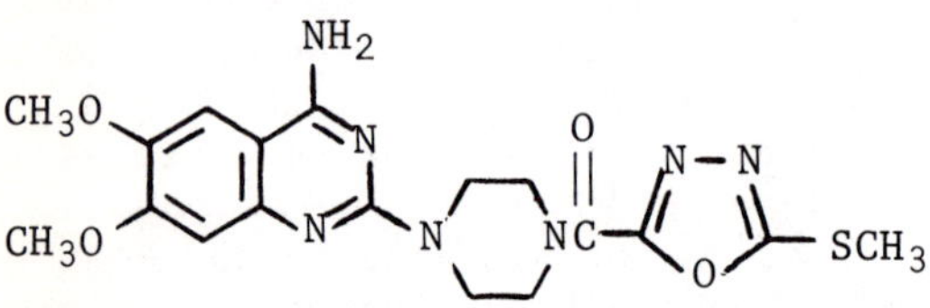

9

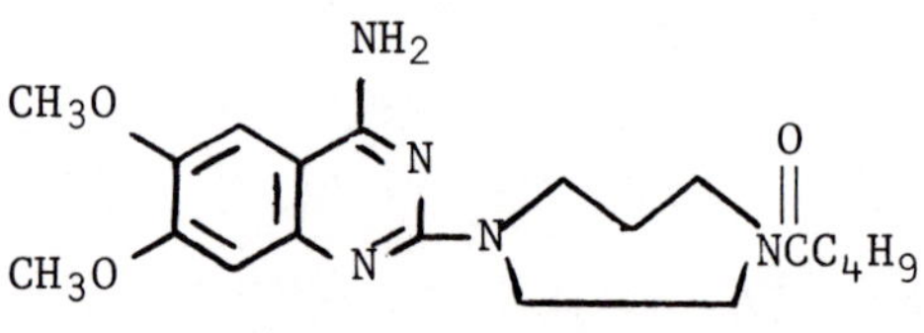

10

More reports have appeared on the efficacy of minoxidil in combination with a β-blocker and diuretic in treating severe hypertension resistant to standard drugs.[81,82] It may induce anginal attacks in patients with coronary artery disease[83] but concern that it may cause pulmonary hypertension seems unwarranted.[84,85] Diazoxide is an excellent drug for hypertensive crises.[86] This compound and analogs block vasoconstriction in isolated aortic rings from hypertensive rats much more than normotensive rats.[87] The clinically effective[88] vasodilator, guancydine, blocks vasoconstriction due to angiotensin II but has no effect on renin secretion.[89] Dihydropyridines, such as nifedipine (11), YC-93[90,91] (12), and niludipine (13) show potent vasodilating actions. Nifedipine was found effective for hypertensive emergencies but not for mild hypertension.[92,93]

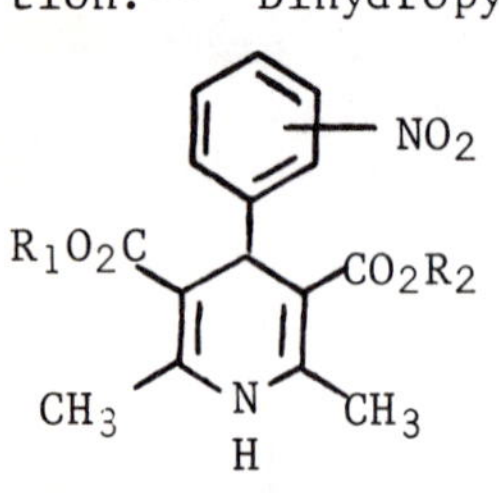

11: $R_1=R_2=CH_3$ ($2\text{-}NO_2$)

12: $R_1=CH_3, R_2=PhCH_2N(CH_3)(CH_2)_2$ ($3\text{-}NO_2$)

13: $R_1=R_2=CH_3(CH_2)_2O(CH_2)_2$ ($2\text{-}NO_2$)

Beta-Adrenergic Blocking Agents - In the U.S.A., FDA approval for β-blockers other than propranolol has been delayed because of the possible carcinogenicity of these agents.[94,95] Metoprolol and at least six other β-blockers have completed the required two-year carcinogenicity testing and may now be used in long-term clinical trials. However, tolamolol, bunolol, and possibly timolol caused an increased incidence of tumors in animals, and tolamolol has been withdrawn from U.S. clinical trials.[95]

The growing importance of β-blockers in the treatment of hypertension is indicated by the proliferation of publications on this subject as well as the marked increase in propranolol use. Reviews and symposia proceedings have appeared on the use of atenolol,[96] pindolol,[97] and metoprolol[98] in hypertension. β-blockers are recommended as first choice drugs[99,100] or as the "step 2" drugs of choice after diuretics.[101] A Veteran's Administration study of propranolol in a large group of mild hypertensives found that it normalized the blood pressure in about half the patients and was more effective in combination with a diuretic and with hydralazine.[102] Other β-blockers compare well with propranolol or methyldopa for treating hypertension. However, β-blockers with intrinsic sympathomimetic activity (i.s.a.) may be less effective at high doses than those without i.s.a. since they show a flat dose-response curve for blocking exercise-induced tachycardia at higher doses.[103]

Cardioselective β-blockers, such as metoprolol and atenolol, and drugs with i.s.a. such as pindolol,[104] are less likely to cause bronchospasm than non-selective agents such as propranolol, but all these drugs may cause bronchoconstriction at higher doses in asthmatics and are contraindicated.[105] Surprisingly, *d*-propranolol increases airway resistance in rats and guinea pigs as much as *dl*-propranolol suggesting that β-blockade is not the only factor responsible for the bronchoconstriction.[106] The effect of β-blockers on blood lipids remains controversial, and any advantage for β_1 or non-selective drugs is uncertain.[107] The β_1-selective drugs may be safer in diabetic patients.[108] Of concern with all β-blockers is their potential to cause the oculomucocutaneous syndrome associated with practolol, but such an effect has not so far been seen with β-blockers other than practolol.[109]

Most β-blockers, with the exception of sotalol[110] and nadolol, have relatively short plasma half-lives.[5] However, several of these drugs[5,97,111] are effective on a once-daily schedule since their hypotensive action in man lasts for many hours after their disappearance from plasma.

How β-blockers lower blood pressure is still unclear. Various central actions of some β-blockers have been demonstrated, but there is little direct evidence that centrally mediated blood pressure lowering occurs in man.[112] Some of the central effects may be mediated by blockade of serotonin uptake.[113] The inhibition of renin secretion by these drugs continues to attract many investigators. However, except in a small number of patients with renin-dependent forms of hypertension, renin lowering does not seem to be the major factor in the hypotensive response.[114] Sotalol decreases norepinephrine release from sympathetic nerve endings by its action on presynaptic β-receptors,[20] but the physiological significance of this action remains uncertain. A new hypothesis concerning the mechanism of β-blockers in hypertension stresses the importance of blocking vascular β_2-receptors thereby allowing adenyl cyclase to regain responsiveness to physiological vasodilators such as histamine and PGE_2.[115] In agreement with this concept, indomethacin, a PG-synthesis inhibitor, blocks the hypotensive action of β-blockers in rabbits and in patients.[116]

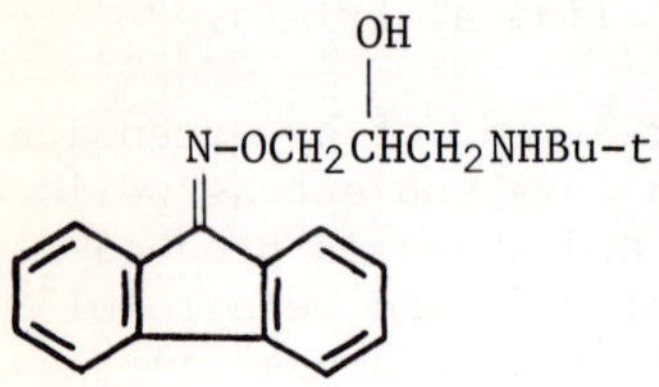

14

The recognized ability of β-blockers to acutely decrease cardiac output and chronically decrease peripheral resistance are still important contributing mechanisms to their lowering of blood pressure. In fact, several of these mechanisms may simultaneously contribute to the hemodynamic profile of β-blockers, and β-adrenergic blockade itself remains the single pharmacologic parameter most predictive of clinical usefulness in lowering blood pressure.

Two new agents, 14[117] (IPS-339) and 15,[118] are selective β_2-receptor blockers. The oxime ether, 14, is an extremely potent β_2-blocker *in vitro* (β_2/β_1=155) and *in vivo*; however, it raised blood pressure in normotensive and hypertensive rats.[119]

In addition to the 18 β-blockers already marketed somewhere in the world,[120] as well as those in advanced clinical trials, new agents continue to be developed. Preclinical pharmacology on the cardioselective agent, bevantolol[121] (16), and the non-selective, bufurolol[122] (17), has appeared. Mepindolol (2-methylpindolol) is even more potent than pindolol but has less inotropic effect on the heart.[123] Carazolol (18) is more potent than 15 well-known β-blockers and has a high therapeutic index.[124] Structural requirements for cardioselectivity in ureido and acylamino analogs of atenolol and practolol have been clarified.[125,126] In *N*-oxyalkyl compounds of the tolamolol type, the oxygen of the N substituent appears to play a major role in determining selectivity.[127]

Ar-X-CH(OH)CH_2NH-R

	Ar	X	R
15	4-benzimidazolyl	OCH_2	i-Pr
16	3-methylphenyl	OCH_2	3,4-dimethoxyphenethyl
17	2-[7-ethylbenzofuranyl]	--	t-Bu
18	4-carbazolyl	OCH_2	i-Pr
19	4-hydroxy-3-[NH_2CO]phenyl	--	1-methyl-3-phenylpropyl
20	4-[4-CF_3-imidazolyl]phenyl	OCH_2	t-Bu
21	5-benzodioxolyl	--	t-Bu/i-Pr
22	3,4-dihydroxyphenyl	OCH_2	t-Bu
23	3-HO-4-CH_3SO_2NH-phenyl	OCH_2	t-Bu

The stage has now been reached where any new β-blocker needs a unique characteristic to justify its development. Labetalol (AH 5138, 19), a drug with both α- and β-antagonist actions,[128,129] has been introduced in the U.K. This drug, given *i.v.*, lowers blood pressure by decreasing vascular resistance and cardiac output with very little negative inotropy.[130] Postural hypotension is common after labetalol *i.v.*[131] but not *p.o.*[132] It is useful for hypertensive emergencies[133] and is an effective antihypertensive agent in some patients not well controlled by other β-blockers;[134] it does not induce bronchoconstriction.[135] A similar concept to labetalol has led to the development of an agent that combines β-blocking and direct vasodilating actions in a single molecule.[136] Compound 20 is as potent as hydralazine in lowering blood pressure in SH rats, it causes cardioselective β-blockade in dogs and increases iliac blood flow in the dog hind limb by a direct vasodilator mechanism. The benzodioxoles[137] (21, R=i-Pr or t-Bu) may have an action in addition to β-blockade since they lower blood pressure in SH rats after single oral doses.

Structural requirements for good β-adrenergic receptor affinity have been determined using "adenyl cyclase coupled" β-receptors on frog erythrocyte membranes labelled with (-)-[^{3}H] alprenolol.[138] These results agree well with SAR's established in whole organ systems and strongly support the existence of the hypothetical β-adrenergic receptors. In membrane systems from rabbit heart, lung, and uterus, the β_1-selectivity of practolol and atenolol compared to propranolol is maintained at the β-receptor-adenyl cyclase level, although to a lesser degree.[139] Although the phenoxypropanolamine structure is usually associated with β-blocking activity, 22 and 23 are potent agonists.[140] Their ability to assume a rigid, bicyclic, hydrogen-bonded conformation may explain the similarity of receptor binding of these agents and phenethanolamines.[140] Surprisingly, 23 shows β_1 selectivity as an agonist.

Peripheral Sympathetic Nerve Inhibitors - The interaction of guanidine antihypertensives with other drugs has been reviewed.[141] New interest has developed in the use of guanethidine in mild hypertension in addition to its traditional use in severe hypertension. It has been found to be more effective than a thiazide diuretic and caused few side effects in mild-moderate hypertension when given in single, daily, low doses.[142] It was superior to bethanidine in a large group of moderate-severe hypertensives.[143] Structural damage to noradrenergic neurones after chronic high doses of guanethidine does not seem to be related to its useful pharmacological actions and is probably unimportant in normal use.[144] The wide variation in the dose of debrisoquin needed to control blood pressure appears due to genetic differences in patients' ability to metabolize it to the 4-hydroxy derivative.[145] Sympathetic blocking drugs should not be used in hypertensive patients particularly prone to exertional hypotension.[146] Several new sympathetic inhibitors including EMD 21192[147] (24) and guanazodine[148] (25) are being tested clinically.

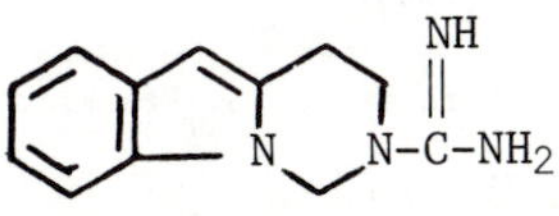

24

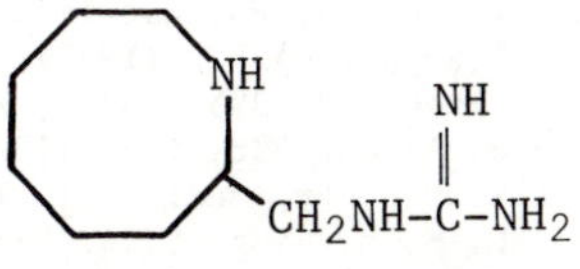

25 guanazodine

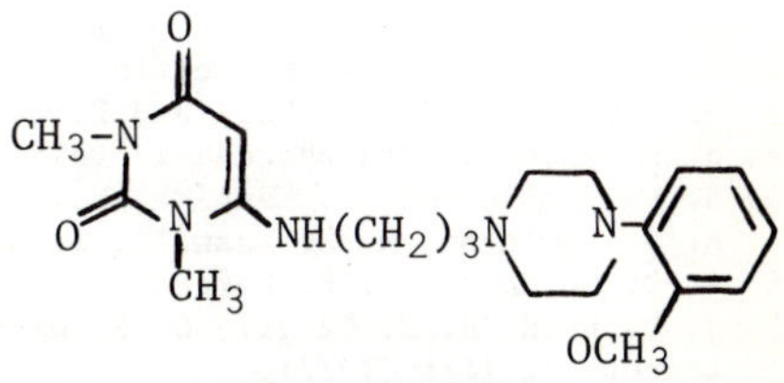

26 urapidil

Miscellaneous Antihypertensives - The recently reported drugs, urapidil[149] (26) and piprofural[150] (27), lower blood pressure by central and complex peripheral effects including α-blockade. The latter drug also has antiarrhythmic properties and inhibits calcium influx into muscle cells. The dopamine derivative, Sandoz 27-403 (28) was identified from a search for a substance that would stimulate vascular dopamine receptors without affecting α- and β-adrenoceptors.[151] It lowers blood pressure in normotensive dogs at 2.5 μg/kg *i.v.*, but not *p.o.*, by dilation of vessels in the mesenteric and renal vascular beds without reflex tachycardia. Its hypotensive action is blocked by the dopamine antagonists, haloperidol and ergometrine. Bromocryptine, another dopamine agonist, has antihypertensive effects in man.[152]

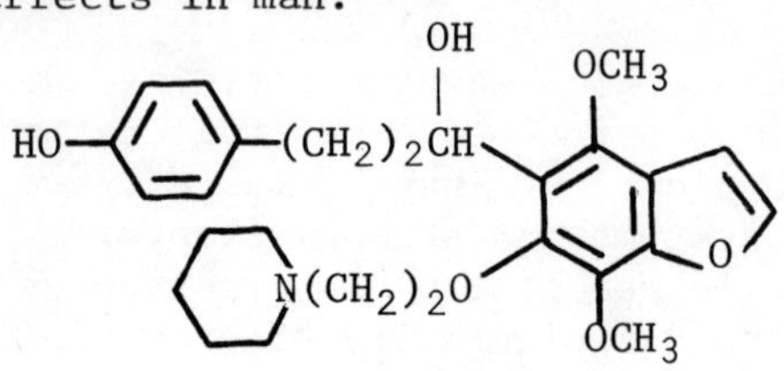

27 piprofural

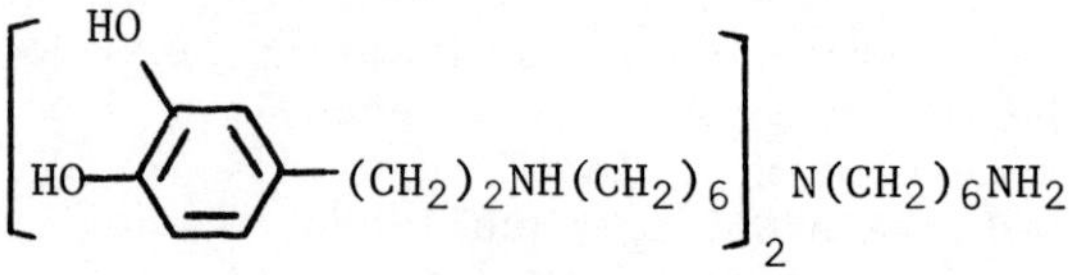

28

References

1. A. S. Nies, Med. Clin. North Am. 61, 675 (1977).
2. J. A. Romankiewicz, Am. J. Hosp. Pharm. 34, 185 (1977).
3. C. T. Dollery, Ann. Rev. Pharmacol. Toxicol. 17, 311 (1977).
4. Report of the Joint National Committee on Detection, Evaluation and Treatment of High Blood Pressure, J. Am. Med. Assoc. 237, 255 (1977).
5. Second Pan American Symposium on Hypertension, Part II, Mayo Clin. Proc. 52, 361 (1977).
6. Editorial, Lancet, 1, 1088 (1977).
7. Basle Hypertension Symposium, Ed., H. Dunér, Acta Med. Scand., Suppl. 606, 7 (1977).
8. K. Iwatsuki, G. J. Cardinale, S. Spector and S. Udenfriend, Science 198, 403 (1977).
9. J. D. Spence, J. Pesout and K. L. Melmon, Stroke, 8, 589 (1977).
10. G. Leonetti, L. Terzoli, A. Morganti, M. Manfrin, C. Bianchini, C. Sala and A. Zanchetti, Am. J. Cardiol. 40, 762 (1977); H. Gavras, I. Gavras, H. R. Brunner and J. H. Laragh, J. Clin. Pharmacol. 17, 372 (1977).
11. B. E. Karlberg, O. Nilsson and K. Tolagen, Curr. Ther. Res. 21, 10 (1977).
12. F. Kersting, J. L. Reid and C. T. Dollery, Clin. Pharmacol. Ther., 21, 547 (1977).
13. M. F. Lokhandwala, J. T. Coats and J. P. Buckley, Eur. J. Pharmacol. 42, 257 (1977).
14. J. W. Wright, P. J. McLeod and W. McCullough, Clin. Pharmacol. Ther. 20, 733 (1976).
15. A. K. Jain, J. R. Ryan, R. Vargas and F. G. McMahon, Clin. Pharmacol. Ther. 21, 382 (1977).
16. P. R. Wilkinson and E. B. Raftery, Br. J. Clin. Pharmacol. 4, 289 (1977).
17. W. A. Pettinger, H. C. Mitchell and H. G. Güllner, Clin. Pharmacol. Ther. 22, 164 (1977).
18. V. G. Tauberger, P.-J. Flory and W. Volkert, Arzneim.-Forsch. 27(II), 1570 (1977).
19. J. L. Reid, L. M. H. Wing, C. J. Mathias and H. L. Frankel, Clin. Exper. Pharmacol. 4, 492 (1977).
20. N. Yamaguchi, J. de Champlain and R. A. Nadeau, Cir. Res. 41, 108 (1977).
21. L. M. H. Wing, J. L. Reid, D. S. Davies, H. J. Dargie and C. T. Dollery, Br. Med. J. 1, 136 (1977).
22. S. Berthelsen and W. A. Pettinger, Life Sci. 21, 595 (1977).
23. H. Karppanen, I. Paakkari and P. Paakkari, Eur. J. Pharmacol. 42, 299 (1977).
24. H. Karppanen, Acta pharmacol. toxicol. 41(Suppl. 4), 20 (1977).
25. S. W. Hoobler and T. Kashima, Mayo Clin. Proc. 52, 395 (1977); F. G. Strauss, S. S. Franklin A. J. Lewin and M. H. Maxwell, J. Am. Med. Assoc. 238, 1734 (1977).
26. A. D. Goldberg, E. B. Raftery and P. Wilkinson, Br. Med. J. 1, 1243 (1977).
27. J. L. Reid, H. J. Dargie, D. S. Davies, L. M. H. Wing, C. A. Hamelton and C. T. Dollery, Lancet, 1, 1171 (1977).
28. G. M. Drew, A. J. Gower and A. S. Marriott, Br. J. Pharmacol. 61, 468P (1977).
29. P. T. S. Putkonen, A. Leppävuori and D. Stenberg, Life Sci. 21, 1059 (1977).
30. M. Vogt, Br. J. Pharmacol. 61, 441 (1977).
31. C. S. Sweet and S. L. Gaul, Can. J. Physiol. Pharmacol. 55, 968 (1977).
32. P. P. M. W. M. Timmermans and P. A. van Zwieten, J. Med. Chem. 20, 1636 (1977); Arch. int. Pharmacodyn. Ther. 228, 237 and 251 (1977); Eur. J. Pharmacol. 45, 229 (1977).
33. B. Rouot, G. Leclerc, C.-G. Wermuth, F. Miesch and J. Schwartz, J. Pharmacol. (Paris), 8, 95 (1977).
34. V. H. Brunner, S. Djawan, W. Dorda, E. Penner and G. Grabner, Arzneim.-Forsch. 27(II), 1599 (1977).
35. F. G. McMahon, J. R. Ryan, A. K. Jain, R. Vargas and S. K. Vanov, Clin. Pharmacol. Ther. 21, 272 (1977).

36. U. C. Dubach, R. Huwyler, P. Radielovic and M. Singeisen, Arzneim.-Forsch. 27(I), 674 (1977).
37. Scrip, p. 24 (Nov. 26, 1977).
38. R. W. Fuller, H. D. Snoddy and W. S. Marshall, J. Pharm. Pharmacol. 29, 375 (1977).
39. N.-E. Anden, C. Gomes, M. Grabowska, B. Persson and G. Trolin, Acta pharmacol. toxicol. 24, (Suppl. 4), 19 (1977).
40. N.-E. Anden and M. Grabowska, Naunyn-Schmiedeberg's Arch. Pharmakol. 298, 239 (1977).
41. J. T. Burke and J. Koch-Weser, Clin. Pharmacol. 21, 99 (1977).
42. W. Kobinger and L. Pichler, Naunyn-Schmiedeberg's Arch. Pharmakol. 300, 39 (1977).
43. M. F. Lokhandwala, H. K. Pariani, J. P. Buckley and B. S. Jandhyala, Eur. J. Pharmacol. 42, 107 (1977).
44. J. Melrose, M. G. Palfreyman, R. H. Poyser and R. L. Whiting, Br. J. Pharmacol. 61, 357 (1977).
45. H. Prozenel, Intl. J. Pharmacol. Biopharm. 15, 31 (1977).
46. Editorial, Lancet, 1, 342 (1977).
47. I. Khatri, N. Uemura, A. Notargiacomo and E. D. Freis, Am. J. Cardiol. 40, 38 (1977).
48. M. Gutkin, B. Das, B.-K. Chin, K. Mezey and R. S. Modlihger, J. Clin. Pharmacol. 17, 509 (1977).
49. T. Talseth, Clin. Pharmacokin. 2, 317 (1977).
50. A. J. McLean, K. W. Barron, B. P. du Souich, K. D. Haegele and J. L. McNay, Clin. Res. 25, 556A (1977).
51. K. Barron, O. Carrier, K. D. Haegele, A. J. McLean, J. L. McNay and P. du Souich, Br. J. Pharmacol. 61, 345 (1977).
52. A. J. McLean, K. Barron, K. D. Haegele, O. Carrier and J. L. McNay, Clin. Pharmacol. Ther. 21, 110 (1977).
53. D. E. Drayer and M. M. Reidenberg, Clin. Pharmacol. Ther. 22, 251 (1977).
54. R. Moroi, K. Ono, T. Saito, T. Akimoto and M. Sano, Chem. Pharm. Bull. 25, 830 (1977).
55. R. Pellegrini and G. Abbondati, Farmaco (Ed. Pract.), 32, 19 (1977).
56. H.-U. Lehmann, E. Witt and H. Hochrein, Med. Klin. (Munich), 72, 1203 (1977).
57. F. Buffoni, G. Ignesti and R. Pirisino, Farmaco (Ed. Sci.), 32, 404 (1977).
58. R. N. Brogden, R. C. Heel, T. M. Speight and G. S. Avery, Drugs, 14, 163 (1977).
59. The Medical Letter, 19, 81 (1977).
60. M. E. Kosman, J. Am. Med. Assoc. 238, 157 (1977).
61. Pfizer Forum on Prazosin and Hypertension: Med. J. Austr. 2 (Suppl. 1 and 2), (1977).
62. Symposium on 'Peripress': Curr. Med. Res. Opin. 4(Suppl. 2), 1 (1977).
63. W. F. Bradley, F. G. Hoffman, J. R. Hutchison, Z. Kalams and S. L. Waldron, Curr. Ther. Res. 21, 28 (1977).
64. A. Schirger and S. G. Sheps, J. Am. Med. Assoc. 237, 989 (1977).
65. M. C. Koshy, D. Mickley, J. Bourgiognie and M. D. Blaufox, Circulation, 55, 533 (1977).
66. Y. K. Seedat, M. A. Seedat and R. Bholla, S. Afr. Med. J. 51, 461 (1977).
67. J. Guevara, H. Collet-Velasco and M. Velasco, Clin. Pharmacol. Ther. 21, 105 (1977).
68. A. S. Turner, O. F. Watson and J. E. Brocklehurst, N. Z. Med. J. 86, 286 (1977).
69. T. Thien, R. A. P. Koene and P. G. A. B. Wijdeveld, Lancet, 1, 363 (1977).
70. G. S. Stokes, R. M. Graham, J. M. Gain and P. R. Davis, Br. Med. J. 1, 1507 (1977).
71. H. F. Oates, R. M. Graham and G. S. Stokes, Arch. int. Pharmacodyn. Ther. 227, 41 (1977).
72. R. M. Graham, H. F. Oates, L. M. Stoker and G. S. Stokes, J. Pharmacol. Exp. Ther. 201, 747 (1977).
73. J. C. Doxey, C. F. C. Smith and J. M. Walker, Br. J. Pharmacol. 60, 91 (1977).
74. I. Cavero, F. Lefevre and A. G. Roach, Br. J. Pharmacol. 61, 469P (1977).
75. S. M. Bentley, G. M. Drew and S. B. Whiting, Br. J. Pharmacol. 61, 116P (1977).
76. T. H. Althuis and H.-J. Hess, J. Med. Chem. 20, 146 (1977).
77. J. A. Taylor, T. M. Twomey and M. S. von Wittenau, Xenobiotica, 7, 357 (1977).
78. W. S. Aronow, J. Tobis, D. Hughes, J. Siegel and J. Easthope, Clin. Pharmacol. Ther. 22, 425 (1977).
79. J. E. Schurig, R. L. Cavanagh, L. E. Roebel and J. P. Buyniski, Pharmacologist, 19, 213, abstr. 485 (1977).
80. T. Igarashi, Y. Nakajima and S. Ohtake, Jpn. Cir. J. 41, 903 (1977).
81. H. J. Dargie, J. Daniel, C. T. Dollery, Lancet, 2, 515 (1977).
82. B. L. Devine, R. Fife and P. M. Trust, Br. Med. J. 2, 667 (1977).
83. G. B. Ambrosio, Lancet, 2, 1087 (1977).
84. J. M. Atkins, H. C. Mitchell and W. A. Pettinger, Am. J. Cardiol. 39, 802 (1977).
85. P. E. Klotman, C. E. Grim, M. H. Weinberger and W. E. Judson, Circulation, 55, 394 (1977).
86. W. J. McDonald, G. Smith, J. W. Woods, H. M. Perry and B. D. Danielson, Am. J. Cardiol. 40, 409 (1977).
87. S. Chona and D. J. Triggle, Can. J. Physiol. Pharmacol. 55, 153 (1977).
88. H. Villarreal, H. Arcila, M. A. Ramirez and P. Sierra, Mayo Clin. Proc. 52, 383 (1977).

89. N. Bernard, D. Benzoni and J. Sassard, J. Pharmacol. (Paris), 8, 149 (1977).
90. T. Seki and T. Takenaka, Int. J. Clin. Pharmacol. 15, 267 (1977).
91. S. Higuchi, H. Sasaki, Y. Shiobara and T. Sado, Xenobiotica, 7, 469 (1977).
92. M. Guazzi, M. T. Olivari, A. Polese, C. Fiorentini, F. Magrini and P. Moruzzi, Clin. Pharmacol. Ther. 22, 528 (1977).
93. V. U. Laaser, K. A. Meurer and W. Kaufmann, Arzneim.-Forsch. 27(I), 676 (1977).
94. J. W. Newberne, P. M. Newberne, J. P. Gibson, K. W. Huffman and F. P. Palopoli, Toxicol. Appl. Pharmacol. 41, 535 (1977).
95. Scrip, P20 (Nov. 12, 1977).
96. Proceedings of a Symposium on Atenolol: Postgrad. Med. J. 53(Suppl. 3), 58 (1977).
97. Symposium on Beta-Blockade in Hypertension: Curr. Med. Res. Opin. 4(Suppl. 5), 1 (1977).
98. R. N. Brogden, R. C. Heel, T. M. Speight and G. S. Avery, Drugs, 14, 321 (1977).
99. D. W. Barritt and A. J. Marshall, Br. Heart J. 39, 821 (1977).
100. R. P. Ahlquist, J. Clin. Pharmacol. 17, 93 (1977).
101. F. A. Finnerty, Clin. Ther. 1, 135 (1977).
102. Veterans Administration Cooperative Study Group on Antihypertensive Agents, J. Am. Med. Assoc. 237, 2303 (1977).
103. D. G. McDevitt, H. C. Brown, S. G. Carruthers and R. G. Shanks, Clin. Pharmacol. Ther. 21, 556 (1977).
104. W. Frishman, M. Stampfer, J. Strom, V. Elkayam, T. LeJemtel, J. Weinstein and E. Sonnenblick, Circulation, 55-56(Suppl. III), III-180 (1977).
105. J. Marché and F. C. Hugues, Thérapie, 32, 81 (1977).
106. J. Maclagan and U. M. Ney, Br. J. Pharmacol. 61, P469 (1977).
107. S. P. Deacon, Br. Med. J., 2, 827 (1977); R. J. Newman, *ibid*, 601 (1977); H. J. Waal-Manning and F. O. Simpson, *ibid*, 705 (1977).
108. S. P. Deacon, A. Karunanayake and D. Barnett, Br. Med. J. 2, 1255 (1977).
109. Editorial, Br. Med. J. 1, 529 (1977).
110. R. Gabriel, Curr. Med. Res. Opin. 4, 739 (1977).
111. J. Tuomilehto, M. Arstila, R. Savilahti and H. Sundquist, Curr. Ther. Res. 21, 668 (1977); W. P. Leary, A. C. Asmal, P. Williams and B. Marivick, *ibid*, 22, 385 (1977).
112. J. L. Reid, C. R. Dean and D. H. Jones, Cardiovas. Med. 2, 1185 (1977).
113. D. N. Middlemiss, L. Blakeborough and S. R. Leather, Nature, 267, 289 (1977).
114. F. Gross, Eur. J. Clin. Invest. 7, 321 (1977).
115. M. S. Amer, Biochem. Pharmacol. 26, 171 (1977).
116. V. Durao, M. M. Prata and L. M. P. Goncalves, Lancet, 2, 1005 (1977).
117. G. Leclerc, A. Mann, C.-G. Wermuth, N. Bieth and J. Schwartz, J. Med. Chem. 20, 1657 (1977).
118. C. R. Crooks, J. Wright, P. S. Callery and J. E. Moreton, Pharmacologist, 19, 244, abstr. 659 (1977).
119. J. L. Imbs, F. Miesch, J. Schwartz, J. Velly, G. Leclerc, A. Mann and C. C. Wermuth, Br. J. Pharmacol. 60, 357 (1977).
120. Scrip, P22 (Nov. 12, 1977).
121. S. G. Hastings, R. D. Smith, R. M. Corey, A. D. Essenburg, C. E. Pettway and D. K. Tessman, Arch. Int. Pharmacodyn. Ther. 226, 81 (1977).
122. T. C. Hamilton and M. W. Parkes, Arzneim.-Forsch. 27(II), 1410 (1977).
123. J. Bonelli, Int. J. Clin. Pharmacol. Biopharm. 15, 325 (1977).
124. W. Bartsch, K. Diétmann, H. Leinert and G. Sponer, Arzneim.-Forsch. 27(I), 1022 (1977).
125. L. H. Smith, J. Med. Chem. 20, 705 (1977).
126. L. H. Smith and H. Tucker, J. Med. Chem. 20, 1653 (1977).
127. L. H. Smith, J. Med. Chem. 20, 1254 (1977).
128. D. A. Richards, B. N. C. Prichard, A. J. Boakes, J. Tuckman and E. J. Knight, Br. Heart J. 39, 99 (1977).
129. J. Mehta and J. N. Cohn, Circulation, 55, 370 (1977).
130. G. Koch, Am. Heart J. 93, 585 (1977).
131. Editorial, Lancet, 1, 890 (1977).
132. A. Breckenridge, T. N. Calvey, G. J. Green, M. McIver, M. L'E. Orme and M. J. Serlin, Lancet, 1, 36 (1977).
133. E. A. Rosei, R. Fraser, J. J. Morton, J. J. Brown, A. F. Lever, J. I. S. Robertson and P. M. Trust, Am. Heart J. 93, 124 (1977).
134. R. Dent and G. S. M. Kellaway, N. Z. Med. J. 86, 213 (1977).
135. J. G. Maconochie, E. P. Woodings and D. A. Richards, Brit. J. Clin. Pharmacol. 4, 157 (1977).
136. J. J. Baldwin, R. Hirschmann, P. K. Lumma, W. C. Lumma, Jr., and G. S. Ponticello, J. Med. Chem. 20, 1024 (1977).
137. H. Tatsuno, K. Goto, K. Shigenobu, Y. Kasuya, H. Obase, Y. Yamada and S. Kudo, J. Med. Chem. 20, 394 (1977).

138. C. Mukherjee, M. G. Caron, D. Mullikin and R. J. Lefkowitz, Mol. Pharmacol. 12, 16 (1976).
139. A. J. Coleman and A. R. Somerville, Br. J. Pharmacol. 59, 83 (1977).
140. C. Kaiser, T. Jen, E. Garvey, W. D. Bowen, D. F. Colella and J. R. Wardell, Jr., J. Med. Chem. 20, 687 and 693 (1977).
141. J. R. Stafford and W. E. Fann, Drugs, 13, 57 (1977).
142. F. M. Howard, Clin. Med. 84, 10 (1977).
143. Veteran's Administration Cooperative Study Group on Antihypertensive Agents, Circulation, 55, 519 (1977).
144. H. Bittiger, L. Maitre, G. Krinke, K. Schnider and R. Hess, Toxicol. 8, 63 (1977); G. D. Nielson, Acta pharmacol. toxicol. 41, 203 (1977).
145. A. Mahgoub, L. G. Dring, J. R. Idle, R. Lancaster and R. L. Smith, Lancet, 2, 584 (1977).
146. S. Talbot and G. W. Gill, Postgrad. Med. J. 52, 487 (1976).
147. H. Grobecker, M. F. Roizen, D. M. Jacobowitz and I. J. Kopin, Eur. J. Pharmacol. 46, 125 (1977).
148. V. W. Reiterer and H. Czitober, Arzneim.-Forsch. 27(II), 2163 (1977).
149. V. W. Schoetensack, P. Bischler, E. Ch. Dittmann and V. Steinijans, Arzneim.-Forsch. 27(II) 1908 (1977).
150. B. Pourrias, D. Garnier and G. Raynaud, J. Pharmacol. (Paris), 8, 125 (1977).
151. B. J. Clark, Acta Med. Scand. Suppl. 606, 95 (1977).
152. K. O. Stumpe, M. Higuchi, R. Kolloch, F. Krüeck and H. Vetter, Lancet, 2, 211 (1977).

Chapter 9. Inhibitors of the Renin-Angiotensin System

Miguel A. Ondetti and David W. Cushman
The Squibb Institute for Medical Research
P.O. Box 4000, Princeton, N.J. 08540

Introduction: The renin-angiotensin system[1-9] consists of blood-borne and tissue-bound peptidases and their protein or peptide substrates that par-

```
 1   2   3   4   5   6   7   8   9   10  11  12  13  14
Asp-Arg-Val-Tyr-Ile-His-Pro-Phe-His-Leu-Leu-Val-Tyr-Ser-R  AO
                     ↓  renin          ▲
Asp-Arg-Val-Tyr-Ile-His-Pro-Phe-His-Leu                    AI
                     ↓  ACE      ▲
Asp-Arg-Val-Tyr-Ile-His-Pro-Phe                            AII
   ▲                 ↓  angiotensinase A
    Arg-Val-Tyr-Ile-His-Pro-Phe                            AIII
              ▲         ▲

                        angiotensinases B and C
```

ticipate in the maintenance of blood pressure in low volume or low sodium states, and in the elevation of blood pressure in certain forms of hypertensive disease. Renin[3-5], the rate-limiting enzyme, is released into the blood from the kidney in response to hyponatremia or low blood pressure; it cleaves a blood glycoprotein angiotensinogen (AO) between leucine residues 10 and 11 to liberate the biologically inactive decapeptide angiotensin I (AI). Circulating AI is converted in lung, kidney and other tissues to the pressor octapeptide angiotensin II (AII) by a peptidyldipeptide hydrolase commonly referred to as angiotensin-converting enzyme (ACE)[6,7]. Circulating AII directly constricts arterioles and produces an immediate elevation of blood pressure; either AII or its des-Asp[1]-heptapeptide derivative angiotensin III (AIII)[8] stimulates release from the adrenal gland of the sodium-retaining steroid aldosterone which causes a more gradual increase in extracellular fluid volume and a sustained increase in blood pressure. Angiotensins I-III are quickly destroyed by blood and tissue enzymes referred to as angiotensinases[9]. Pharmacological interruption of the renin-angiotensin system has been a powerful tool for elucidating its role in hypertensive disease. In this brief review we will discuss various approaches to the inhibition of different components of this system, but we will concentrate on recent developments concerning those agents that have the greatest potential for therapeutic use.

Renin Inhibitors: Renin is inhibited *in vitro* by high concentrations (0.4 to 2 mM) of naturally-occurring renal lysophosphatidylethanolamines[10,12], synthetic phosphatidylethanolamines[11] and lysophosphatidylethanolamine analogs[12,13], and also by neutral lipids and phosphatidylcho-

ISBN 0-12-040513-X

line derivatives[14]. In spite of their weak inhibitory activity *in vitro*, several of these compounds significantly lower blood pressure in the Goldblatt two-kidney renal hypertensive rat (RHR), a renin-mediated hypertensive model in which one renal artery is constricted and the other kidney is left intact. The renal phospholipid and synthetic analogs 1 and 2 given by daily intramuscular injections (7-50 mg/kg) produced a progressive lowering of blood pressure that reached a maximum of 40-50 mm Hg within 2-4 days[10,12]. Analog 2 also produced an 85% inhibition of plasma renin activity in the RHR[12]. The phosphorylethanolamine analog PE-104 (3) was shown to be a specific competitive inhibitor of renin *in vitro* (K_i=2 mM). Upon intravenous infusion at a total dose of 200 mg/kg, it produced a 26 mm Hg lowering of blood pressure and a partial

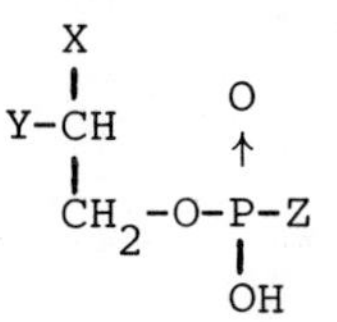

	X	Y	Z
1	$-CH_2O_2C(CH_2)_{16}CH_3$	$CH_3(CH_2CH{=}CH)_3(CH_2)_7CO_2-$	$-OCH_2CH_2NH_2$
2	$-CH_2CH_2(CH{=}CHCH_2)_4(CH_2)_3CH_3$	H-	$-CH_2CH_2NH_2$
3	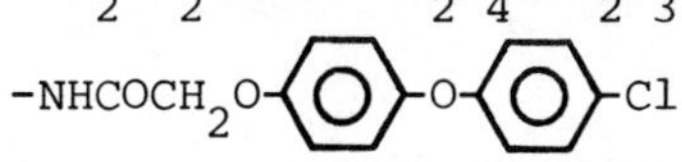	H-	$-OCH_2CH_2NH_2$

inhibition of renin activity in RHR[13]; its renin inhibitory activity was reported to be of short duration. It remains to be conclusively demonstrated whether or not the antihypertensive actions of analogs 1-3 are related to their weak renin inhibitory activity.

4: X=OH

5: X=H

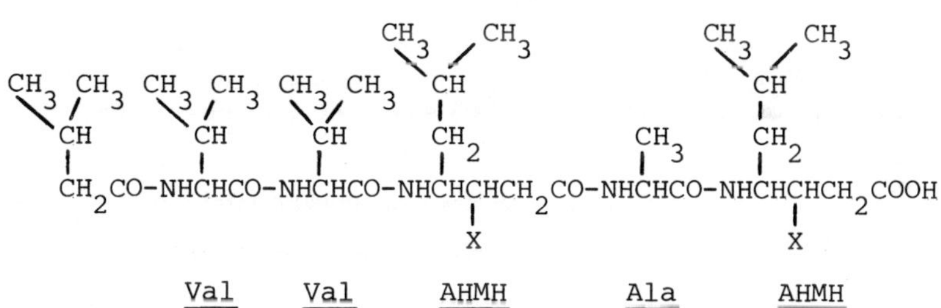

Pepstatin A (4) is an N-acetylated pentapeptide of microbial origin that contains two residues of the unusual amino acid 4-amino-3-hydroxy-6-methylheptanoic acid (AHMH) and is a potent inhibitor of acid proteases such as pepsin, cathepsin D, and renin[15-17]. Structure-activity studies[17,18] indicate that the hydrophobic side-chains and the first AHMH residue of pepstatin are important for its inhibitory activity. Such results have led to the suggestion that pepstatin is a transition-state analog, with the hydroxyl group of the first AHMH residue mimicking the tetrahedral transition state of the scissile peptide carbonyl. In apparent support of this concept, the dideoxy analog 5 is a competitive inhibitor of pepsin, with a 1000-fold lower inhibitory action than pepstatin[18]. In rats, intravenous doses of 0.2 to 0.8 mg/kg (limited by the poor aqueous solubility of pepstatin) inhibit the pressor response to infused renin, and lower blood pressure in RHRs[16,19], but with a duration of only 10 to 15 minutes.

Several structural analogs of the renin substrate are reasonably potent competitive inhibitors of renin *in vitro*; but none has yet been shown to inhibit significantly the action of renin *in vivo*. Tetrapeptide ester 6 and similar analogs[20] were shown to be weak competitive inhibitors of renin at pH 6.4 (I_{50}=0.5 to 1.0 mM), and inhibited only partially

6	Leu-Leu-Val-Phe-OEt	
7	His-Pro-Phe-His-Leu-*Leu*-Val-Tyr	*Leu* = D-Leu
8	Arg-Val-Tyr-Ile-His-Pro-Phe-His-Leu-*Leu*-Val-Tyr-Ser	
9	Pro-His-Pro-Phe-His-Phe-Phe-Val-Tyr	

the blood pressure response to renin at a total intravenous dose of 50 mg in rabbits. Octapeptide analog 7 and tridecapeptide analog 8, with D-leucine incorporated into the bond normally cleaved by renin, are potent inhibitors of renin at pH 5.5 (K_i=3 μM and 7 μM, respectively)[21,22]; analog 7, however, was shown to be inactive at neutral pH[23]. Recently the phenylalanine substituted analog (9) was shown to be a potent inhibitor of human renin at physiological pH (K_i=1.0 μM), but a poor inhibitor of non-primate renins[23,24].

Inhibitors of Angiotensin-Converting Enzyme: The peptidyldipeptide hydrolase usually referred to as angiotensin-converting enzyme (ACE) also inactivates the vasodepressor nonapeptide bradykinin (BK)[25]; for this reason, all inhibitors of ACE have two different but related biological activities: inhibition of AI actions and augmentation or prolongation of BK actions. Both of these activities, however, can lead to lowering of blood pressure. Two distinct classes of specific competitive inhibitors of ACE have been useful in clinical studies: peptides originally isolated from snake venoms, and acylamino acids designed for specific interaction with ACE.

10 (BPP_{5a}) <Glu-Lys-Trp-Ala-Pro

11 (teprotide) <Glu-Trp-Pro-Arg-Pro-Gln-Ile-Pro-Pro

<Glu- =

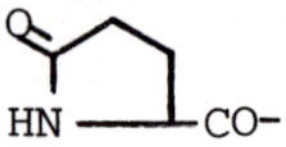

A mixture of bradykinin-potentiating peptides (BPP) from the venom of the Brazilian pit viper *Bothrops jararaca*[26] was shown in 1968 to inhibit ACE[27]. A number of peptides were isolated from this venom as bradykinin potentiators[28] or as ACE inhibitors[29]; and similar bradykinin potentiating peptides were isolated from the Asian viper *Agkistrodon halys Blomhoffii*[30]. One of the bradykinin-potentiating peptides from *B. jararaca* (BPP_{5a}, 10) was sequenced, synthesized, and shown also to be a potent inhibitor of ACE[28,31]. Six of the ACE inhibitors from *B. jararaca* were also sequenced, synthesized, and shown to be bradykinin-potentiating peptides as well as competitive inhibitors of ACE[29,32,33]; the most potent and thoroughly characterized of these was the nonapeptide SQ 20,881 (11). Peptide 11, employed as a bradykinin-potentiating peptide, has also been referred to as BPP_{9a} (see Table II of reference 33), or sometimes as CEI (converting enzyme inhibitor)[34]. Structure-activity studies with analogs of 10 and 11 have revealed the importance of the free carboxyl group and the C-terminal tripeptide sequence for competitive binding at the active site of ACE; certain of the other (N-terminal) amino acid residues also apparently bind to the enzyme and contribute to the overall inhibitory potency[35]. Replacement of the glutamine in 11 by lysine appears to increase tissue binding *in vitro*[36].

The *Agkistrodon* peptides[30,37] have not been extensively tested *in vivo*. The pentapeptide 10 was found to inhibit vasopressor responses to AI and augment vasodepressor responses to BK in rats, and also to lower blood pressure in two-kidney RHR; but its potency and duration of action were much less than those of the nonapeptide 11, which has been the only peptidic inhibitor of ACE used in clinical studies. At intravenous doses of 3 to 25 mg/kg, 11 produced a dramatic and prolonged lowering of blood pressure in two-kidney RHR[32]. Similar doses lowered blood pressure of dogs made hypertensive by constriction of one renal artery[34], and produced marked increases in plasma renin activity, presumably by interrupting a direct negative feedback action of AII on renin release. The nonapeptide 11 was not hypotensive in normal animals, but significantly lowered blood pressure in sodium depleted rats[34,38,39] and prevented the increase in plasma aldosterone that normally results from sodium depletion[38,39].

Compound 11 was also not hypotensive in normal human volunteers; but at an intravenous dose of 0.25 mg/kg a marked hypotensive response was obtained in sodium depleted subjects after a rapid 70° tilt. Plasma renin activity rose dramatically, but the normal increase in aldosterone was blocked[34]. In 65 hypertensive patients of various etiologies including renovascular, malignant, and essential, all high-renin patients and more than 90% of the "normal-renin" patients showed a lowering of blood pressure after intravenous administration of 11 at 1 mg/kg[40]. In earlier studies[41], its duration of action, at doses of 1-4 mg/kg, was shown to be as great as 16 hours, and the antihypertensive action was shown to be potentiated by mild sodium depletion.

Since the renin-angiotensin and kallikrein-kinin systems may increase in parallel in response to stimuli such as sodium depletion, it is not easy to assess the relative contributions of AII inhibition and BK augmentation to the antihypertensive action of 11. No increase in plasma BK was found during the hypotension produced by 11 in sodium depleted subjects[42], but a 2.3-fold increase in plasma BK was observed in sodium depleted essential hypertensive patients[43]. Unlike most antihypertensive drugs, this nonapeptide increased renal blood flow in spite of its lowering of blood pressure[43,44]; this intrarenal effect was not associated with an increase in BK[44].

Other potential uses of ACE inhibitors have been explored. Several investigators (see reference 45) have suggested the possible use of the nonapeptide 11 for treatment of shock. At 1 mg/kg, 11 protected dogs from death following hemorrhagic shock; AII levels during shock were decreased 10-fold, and increases in vasopressin were unaffected. Studies with 11 have also indicated that the renin-angiotensin system is essential for the compensatory response to circulatory insufficiency in an animal model of congestive heart failure[46]. In patients with established heart failure, this nonapeptide improved cardiac function by decreasing peripheral resistance and afterload on the heart[47].

Recently, a second class of potent and specific inhibitors of ACE has been developed that has the additional advantage of oral activity[48]. These compounds, carboxyalkanoyl and mercaptoalkanoyl amino acid derivatives, were designed for optimal binding to the active site of ACE as visualized in a hypothetical model based on the known active site of a similar exopeptidase, carboxypeptidase A[48,49], which, like ACE, has a Zn ion at the active site. The most potent inhibitor of this class is SQ 14,225 [D-3-mercapto-2-methylpropanoyl-L-proline (S,S), 12], a competitive inhibitor with a K_i value of 1.7×10^{-9} M. The sulfhydryl function, amide carbonyl, and carboxylic acid group of 12 are thought to bind to the zinc ion, a hydrogen bonding group, and a positively charged residue, respectively, at the active site of ACE[48,49]. Structure-activity studies[49] have confirmed the great importance of these three structural features of this inhibitor and have also indicated that the acyl chain length, the 2-methyl substituent, and the pyrrolidine ring are optimal for binding to the enzyme. Hydroxamic acid derivatives related to 12[50] and ureidoacetohydroxamates (13)[51] have also been described as ACE inhibitors. In the interaction of these compounds with the enzyme, the hydroxamic acid functionality probably binds to the Zn ion.

12 (captopril)

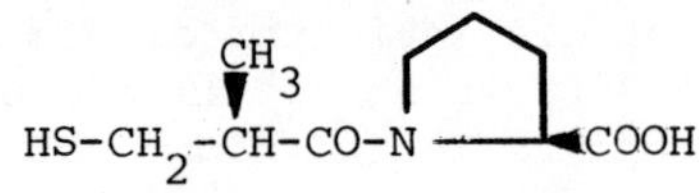

13

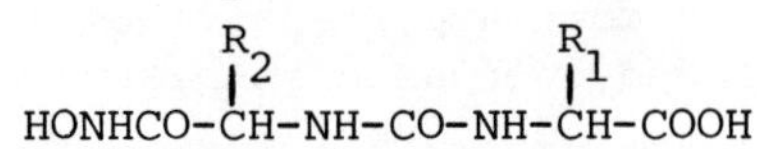

In rats, 12 administered orally was at least ten times more inhibitory, on a weight basis, than the nonapeptide 11 administered parenterally[52]; it specifically inhibited AI vasopressor activity and augmented BK vasodepressor activity in rats, cats, dogs, and rabbits[52-55]. Administered centrally, 12 did not affect blood pressure, but did inhibit central effects of AI; the compound, however, did not readily cross the blood-brain barrier[55]. At 3-30 mg/kg oral doses, it rapidly lowered blood pressure by 50 to 60 mm Hg in two-kidney RHR. At the higher dose, blood pressure did not return to normal in 24 hours[56]. The drug lowered more slowly the blood pressure of spontaneously hypertensive rats (SHR)[56,57], with about a 30 mm Hg drop, but did not appreciably affect pressures of normotensive rats. Only a mild tachycardia was observed with 12; this was not related to the degree or suddenness of the blood pressure drop. After 11 days of treatment in spontaneously hypertensive rats, no evidence was obtained for decreased responsiveness[56]. Compound 12 also inhibited the vasopressor activity of AI in human volunteers[58]; total blockade for 2 hours was obtained at an oral dose of 0.3 mg/kg. No untoward side effects or changes in biochemical parameters were observed in this first clinical study.

Angiotensin-Receptor Antagonists: Extensive structure-activity studies on analogs of AII carried out since its original synthesis in 1957 led in 1970 to the development of specific AII receptor antagonists: [Ile^5, Ala^8]-AII was shown to inhibit the contractile response of guinea pig ileum to AII[59], and [Phe^4, Val^5, Tyr^8]-AII was shown to be a competitive inhibitor of the AII actions *in vitro* and *in vivo*[60]. The Ala^8 analogs of

Ile^5-AII and Asn^1-Val^5-AII were later reported to inhibit the vasopressor action of AII in rats[61,62] but not in cats[63].

A major development in the search for useful AII antagonists was the observation that replacement of the asparagine residue in position 1 of the Asn^1-Val^5-Ala^8-AII analog by sarcosine[64] led to a substantial increase in the antagonistic activity. Subsequently, similar observations were made with the Ile^8, Leu^8, and Phg^8 analogs[65-67]. Since that time, a considerable effort has been devoted to the development of new and more specific antagonists and to the reduction of the intrinsic agonistic activity of these compounds. Structure-activity studies have been recently reviewed[37,68], and several papers have appeared since these reviews that have further refined our understanding of the interactions between AII receptors and agonists or antagonists[69-71]. Based on these studies the following conclusions can be drawn. 1) Replacement of the Phe^8 residue of AII by an aliphatic amino acid is the single most important modification required to obtain an antagonist or to decrease substantially the agonistic activity. 2) Replacement of the N-terminal aspartic acid residue with sarcosine increases the agonistic or antagonistic potency *in vitro* and *in vivo*, mostly due to a stronger binding to, and a slower dissociation from, the receptor, but also and to a smaller extent by increasing resistance to enzymatic degradation[72]. 3) None of the antagonists developed so far is completely devoid of agonistic activity[73], and some authors[74] have emphasized that these compounds should be more correctly referred to as weak competitive agonists. 4) Some of the most commonly studied AII antagonists are Ile^5 analogs, and some are Val^5 analogs. Where this substitution was specifically examined[75,76], no major differences were observed, even though minor ones do appear to exist[76].

<u>14</u> (saralasin)	Sar-Arg-Val-Tyr-Val-His-Pro-Ala
<u>15</u> (Sar^1-Ala^8-AII)	Sar-Arg-Val-Tyr-Ile-His-Pro-Ala
<u>16</u> (Sar^1-Ile^8-AII)	Sar-Arg-Val-Tyr-Ile-His-Pro-Ile
<u>17</u> (Sar^1-Thr^8-AII)	Sar-Arg-Val-Tyr-Ile-His-Pro-Thr
<u>18</u> (Ile^0-AIII)	Arg-Val-Tyr-Ile-His-Pro-Ile

The angiotensin antagonists that have been most thoroughly studied *in vivo* are saralasin (<u>14</u>), Sar^1-Ala^8-AII (<u>15</u>), Sar^1-Ile^8-AII (<u>16</u>), and Sar^1-Thr^8-AII (<u>17</u>). The Sar^1-Ile^8 and Sar^1-Thr^8 analogs are the most potent antagonists of the blood pressure increase induced by exogeneous AII[65,77,78]. Sar^1-Ile^8-AII has equal or more agonistic activity than Sar^1-Ala^8-AII, but Sar^1-Thr^8-AII has significantly less agonistic activity than either[77,78]. A more recently synthesized analog [Sar^1-$Thr(Me)^8$]-AII, has an even higher antagonist activity than the Thr^8 analog, but this modification unfortunately also increases significantly the agonistic activity[79]. The same comparative degree of agonistic activity of these analogs can be also observed in their stimulation of aldosterone release from the adrenal cortex[39,78] and catecholamine release from adrenal medulla[79]. All AII antagonists developed so far have a comparatively short duration of action *in vivo* and must be administered by continuous infusion.

Angiotensin antagonists (saralasin, Sar^{1}-Ile^{8}-AII, and Sar^{1}-Thr^{8}-AII) have been shown to lower blood pressure in the acute hypertensive phase of two-kidney RHR[64,80,81] and one-kidney RHR (unclipped kidney removed)[81] when infused at a maximal dose of 10 to 60 μg/kg/min. The acute (renin dependent) hypertensive phase in the one-kidney model is so short that in many cases angiotensin antagonists and other renin-angiotensin system blockers have been found inactive in this model. In the chronic phase of both models the renin dependency disappears, and angiotensin antagonists are inactive[64,80,81]. Similar results were obtained in a new model of two-kidney hypertension in conscious dogs[82]. Renin dependency and, therefore, response to angiotensin antagonists in these models can be reinstated by sodium depletion[80]. In the SHR, saralasin[64] and several analogs of Phg^{8}-AII[67] have been found inactive. However, Sar^{1}-Ile^{8}-AII (5.5 μg/kg/min)[83] and Sar^{1}-Thr^{8}-AII (1 μg/kg/min)[84] lower blood pressure in this model, and, in the case of Sar^{1}-Thr^{8}-AII, this effect appeared to be dependent on the age of the rats.

The availability of saralasin has prompted a considerable number of clinical studies with this angiotensin antagonist in normal subjects and hypertensive patients. Saralasin is usually administered by infusion, but bolus intravenous injection has been studied[85,86] for diagnostic purposes in hypertensive patients. In normal man, saralasin (10-20 μg/kg/min) has generally been found to lower blood pressure significantly only under the combined stimulus of sodium restriction and upright posture[87-89], and this response depended on the degree of sodium balance[90]. When Sar^{1}-Ile^{8}-AII and Sar^{1}-Ala^{8}-AII were compared in normal subjects[91] in the supine position, it was found that both analogs had vasopressor activity after salt repletion or regular diet, and that Sar^{1}-Ile^{8}-AII had vasopressor activity even in salt depleted subjects, thus confirming the higher agonistic activity of this analog found in animals.

In hypertensive patients, saralasin has been shown to produce consistent lowering of blood pressure only in those patients with high plasma renin activity[74,92-95], and similar results were obtained with Sar^{1}-Ile^{8}-AII[96,97]. Low-renin hypertensive patients showed vasopressor responses after saralasin infusion[74,88-90], and normal-renin patients have shown either no response, or a mildly vasopressor response[74]. Due to their residual agonistic activity, the angiotensin antagonists so far available for clinical studies can only be used reliably in the diagnosis of the renin component of hypertension in those cases where a clear vasodepressor response has been obtained. The usefulness of prior sodium depletion for this diagnosis has been proposed[92], and questioned[74].

The analogs obtained by replacing the Phe^{8} residue of the heptapeptide AIII by an aliphatic amino acid residue are more specific antagonists of the AII-stimulated aldosterone secretion than the corresponding octapeptide analogs[68]. The Ile^{8}-AIII analog (<u>18</u>) has now been shown to have both agonistic and antagonistic activities on blood pressure and aldosterone secretion in normal human subjects[98], even though its effect is more pronounced on the adrenal function than on the peripheral vasculature. The data gathered so far utilizing this new heptapeptide inhibitor have not provided conclusive evidence for the hypothesis that the conversion of AII to AIII is a necessary step in the stimulation of aldosterone biosynthesis[73]. The recent finding[99] that rat adrenal tissue has binding sites with high affinity, specific only for AIII and sites with lower affinity that can bind both AII and AIII, suggests, however, that under physiological conditions AIII may be the normal stimulus for aldosterone secretion.

Conclusions: Renin inhibitors have a unique potential for studying the pathophysiological function of the renin-angiotensin system, since they lack the ambiguity of angiotensin antagonists (partial agonism) or ACE inhibitors (bradykinin potentiation). However, none of the inhibitors of renin that have been developed to date have been thoroughly evaluated *in vivo*. Parenterally administered AII antagonists and ACE inhibitors have contributed significantly to our understanding of the renin angiotensin system and its role in human hypertension. The orally active ACE inhibitors show great promise as a novel type of antihypertensive drug.

References

1. S. Oparil, "Renin 1976", Eden Press, Montreal, 1976.
2. M. J. Peach, Physiol. Rev., 57, 313 (1977).
3. L. T. Skeggs, F. E. Dorer, J. R. Kahn, K. E. Lentz, and M. Levine, Am. J. Med., 60, 737 (1976).
4. L. T. Skeggs, M. Levine, K. E. Lentz, J. R. Kahn, and F. E. Dorer, Fed. Proc., 36, 1755 (1977).
5. E. Haber, Circulation, 54, 849 (1976).
6. R. L. Soffer, Ann. Rev. Biochem., 45, 73 (1976).
7. E. G. Erdös, Fed. Proc., 36, 1760 (1977).
8. J. O. Davis and R. H. Freeman, Biochem. Pharmacol., 26, 93 (1977).
9. P. A. Khairallah and M. M. Hall in "Hypertension: Physiopathology and Treatment", J. Genest, E. Koiw, O. Kuchel, Eds., McGraw-Hill, New York, N.Y., 1977, p. 179.
10. S. Sen, R. R. Smeby, and F. M. Bumpus, Biochemistry, 6, 1572 (1967).
11. M. Miyazaki and K. Yamamoto, Proc. Soc. Exp. Biol. Med., 155, 468 (1977).
12. J. C. Turcotte, C. S. Yu, H. L. Lee, S. K. Pavanaram, S. Sen, and R. R. Smeby, J. Med. Chem., 18, 1184 (1975).
13. K. Hosoki, M. Miyazaki, and K. Yamamoto, J. Pharmacol. Exp. Therap., 203, 485 (1977).
14. M. Overturf, E. R. Druilhet, and W. M. Kirkendall, Biochem. Pharmacol., 25, 2443 (1976).
15. F. Gross, J. Lazar, and H. Orth, Science, 175, 656 (1972).
16. R. P. Miller, C. J. Poper, C. W. Wilson, and E. DeVito, Biochem. Pharmacol., 21, 2941 (1972).
17. T. Aoyagi, H. Morishima, R. Nishizawa, S. Kunimoto, T. Takeuchi, and H. Umezawa, J. Antibiot., 25, 689 (1972).
18. D. H. Rich, E. Sun, and J. Singh, Biochem. Biophys. Res. Commun., 74, 762 (1977).
19. B. A. Schölkens and W. Jung, Arch. Int. Pharmacodyn., 208, 24 (1974).
20. T. Kokubu, K. Hiwada, T. Ito, E. Ueda, Y. Yamamura, T. Mizoguchi, and K. Shigezane, Biochem. Pharmacol., 22, 3217 (1973).
21. K. Poulsen, J. Burton, and E. Haber, Biochemistry, 12, 3877 (1973).
22. I. Parikh and P. Cuatrecasas, Biochem. Biophys. Res. Commun., 54, 1356 (1973).
23. K. Poulsen, J. Burton, and E. Haber, Prog. Biochem. Pharmacol., 12, 135 (1976).
24. K. Poulsen, E. Haber, and J. Burton, Biochim. Biophys. Acta, 452, 533 (1976).
25. E. G. Erdös, Biochem. Pharmacol., 25, 1563 (1976).
26. S. H. Ferreira, Brit. J. Pharmacol., 24, 163 (1965).
27. Y. S. Bakhle, Nature, 220, 919 (1968).
28. S. H. Ferreira, D. C. Bartelt, and L. J. Greene, Biochemistry, 9, 2583 (1970).
29. M. A. Ondetti, N. J. Williams, E. F. Sabo, J. Pluščec, E. R. Weaver, and O. Kocy, Biochemistry, 10, 4033 (1971).
30. H. Kato and T. Suzuki, Biochemistry, 10, 972 (1971).
31. L. J. Greene, A. C. M. Camargo, E. Krieger, J. M. Stewart, and S. H. Ferreira, Circ. Res., 30, II-62 (1972).

32. S. L. Engel, T. R. Schaeffer, M. H. Waugh, and B. Rubin, Proc. Soc. Exp. Biol. Med., 143, 483 (1973).
33. H. S. Cheung and D. W. Cushman, Biochim. Biophys. Acta, 293, 451 (1973).
34. E. Haber and C. Barger, Prog. Biochem. Pharmacol., 12, 16 (1976).
35. D. W. Cushman, J. Pluščec, N. J. Williams, E. R. Weaver, E. F. Sabo, O. Kocy, H. S. Cheung, and M. A. Ondetti, Experientia, 29, 1032 (1973).
36. E. B. Sabia, M. Tomenaga, A. C. M. Paiva, and T. B. Paiva, J. Med. Chem., 20, 1679 (1977).
37. G. R. Marshall, Fed. Proc., 35, 2494 (1976).
38. G. A. Stephens, J. O. Davis, R. H. Freeman, B. E. Watkins, and M. C. Khosla, Endocrinology, 101, 378 (1977).
39. R. E. McCaa, Circ. Res., 40, I-157 (1977).
40. D. B. Case, J. M. Wallace, H. J. Keim, M. A. Weber, J. E. Sealey, and J. H. Laragh, New Eng. J. Med., 296, 641 (1977).
41. H. Gavras, H. R. Brunner, J. H. Laragh, J. E. Sealey, I. Gavras, and R. Vukovich, New Eng. J. Med., 291, 817 (1974).
42. J. Sancho, R. Re, J. Burton, A. C. Barger, and E. Haber, Circulation, 53, 400 (1976).
43. G. H. Williams and N. K. Hollenberg, New Eng. J. Med., 297, 184 (1977).
44. N. K. Hollenberg, G. H. Williams, K. J. Taub, I. Ishikawa, C. Brown, and D. F. Adams, Kidney Int., 12, 285 (1977).
45. J. J. Morton, P. F. Semple, I. M. Ledingham, B. Stuart, M. A. Tehrani, A. R. Garcia, and G. McGarrity, Circ. Res., 41, 301 (1977).
46. A. C. Barger, Agents and Actions, 6, 538 (1976).
47. P. Faxon, J. Berkoben, H. Gavras, P. Flessas, and T. J. Ryan, Circulation, 56, 117, (1977).
48. M. A. Ondetti, B. Rubin, and D. W. Cushman, Science, 196, 441 (1977).
49. D. W. Cushman, H. S. Cheung, E. F. Sabo, and M. A. Ondetti, Biochemistry, 16, 5484 (1977).
50. M. A. Ondetti, E. F. Sabo, K. A. Losee, H. S. Cheung, D. W. Cushman, and B. Rubin, "Peptides, Proceedings of the Fifth American Peptide Symposium", M. Goodman and J. Meienhofer, Eds., John Wiley & Sons, New York, N.Y., 1977, p. 576.
51. D. C. Fessler, G. A. Heavner, and T. H. Massay, U.S. Patent #4,028,401, June 7, 1977.
52. B. Rubin, R. J. Laffan, D. G. Kotler, E. H. O'Keefe, D. DeMaio, and M. E. Goldberg, J. Pharmacol. Exp. Therap. (In Press).
53. V. S. Murthy, T. L. Waldron, M. E. Goldberg, and R. R. Vollmer, Eur. J. Pharmacol., 46, 207 (1977).
54. V. S. Murthy, T. L. Waldron, and M. E. Goldberg, Proc. Soc. Exp. Biol. Med., 157, 121 (1978).
55. R. R. Vollmer and J. A. Boccagno, Eur. J. Pharmacol., 45, 117 (1977).
56. R. J. Laffan, M. E. Goldberg, J. P. High, T. R. Schaeffer, M. H. Waugh, and B. Rubin, J. Pharmacol. Exp. Therap. (In Press).
57. E. E. Muirhead, R. L. Prewitt, B. Brooks, and W. L. Brosius, Clin. Res., 25, A603 (1977).
58. R. K. Ferguson, G. A. Turini, H. R. Brunner, H. Gavras, and D. McKinstry, Lancet, 775, (1977).
59. P. A. Khairallah, A. Toth, and F. M. Bumpus, J. Med. Chem., 13, 181 (1970).
60. G. R. Marshall, W. Vine, and P. Needleman, Proc. Nat. Acad. Sci., 67, 1624 (1970).
61. W. K. Park and D. Regoli, Brit, J. Pharmacol., 43, 418P (1971).
62. D. T. Pals, F. D. Masucci, F. Sipös, and G. S. Denning, Jr., Circ. Res., 29, 664 (1971).
63. R. K. Türker, M. Yamamoto, P. A. Khairallah, and F. M. Bumpus, Eur. J. Pharmacol., 15, 285 (1971).
64. D. T. Pals, F. D. Masucci, G. S. Denning, Jr., F. Sipos, and D. C. Fessler, Circ. Res., 29, 673 (1971).
65. R. K. Türker, M. M. Hall, M. Yamamoto, C. S. Sweet, and F. M. Bumpus, Science, 177, 1203 (1972).
66. D. Regoli, F. Rioux, and N. K. Park. Rev. Can. Biol., 31, 73 (1972).
67. B. A. Schoelkens, Clin. Sci. Mol. Med., 48, 19s (1975).
68. F. M. Bumpus and M. C. Khosla in "Hypertension: Physiopathology and Treatment", J. Genest, E. Koiw, O. Kuchel, Eds., McGraw-Hill, New York, N.Y., 1977, p. 183.
69. M. C. Khosla, M. M. Hall, H. Muñoz-Ramírez, P. A. Khairallah, F. M. Bumpus, J. H. Seely, and A. M. Thomas, J. Med. Chem., 20, 253 (1977).
70. M. C. Khosla, H. Muñoz-Ramírez, M. M. Hall, P. A. Khairallah, and F. M. Bumpus, J. Med. Chem., 20 , 1051 (1977).
71. A. C. M. Paiva, V. L. A. Nouailhetas, and T. B. Paiva, J. Med. Chem., 20, 898 (1977).
72. D. Regoli, F. Rioux, W. K. Park, and C. Choi, Can. J. Physiol. Pharmacol., 52, 39 (1974).

73. F. M. Bumpus, Fed. Proc., 36, 2128 (1977).
74. D. B. Case, J. M. Wallace, H. J. Keim, J. E. Sealey, J. H. Laragh, Am. J. Med., 60, 825 (1976).
75. D. Regoli, W. K. Park. F. Rioux, Pharmacol. Rev., 26, 69 (1974).
76. B. A. Schoelkens, H. Wissmann, E. Lindner, R. Geiger, Z. Physiol. Chem., 357, 825 (1976).
77. H. Muñoz-Ramírez, M. C. Khosla, M. M. Hall, F. M. Bumpus, and P. A. Khairallah, Res. Commun. Chem. Path. Pharmacol., 13, 649 (1976).
78. E. L. Bravo, M. C. Khosla, and F. M. Bumpus, Prog. Biochem. Pharmacol., 12, 33 (1976).
79. M. C. Khosla, H. Muñoz-Ramírez, M. M. Hall, R. R. Smeby, P. A. Khairallah, F. M. Bumpus, and M. J. Peach, J. Med. Chem., 19, 244 (1976).
80. H. Gavras, H. R. Brunner, H. Thurston, and J. H. Laragh, Science, 188, 1316 (1975).
81. C. M. Ferrario, F. M. Bumpus, Z. Masaki, M. C. Khosla, and J. W. McCubbin, Prog. Biochem. Pharmacol., 12, 86 (1976).
82. Z. Masaki, C. M. Ferrario, F. M. Bumpus, E. L. Bravo, and M. C. Khosla, Clin. Sci. Mol. Med., 52, 163 (1977).
83. T. G. Dimitrov, D. I. Kiprov, A. I. Maleeva, and S. A. Terziyska, Compt. Rend. Acad. Bulg. Sci., 30, 771 (1977).
84. H. Muñoz-Ramírez, M. C. Khosla, F. M. Bumpus, and P. A. Khairallah, Pharmacologist, 18, 229 (1976).
85. L. S. Marks, M. H. Maxwell, and J. J. Kaufman, Lancet, 2, 784 (1975).
86. D. H. P. Streeton, G. H. Anderson, Jr., and T. G. Dalakos, Am. J. Med., 60, 817 (1976).
87. R. H. Noth, S. Y. Tan, P. J. Mulrow, J. Clin. Endocrinol. Metab., 45, 10 (1977).
88. G. A. MacGregor and P. M. Dawes, Clin. Sci. Mol. Med., 51, 193s (1976).
89. J. J. Brown, W. C. B. Brown, R. Fraser, A. F. Lever, J. J. Morton, J. I. S. Robertson, E. A. Rosei, and P. M. Trust, Aust. N.Z. J. Med., 6, Suppl. 3, 48 (1976).
90. H. R. Brunner, H. Gavras, A. B. Ribeiro, L. Posternak, Prog. Biochem. Pharmacol., 12, 145 (1976).
91. T. Ogihara, T. Hata, H. Mikami, T. Mandai, and Y. Kumahara, Life Sci., 20, 1855 (1977).
92. D. H. P. Streeten, T. G. Dalakos, and G. H. Anderson, Jr., Prog. Biochem. Pharmacol., 12, 214 (1976).
93. Th. Philipp, H. Zschiedrich, and A. Distler, Klin, Wochensch., 55, 917 (1977).
94. R. Fagard, A. Amery, P. Lijnen, and T. Reybrouck, Eur. J. Clin. Pharmacol., 12, 1 (1977).
95. W. A. Pettinger, H. C. Mitchell, Fed. Proc., 35, 2521 (1976).
96. T. Yamamoto, T. Ogihara, T. Hata, K. Ichihara, Y. Kumahara, Jap. J. Med., 16, 117 (1977).
97. M. Yasujima, K. Abe, N. Irokawa, K. Ritsu, M. Seino, K. Saito, Y. Sakurai, S. Chiba, T. Ito, and K. Yoshinaga, Tohuka J. Exp. Med., 122, 191 (1977).
98. T. Kono, F. Oseko, F. Ikeda, M. Nanno, and J. Endo, Acta Endocrinol., 86, 156 (1977).
99. M. Devynck, M. Pernollet, P. G. Matthews, M. C. Khosla, F. M. Bumpus, and P. Meyer, Proc. Nat. Acad, Sci., 74, 4029 (1977).

Chapter 10. Agents for the Treatment of Heart Failure

Simon F. Campbell and John C. Danilewicz

Pfizer Central Research, Sandwich, Kent, England

Introduction - Heart failure exists when cardiac function is compromised to a point that the needs of peripheral organs are not satisfied. Wagner and Cohn[1] offer the following classification:- systolic failure, in which the left ventricle fails to contract adequately, diastolic failure, in which the left ventricle fails to relax sufficiently and overload of the heart, which includes volume overload states. Burch[2] points out that cardiac failure should not be viewed solely as a low output state and stresses the importance of an appropriate balance between right and left heart function. This interesting view has been the subject of very recent comment.[3]

Drugs used for treating heart failure are primarily the cardiac glycosides and diuretics. The cardiac glycosides are positive inotropic agents, i.e. increase the force of myocardial contraction, though their effect on cardiac rhythm may also be important. Diuretics relieve symptoms of congestion by reducing plasma volume but are not considered in this review. Recently, attention has been turning to the response of the peripheral vasculature to the failing heart and vasodilators are being increasingly investigated. A number of new inotropic agents also appear to be in various stages of development. This review is primarily concerned with developments over the last two years.

Cardiac Glycosides - The side effects of cardiac glycosides are well recognised[4] though in a prospective study involving 649 patients on maintenance therapy with digitoxin, a low incidence (5.8%) was found.[5] This was ascribed to careful usage of the glycoside. Cardiac glycosides are particularly effective in cases where cardiac rhythm is accelerated.[6] Indeed, their use in failure accompanied by normal sinus rhythm has been questioned.[6-9]

Currently there is a debate of considerable interest on the mechanism of action of cardiac glycosides. One view is that the positive inotropic activity of these agents is due to the inhibition of myocardial cell membrane Na^+-K^+ transport ATPase (Na^+-pump). The function of this system is to exchange intracellular Na^+ for extracellular K^+, which is achieved in a ratio of approximately 3:2. The trans-membrane ion fluxes involved in the excitation-contraction process are complex and have been recently discussed.[10,11] Considering only Na^+, the process is visualised to function as follows: (a) Na^+ rapidly enters the cell on excitation, (b) increasing intracellular $[Na^+]$ progressively activates the pump to the point when Na^+ extrusion balances entry and peak $[Na^+]$ is achieved, (c) the pump, by then fully activated, coupled with reduced passive membrane permeability to Na^+, repolarises the cell by returning $[Na^+]$ to resting levels. The

ISBN 0-12-040513-X

temporary increase in intracellular $[Na^+]$ is termed the "Na^+ transient". Pump inhibition will allow Na^+ entry to persist at a higher rate, reach a greater maximum concentration and reduce its rate of extrusion from the cell. The Na^+ transient is thus increased, resulting in a greater mobilisation of Ca^{++}, which controls contraction.[12,13] With only partial inhibition, it is not necessary to invoke net Na^+ accumulation at therapeutic doses of cardiac glycosides. However, as doses increase, the pump will be inhibited to a degree that the extrusion of Na^+ will be incomplete before the beginning of the next depolarisation cycle. This results in progressive Na^+ accumulation and eventually to myocardial intoxication. Toxicity and therapeutic effect are seen therefore to depend on the same biochemical mechanism and this poses considerable problems when searching for agents of this class with a greater margin of safety.

The alternative view is that the positive inotropic activity of the cardiac glycosides can be achieved independently of Na^+-pump inhibition. In cardiac tissue exposed to ouabain, the inotropic effect disappears in minutes after wash-out whilst cardiac toxicity persists for several hours.[14,15] In isolated guinea-pig atria, starting with low doses (10^{-9}-10^{-8}M) of ouabain, inotropism is associated with stimulation of the Na^+-pump. Concentrations above this range cause further increases in systolic tension but with pump inhibition.[16] Furthermore, in the same tissue there are high and low affinity ouabain-specific binding sites linked to pump stimulation and inhibition respectively.[17] Positive inotropic activity has been demonstrated with ouabain in vivo in the dog without pump inhibition,[18] whilst measurement of myocardial K^+ content during the development of digoxin positive inotropism suggests pump stimulation.[19] How pump stimulation results in a greater mobilisation of Ca^{++} remains to be explained but the demonstration that an inotropic effect is possible without pump inhibition, which is known to be associated with toxicity, should give encouragement for a more vigorous search for safer agents.[20]

A complicating factor in the interpretation of the mode of action of the cardiac glycosides in vivo is that they have neuroexcitatory activity. A significant vagomimetic action has been demonstrated at therapeutic doses[21-23] and this probably accounts for their effectiveness in atrial flutter and fibrillation.[24] Additionally, sympathetic nerve stimulation has been shown to coincide with the onset of arrhythmia in animals.[25] One group conclude that the primary site of action is within the peripheral nervous system,[26] whilst another find it to be central in origin.[25] Reserpine, guanethidine and β-blockers[27] as well as clonidine[25] protect against cardiac glycoside-induced arrhythmias in animals, thus implicating the involvement of the sympathetic nervous system. It has been suggested therefore that a cardiac glycoside which does not enter the brain may have a safety advantage.[24]

Cardiac Glycoside Analogues - An aminosugar cardiac glycoside , ASI-222 (1) produced a greater maximum increase in contractile force than ouabain and digoxin in the dog with a more rapid onset of activity, greater potency and less evidence of toxicity.[28-30] A study including a close analogue, ASI-254 (2), showed that the greater therapeutic index of these compounds is not

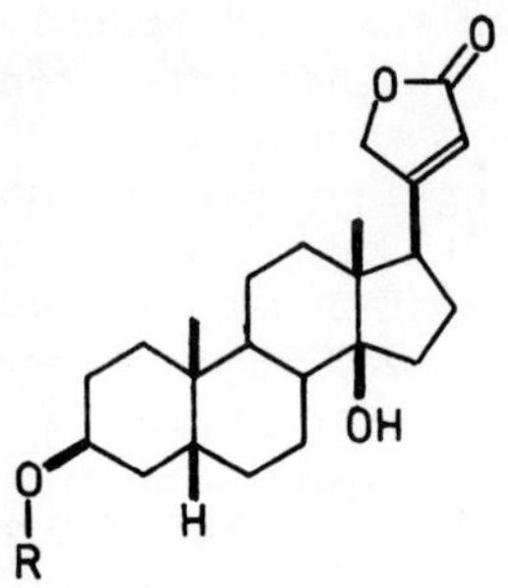

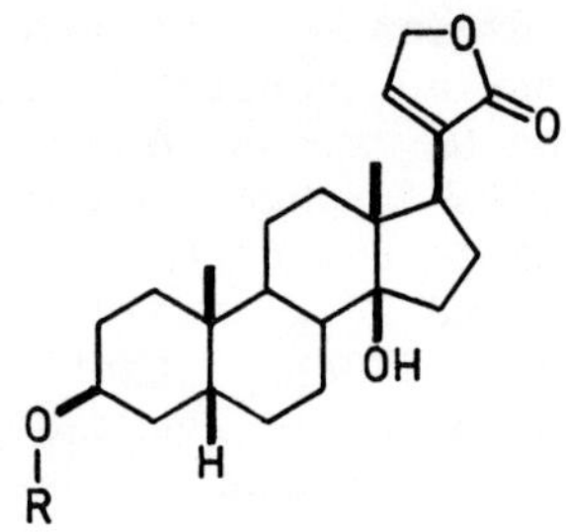

1 ASI-222, R=4-amino-4,6-dideoxy-β-D-galactopyranosyl.

2 ASI-254, R=4-amino-4,6-dideoxy-β-D-glucopyranosyl.

3 AY-22,241 R=β-D-glucopyranosyl.

associated with reduced inhibition of Na^+-K^+ATPase.[31] In the rat 3β-acetylthio-3-deoxydigitoxigenin may have a toxicity advantage over 3-O-acetyl-digitoxigenin.[32] In a comparative study with ouabain in anaesthetised dogs, Actinogen (actodigin, AY-22,241) (3) was inotropic at lower fractions of the toxic dose. The onset of activity and recovery from toxicity were also more rapid.[33] This paralleled results obtained with the isolated Na^+-K^+ATPase enzyme[34] and though not effective on acute administration to patients with congestive heart failure, actodigin proved very effective in controlling atrial fibrillation.[35] In a volunteer study, AQM-263 (4)[36] has shown slightly greater potency than digoxin.[37] This follows from the earlier demonstration that the activity of digitoxigenin could be essentially retained by replacing the lactone ring by some open chain α,β-unsaturated systems.[38] However, it is now clear that the presence of an α,β-unsaturated system is not necessary for inotropic or Na^+-K^+ATPase inhibitory activity. The furan analogue (5) shows comparable inotropic activity to digitoxin in isolated guinea-pig atria[39] and a greater margin of safety than digitoxin in the anaesthetised dog.[40] A compound, SC-4453, in which the 17β-lactone ring of digoxin is replaced

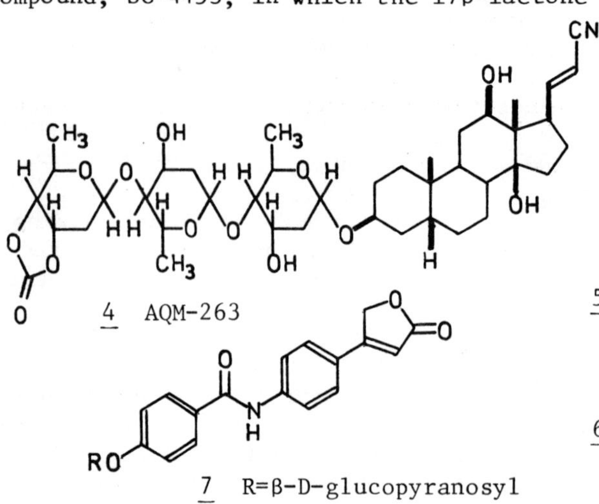

4 AQM-263

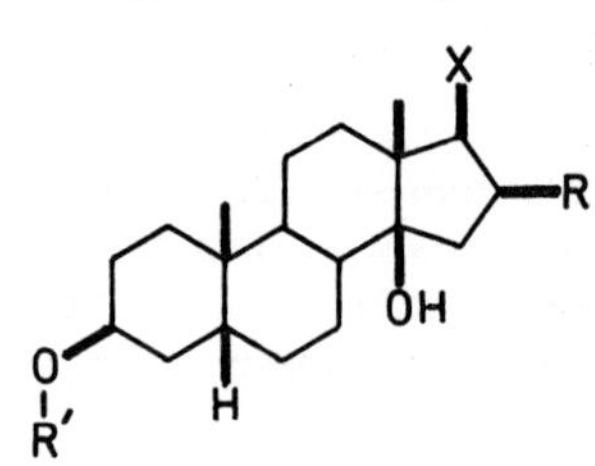

5 R=OH, X=3-furyl, R'=4-O-(2,6-dideoxy-D-ribohexopyranosyl)-2,6-dideoxy-D-ribohexopyranosyl.

6 R=H, X=4-pyridazinyl, R'=6-deoxy-3-O-methyl-α-L-glucopyranosyl.

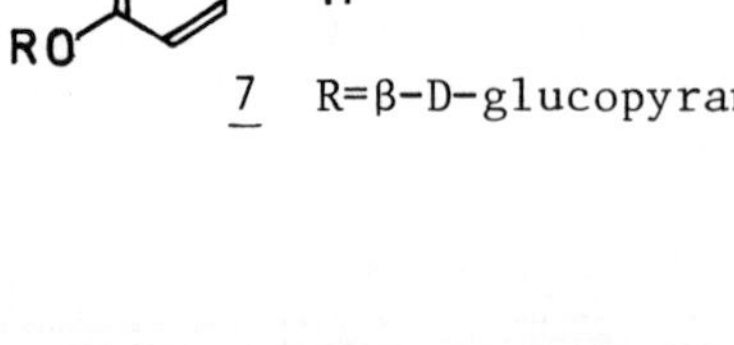

7 R=β-D-glucopyranosyl

by a 4-pyridazinyl group, has shown similar Na^{+}-K^{+}ATPase inhibitory activity to digoxin.[41] An analogue, SC-4362 (6) is a tenth as potent and is claimed to have been effective in a case of cardiac failure.[42] Replacement of the steroid system in cardiac glycosides by alternative simplified structures has been disappointing. An interesting exception is compound (7) which has shown greater inotropic efficacy than ouabain in isolated hearts with considerably less evidence of toxicity.[43]

Vasodilators - The use and mechanism of vasodilators in the treatment of heart failure have been extensively reviewed in 1977.[44-48] Their mode of action is interpreted by considering three points:- preload, which determines ventricular filling pressure, the inotropic state of the heart, that is the ability to perform work and afterload, which is a measure of arterial impedance to the ejection of blood during systole.[48] In health, stroke volume can be maintained within limits in the face of varying outflow impedance and, therefore, vasodilatation may produce hypotension if cardiac output is not sufficiently augmented by the reflex increase in heart rate. In decompensated heart failure, however, where no cardiac reserve exists, stroke volume bears a much accentuated inverse relationship to output impedance so that a reduction in peripheral resistance causes an increase in stroke volume. Cardiac output can therefore be increased with little effect on blood pressure and heart rate under optimum conditions. Thus, by reducing output impedance, which is generally raised in heart failure, vasodilators exert a salutary effect on cardiac performance. Most dilators also cause venodilatation to varying degrees and so by reducing preload, will relieve symptoms of pulmonary congestion and decrease myocardial oxygen consumption by reducing heart size. However, if venous pooling predominates, as with the nitrates, the advantages gained in reducing afterload will be lost, with little overall change in stroke volume unless left ventricular end diastolic pressure is markedly raised, when the heart is presumably functioning on the descending part of the Frank-Starling curve. Therefore, in analysing the effects of vasodilators, it is important to consider both the overall haemodynamic effect and the pathophysiological state of the patient.[49,50]

The current position with respect to sodium nitroprusside, nitroglycerin and isosorbide dinitrate is summarised in the recent reviews.[44-48] The principal action of the nitrates appears to be on the venous circulation and though a reduction in preload is observed, the effect on cardiac output is variable. Sodium nitroprusside has a rather more balanced action on preload and afterload but its use is limited to parenteral administration. Oral phentolamine has shown a beneficial effect extending to four hours, though tachycardia may be a problem.[51] However, most of 40 patients benefited from a slow release formulation acting over 12 hours.[52] Ten patients with refractory heart failure have shown clinical improvement with hydralazine[53] and in a further report, cardiac output was shown to increase without alteration in venous compliance.[54] In fact, the relative lack of effect of hydralazine on the venous circulation may limit its utility in congestive heart failure and its beneficial combination with nitrates administered over a 3-10 month period has been reported.[55] Relevant in this context is that hydralazine has a direct cardiac stimulant action which is mediated by β-adrenoceptors.[56] A patient who was unresponsive to nitrates responded to minoxidil with a significant increase in cardiac output without tachycardia or hypotension.[57] Oral trimazosin increased stroke volume in six patients, reducing both systemic and pulmonary vascular resistance.[58] Ten patients treated with prazosin showed beneficial effects persisting at least six hours, increased cardiac index being accompanied by a reduction both in arterial and venous tone.[59] The compound has also shown substantial benefit on daily administration over a two week period.[60] Its haemodynamic action on oral administration appears to be similar to that of parenteral sodium nitroprusside.[61]

Beta-Adrenoceptor Stimulants - Myocardial noradrenaline levels are markedly reduced in heart failure and there may also be a depressed inotropic response to released transmitter.[62,63] β-1 adrenoceptor agonists may therefore find use in heart failure but selective stimulation of force rather than rate of contraction is paramount. Controversy continues over the further sub-division of cardiac β-receptors into inotropic and chronotropic types, while in the whole animal any intrinsic force- or rate-selectivity of an agonist can be greatly modified by a whole range of compensatory mechanisms.[64-66]

Dobutamine (Dobutrex) (8) was launched onto the UK hospital market in 1977 for use after myocardial infarction and cardiac surgery. The use of dopamine (Intropin) and dobutamine in heart failure has been reviewed.[67] The cardiac effects of both compounds are blocked by propranolol indicating β-receptor mediation. There is little evidence for the involvement of dopamine receptors. Dobutamine is reported to be superior to dopamine in low output patients[68,69] although its force/rate selectivity has been questioned.[70] Both catecholamines have to be given by intravenous infusion and have a short duration of action, although clinical improvement was maintained for at least one week after a 72 hr infusion of dobutamine.[71] Dopamine and nitroprusside have been combined advantageously.[72] The metabolism of dobutamine in dogs has been reported.[73]

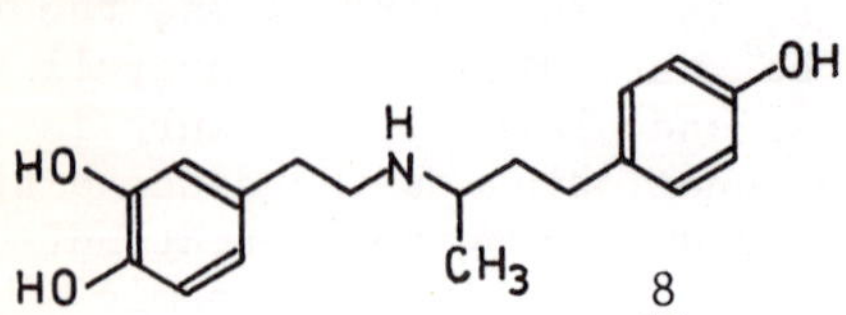

8

dobutamine

Intragastric administration of tazolol (9) to conscious dogs produced a marked increase in right ventricular contraction with little effect on heart rate.[74] The cardiac stimulant from aconite root, long used in Chinese medicine, has been identified as the β-agonist, higenamine (10)

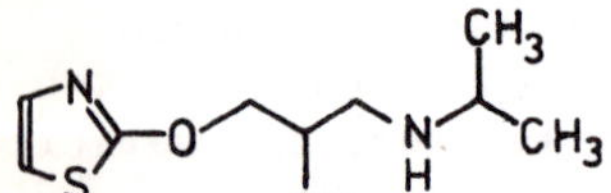

9

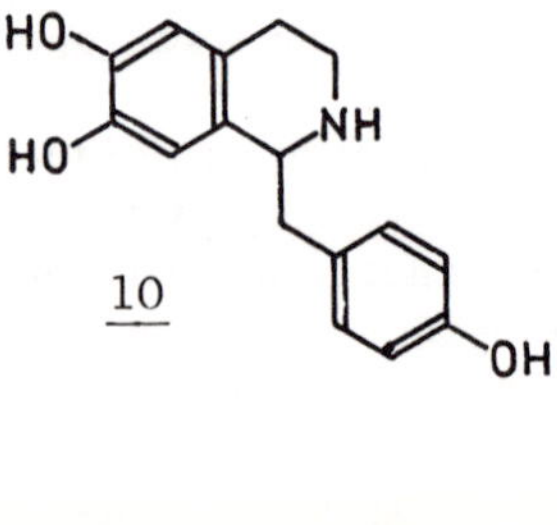

10

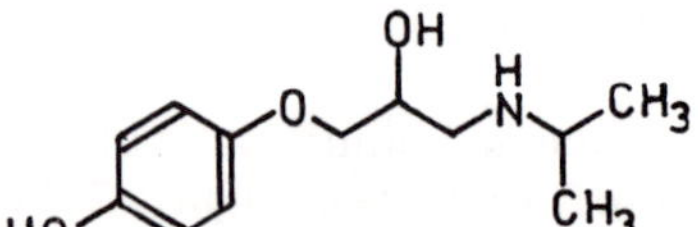

11

and the crystal structure has been determined.[75,76] H 80/62 (11) is said to produce inotropic stimulation in man with only little change in heart rate and peripheral vascular resistance[77] while oxyfedrine, a weak β-receptor agonist, also showed a positive inotropic action in volunteers.

Phosphodiesterase Inhibitors (PDEIs) - Although there are numerous examples of potent PDEIs, little success has been achieved in the past in developing a useful inotropic agent. Both theophylline and papaverine have cardiac stimulant activity but their use is limited by a range of additional pharmacological properties resulting probably from poor tissue and iso-enzyme selectivity.[79] Additionally, other mechanistic effects not related to PDEI often intrude.[80-82] In view of the opposing effects of cAMP and cGMP on myocardial contractility,[83,84] a basic requirement for a useful cardiac stimulant from this mechanistic class would be marked selectivity for cAMP- rather than cGMP-PDE.

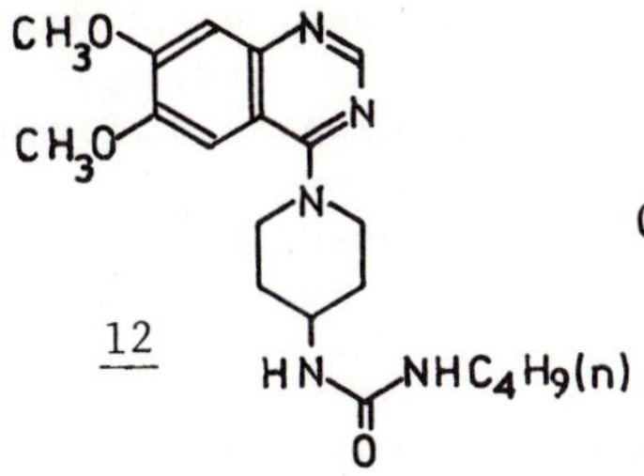

12

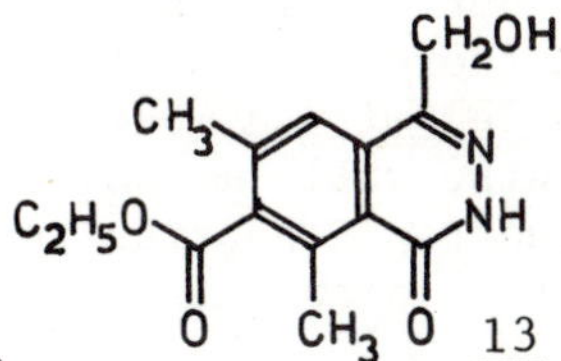

13

phthalazinol

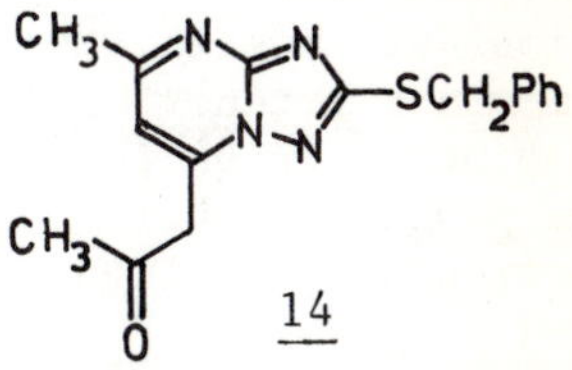

14

Interest in this area may be stimulated by UK-14,275 (12) which is some twenty times more potent than theophylline as an inhibitor of cAMP-PDE and which is an orally active, selective inotropic agent.[85] Infusion into normal volunteers[86] or patients with coronary heart disease[87] resulted in increased myocardial contractility without hypotension, tachycardia or subjective side effects being observed. Phthalazinol (EG 626) (13) is a potent selective inhibitor of human platelet cAMP-PDE.[88] Administration (300mg p.o.) to patients with ischaemic heart disease resulted in an increase in cardiac output but this could not be attributed unambiguously to a positive inotropic effect.[89] The s-triazolo(1,5a) pyrimidine derivative (14) is one of a related series of PDEIs which increased cardiac output in the dog with little effect on heart rate.[90]

Cyclic Nucleotide Analogues - SQ 80,122 (15) is superior to dibutyryl-cAMP as an inotropic agent, possibly acting by stimulation of a cAMP-dependent protein kinase.[91] In the dog, SQ 80,122 produced a positive inotropic effect not attenuated by β-blockade, with little effect on blood pressure and heart rate.

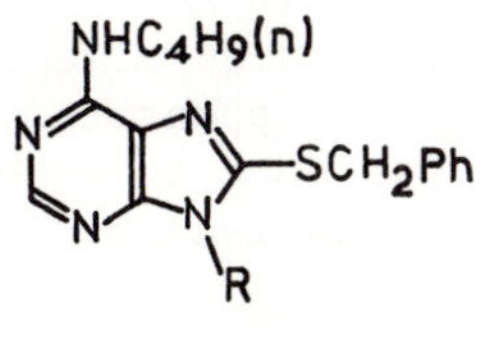

15

SQ 80,122

R=β-D-ribofuranosyl-3',5'-cyclicphosphate

Ionophores - The investigation of ionophores as cardiac stimulants has proved attractive over the past few years due to the availability of a range of compounds which transport mono- and di-valent cations across biological membranes.[92] Various ionophores have shown marked inotropic activity both in vitro and in vivo but these effects are reduced after β-blockade,[93,94] suggesting an indirect mechanism heavily dependent on catecholamine release.[95] This mode of action, together with the wide range of biological activities these compounds possess, may well limit clinical usefulness.

Cardiac Stimulant Peptides - The exciting development in this area, which may have a profound impact on our understanding of the mechanisms of cardiac contraction, has been the isolation and identification of a cardiac stimulant polypeptide from the sea anemone *Anthopleura xanthogrammica*.[96,97] The compound, anthopleurin A (AP-A), a fortynine unit polypeptide, is some thirty times more potent than digoxin as a cardiac stimulant in the anaesthetised dog and has a better therapeutic ratio.[98] Interestingly, the amino acid sequence is remarkably similar to the so-called toxin II isolated from *Anemonia sulcata* but the latter is a less effective cardiac stimulant, possibly having a different mode of action.[99] The cardiac stimulant potency of AP-A, coupled with a mode of action which is different from other known inotropic agents, will no doubt stimulate speculation on the possibility of a natural inotropic peptide receptor/transmitter system, particularly in light of recent developments in the morphine/enkephalin area.

Alpha-Adrenergic and Histamine Agonists - The predominant role of myocardial β-receptors is well established but evidence is now accumulating for the additional presence, in some species, of α, H-1 and H-2 receptors although their physiological significance still awaits clarification. The α-agonists methoxamine and phenylephrine produce positive inotropic effects in cat papillary muscle[100] and rat heart[101] respectively without activation of the adenyl cyclase/cAMP system. Indeed, it has been suggested that stimulation of α-receptors in rat heart leads to a decrease in cAMP[102] and an increase in cGMP.[103] The suggestion that cardiac α- and β-receptors are interconvertible under certain conditions[104,105] has been questioned.[106]

Histamine has been known since Dale's work to produce an inotropic effect but it is only recently that cardiac histamine receptors have been classified.[107,108] The situation is complex, however, as in guinea-pig heart, H-1 receptors are present in the left atrium and right ventricle with H-2 receptors in the right atrium and ventricle. Stimulation of either receptor can produce a positive inotropic effect but only H-2 activation is associated with an increase in cAMP.[109] The cardiac effects of both clonidine and tolazoline in isolated guinea-pig heart appear to involve histamine receptors[110,111] but the relevance of this data to other species is not clear.[112] Histamine receptors have been identified in human heart.[113]

Miscellaneous - In volunteers, the imidazo(4,5-b)pyridine derivative[114] AR-L57CL (16) produced a positive inotropic effect of short duration accompanied by subjective side effects.[115,116] Both amrinone (Win 40,680) (17) and Win 35,020 (18) produced a long-lasting inotropic effect after oral administration in the dog.[117,118] 9-Hydroxyellipticine (19)

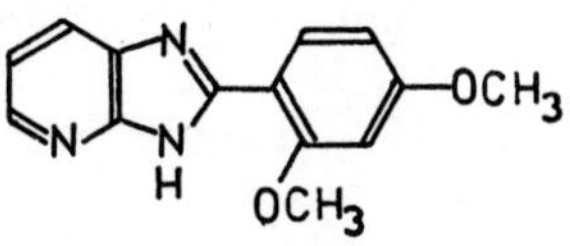

16 AR-L57CL

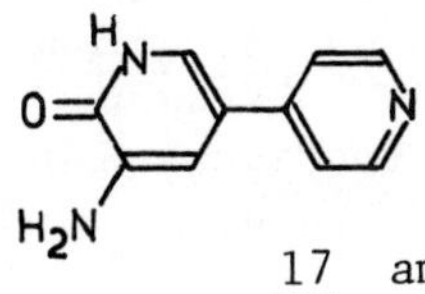

17 amrinone

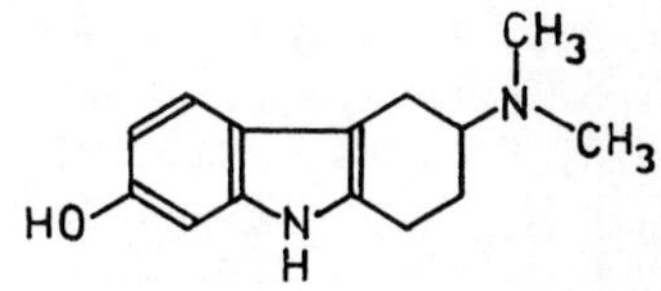

18 Win 35,020

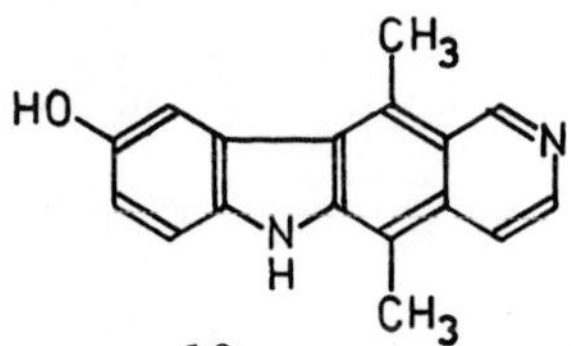

19

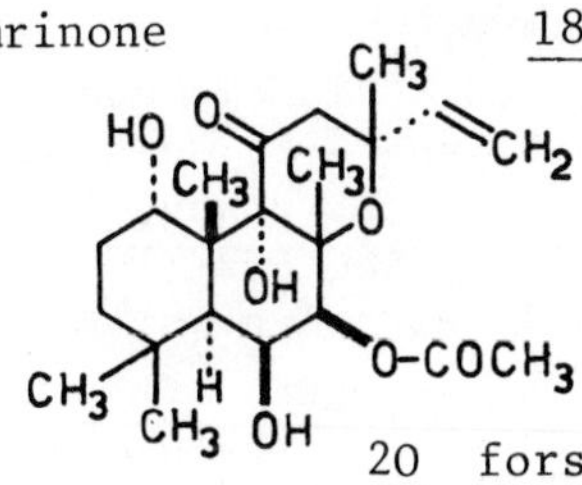

20 forskolin

increased contractile force in anaesthetised dogs but like (18), relies heavily on catecholamine release.[119] Forskolin (20), a diterpene derivative from the Indian plant Coleus forskohli, has dose-dependent positive inotropic and blood pressure lowering activity in animals. The mechanism of action has not been elucidated as yet but does not depend on either catecholamines or inhibition of cAMP-PDE or Na^+-K^+ATPase.[120] Interestingly, inosine produces a positive inotropic effect in the dog and may also exert a modulatory action on β-adrenoceptors.[121]

References

1. S. Wagner and K. Cohn, Arch. Intern. Med., 137, 675 (1977).
2. G.E. Burch, Am. Heart J., 94, 269 (1977).
3. Editorial, Br. Med. J., 1, 324 (1978).
4. S.M. Deglin, J.M. Deglin and E.K. Chung, Drugs, 14, 29 (1977).
5. O. Storstein, V. Hansteen, L. Hatle, L. Hillestad and L. Storstein, Am. Heart J., 93, 434 (1977).
6. J. Hamer, Br. Med. J., 2, 220 (1976).
7. Lord Platt, World Med., 39 (1975).
8. J.R. Sewell, Br. Med. J., 1, 454 (1976).
9. Editorial, Br. Med. J., 1, 49 (1975).
10. G.W. Beeler, Fed. Proc., 36, 2209 (1977).
11. G.A. Langer, Fed. Proc., 36, 2231 (1977).
12. T.M. Brody and T. Akera, Fed. Proc., 36, 2219 (1977).
13. T. Akera, Science, 198, 569 (1977).
14. G.T. Okita, Fed. Proc., 36, 2225 (1977).
15. B.E. Blood and D. Noble, J. Physiol. (London), 266, 76P (1977).
16. J. Ghysel-Burton and T. Godfraind, Br. J. Pharmacol., 55, 249P (1975).
17. T. Godfraind and J. Ghysel-Burton, Nature, 265, 165 (1977).
18. H.M. Rhee, S. Dutta and B.H. Marks, Eur. J. Pharmacol., 37, 141 (1976).
19. E. Steiness and N. Valentin, Br. J. Pharmacol., 58, 183 (1976).
20. Th. W. Güntert and H.H.A. Linde, Experientia, 33, 697 (1977).
21. R.A. Gillis, J.A. Quest, H. Thibodeaux, M.M. Clancy and D.E. Evans, J. Pharmacol. Exp. Ther., 193, 336 (1975).
22. R.J. McRitchie and S.F. Vatner, Circulation Res., 38, 321 (1976).
23. D.J. Goodman, R.M. Rossen, D.S. Cannom, A.K. Rider and D.C. Harrison, Circulation, 51, 251 (1975).
24. R.A. Gillis, D.L. Pearle and B. Levitt, Circulation, 52 739 (1975).

25. D.G. Pace and R.A. Gillis, J. Pharmacol. Exp. Ther., 199, 583 (1976).
26. L.C. Weaver, T. Akera and T.M. Brody, J.Pharmacol.Exp.Ther.,197,1(1976).
27. J. Roberts, G.J. Kelliher and C.M. Lathers, Life Sci., 18, 665 (1976).
28. R.W. Caldwell and C.B. Nash, J. Pharmacol.Exp.Ther., 197, 19 (1976).
29. L.S. Cook, R.W. Caldwell and C.B. Nash, Arch. Int. Pharmacodyn. Ther., 227, 220 (1977).
30. L.S. Cook, R.W. Caldwell and C.B. Nash, Clin. Res., 24, 604A (1976).
31. R.W. Caldwell and C.B. Nash, Am. J. Cardiol., 39, 291 (1977).
32. H.N. Abramson, C.L. Huang, Chiu-Chung Ho, L.L. Walny and You-Meei Hsu, J. Pharm. Sci., 66, 602 (1977).
33. R. Mendez, G. Pastelin and E. Kabela, J. Pharmacol. Exp. Ther., 188, 189 (1974).
34. C.R. Ross and N.I. Pessah, Eur. J. Pharmacol., 33, 223 (1975).
35. N.A. Cagin, S. Naidu, S. Arvan, I. Goldman, J. Somberg and B. Levitt, Clin. Pharmacol. Ther., 22, 274 (1977).
36. G. Bodem and K. Wirth, Arzneim-Forsch, 26, 1253 (1976).
37. J. Gerloff and G. Bodem, Naunyn-Schmiedeberg's Arch. Pharmacol., Suppl. II, 297, R59 (1977).
38. R. Thomas, J. Boutagy, A. Gelbart, J. Pharm. Sci., 63, 1649 (1974).
39. S. Matsumura, S. Kimoto, O. Uno, T. Minesita and M. Ueda, Arch. Int. Pharmacodyn. Ther., 225, 246 (1977).
40. S. Matsumura, E. Morishige, O. Uno, T. Minesita and M. Ueda, Jap. J. Pharmacol., 26 Suppl., 134P (1976).
41. N.T. Lutete, F. Noel, A. De Pover and T. Godfraind, Arch. Int. Pharmacodyn. Ther., 227, 166 (1977).
42. British Patent GB-1484655.
43. A-F. Prigent, M. Roche and H. Pacheco, Eur.J.Med.Chem., 10, 498 (1975).
44. K. Chatterjee and W.W. Parmley, Br. Heart J., 39, 706 (1977).
45. K. Chatterjee and W.W. Parmley, Prog. Cardiovas. Dis., 19 301 (1977).
46. J.N. Cohn and J.A. Franciosa, New Eng. J. Med., 297, 27 (1977).
47. P.K. Shah, Am. Heart J., 93, 256, 403 (1977).
48. E. Braunwald, New Eng. J. Med., 297, 331 (1977).
49. D.O. Williams, W.J. Bommer, R.R. Miller, E.A. Amsterdam and D.T. Mason, Am. J. Cardiol., 39, 84 (1977).
50. R.R. Miller, L.A. Vismara, D.O. Williams, E.A. Amsterdam and D.T. Mason, Circ. Res., 39, 127 (1976).
51. R. Schreiber, H. Loeb and R. Gunnar, Am. J. Cardiol., 39, 297 (1977).
52. P. Imhof, Schweiz Med. Wochenschr., 107, 1041 (1977).
53. K. Chatterjee, W.W. Parmley, B. Massie, B. Greenberg, J. Werner, S. Klausner and A. Norman, Circulation, 54, 879 (1976).
54. J.A. Franciosa, G. Pierpont and J.N. Cohn, Ann. Intern. Med., 86, 388 (1977).
55. B. Massie, K. Chatterjee, J. Werner, B. Greenburg, R. Hart and W.W. Parmley, Am. J. Cardiol., 40, 794 (1977).
56. I. Khatri, N. Uemura, A. Notargiacomo and E.D. Freis, Am. J. Cardiol., 40, 38 (1977).
57. K. Chatterjee, D. Drew, W.W. Parmley, S.C. Klausner, J. Polansky and B. Zacherle, Ann. Int. Med., 85, 467 (1976).
58. J.A. Franciosa and J.N. Cohn, Clin. Pharmacol. Ther., 21, 102 (1977).
59. R.R. Miller, N.A. Awan, K.S. Maxwell and D.T. Mason, New Eng. J. Med., 297, 303 (1977).

60. N.A. Awan, R.R. Miller, A.N. DeMaria, K.S. Maxwell, A. Neumann and D.T. Mason, Circulation, 56, 346 (1977).
61. N.A. Awan, R.R. Miller and D.T. Mason, Circulation, 57, 152 (1978).
62. H.L. Rutenberg and J.F. Spann in 'Congestive Heart Failure, Mechanisms, Evaluation and Treatment', Dean T. Mason Ed., Dun-Donnelly Publishing Corporation, New York, 1976, p.85.
63. W.H. Newman, Am. Heart J., 93, 216 (1977).
64. P. Lumley and K.J. Broadley, J. Pharm. Pharmacol., 29, 598 (1977).
65. D.F. Colella, A.J. Tobia, R.A. Hahn, J.W. Wilson and J.R. Wardell, 2nd Joint Conference CIC/ACS, (Montreal, June 1977) Abs. Medi. No. 33.
66. J. Bonelli, D. Magometschnigg and G. Hitzenberger, Intern. J. Clin. Pharmacol. Biopharm., 14, 231 (1976).
67. L.I. Goldberg, Y.Y. Hsieh and L. Resnekov. Prog. Cardiovas. Dis., 19, 327 (1977).
68. J.D. Stoner, J.L. Bolen and D.C. Harrison, Br. Heart J., 39 536 (1977).
69. H.S. Loeb, J. Bredakis and R.M. Gunnar, Circulation, 55, 375 (1977).
70. F. Kersting, F. Follath, R. Moulds, J. Mucklow, R. McCloy, J. Sheares and C. Dollery, Br. Heart J., 38, 622 (1976).
71. C.V. Leier, J. Webel and C.A. Bush, Circulation, 56, 468 (1977).
72. R.R. Miller, N.A. Awan, J.A. Joye, K.S. Maxwell, A.N. DeMaria, E.A. Amsterdam and D.T. Mason, Circulation, 55, 881 (1977).
73. P.J. Murphy, T.L. Williams and D.L.K. Kau, J. Pharmacol. Exp. Ther., 199, 423 (1976).
74. A.M. Strosberg, Arch. Int. Pharmacodyn. Ther., 222, 200 (1976).
75. T. Kosuge and M. Yokota, Chem. Pharm. Bull., 24, 176 (1976).
76. N. Masaki, H. Iizuka, M. Yokota and A. Ochiai, J. Chem. Soc. Perkin Trans., 1, 717 (1977).
77. E. Carlsson, C-G. Dahlöf, A. Hedberg, H. Persson and B. Tangstrand, Naunyn Schmiedeberg's Arch. Pharmacol., 300, 101 (1977).
78. C.L. Papadopoulos, N.P. Lefkos and L.P. Concouris, Arzneim-Forsch., 26, 93 (1976).
79. B. Weiss and W.N. Hait, Ann. Rev. Pharmacol. Toxicol., 17, H.W. Elliot, R. George and R. Okun Eds., Annual Reviews Inc., Palo Alto, Calif., 1977 p.441.
80. M. Huang and G.I. Drummond, Biochem. Pharmacol., 25, 2713 (1976).
81. D.F. Horrobin, M.S. Manku, D.J. Franks and P. Hamet, Prostaglandins, 13, 33 (1977).
82. T.T. Martinez and J.H. McNeill, Can.J.Physiol.Pharmacol., 55, 98 (1977).
83. G.D. Fink, R.J. Paddock, G.M. Rodgers, R.W. Busuttil and W.J. George, Proc. Soc. Exp. Biol. Med., 153, 78 (1976).
84. H. Nawrath, Nature, 262, 509 (1976).
85. C.T. Alabaster, K.J. Blackburn, J.R. Joice, R. Massingham and P.C. Scholfield, Br. J. Pharmacol., 60, 284P (1977).
86. F. Follath, F. Kersting, G.R.J. Lewis, R.J. Walden, N.M. Woolhouse and C.T. Dollery, Clin. Pharmacol. Therap., 20, 24 (1976).
87. I. Hutton, W.S. Hillis, C.E. Langhan, J.M. Conely and T.D.V. Lawrie, Br. J. Clin. Pharmacol., 4, 513 (1977).
88. T. Asano, Y. Ochiai and H. Hidaka, Mol. Pharmacol., 13, 400 (1977).
89. T. Motomiya, T. Sano and T. Shimamoto, Angiology, 28, 346 (1977).
90. U.S. Patent, 4,036,840.

91. D.B. Evans, C.S. Parham, M.T. Schenck and R.J. Laffan, J. Cyclic Nucleotide Res., 2, 307 (1976)
92. B.C. Pressman, Ann. Rev. Biochem., 45, E.S. Snell, P.D. Boyer, A. Meister and C.C. Richardson Eds., Annual Reviews Inc. Palo Alto, Calif., 1976, p.501.
93. G. Haeusler, Experientia, 32, 779 (1976).
94. M.W. Osborne, J.J. Wenger and M.T. Zanko, J. Pharmacol. Exp. Ther., 200, 195 (1977).
95. B.C. Pressman and N.T. deGuzman, The Pharmacologist, 18, 122 (1976).
96. M. Tanaka, M. Haniu, K.T. Yasunobu and T.R. Norton, Biochemistry, 16, 204 (1977).
97. S. Shibata, T.R. Norton, T. Izumi, T. Matsuo and S. Katsuki, J. Pharmacol. Exp. Ther., 199, 298 (1976).
98. A. Scriabine, C.G. Van Arman, A.A. Morris, G. Morgan and C.D. Bennett, Fed. Proc., 36, 973 (1977).
99. U. Ravens, Naunyn-Schmiedeberg's Arch. Pharmacol., 296, 73 (1976).
100. B. Rabinowitz, L. Chuck, M. Kligerman and W.W. Parmley, Am. J. Physiol., 229, 582 (1975).
101. J.B. Osnes, Acta. Pharmacol. Toxicol., 39, 232 (1976).
102. A.M. Watanabe, D.R. Hathaway, H.R. Besch, B.B. Farmer and R.A. Harris, Circ. Res., 40, 596 (1977).
103. S.L. Keely, J.D. Corbin and T. Lincoln, Mol.Pharmacol., 13, 965 (1977).
104. G. Kunos, Br. J. Pharmacol., 59, 177 (1977).
105. M. Nickerson and G. Kunos, Fed. Proc., 36, 2580 (1977).
106. B.G. Benfey, Fed. Proc., 36, 2575 (1977).
107. R. Levi, G. Allan and J.H. Zavecz, Fed. Proc., 35, 1942 (1976).
108. D.A.A. Owen, Gen. Pharmacol., 8, 141 (1977).
109. S.C. Verma and J.H. McNeill, J.Pharmacol.Exp.Ther., 200, 352 (1977).
110. S.C. Verma and J.H. McNeill, J.Cyclic Nucleotide Res., 3, 95 (1977).
111. S.C. Verma and J.H. McNeill, Agents and Actions, 7, 191 (1977).
112. J.R. Powell and M.J. Brody, J. Pharmacol.Exp.Ther., 196, 1 (1976).
113. J.G. Papp and B.A. Resch, Agents and Actions, 5, 463 (1975).
114. Netherland Patent 7401-254.
115. G.G. Belz, H. Nübling and A. Zimmer, Europ. J. Clin. Pharmacol., 10, 319 (1976).
116. A. Schinz, K. Schnelle and G. Klein, Z.Kardiol. Suppl.3, 179 (1976).
117. U.S. Patent 4,004,012.
118. A. Mooradian, A.G. Hlavac, P.E. Dupont, M.R. Bell and A.A. Alousi, J. Med. Chem., 18, 640 (1975).
119. P-H-Chanh, N-D-Xuong, J.B. LePecq and C. Paoletti, Pharmacology, 14, 490 (1976).
120. E. Lindner, A.N. Dohadwalla and B.K. Bhattacharya, Arzneim-Forsch., 28, 284 (1978).
121. A. Juhász-Nagy and D.M. Aviado, J. Pharmacol. Exp. Ther., 202, 683 (1977).

Section III - Chemotherapeutic Agents

Editor: George B. Whitfield, The Upjohn Company, Kalamazoo, Michigan

Chapter 11. Antibiotics

Herman Hoeksema and Lorraine C. Davenport
The Upjohn Company, Kalamazoo, Michigan

This chapter will be limited to those antibiotics for which antibacterial activity has been demonstrated. Antibiotics which are described exclusively as antitumor, antifungal and antiviral agents as well as subjects related to biosynthesis are excluded. Included is a very limited section on β-lactam antibiotics.

General - The 17th Interscience Conference on Antimicrobial Agents and Chemotherapy, for which abstracts were published,[1] was concerned with its usual wide variety of antibiotic subjects. Zurich hosted the 10th International Congress of Chemotherapy which emphasized clinical topics in the antibiotic field.[2] The pilot volume of a projected new series, called *Topics in Antibiotic Chemistry*, was published.[3]

Aminocyclitols - Large numbers of clinical reports on experiences with aminocyclitol antibiotics continued to appear, including a rather extensive review[4] on various aspects of their use. Clinical effort on new aminocyclitols appeared to center on netilmicin, 1, 1-N-ethylsisomicin, which is active against some of the gentamicin-resistant organisms. In general the preliminary information which was reported last year held up in the current expanded studies. In comparative pharmacological studies[5] of gentamicin, 2, and netilmicin, the latter appeared to produce more predictable blood levels. Another study[6] reported favorable clinical responses for 70% of patients infected with susceptible strains of *Enterobacteriaceae* and *Pseudomonas aeruginosa*. Despite lower nephrotoxicity in experimental animals, some of these patients displayed some renal involvement, as suggested by elevated BUN and serum creatinine and the appearance of granular casts. Several other reports[7,8,9,10] only showed very low incidences of toxicity. A new high-pressure liquid chromatographic assay of netilmicin in plasma[11] gave results which correlated well with microbiological assays.

Synthetic modifications of gentamicin and kanamycin afforded a number of active compounds. Hydroxy-amino-acylates of gentamicin B, 3 and 4, had greatly enhanced antimicrobial activity, but their toxicities were correspondingly higher.[12] Two laboratories reported[13,14] conversions of kanamycin B, 5, to kanamycin C, 6, and 6'-deoxykanamycin C, 7, utilizing nitrous acid deamination at the 6' position of suitably protected intermediates. Only weak activity was shown by 7 against most of the microorganisms tested. A novel derivative, 1-N-[(S)-4-amino-2-hydroxybutyl]

ISBN 0-12-040513-X

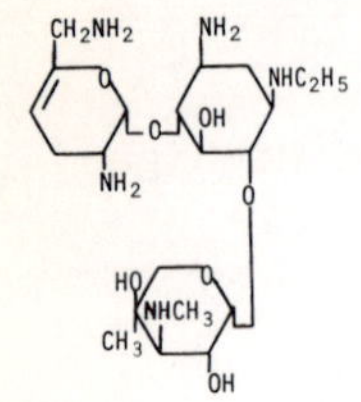

1

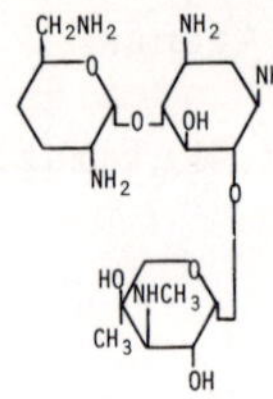

2

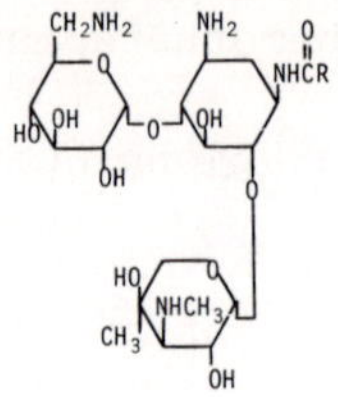

3 R=$CH_2(NH_2)CH_2CH(OH)$-
4 R=$CH_2(NH_2)CH(OH)$-

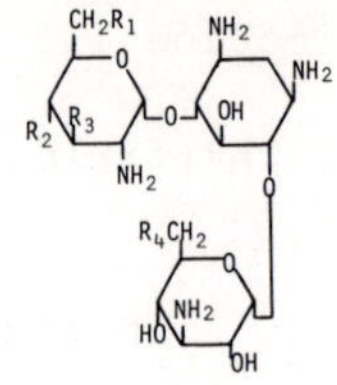

Compound	R_1	R_2	R_3	R_4
5	NH_2	OH	OH	OH
6	OH	OH	OH	OH
7	H	OH	OH	OH
9	NH_2	H	OH	OH
10	NH_2	OH	H	H

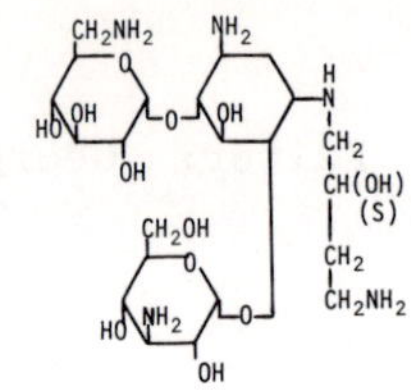

8

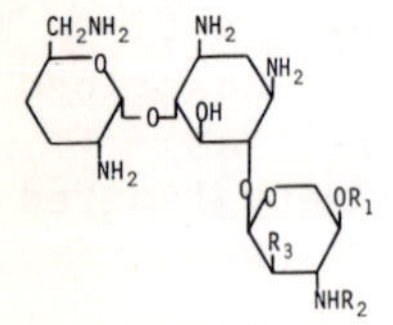

	R_1	R_2	R_3
11	CH_3	H	NH_2
12	H	CH_3	OH

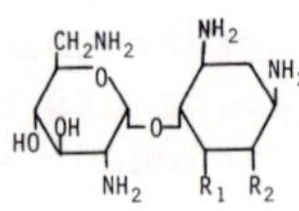

	R_1	R_2
13	H	OH
14	OH	H

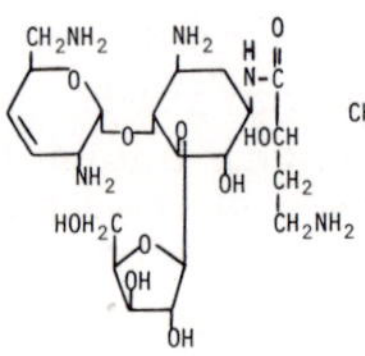

15

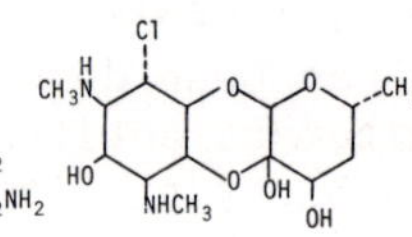

16

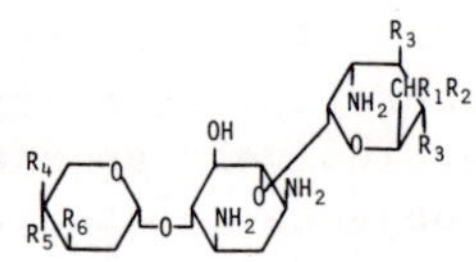

	R_1	R_2	R_3	R_4	R_5	R_6
17	CH_3	OH	OH	H	OH	$NHCH_3$
18	CH_3	OH	OH	OH	H	$NHCH_3$
19	CH_3	NH_2	H	OH	CH_3	NH_2
20	CH_3	$NHCH_3$	H	OH	H	$NHCH_3$
21	CH_3	NH_2	H	OH	H	$NHCH_3$
22	H	NH_2	H	OH	H	$NHCH_3$

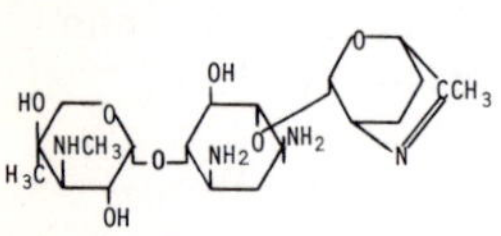

23

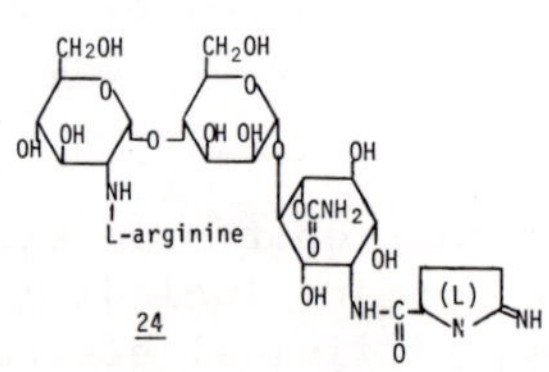

24

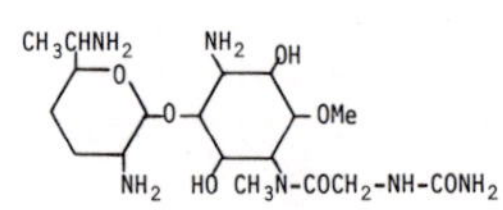

25

kanamycin A, 8, was synthesized by a diborane reduction of a trifluoroacetate salt of the corresponding butyryl derivative of kanamycin A.[15] Clinical evaluation is underway for this compound, UK-18892, which demonstrates an order of activity like that of amikacin. Newly synthesized 4'-deoxykanamycin B, 9,[16,17] displayed varied activity against strains of *Staphylococcus aureus*, *S. epidermis*, and *Bacillus brevis* which had been reported to produce aminoglycoside-4'-adenyltransferase. The activity of 6"-deoxytobramycin, 10, was similar to that of tobramycin.[18] Since enzymatic 3-O-phosphorylation inactivates seldomycin factor 5, the 3'-deoxy analog, 11, was prepared in two laboratories.[19,20] Enhanced activity was seen against Gram-negative sensitive strains as well as the target resistant ones. Attachment of gentosamine to 3',4'-dideoxyneamine gave a broad spectrum antibiotic, 12, which was, however, less active than the gentamicin C complex.[21] The 1-*epi*-derivatives of sisomicin, netilmicin and gentamicin C were found to be potent broad spectrum antibiotics which were less toxic than the parent antibiotics.[22] Replacement of the C-6 hydroxyl of neamine with hydrogen as in 14 diminished its antibacterial effect but 5-deoxyneamine, 13, had enhanced activity, especially against kanamycin-resistant strains.[23] While less active than 3',4'-dideoxybutirosin, newly synthesized 3',4'-dideoxy-3'-enobutirosin A, 15,[24] was active against a broad range of sensitive and aminoglycoside-resistant organisms.

A novel approach to aminocyclitol modification sequenced the use of inactivating enzymes with synthetic organic procedures.[25] An enzyme from

Pseudomonas aeruginosa GN573 was used in the presence of ATP and $MgSO_4$ to phosphorylate kanamycin B specifically at the 3' position. Treatment with silylating agents gave the chloride which was subsequently hydrogenated to give kanamycin B.

Since inactivation of spectinomycin occurs by adenylation at the 9-position, the analogs 9-chloro-9-deoxy-4(R)-dihydrospectinomycin, 16, and its 9-epimer, and 9-deoxy-8,9-epimino-4(R)-dihydrospectinomycin were prepared.[26] All three were devoid of antibacterial activity. A spectinomycin resistant *Neisseria gonorrhoeae* was studied[27] with no finding of spectinomycin inactivation. Chromosomal mutation was suggested as causative.

More inactivating enzymes have been found. Strains of *Staphylococcus aureus* elaborated both kanamycin-neomycin[28] and gentamicin[29] phosphotransferases. Another strain of that organism also produced an amikacin-modifying 3'-phosphotransferase while remaining sensitive to the antibiotic.[30] Five strains of *Escherichia coli* have been isolated which inactivate extracellular streptomycin in large quantities.[31] Alkaline phosphotase liberated inorganic phosphate from the inactive compound but the remaining streptomycin-like compound had no activity. Plasmid-induced resistance of a clinically isolated *Pseudomonas aeruginosa* strain to kanamycin, tetracycline, chloramphenicol, and streptomycin was related to decreased cell permeability rather than to inactivating derivatization.[32]

Among the new microbially produced aminocyclitols were seven gentamicin-related substances, 17-23, in the broth of a *Micromonospora* species which produced eighteen additional known antibiotics.[33] Biological details were not reported beyond a mention of broad antibacterial activity. LL-BM123α, 24, a *Nocardia*-produced aminocyclitol, had *myo*-inosamine as the aminocyclitol moiety.[34]

Fortimicin C, 25, elaborated by *Micromonospora olivoasterospora* was active against kanamycin-, gentamicin-, and tobramycin-resistant *E. coli* strains.[35]

Neomycin C has now been synthesized by regioselective glycosidation between suitably protected ribostamycin and neosamine C.[36]

β-Lactams - Clinical evaluation studies were initiated for SCE-963, 26, a new broad spectrum parenteral cephalosporin.[37,38] Another new parenteral cephalosporin for clinical investigation is CGP 7174E (SCE-129), 27, a compound which compared favorably with gentamicin in the treatment of experimental *Pseudomonas aeruginosa* infections.[39,40] FR13301 is a third parenteral cephalosporin receiving

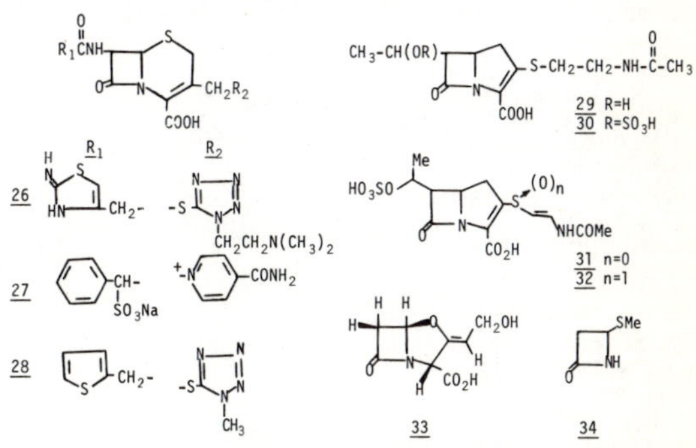

clinical attention. It is most active against Gram-negative organisms[41] as is a fourth clinical candidate, FR10024, 28.[42]

Reports on new microbially-produced β-lactam antibiotics included N-acetyl thienamycin, 29, from *Streptomyces cattleya*,[43] three compounds from *Streptomyces olivaceus* (MM 17880, 30,[44] MM 13902, 31,[45] and MM 4550, 32[45]), and four epithienamycins from *Streptomyces flavogriseus*.[46] The epithienamycins showed antimicrobial activities and β-lactamase susceptibilities which vary widely amongst each other.[47] The thienamycins share a characteristic instability.[48] The first total synthesis of the β-lactamase inhibitor, clavulanic acid, 33, was reported.[49] The starting compound was (±)-4-methylthioazetidin-2-one, 34.

Macrolides - In a symposium on the macrolide antibiotics held at the 173rd Meeting of the American Chemical Society,[50] biological activities were correlated with structure. Rosamicin, a basic macrolide with a 16-membered ring, has shown some clinical promise in the treatment of bacterial prostatitis.[51] SP127, a protein, has been found to enhance the activity of macrolide antibiotics by promoting their ability to penetrate the bacterial cell.[52,53]

The production by *Micromonospora capillata* of three new macrolides, 35, 36, 37, with 16-membered rings was reported.[54,55] These antibiotics, M-4365A_1,G_1, and G_2 generally inhibited the same organisms that were sensitive to rosamicin and the juvenimicins which were coproduced in the fermentation. The revision of the structures of oligomycins A and C 38, 39, showed them to be closely related to oligomycin B and rutamycin.[56]

A review on the synthesis of macrolide compounds[57] included not only the macrolide antibiotics but ansamycins, macrotetralides, macrodilides, etc. None of the major 14 or 16-membered macrolide antibiotics has yet been synthesized, although a semisynthesis of carbomycin B, 40, from carbonolide B and the two carbohydrate fragments was accomplished.[58] Cladinose analogs of carbomycin B 41, 42, were prepared and found to approximate the *in vitro* antibacterial action of carbomycin B.[59]

A study correlating the structure and activity of the acylated leucomycins, 43, showed that a free 9-hydroxyl group is not essential for ribosomal binding. However, 4"-O-acylation did affect binding which decreased

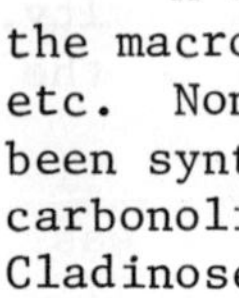

35 M-4365A_1

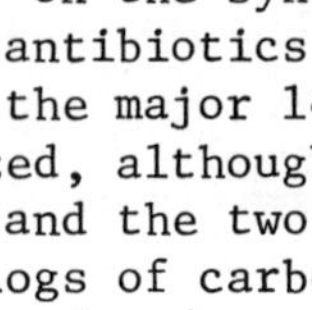

36 M-4365G_1 R=-CH_3

37 M-4365G_2 R=-CHO

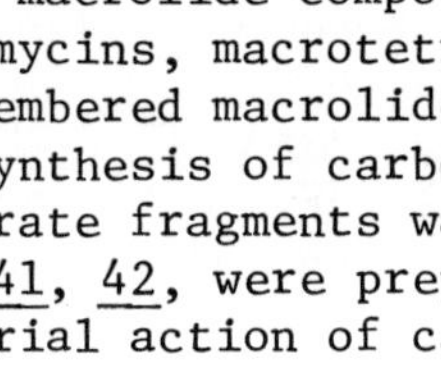

38 R_1=OH

39 R_1=H

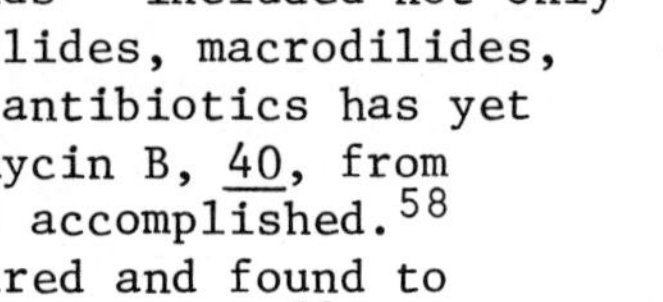

40 R_1=R_2=H

41 R_1=CH_3, R_2=H

42 R_1=CH_3, R_2=Br

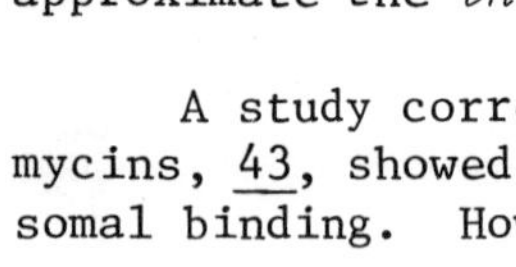

43 R=H or acyl

with decreasing acyl size . Incubation with the test microorganism caused hydrolysis of the 2'-O-acyl groups.[60]

Peptides - Several new microbially produced members of the largest class of antibiotics were described. The chemistry, biogenesis, and functions of these peptides were recently reviewed.[61] Polymyxin F from *Bacillus circulans*,[62] and polymyxins S_1, 44, and T_1, 45, from *Bacillus polymyxa*[63,64] were recently isolated and reported to have the usual polymyxin antibacterial spectra, although T_1 is more active against Gram-positive organisms. Tallysomycins[65,66] are bleomycin-like, while nosiheptide[67] and micrococcin P[68] are related to thiostrepton, plauracin is in the virginiamycin sub-group.[69] Structures are unavailable for several other new peptides, NRC-501,[70] compound 41,012,[71] and FCRC-53.[72] Two unique dipeptides were isolated, plumbemycin A, 46,[73] and cairomycin B, 47.[74] The latter had antifungal and antibacterial properties. LL-BM547, viomycin-like, is an antitubercular antibiotic produced by a *Nocardia* species.[75] New or revised structures appeared for a number of the older antibiotics such as the bacillomycins L, 48,[76] the cyclosporins, 49-51,[77,78] and berninamycin, 52.[79] Sulfomycin I was found to contain 2,5-berninamycinic acid.[80] Structures for the peptaibophol[81] sub-group, alamethicin I and II, 53, 54,[81] emericins IV and III, 55, 56,[82] and antiamoebin I, 57,[83] were elucidated. Stenothricin was found to be a complex of peptides varying in the ketoacyl moiety of the general formulas, β-ketoacyl-D-cys(O_3H)-L-Val-DSer-LLys-Sar-DαThr-LSer-LDap-OH.[84]

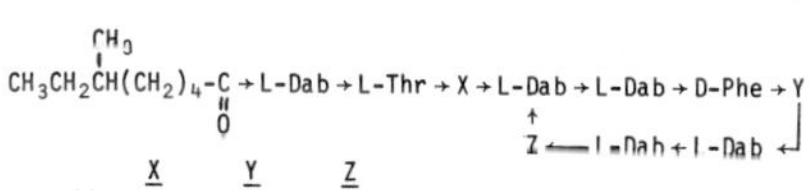

	X	Y	Z
44	D-Ser	L-Thr	L-Thr
45	L-Dab	L-Leu	L-Leu

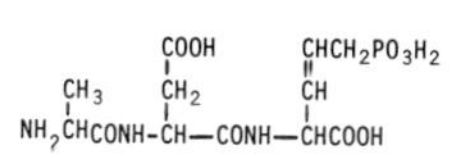

46

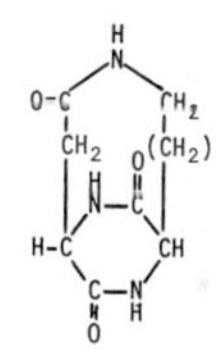

47

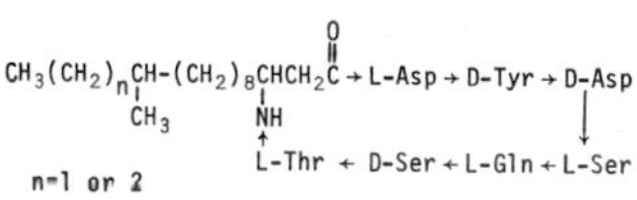

48

n=1 or 2

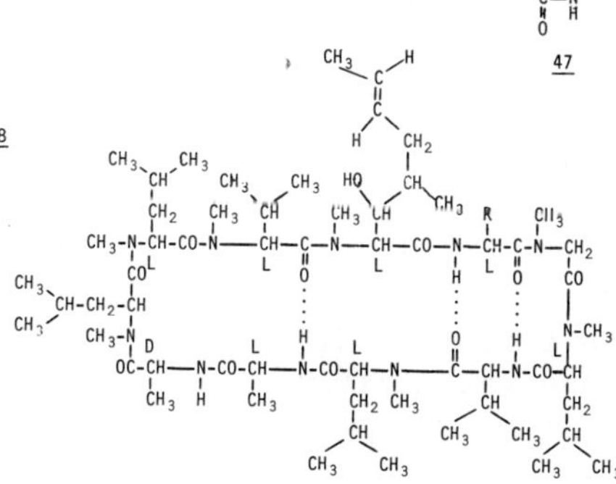

49 R=-CH_3 Cyclosporin B
50 R=CH(OH)-CH_3 Cyclosporin C
51 R=$CH(CH_3)_2$ Cyclosporin D

52

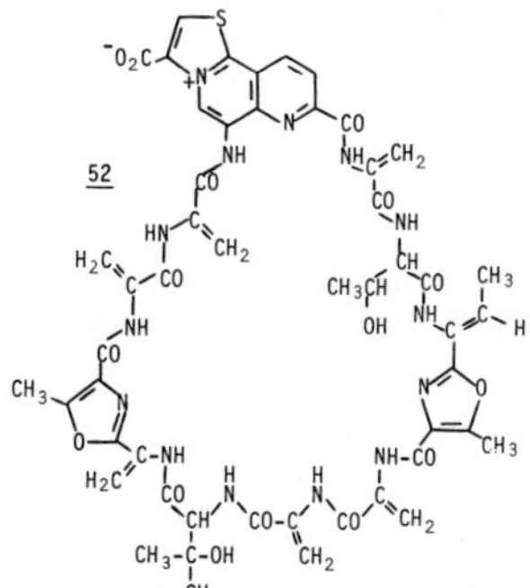

Ac → Aib → L-Pro → Aib → L-Ala → Aib → L-Ala → (Aib)
→ L-Gln → Aib → L-Val → Aib → Gly → L-Leu → Aib →
→ L-Pro → L-Val → Aib → Aib → L-Glu →(a) L-Gln → L-Phol

53 (54)

55 (Emerimicin IV): Ac-L-Phe-Aib-Aib-Aib-L-*Val*-Gly-L-Leu-Aib-Aib-L-Hyp-L-Gln-L-Iva-L-Hyp-*Aib*-L-Phol
56 (Emerimicin III): Ac-L-Phe-Aib-Aib-Aib-L-*Val*-Gly-L-Leu-Aib-Aib-L-Hyp-L-Gln-L-Iva-L-Hyp-L-*Ala*-L-Phol
57 (Antiamoebin I): Ac-L-Phe-Aib-Aib-Aib-L-Iva-Gly-L-Leu-Aib-Aib-L-Hyp-L-Gln-L-Iva-L-Hyp-*Aib*-L-*Pro*-L-Phol

A 19-residue peptide with alamethicin-like activity in liquid bilayer membranes has been synthesized and tested.[85] Virginiamycin S reduction products were prepared, but they were less active than virginiamycin S.[86] EM-49 was converted to a number of active derivatives by acylation and alkylation of the terminal amino groups of the 2,4-diaminobutyric acid residues.[87] Good activity was frequently seen in the Gram-positive areas with decreased antipseudomonal activity. Plasmid-mediated pristinamycin acetyltransferase, produced by a *Staphylococcus* strain, O-acetylated that antibiotic, thereby inactivating it.[88]

When polymyxin B, immobilized on agarose beads, was used to specifically disrupt the outer membrane of Gram-negative bacteria, synergism with bacitracin, rifamycin, or lysozyme was still in effect. Thus polymyxin B plays its role in these combinations at the outer membrane.[89, 90]

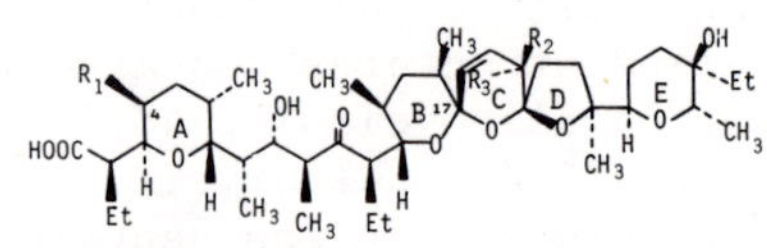

58 R_1=CH_3; R_2=OH; R_3=H
59 R_1=R_3=H; R_2=OH
60 R_1=CH_3; R_2, R_3=O
61 R_1=R_2=R_3=H

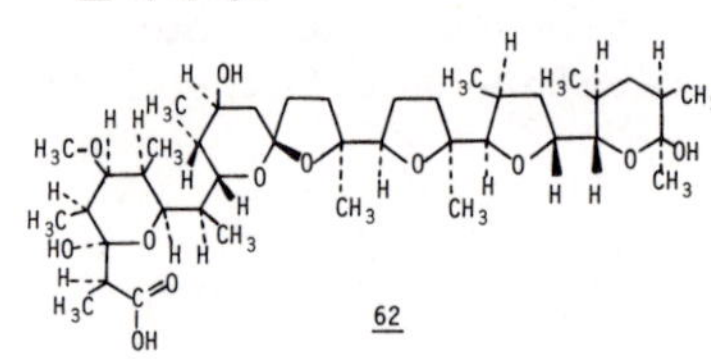

62

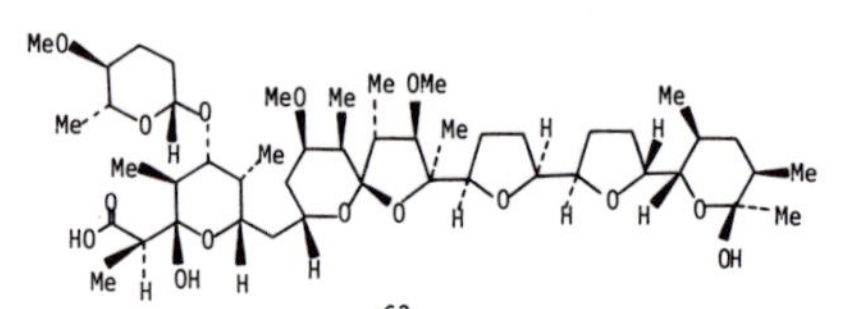

63

Polyethers - Mass spectral data[91] required the assignment of the 4-methylsalinomycin structure to narasin, 58. Analyses of the ^{13}C-NMR spectra of salinomycin, 59,[92] and narasin[93] indicated an equatorial orientation for the new methyl group. Another ionophore, A28086B, 60, differs from narasin in the C-ring only, with a keto function replacing the secondary hydroxyl.[91] *Streptomyces albus* (ATCC12838) elaborated deoxy-(O-8) salinomycin, 61, and a second polyether differing from 61 by epimerization at position 17.[94] Mutalomycin, 62, produced by *Streptomyces mutabilis* (NRRL 8088), is active against Gram positive bacteria and *Eimeria tenella*.[95] Carriomycin, 63, another new polyether, contains the sugar residue that is present in septamycin, A130A (lenoremycin) and A-204A according to a crystallographic structure analysis of the thallium salt.[96] The aglycone was similar to lonomycin.

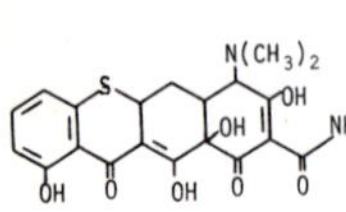

64

Tetracyclines - EMD33,330, 64, was one of a number of 6-thiatetracyclines of synthetic origin.[97] Its minimum inhibitory concentrations for a broad range of organisms were lower than those of doxycycline and tetracycline, except for *Pseudomonas aeruginosa* where it was less active. Tetracycline-resistant strains were sensitive. High and prolonged serum concentrations were seen in mice and dogs, with peaks 2-3 times those of doxycycline.

Miscellaneous Antibiotics - The search for new antibiotics again afforded a number of new activities which are summarized in Table 1.

TABLE 1: NEW ANTIBIOTIC ENTITIES

Antibiotic	Producing Organism	Activity	Structure or Structure/Type	Reference
A-35512	*Streptomyces candidus*	G^+	Glycopeptide/Vancomycin	98
Baumycins	*Streptomyces coerulerorubidus*	G^+, AT	Anthracycline	99
Chloquinomycin	*Streptomyces californicus* var. *rivalis*	G^+	—	100
CP-41043, CP-41494	*Pseudonocardia fastidiosa*	G^+, G^-	Thiostrepton	101
CP-42752, CP-43038, CP-43139	*Micromonospora saitamica*	G^+, G^-	—	102
Demethylblasticidin S	*Streptomyces griseochromogenes*	G^+, AF	Nucleoside	103
3-*epi*-Deoxynegamycin	*Streptomyces goshikiensis*	G^+, G^-	Hydrazide/Amino Acid	104
Dihydrogranaticin	*Streptomyces thermoviolaceus*	G^+	65	105
Dihydromocimycin	*Streptomyces ramocissimus*	G^+, G^-, AP	Mocimycin	106
Frustulosinol	*Stereum frustulosum*	G^+, *Vibrio sp.*	66	107
G-7063-2	*Streptomyces sp.*	G^+, G^-, AF	67	108
Glycinothricin	*Streptomyces griseus*	G^+, G^-	Streptothricin	109
Hydroxynybomycin	*Streptomyces sp.* D-57	G^+, G^-	Nybomycin	110
K-52B	*Streptoverticillium roseoverticillatum* subsp. *albosporum*	G^+, G^-	—	111
Leucyl-3-*epi*-deoxynegamycin	*Streptomyces goshikiensis*	G^+, G^-	Amino Acid/Hydrazide	104
MA-144 Complex	*Streptomyces galilaeus*	G^+, AF, AT	Anthracycline	112
Marcellomycin	*Actinosporanguin sp.* C-36145	G^+, G^-, AT	Anthracycline	113,114
Musettamycin	*Actinosporanguin sp.* C-36145	G^+, G^-, AT	Anthracycline	113,114
Nocamycin	*Nocardiopsis syringae*	G^+, AT	—	115
Norplicacetin	*Streptomyces plicatus*	G^+, *Mycobacteria*	68	116
OS-1804	*Streptomyces michiganensis*	G^+, G^-, AF	—	117
OS-4742	*Streptomyces matensis* subsp. *vineus*	G^+, AT	Anthracycline	118
Pseudomonic Acid B	*Pseudomonas fluorescens*	G^+	69	119
Rhodirubins A, B	*Streptomyces sp.*	G^+, *Mycobacteria*, AT	Anthracycline	120
Saframycins	*Streptomyces lavendulae*	G^+, G^-	—	121
SC30532	*Spicaria divaricata*	G^+, G^-, AP, AF	70	122
Secalonic Acid F	*Aspergillus aculeatus*	G^+	Secalonic Acids	123
Striatins	*Cyathus striatus*	G^+, G^-, AF	—	124
T-41348	*Streptomyces sp.*	G^+, G^-	Phenazine	125
Trichorin A	*Trichoderma sp.* strain K472	G^-	*epi*Polythiadiketopiperazine	126
Zg	*Streptomyces thermoviolaceus*	G^+	71	105
Zgg (Bisanhydrogranaticin)	*Streptomyces thermoviolaceus*	G^+	72	105
792	*Streptomyces bottropensis*	G^+, G^-, AF, AT	—	127

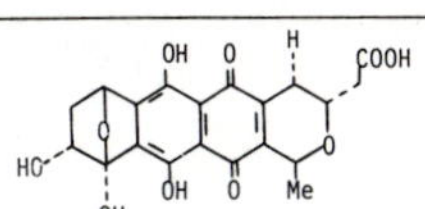
65

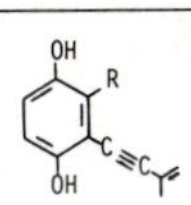
66 R=CH_2OH

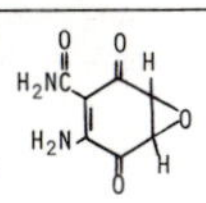
67

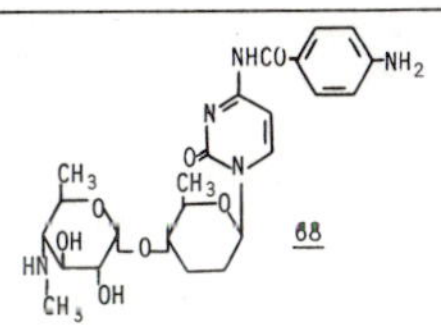
68

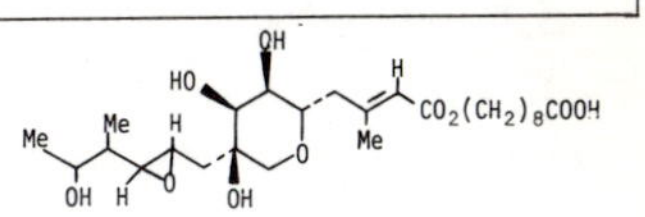
69

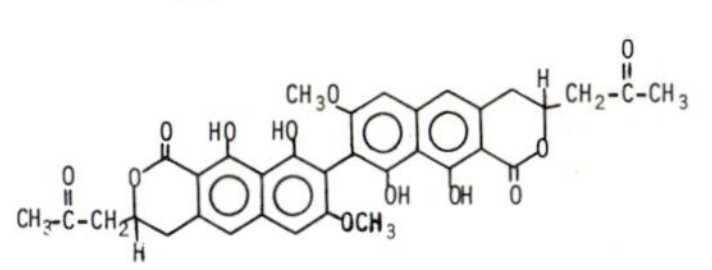
70

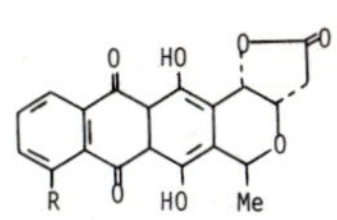
71 R=$CHOHCH_3$, R_2=H
72 R=$COCH_3$, R_2=H

Structures were published for a number of antibiotics which have been known for some time including nogalamycin, 73[128] steffimycin and steffimycin B, 74, 75,[129] pluramycin A, and neopluramycin, 76, 77,[130] all of which show both antibacterial and antitumor activity. Elucidations of the structures of neothramycins A and B, 78, 79,[131] LA-1 80,[132] griseorhodin A 81,[133] melinacidins II, III 82, 83,[134] and ambruticin, 84, (formerly acid S)[135] were also disclosed. Halomicins A and C, 85, 86,[136] are ansamycins and the silver salt of aplasmomycin, 87, was shown by crystallography to be a macrocyclic dilactone with boron in the center.[137] The configurational assignments of albonoursin, 88, were made by synthesizing the four possible isomers.[138] Revisions of structures for everninomicin[139] at the C-3 of evernitrose, 89, anthelmycin (hikizimycin), 90,[140] rimocidin, 91,[141] and frustulosin, 92,[107] were published.

Total syntheses for miscellaneous antibiotic substances were reported for the first time. These included oxazinomycin,[142] elaiomycin,[143] dl-cerulenin,[144,145,146] (±)-methylenomycin A,[147] minosaminomycin,[148] lydimycin (α-dehydrobiotin),[149] dl-porfiromycin,[150] mitomycins A and C,[151] vermiculine[152] and mimosamycin.[153]

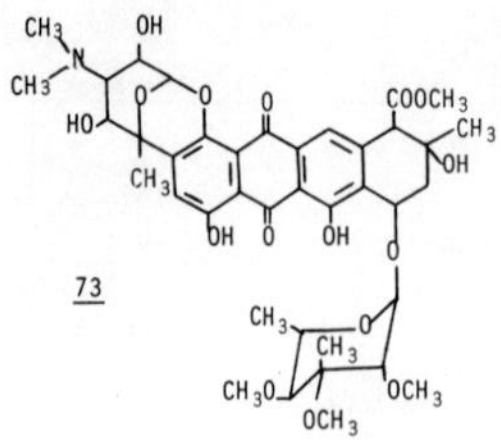

73

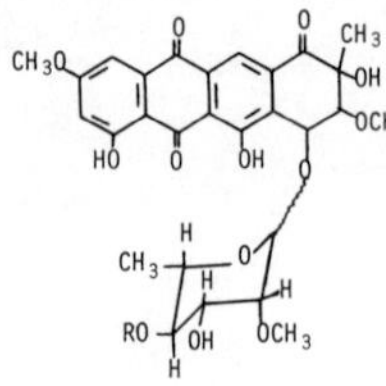

74 R=H
75 R=CH_3

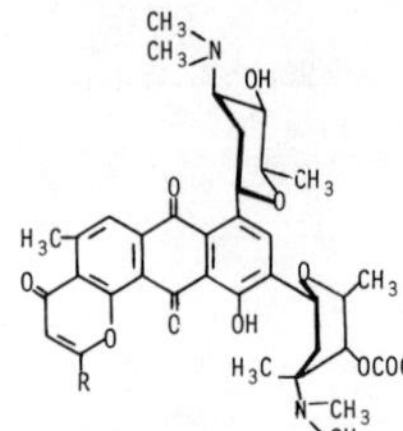

76 R=-C(=O)-CH(CH$_3$)-CH=CH-CH$_3$
77 R=-C(CH$_3$)=CH-CH$_3$

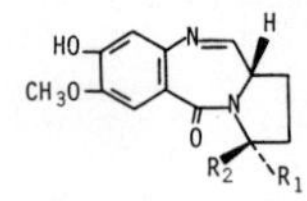

78 R_1=OH; R_2=H
79 R_1=H; R_2=OH

CH_3-C(=O)-CH=CH-CH=C=CH-CH=CH-C(=O)-OH

80

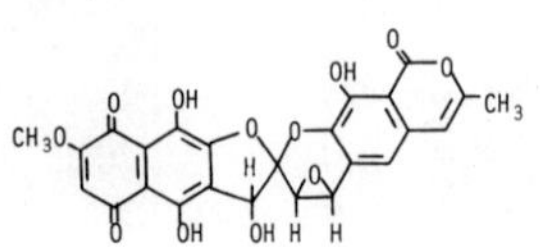

81

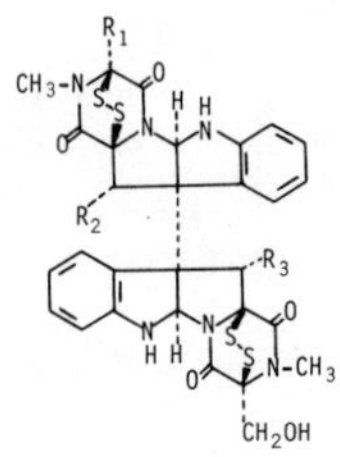

	R_1	R_2	R_3
82	-CH_3 or -CH_3	-H / -OH	-OH / -H
83	-CH_2OH	-OH	-H

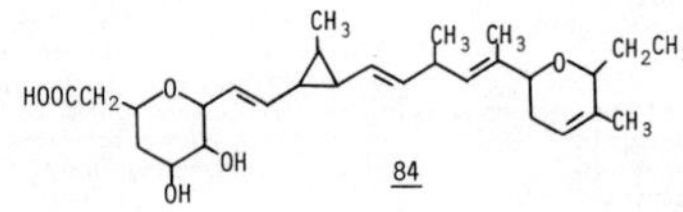

84

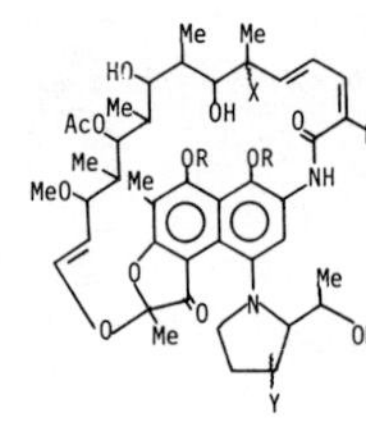

85 X=R=H; Y=OH
86 X=OH; Y=R=H

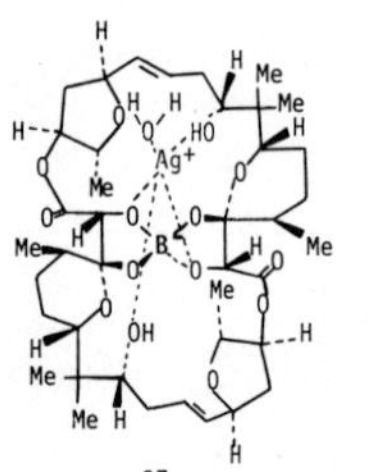

87

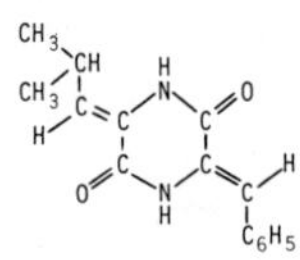

88

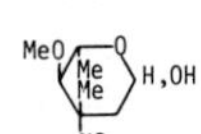

89

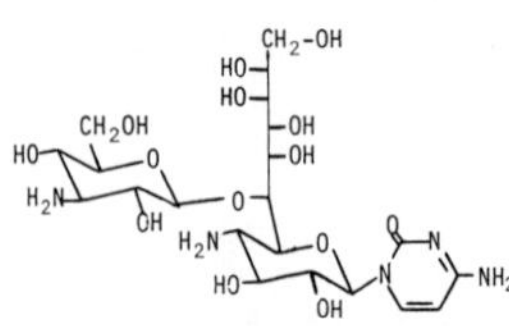

90

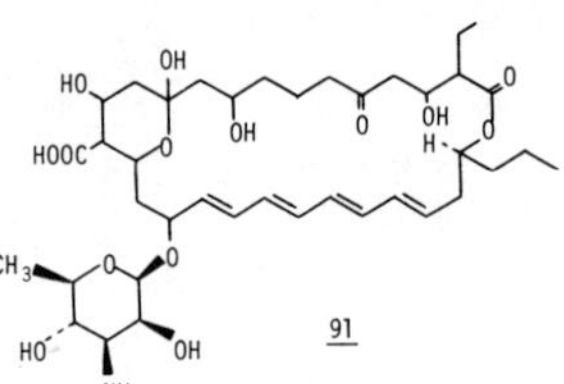

91

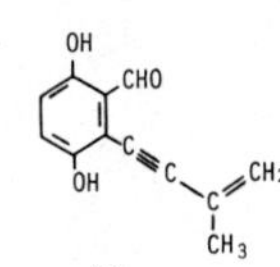

92

Various studies forecasted potential benefits for the use of antibiotics in combination. Benzylpenicillin displayed remarkable activity against a number of *Bacteroides fragilis* strains when combined with clavulanic acid.[154] Clinical trials for a mixture of rifamycin and trimethoprim were recommended on the basis of *in vitro* studies showing that the mixture decreased the incidence of resistance.[155] Another report stated that novobiocin effectively eliminated plasmids from several bacterial species.[156] Polymyxin B and rifamycin was an effective combination for 8 out of 12 patients with resistant nosocomial *Serratia marcescens* infections.[157] Novobiocin demonstrated a "probenicid effect" with β-lactam antibiotics in the treatment of experimental *Salmonella schottmuelleri* infections in mice.[158] Combinations of fosfomycin with chloramphenicol or ampicillin were effective in the treatment of *Salmonella typhi* infections in humans.[159] Fosfomycin, alone, was also shown to be particularly effective in the treatment of humans infected with Gram-negative bacilli and Gram-positive cocci.[160]

REFERENCES

1. Abstracts, 17th Interscience Conference on Antimicrobial Agents and Chemotherapy (17th ICAAC), New York, New York, October 12-14, 1977.
2. Abstracts, 10th International Congress of Chemotherapy, Zurich, Switzerland, September 18-23, 1977.
3. *Topics in Antibiotic Chemistry*, Peter Sammes, Ed., Ellis Horwood Ltd. Chichester, Sussex, England, 1977.
4. M. Barza and R. T. Scheife, Am. J. Hosp. Pharm. 34, 723 (1977).
5. L. J. Riff and G. Moreschi, Antimicrob. Ag. Chemotherap. 11, 609 (1977).
6. J. Klastersky, F. Meunier-Carpentier, L. Coppens-Kahan, D. Daneau and J. M. Prevost, ibid. 12, 503 (1977).
7. P. Christensson, T. Eden, I. Frolov, M. Jonsson, I. Juhlin, I. Julander, L. Nordstrom, P. Skansberg, O. Tjernström, G. Tunevall, O. Tjernstrom and E. Wallmark, 10th Intl. Cong. Chemother., 383 (1977).
8. P. O. Madsen and U. Hoyme, ibid. 384 (1977).
9. P. H. Edelštein and R. D. Meyer, ibid. 381 (1977).
10. F. J. Buckwold, A. R. Ronald, B. Lank, L. Fox, G. Harding, and M. Gurwith, ibid. 382 (1977).
11. G. W. Peng, G. C. Jackson and W. L. Chiou, Antimicrob. Ag. Chemotherap. 12, 707 (1977).
12. T. L. Nagabhushan, A. B. Cooper, H. Tsai and P. J. L. Daniels, 17th ICAAC, 249 (1977).
13. S. Toda, S. Nakagawa and T. Naito, J. Antibiot. 30, 1002 (1977).
14. S. Kondo, T. Miyasaka, K. Yoshida, K. Iinuma and H. Umezawa, ibid. 30, 1150 (1977).
15. K. Richardson, S. Jevons, J. W. Moore, B. C. Ross and J. R. Wright, ibid. 843 (1977).
16. Y. Abe, S. Nakagawa, K. Fujisawa, T. Naito and H. Kawaguchi, ibid. 30, 1004 (1977).
17. T. Miyake, T. Tsuchiya, S. Umezawa and H. Umezawa, Bull. Chem. Soc. Jap. 50, 2362 (1977).
18. United States Patent 4,051,315, September 27, 1977.
19. H. Matsushima, Y. Mori and K. Kitaura, J. Antibiot. 30, 890 (1977).
20. R. E. Carney, J. B. McAlpine, 17th ICAAC, 155 (1977).
21. R. D. Sitrin, D. J. Cooper and J. A. Weisbach, J. Antibiot. 30, 836 (1977).
22. A. K. Mallams, D. H. Davies, D. L. Boxler, H. F. Vernay and P. Reichert, 17th ICAAC, 251 (1977).
23. T. Suami, S. Nishiyama, Y. Ishikawa and S. Katsura, Carbohyd. Res. 53, 239 (1977).
24. T. Hayashi, N. Takeda, H. Saeki and E. Ohki, Chem. Pharm. Bull. 25, 2134 (1977).
25. T. Okutani, T. Asako, K. Yoshioka, K. Hiraga and M. Kida, J. Am. Chem. Soc. 99, 1278 (1977).
26. R. E. Carney and W. Rosenbrook, Jr., J. Antibiot. 30, 960 (1977).
27. C. Thornsberry, H. Jaffee, S. T. Brown, T. Edwards, J. W. Biddle and S. E. Thompson, J. Am. Med. Assoc. 237, 2405 (1977).
28. F. H. Kayser, M. Devaud and J. Biber, Experientia 33, 132 (1977).
29. J. E. Dowding, Antimicrob. Ag. Chemotherap. 11, 47 (1977).
30. P. Courvalin and J. Davies, ibid. 11, 619 (1977).
31. A. Diedrichsen, J. Bang and H. Heding, J. Antibiot. 30, 83 (1977).
32. M. Kono and K. O'Hara, ibid. 30, 688 (1977).
33. J. Berdy, J. K. Pauncz, Zs. M. Vajna, Gy. Horvath, J. Gyimesi and I. Koczka, ibid. 30, 945 (1977).
34. G. A. Ellestad, J. H. Martin, G. O. Morton, M. L. Sassiver and J. E. Lancaster, ibid. 30, 678 (1977).
35. Belgian Patent 844,756, January 31, 1977.
36. S. Umezawa and Y. Nishimura, J. Antibiot. 30, 189 (1977).
37. M. Numata, I. Minamida, M. Yamaoka, M. Shiraishi, T. Miyawaki and T. Nishimura, 17th ICAAC, 44 (1977).
38. I. Nakayama, H. Iwamoto, S. Iwai, T. Kawabe, H. Mizuashi and S. Ishiyama, ibid. 46 (1977).
39. E. A. Konopka, H. C. Zoganas, E. F. Kimble, E. R. Lasinski, W. L. Tobia and H. Heymann, ibid. 244 (1977).
40. H. Nomura, I. Minami, T. Hitaka and T. Fugono, J. Antibiot. 30, 928 (1977).
41. Y. Mine, T. Murakawa, T. Kamimura, T. Takaya, M. Nishida, S. Goto and S. Kuwahara, 17th ICAAC, 147 (1977).
42. M. Nishida, T. Murakawa, T. Kamimura, N. Okada, S. Fukada, H. Sakamoto, S. Nakamoto, Y. Yokota and Y. Kono, Antimicrob. Ag. Chemotherap. 11, 51 (1977).
43. Belgian Patent 848,346, May 16, 1977.
44. British Patent 1,483,142, August 17, 1977.
45. A. G. Brown, D. F. Corbett, A. J. Eglington and T. T. Howarth, J.C.S. Chem. Comm. 523 (1977).
46. P. J. Cassidy, E. O. Staphley, R. Goegelman, T. W. Miller, B. Arison, G. Albers-Schönberg, S. B. Zimmerman and J. Birnbaum, 17th ICAAC, 81 (1977).
47. E. O. Staphley, P. Cassidy, S. A. Currie, D. Daust, R. Goegelman, S. Hernandez, M. Jackson, J. M. Mata, A. K. Miller, R. I. Monaghan, J. B. Tunac, S. B. Zimmerman and D. Hendlin, ibid. 80 (1977).
48. K. Maeda, S. Takahashi, M. Sezaki, K. Iinuma, H. Naganawa, S. Kondo, M. Ohno, H. Umezawa, J. Antibiot. 30, 770 (1977).
49. P. H. Bentley, P. D. Berry, G. Brooks, M. L. Gilpin. E. Hunt and I. Zomaya, J.C.S. Chem. Comm. 748 (1977).
50. L. A. Mitscher, 173rd ACS, Medi.1 (1977).
51. A. Baumueller, U. Hoyme and P. O. Madsen, Antimicrob. Ag. Chemotherap. 12, 240 (1977).
52. M. Kikuchi and Y. Nakao, J. Antibiot. 30, 209 (1977).
53. M. Kikuchi and Y. Nakao, ibid. 30, 215 (1977).
54. T. Furumai, I. Maezawa, N. Matsuzawa, S. Yano, Y. Yamaguchi, K. Takeda and T. Okuda, ibid. 30, 443 (1977).
55. A. Kinumaki, K. Harada, T. Suzuki, M. Suzuki and T. Okuda, ibid. 30, 450 (1977).
56. G. T. Carter, Dissert. Abstr. Intl. B. 37, 766 (1976).
57. K. C. Nicolaou, Tetrahedron 33, 683 (1977).
58. K. Tatsuta, A. Tanaka, K. Fujimoto, M. Kinoshita and S. Umezawa, J. Am. Chem. Soc. 99, 5826 (1977).
59. K. Tatsuta, A. Tanaka, M. Kinoshita and S. Umezawa, Chemistry Letters, 769 (1977).
60. S. Omura, A. Nakagawa, H. Sakakibara, O. Okekawa, R. Brandsch and S. Pestka, J. Med. Chem. 20, 732 (1977).
61. E. Katz and A. L. Demain, Bacteriological Reviews 41, 449 (1977).
62. W. L. Parker, M. L. Rathnum, L. D. Dean, M. W. Nimeck, W. E. Brown and E. Meyers, J. Antibiot. 30, 767 (1977).
63. J. Shoji, H. Hinoo, Y. Wakisaka, K. Koizumi, M. Mayama and S. Matsuura, ibid. 30, 1029 (1977).
64. J. Shoji, T. Kato and H. Hinoo, ibid. 30, 1042 (1977).
65. H. Kawaguchi, H. Tsukiura, K. Tomita, M. Konishi, K. Saito, S. Kobaru, K. Numata, K. Fujisawa, T. Miyaki, M. Hatori and H. Koshiyama, ibid. 30, 779 (1977).
66. M. Konishi, K. Saito, K. Numata, T. Tsuno, K. Asama, H. Tsukiura, T. Naito and H. Kawaguchi, ibid. 30, 789 (1977).
67. T. Prange, A. Ducruix, C. Pascard and J. Lunel, Nature 265, 189 (1977).
68. J. Walker, A. Olesker, L. Valente, R. Rabanal and G. Lukacs, J.C.S. Chem. Comm. 706 (1977).
69. C. E. Moppett and E. B. Whipple, 17th ICAAC, 243 (1977).
70. A. A. Abou-Zeid, M. M. Abd El-Hamid and Y. M. Shehata, Z. Allg. Mikrobiol. 16, 337 (1976).
71. United States Patent 4,001,397, January 4, 1977.
72. J. A. Chan, T. T. Wei, C. C. Kalita, D. J. Warnick, A. L. Garretson and A. A. Aszalos, J. Antibiot. 30, 1140 (1977).
73. B. K. Park, A. Hirota and H. Sakai, Agric. Biol. Chem. 41, 573 (1977).
74. I. R. Shimi, N. Abedallah and S. Fathy, Antimicrob. Ag. Chemotherap. 11, 373 (1977).
75. W. J. McGahren, G. O. Morton, M. P. Kunstmann and G. A. Ellestad, J. Org. Chem. 42, 1282 (1977).
76. F. Besson, F. Peypoux, G. Michel, and L. Delcambe, Eur. J. Biochem. 77, 61 (1977).
77. R. Traber, M. Kuhn, H. Loosli, W. Pache and A. vonWartburg, Helv. Chim. Acta 60, 1568 (1977).
78. R. Traber, M. Kuhn, A. Rüegger, H. Lichti, H. Loosli and A. vonWartburg, ibid. 60, 1247 (1977).
79. J. M. Liesch and K. L. Rinehart, Jr., J. Am. Chem. Soc. 99, 1645 (1977).
80. H. Abe, M. Ikeda, T. Takaishi, Y. Ito and T. Okuda, Tetrahedron Lett. 735 (1977).
81. R. C. Pandey, J. C. Cook, Jr. and K. L. Rinehart, Jr., J. Am. Chem. Soc. 99, 8469 (1977).
82. R. C. Pandey, J. C. Cook, Jr. and K. L. Rinehart, Jr., ibid. 99, 5205 (1977).
83. R. C. Pandey, H. Meng, J. C. Cook, Jr. and K. L. Rinehart, Jr., ibid. 99, 5203 (1977).

84. W. A. König and C. Engelfried, H. Hagemaier, H. Kneifel, J. Liebigs, Ann. Chem., 2011 (1976).
85. B. F. Gisin, S. Kobayashi and J. E. Hall, Proc. Natl. Acad. Sci. 74, 115 (1977).
86. G. Janssen, J. Anne and H. Vanderhaeghe, J. Antibiot. 30, 141 (1977).
87. J. Pluscec, E. F. Sabo, R. O. Neubeck, E. R. Weaver, H. Basch and M. A. Ondetti, ibid. 30, 756 (1977).
88. F. Le Goffic, M. Capmau, D. Bonnet, C. Cerceau, C. Soussy, A. Dublanchet and J. Duval, ibid. 30, 665 (1977).
89. D. C. LaPorte, K. S. Rosenthal and D. R. Storm, Biochemistry 16, 1642 (1977).
90. K. S. Rosenthal and D. R. Storm, J. Antibiot. 30, 1087 (1977).
91. J. L. Occolowitz, D. H. Berg, M. Debono and R. L. Hamill, Biomed. Mass Spectrom. 3, 272 (1976).
92. H. Seto, Y. Miyazaki, K. Fujita and N. Otake, Tetrahedron Lett., 2417 (1977).
93. H. Seto, T. Yahagi, Y. Miyazaki and N. Otake, J. Antibiot. 30, 530 (1977).
94. J. W. Westley, J. F. Blount, R. H. Evans, Jr. and C. Liu, ibid. 30, 610 (1977).
95. T. Fehr, H. D. King and M. Kuhn, ibid. 30, 903 (1977).
96. N. Otake, H. Nakayama, H. Miyamae, S. Sato and Y. Saito, J.C.S. Chem. Comm., 590 (1977).
97. E. Dingeldein and H. Wahlig, 17th ICAAC, 71 (1977).
98. H. K. Michel, R. M. Shah and R. L. Hamill, ibid. 41 (1977).
99. T. Komiyama, Y. Matsuzawa, T. Oki, T. Inui, Y. Takahashi, H. Naganawa, T. Takeuchi and H. Umezawa, J. Antibiot. 30, 622 (1977).
100. Ger. Offen. 2,541,101, March 24, 1977.
101. United States Patent 4,031,206, June 21, 1977.
102. United States Patent 4,032,631, June 28, 1977.
103. H. Seto and H. Yonehara, J. Antibiot. 30, 1022 (1977).
104. S. Kondo, K. Yoshida, T. Ikeda, K. Iinuma, Y. Honma, M. Hamada and H. Umezawa, ibid. 30, 1137 (1977).
105. J. St. Pyrek, O. Achmatowicz, Jr. and A. Zamojski, Tetrahedron 33, 673 (1977).
106. Ger. Offen. 2,621,615, November 25, 1976.
107. M. S. R. Nair and M. Anchel, Phytochemistry 16, 390 (1977).
108. M. Noble, D. Noble and R. B. Sykes, J. Antibiot. 30, 455 (1977).
109. Y. Sawada, S. Kawakami, H. Taniyama, K. Hamano, R. Enokita, S. Iwado and M. Arai, ibid. 30, 460 (1977).
110. A. M. Nadzan, K. L. Rinehart, Jr. and W. T. Sokolski, ibid. 30, 523 (1977).
111. M. Shibata, M. Uyeda, Y. Kido, M. Kinoshita, F. Ishimaru and I. Hatanaka, Agric. Biol. Chem. 41, 1407 (1977).
112. T. Oki, N. Shibamoto, Y. Matsuzawa, T. Ogasawara, A. Yoshimoto, I. Kitamura, T. Inui, H. Naganawa, T. Takeuchi and H. Umezawa, J. Antibiot. 30, 683 (1977).
113. D. E. Nettleton, Jr., W. T. Bradner, J. A. Bush, A. B. Coon, J. E. Moseley, R. W. Myllymaki, F. A. O'Herron, R. H. Schreiber and A. L. Vulcano, ibid. 30, 525 (1977).
114. W. T. Bradner and M. Miseik, ibid. 30, 519 (1977).
115. G. F. Gauze, M. A. Sveshnikova, R. S. Ukholina, G. N. Komarova and V. S. Bazhanov, Antibiotiki 22, 483 (1977).
116. J. R. Evans and G. Weare, J. Antibiot. 30, 604 (1977).
117. M. Shimada, H. Honda, J. Awaya and S. Omura, ibid. 30, 330 (1977).
118. S. Omura, H. Tanaka, R. Oiwa, S. Awaya, R. Masuma and K. Tanaka, ibid. 30, 908 (1977).
119. E. B. Chain and G. Mellows, J.C.S. Perkin I, 318 (1977).
120. I. Kitamura, N. Shibamoto, T. Oki, T. Inui, H. Naganawa, M. Ishizuka, T. Masuda, T. Takeuchi and H. Umezawa, J. Antibiot. 30, 616 (1977).
121. T. Arai, K. Takahashi and A. Kubo, ibid. 30, 1015 (1977).
122. S. Mizuba, C. Hsu and J. Jiu , ibid. 30, 670 (1977).
123. R. Andersen, G. Büchi, B. Kobbe, A. L. Demain, J. Org. Chem. 42, 352 (1977).
124. T. Anke, F. Oberwinkler, W. Steglich and G. Hofle, J. Antibiot. 30, 221 (1977).
125. Japanese Patent 52 083,357, July 13, 1977.
126. T. Katayama, H. Minato, K. Ishi and E. Kondo, J. Antibiot. 30, 430 (1977).
127. G. B. Fedorova, M. F. Lavrova, N. N. Lomakina, L. P. Terekhova, L. P. Ivanitskaya and L. V. Makukho, Antibiotiki 22, 3 (1977).
128. P. F. Wiley, R. B. Kelly, E. L. Caron, V. H. Wiley, J. H. Johnson, F. A. MacKellar and S. A. Mizsak, J. Am. Chem. Soc. 99, 542 (1977).
129. R. C. Kelly, I. Schletter, J. M. Koert, F. A. MacKellar and P. F. Wiley, J. Org. Chem. 42, 3591 (1977).
130. S. Kondo, M. Miyamoto, H. Naganawa, T. Takeuchi and H. Umezawa, J. Antibiot. 30, 1143 (1977).
131. M. Miyamoto, S. Kondo, H. Naganawa, K. Maeda, M. Ohno and H. Umezawa, ibid. 30, 340 (1977).
132. S. Omura, H. Imai, H. Takeshima and A. Nakagawa, Chem. Pharm. Bull. 24, 3139 (1976).
133. K. Eckardt, D. Tresselt and W. Ihn, Z. Chem. 16, 486 (1976).
134. A. D. Argoudelis and S. A. Mizsak, J. Antibiot. 30, 468 (1977).
135. S. M. Ringel, R. C. Greenough, S. Roemer, D. Connor, A. L. Gutt, B. Blair, G. Kanter and M. vonStrandtmann, ibid. 30, 371 (1977).
136. A. K. Ganguly, Y. T. Liu, O. Z. Sarre and S. Szmulewicz, ibid. 30, 625 (1977).
137. H. Nakamura, Y. Iitaka, T. Kitahara, T. Okazaki and Y. Okami, ibid. 30, 714 (1977).
138. C. Shin, M. Hayakawa, K. Mikami and J. Yoshimura, Tetrahedron Lett., 863 (1977).
139. A. K. Ganguly, O. Z. Sarre, A. T. McPhail and K. D. Onan, J.C.S. Chem. Comm., 313 (1977).
140. S. Ennifar and B. C. Das, S. M. Nash, R. Nagarajan, ibid. 41 (1977).
141. R. C. Pandey and K. L. Rinehart, Jr., J. Antibiot. 30, 146 (1977).
142. S. DeBernardo and M. Weigele, J. Org. Chem. 42, 109 (1977).
143. R. A. Moss and M. Matsuo, J. Am. Chem. Soc. 99, 1643 (1977).
144. R. K. Boeckman, Jr. and E. W. Thomas, ibid. 99, 2805 (1977).
145. A. A. Jakubowski, F. S. Guziec, Jr. and M. Tishler, Tetrahedron Lett., 2399 (1977).
146. E. J. Corey and D. R. Williams, ibid. 3847 (1977).
147. R. M. Scarborough, Jr. and A. B. Smith, III, J. Am. Chem. Soc. 99, 7085 (1977).
148. K. Inuma, S. Kondo, K. Maeda and H. Umezawa, Bull. Chem. Soc. Jap. 50, 1850 (1977).
149. G. F. Field, W. J. Zally, L. H. Sternbach and J. F. Blount, J. Org. Chem. 41, 3853 (1976).
150. F. Nakatsubo, T. Fukuyama, A. J. Cocuzza and Y. Kishi, J. Am. Chem. Soc. 99, 8115 (1977).
151. T. Fukuyama, F. Nakatsubo, A. J. Cocuzza and Y. Kishi, Tetrahedron Lett., 4295 (1977).
152. D. Seebach, B. Seuring, H. Kalinowski, W. Lubosch and B. Renger, Angew. Chem. Int. Ed. Engl. 16, 264 (1977).
153. H. Fukumi, H. Kurihara, T. Hata, C. Tamura and H. Mishima, A. Kubo, T. Arai, Tetrahedron Lett., 3825 (1977).
154. R. Wise, Lancet 2, 145 (1977).
155. V. Arioli, M. Berti, G. Carniti, E. Rossi and L. G. Silvestri, J. Antimicrob. Chemother. 3, 87 (1977).
156. G. L. McHugh and N. M. Swartz, Antimicrob. Ag. Chemotherap. 12, 423 (1977).
157. R. C. Ostenson, B. T. Fields and C. M. Nolan, ibid. 12, 655 (1977).
158. A. K. Miller, E. Celozzi and B. A. Pelak, J. Antibiot. 30, 893 (1977).
159. A. Rodriguez, A. Gallego, T. Olay and J. M. Mata, Chemotherapy 23, Suppl. 1, 247 (1977).
160. R. Fujii, ibid. 23, Suppl. 1, 234 (1977).

Chapter 12. Antifungal Agents

R.Y. Cartwright, Public Health Laboratory, St. Luke's
Hospital, Guildford, Surrey, England.

Introduction - Since the last review two years ago there have been no new major antifungal drugs introduced into clinical practice. Clotrimazole, 1, and miconazole, 2, are regarded as promising advances in two editorials.[1,2] The possibilities of miconazole for the treatment of systemic mycoses including reports on its experimental and clinical evaluation was the subject of a symposium.[3] The use of and the mode of action of 5 fluorocytosine (5FC), 3, was comprehensively reviewed.[4]

It was suggested that the synthesis of chitin might be a suitable site for a future antifungal drug. Chitin is specific to fungal cells, is essential to their structure, is produced precisely at the site of invasion of tissue - the hyphal apex and its synthesis is accomplished by one enzyme - chitin synthase.[5]

New Antifungal Agents - A series of 1 - (2-alkyl-2-phenylethyl)-1H-imidazole derivatives were synthesized from corresponding phenylacetonitriles, 4,[6].

Most activity was found in analogues with ortho-para distribution on the phenyl ring. Significant broad-spectrum activity was associated with at least four carbon atoms in the alkyl chain. Trichostatin, 5, an analogue of a primary hydroxamic acid was isolated from *Streptomyces hygroscopicus.* It was active *in vitro* against dermatophytes but not yeasts.[7] A non-polyene antibiotic (H537 SY2) isolated from *Streptomyces yokosukanensis* was active against *Candida* spp.[8] The structure has not yet been elucidated but appears to contain three amino sugars and a carbonyl group. A group of quinolizidine-derived hemiaminals and beta-tert-amino

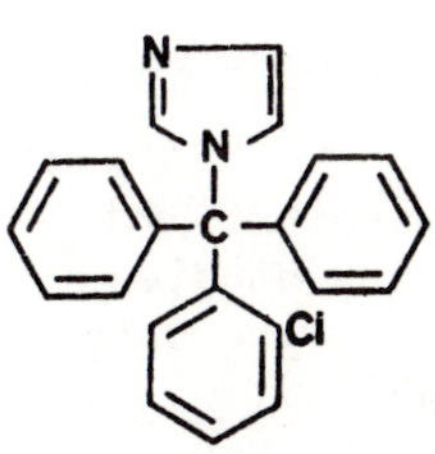

1

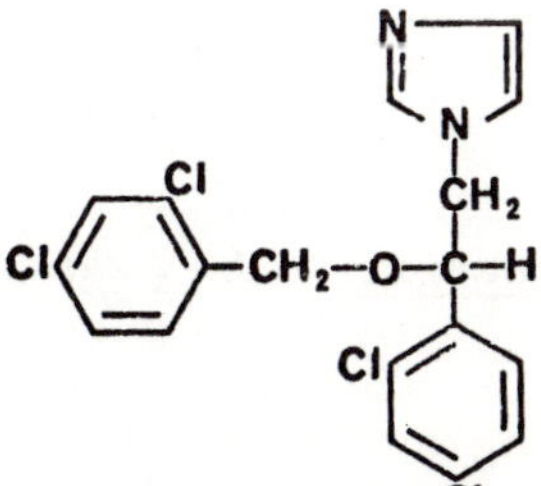

2

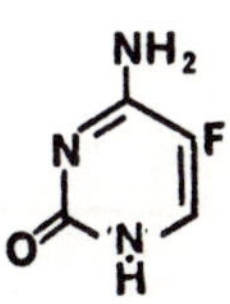

3

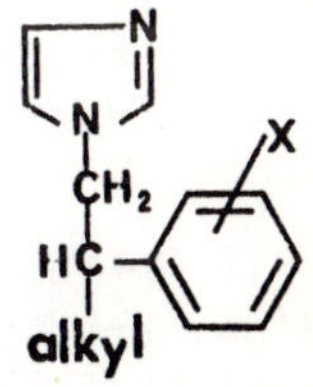

4

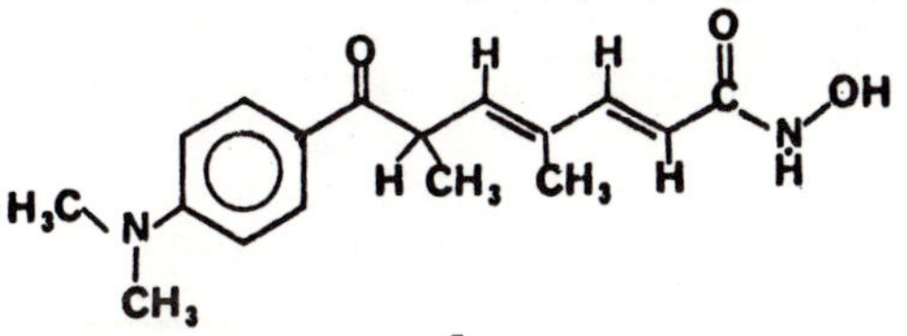

5

ISBN 0-12-040513-X

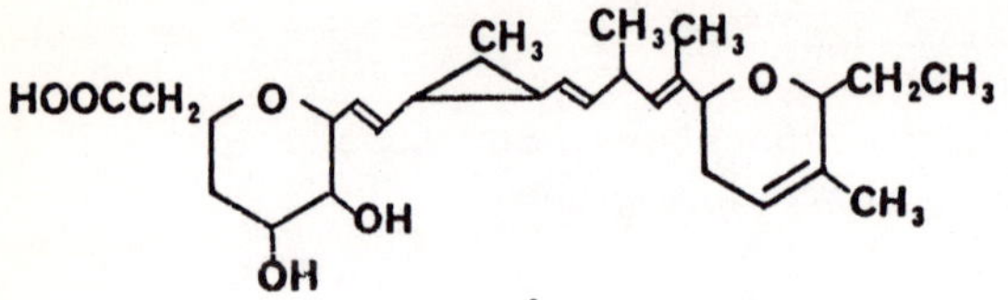

6

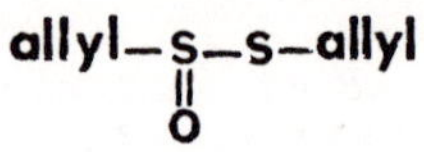

7

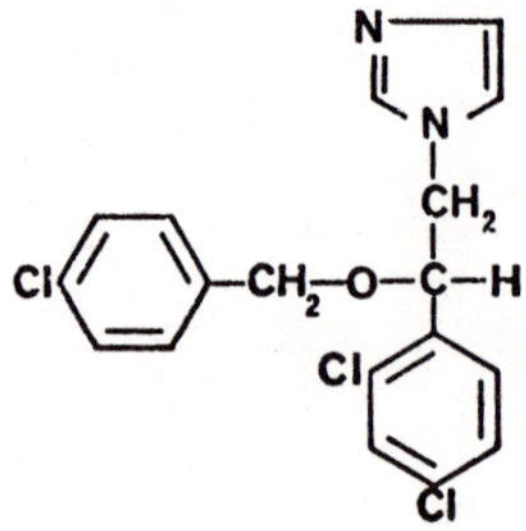

8

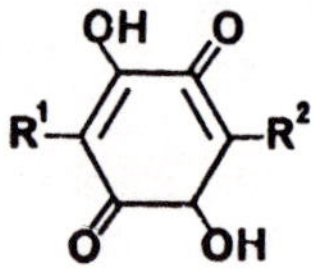

9

sulfides were prepared.[9] Only those α-thiohemiaminals possessing the C-1 equatorial methyl and the C-4 equatorial 3-furyl groups were active antifungal agents and their in vitro activity was greater than amphotericin B. Four thiocyanatopyrazole derivatives were synthesized and in vitro activity was demonstrated against a number of dermatophytic fungi. Electron microscopic studies on Trichophyton mentagrophytes exposed to 1, 3-dimethyl -4-thiocyanato-5-amino-pyrazole showed an increase of the plasma membrane with intra and extra cytoplasmic processes. The nuclear and mitochondrial membranes deteriorated and there was final plasmolysis.[10] Inhibition of T.mentagrophytes was inhibited by some 7-alkyl amino pyrazolo (1, 5-a) pyrimidines. The degree of inhibition increased with the length of 7-alkylamino chain up to C_8 units then decreased. Unsaturated chains had greater activity than saturated chains.[11] Aculeacin, the structure of which has not yet been elucidated, is a peptide antibiotic containing palmitic acid, isolated from Aspergillus aculeatus. It was active against yeasts, dermatophytes and phytopathogenic fungi, and although not strongly fungicidal, inhibited filamentous fungi. Toxicity for mice was low.[12]

A metabolite of Aspergillus tamarii A30641 was active against candida, cryptococci and gram-positive bacteria.[13] Preliminary studies suggest that the structure includes a phenolic hydroxyl and the presence of the epidithiodiketopiperazine ring system. Ambruticin (W7783), 6, was isolated from Polyangium cellulosum var fulvum. A cyclopropyl-polyene-pyran acid, it was highly active against Coccidioides immitis, Histoplasma capsulatum and Blastomyces dermatitidis.[14] Allicin, 7, an extract from Allium sativum, was active in vitro against yeasts and dermatophytes but not against aspergilli.[15] The observed effect was dependent on the inoculum size.

Laboratory Methods - A potential bioassay for nystatin depending on nystatin-induced potassium efflux from Saccharomyces cerevisiae, measured by flame photometry, was described.[16] Polyenes were assayed by two methods involving the replacement of intracellular potassium by rubidium and measuring its subsequent release from cells exposed to a polyene antibiotic. Using S. cerevisiae as the test organism, the release rubidium was measured by atomic absorption spectrophotometry.[17] A radiometric approach used ^{86}Rb to replace the potassium in a strain of Candida parapsilosis. This method enabled amphotericin B to be assayed within the range 0.06 - 2.9 μg/ml.[18] The rapid assay of amphotericin B, 8, in less than thirty minutes was achieved with the use of high-pressure liquid chromatography.[19] Absorption was at 405 nm and the lower level of sensitivity was 0.02 μg/ml. There was no interference from 5FC. 5FC was assayed in the presence of amphotericin B after heating the serum sample at 100°C for forty-five minutes which inactivated the polyene.[20] C.stellatoidea was used in the bioassay of miconazole by radial diffusion.[21] Difficulties in assessing the susceptibility testing of yeasts to imidazoles were recognized and a turbimetric technique independent of inoculum size was developed.[22] A Coulter counter was used to assess the ED_{50} and the MIC of a wide range of antifungal agents against strains of S.cerevisiae and C. albicans. The degree of inhibition of cell division and of protein synthesis could be compared.[23] Econazole, 9, was compared to other agents by the Warburg assay.[24] The antifungal activity of 5FC was measured by disc diffusion susceptibility testing against 216 yeasts using 1 μg and 10 μg discs.[25] The 10 μg disc was preferred. Disc diffusion susceptibility was used to determine the MIC of yeasts against amphotericin B, nystatin and 5FC.[26] It was demonstrated that the antifungal activity of imidazoles was reduced by complex media - Sabouraud's glucose and brain heart infusion - but not by a synthetic amino acid medium or modified yeast nitrogen broth. No inhibition was shown with any of the media by amphotericin B methyl ester.[27]

In vitro and animal studies - 15-Aza-24-methylene-D-homocholestadiene, a naturally occurring azasterol with antimycotic properties was shown to competitively inhibit sterol 24 (28) methylene reductase in S.cerevisiae.[28] 2, 5-Dihydroxy-1, 4 benzoquinones were shown to decrease the vegetative growth and inhibit spore germination in twelve fungal species. Substitution at 3 and 6 in the quinone ring affected these properties; the most active compounds generally had a low polarity.[29] The antibiotic phacidin was inhibitory against T.mentagrophytes, T. rubrum and Epidermophyton floccosum.[30] 2, 4-Diamino-6-{2-(3,4-dichlorophenyl) acetamido} quinazoline inhibited the incorporation of labelled precursors into the RNA and protein of C. neoformans. Experimental infections in mice responded to intraperitoneal therapy.[31] In vitro, tolciclate was more active against dermatophytes than clotrimazole or miconazole.[32] Versicolin was active against T. rubrum both in vitro and in experimental infections of mice and guinea pigs.[33] The activity of amphotericin B was prolonged using the antioxidant propyl gallate.[34] The inhibitory effect of amphotericin B methyl ester on protoplasts of C. albicans was inhibited by the presence of 85 mM KCl or 45 mM $MgCl_2$.[35] Amphotericin B inhibited phosphate uptake in C. albicans, especially in young (2h) cells and this effect was stronger than growth inhibition.[36] The sterol structure of two polyene-resistant mutants of C. albicans showed that one accumulated lichesterol and fecosterol, and the other eburicol and lanosterol.[37] In polyene-resistant strains of C. krusei, C. parakrusei and C. tropicalis isolated from patients, the sterols were the same as in the wild types but present in lower concentrations.[38] In an auxotroph of C. albicans, the resistance to polyenes was related to fatty acid composition rather than sterols. Greatest resistance was shown when the strain was grown in the presence of oleic or linoleic acid.[39] The action of candicidin on C. albicans at various stages of the growth cycle was related to differing fatty acid composition of the cells.[40] It was suggested that the divalent ions Ca++ and Mg++ can interact with membrane sterols in C. albicans creating steric hinderance to the absorption of candicidin. K+ and NH_4+ reversed the inhibition of glycolysis by candicidin but did prevent antibiotic absorption.[41] Ultrastructural changes were observed in the cells of A. fumigatus from infected mice treated with clotrimazole.[42] Miconazole was highly active against Histoplasma capsulatum and Blastomyces dermatitidis and serum levels in man could be expected to exceed the MIC. C. immitis, Sp.schenckii, C. neoformans, C. albicans and A. fumigatus were less sensitive and Fusarium spp. were resistant.[43]

The mode of action of miconazole against C. albicans was studied by biochemical, cytochemical and ultrastructural techniques.[44, 45, 46]. Changes were observed in oxidative and peroxidative enzymes and it was suggested that fungistatic levels of miconazole produce an increase in the production of intracellular hydrogen peroxide which is broken down by catalase. At fungicidal levels, the catalase was inhibited leading to lethal levels of hydrogen peroxide. Miconazole is also a potent inhibitor of demethylation at the C-14 position in ergosterol biosynthesis. The emergence of miconazole-resistant candida during treatment was reported.[46] Econazole inhibited fungal growth by its damaging effects on the various membrane systems of fungal cells.[48] Ultrastructural changes in the cell wall followed the exposure of C. albicans to econazole.[49] Econazole was more active than miconazole in vitro against filamentous fungi.

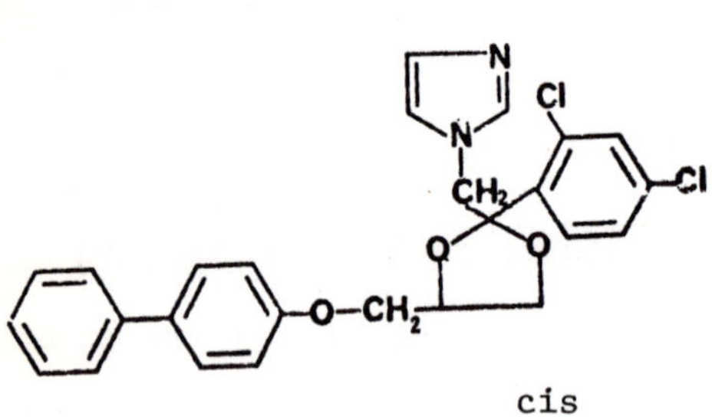

cis

10

R34,000, 10, was effective orally in controlling murine coccidioidomycosis.[51] 5FC sensitive cells of candida possess an electron dense layer dividing the inner layer of the cell wall. The dense layer is absent in resistant strains.[52] Following exposure to 5FC, yeast cells enlarge. Ultrastructure studies of treated cells show an enlarged nucleus and a thin cell comparative to the changes caused by DNA synthesis inhibitors in mammalian cells.[53] Studies on the influence of 5FC on nucleic and synthesis in yeasts suggested that it may act by the formation of 5-fluorodeoxyuridine monophosphate which inhibits thymidylate synthetase and also by the incorporation of fluorouridylic acid into RNA.[54] A wide range of purines and pyrimidines except thymidine inhibited the action of 5FC.[55]

Griseofulvin was shown to interfere with the normal polymerization of microtubule protein; it also acted directly on tubulin in common with other mitotic drugs.[56]

Drug Combinations:- Minocyline at 10 μg/ml or less was synergistic with amphotericin B. Doxycycline had a reduced effect but demeclocycline and tetracycline were ineffective.[57] *In vitro* synergism between amphotericin B and rifampin was demonstrated against *Candida* spp.[58] and *C. immitis*.[59] The combination however, was not superior to amphotericin B alone in murine coccidioidomycosis. Therapy of murine aspergillosis with amphotericin B in combination with rifampin or 5FC was more effective than amphotericin B alone but did not result in complete cure.[60] Amphotericin B and rifampin were used successfully for pulmonary aspergillosis in a leukemic patient.[61] *In vitro* inhibition of aspergilli was increased by the combination of amphotericin B with 5FC and rifampin.[62] Five patients with systemic infection due to candida or *Torulopsis glabrata* were successfully treated by amphotericin B in combination with 5FC.[63, 64] The effect of the combination of amphotericin B and 5FC on *C. albicans* appeared to be sequential, amphotericin B acting first.[65]

The combination of amphotericin B and griseofulvin was used with success in a diabetic with pulmonary and rhinocerebral mucormycosis.[66] Sulfamethoxazole acted synergistically with both clotrimazole[67] and miconazole[68] against *Candida* spp. *In vitro* synergism was shown between clotrimazole and both amphotericin B and 5FC[69] but there was antagonism between miconazole and amphotericin B.

Therapeutic and Pharmacologic Studies:- In a double blind study, a 1% solution of ciclopirox was effective against *T. rubrum*, *T. violaceum*, *T. mentagrophytes* and *Malassezia furfur*.[71] Tolciclate treatment produced a 78% cure rate in a multicentre trial against dermatophytes.[72] Three patients with indwelling catheters and a candidal urinary tract infection were successfully treated with oral nifuratel.[73] The value of intravenous 5FC was illustrated by the case report of a patient with candida septicemia following severe trauma.[74] Four out of fifteen patients receiving 5FC had evidence of bone marrow toxicity which was related to serum levels above 125 μg/ml.[75] The nephrotoxicity of amphotericin B was reduced by the infusion of 25 gram of mannitol with each dose.[76] In a double blind study involving eleven patients, no difference was observed whether or not mannitol was given with the amphotericin B. Renal biopsies showed a hitherto undescribed vacuolization of smooth muscle cells in the media of arterioles and arteries associated with amphotericin B.[77] Miconazole and clotrimazole were both effective topically against dermatophytes, pityriasis, candida and erythrasma.[78]

The topical pharmacology of chlormidazole, clotrimazole, miconazole and econazole and the relative value of topical antifungal drugs was discussed.[79] The general pharmacology of imidazoles was reviewed.[80] Pharmacologic studies of intravenous miconazole in patients with coccidioidomycosis revealed a biphasic clearance from the blood. Passage into cerebrospinal fluid did not occur in therapeutic amounts.[81] A more detailed study in normal subjects and patients with renal failure showed an initial serum half life of 0.38 h., then 2.08 h and finally a prolonged phase of 24.1 h. Renal insufficiency did not affect the rate of elimination from the body.[82] Five of the patients with coccidioidal meningitis responded to miconazole intravenously and four more intrathecally.[83] No response was recorded in two patients with cryptococcal meningitis. A leukemic patient with disseminated candidiasis was successfully treated with miconazole.[84] Intravenous miconazole was also used with success in a patient with chronic esophageal candidiasis[85] and a patient with an extensive cavitatory infection with Sporotrichum schenckii.[86] The latter patient had received amphotericin B alone and in combination with 5FC without effect. The failure of oral polyenes in the management of candidiasis of the digestive tract was followed successfully by oral miconazole.[87] Preliminary studies indicate the value of long term miconazole for patients with paracoccidioidomycosis.[88] The use of intravenous miconazole should be accompanied by careful hematologic studies as six consecutive patients showed an anemia and thrombocytosis. The effect was dose related and reversible. There were no hemorrhagic or thrombotic episodes.[89]

References

1. P.S. Lietman, J. Pediat. 88, 908,(1976).
2. Editorial. Brit. Med. J. ii, 347,(1977).
3. Proc. R. Soc. Med. 70, Suppl. 1. (1977).
4. H.J. Schöler, Proc. 10th. Int. Cong. Chemother.,Zurich (1977).
5. G.W. Goodhay, J. Gen. Microbiol., 99, 1,(1977).
6. J. Heeres, L.J. Back and J.M. Van Cutsem, J. Med. Chem. 19, 1148,(1976).
7. N. Tsuji, M. Kobayashi, K. Nagashima, Y.Wakisaka and K.Koizumi.,J. Antibiot.(Tokyo)29,1, (1976).
8. H. Kondo, M.Vehara, S.Nakama, T.Otani and S.Nakamura, ibid., 29, 847,(1976).
9. R.T. LaLonde, A.I. Tsai, C.J.Wang, C.Wong and G.Lee, J.Med. Chem., 19, 214,(1976).
10. G.L. Vannini, G. Dall'Olio and P.Giori, Mycopathologia, 58, 39,(1976).
11. T. Novinson, R.K. Robins and T.R. Mathews, J.Med. Chem., 20, 296,(1977).
12. K. Mizuno, A. Yagi, S. Satoi, M. Takada, M. Hayashi, K.Asano and T.Matsuda, J.Antibiot.(Tokyo) 30, 297,(1977).
13. D.H. Berg, R.P.Massing, M.M.Hoehn, L.D.Boeck and R.L.Hamill, ibid. 29, 394,(1976).
14. S.M. Ringel, R.C. Greenough, S.Roemer, D.Connor, A.L.Gutt, B.Blair,G.Kanter and M.von Strandtmann, ibid. 30, 371, (1977).
15. Y.Yamada and K. Azuma, Antimicrob. Ag. Chemother. 11, 743,(1977).
16. S. Clements-Jewery, ibid. 8, 585,(1976).
17. R.F. Cosgrove and J.E. Fairbrother, ibid. 11,31, (1977).
18. R.E. Drazin and R.I. Lehrer, J.Infect. Dis. 134, 238,(1976).
19. I. Nilsson-Ehle, T.T. Yoshikawa, J.E. Edwards, M.C.Schotz and L.B. Guze, ibid. 135, 414,(1977).
20. C.A. Kauffman, J.A. Carleton and P.T. Frame, Antimicrob. Ag. Chemother. 9, 381, (1976).
21. A. Espinel-Ingroff, S. Shadomy and J.F. Fisher, ibid. 11, 365 (1977).
22. J.N. Galgiani and D.A. Stevens, ibid. 10, 721, (1976).
23. J. Brotherton, Mykosen, 19, 361,(1976).
24. W. Raab and B. Gmeiner, ibid. 19, 238, (1976).
25. C.J. Utz and S. Shadomy, J. Infect. Dis. 135, 970, (1977).
26. J.M. Boyer, Antimicrob. Ag. Chemother. 9, 1070, (1976).
27. P.D. Hoeprich and A.C. Huston, J. Infect. Dis. 134, 336, (1976).
28. P.R. Hays, W.D. Neal and L.W. Parks, Antimicrob. Ag. Chemother. 12, 185,(1977).
29. D. Brewer, W.S. Maass and A. Taylor, Can. J. Microbiol. 23, 845, (1977).
30. A.S. Sekhon and A. Funk, J. Antimicrob. Chemother. 3, 95, (1977).
31. A.R. Harari and H.W. Larsh, Proc. Soc. Exp, Biol. Med. 151, 173,(1976).
32. A. Bianchi, G. Monti and I. de Carneri, Antimicrob. Chemother. 12, 429, (1977).
33. J. Nandi and S.K. Bose, J. Antibiot(Tokyo), 29, 50, (1976).
34. F.A. Andrews, W.H. Beggs and G.A. Sarosi, Antimicrob. Ag. Chemother. 11, 615, (1977).
35. D. Kerridge, T.Y. Koh and A.M. Johnson, J. Gen. Microbiol. 96, 117, (1976).
36. I. Berdicevsky and N. Grossowicz, ibid. 102, 299, (1977).
37. R.E. Subden, L. Safe, D.C. Morris, R.G.Brown and S. Safe, Can. J. Microbiol. 23, 751, (1977).
38. L.M. Safe, S.H.Safe, R.E. Subden and D.C. Morris, ibid. 23, 398, (1977).
39. T.Y. Koh, M.S. Marriott, J.Taylor and E.F. Gale, J. Gen. Microbiol. 102, 105, (1977).
40. S.M. Hammond, B.N. Kliger, Antimicrob. Ag. Chemother. 9, 561, (1976).
41. S.M. Hammond and B.N. Kliger, J. Appl. Bacteriol. 41, 59, (1976).
42. W.H. Voigt, Mykosen, 19, 345, (1976).

43. S. Shadomy, L. Paxton, A. Espinel-Ingroff and H.J. Shadomy, J. Antimicrob. Chemother. 3, 147, (1977).
44. S. de Nollin and M. Borgers, Mykosen, 19, 317, (1976).
45. S. de Nollin, H. Van Belle, F. Goossens, F. Thone and M. Borgers, Antimicrob. Ag. Chemother. 11, 500 (1977).
46. H. Van den Bossche, G. Willemsens and W.F.J. Lavers, Abst. 10th. Int.Cong.Chem., 155. (Zurich).
47. R.J. Holt and A. Azmi, Lancet, 1, 50, (1978).
48. R. Kern and F.K. Zimmermann, Mykosen, 20, 133, (1977).
49. H-J. Preusser, ibid. 19, 304, (1976).
50. G. Shar, F.H. Kayser and M.C. Dupont, Chemotherapy, 22, 211, (1976).
51. H.B. Levine, Chest, 70, 755, (1976).
52. S. Montplaisir, B. Nabarra and E. Drouhet, Antimicrob. Ag. Chemother. 9, 1028, (1976).
53. T. Arai, Y. Mikami, K. Yokoyama, T. Kawata and K.Masuda, ibid. 12, 255, (1977).
54. A. Polak and W.H. Wain, Chemotherapy, 23, 243, (1977).
55. G.E. Wagner and S. Shadomy, Antimicrob. Ag. Chemother. 11, 229, (1977).
56. J. Wehland, W. Herzog and K. Weber, J. Mol.Biol.111, 329, (1977).
57. M.A. Lew, K.M. Beckett and M. J. Levin, J. Infect. Dis. 136, 263, (1977).
58. W.H. Beggs, G.A. Sarosi and M.I. Walker, ibid., 133, 206, (1976).
59. M. Huppert, D. Pappagianis, S.H. Sun, I. Gleason-Jordon, M.S.Collins and K.R.Vukovich, Antimicrob. Ag. Chemother. 9, 406, (1976).
60. L.Arroyo, G. Medoff and G.S. Kobayashi, ibid. 11, 21, (1977).
61. B. Ribner, G.T. Keusch, B.A. Hanna and M. Perloff, Chest, 70, 681, (1976).
62. M. Kitahara, V.K. Seth, G. Medoff and G.S. Kobayashi, Antimicrob. Ag. Chemother. 9, 915, (1976).
63. T. Eilard, D. Beskow, R. Norrby, P. Wåhlén and K. Alestig, J. Antimicrob. Chemother. 2, 239, (1976).
64. P.J. Chesney, K.C. Teets, J.J. Mulvihull, I.E. Salit and M.I. Marks, J. Pediat. 89, 1017, (1976).
65. J.F. Brown, L.S. Gottlieb and R.A. McCormick, Arch. Intern. Med. 137, 936, (1977).
66. W.H. Beggs, F.A. Andrews and G.A. Sarosi, Res. Commun. Chem. Pathol. Pharmacol. 16, 557, (1977).
67. W.H. Beggs, G.A. Sarosi and N.M. Steele, Curr. Ther. Res. 20, 623, (1976).
68. W.H. Beggs and G.A. Sarosi, ibid. 21, 547, (1977).
69. W.H. Beggs, G.A. Sarosi and N.M. Steele, Antimicrob. Ag. Chemother. 9, 863, (1976).
70. L.P. Schacter, R.J. Owellen, H.K.Rathbun and B. Buchanan, Lancet, 2, 318, (1976).
71. V.N. Sehgal, Br. J. Dermatol. 95, 83, (1976).
72. V. Mandelli, Arzneim. Forsch. 26, 769, (1976).
73. R.N. Grüneberg and A. Leakey, Br. Med. J. ii, 908, (1976).
74. M. Starorovsky, S. Wientraub and A. Iellim, Int. Surg., 61, 426, (1976).
75. C.A. Kauffman and P.T. Frame, Antimicrob. Ag. Chemother. 11, 244, (1977).
76. J.M. Rosch, G.J. Pazin and D. Fireman, JAMA., 235, 1995, (1976).
77. W.E. Bullock, R.G. Luke, C.E. Nuttall and D. Bhathena. Antimicrob. Ag. Chemother. 10, 555, (1976).
78. Y.M. Clayton and A.G. Knight, Clin. Exp. Dermatol. 1, 225, (1976).
79. R.J. Holt, J. Cutan, Pathol. 3, 45, (1976).
80. R.Y. Cartwright, Mykosen, 21, Suppl. 1.,(1978).
81. D.A. Stevens, H.B. Levine and S.C. Deresinksi, Am. J. Med. 60, 191, (1976).
82. P.J. Lewi, J. Boelaert, R. Deneels, R. De Meyere, H. Van Landuyt, J.J.D. Heykants, J. Symoens and J. Wynants, Eur. J. Clin. Pharmacol. 10, 49, (1976).
83. S.C. Deresinski, R.D. Lilly, H.B. Levine, J.N. Galgiani and D.A. Stevens, Arch. Intern. Med. 137, 1180,(1977).
84. M.E. Katz and P.A. Cassileth, JAMA., 237, 1124, (1977).
85. L. Rutgeerts and H. Verhaegen, Gastroenterology, 72, 316, (1977).
86. J.J. Rohwedder and G. Archer, Am. Rev. Respir. Dis. 114, 403, (1976).
87. E. Svejgaard, Act. Derm. Venereol. 56, 303, (1976).
88. R. Negroni, E. Libonatti, P. Rubenstein, H. Ramo, O. Palmieri, M. Waismann, M. Elder and E.Cablinsky, Castellanis, 4, 11, (1976).
89. L.C. Marmion, K.B. Desser, R.B. Lilly and D.A. Stevens, Antimicrob. Ag. Chemother. 10, 447, (1976).

Chapter 13. Antineoplastic Agents

Allen R. Kraska and J.S. Wolff, Pfizer Inc., Groton, Connecticut 06340

Introduction — A survey of the 1977 literature revealed no truly significant breakthrough in the design or discovery of agents for cancer therapy. With the exception of drugs for enzyme and hormonal therapy, the search for new drugs has continued to rely on antibiotic screening, empirical compound screening, and molecular modifictions of existing agents. One of the most comprehensive treatises on chemotherapy published to date discussed general principles that have led to progress and explained difficulties in achieving a quantum improvement in therapy.[1] The mechanisms of action (MOA) of the various classes of antitumor agents were described, with details covering the most effective in the clinic. General reviews on cancer chemotherapy and immunotherapy[2-6] were published, as well as specific reviews on anthracyclines,[7] antineoplastic agents from plants,[8,9] pharmacokinetics of 5-fluorouracil (5-FU),[10] methotrexate (MTX),[11] levamisole,[12] bleomycin,[13] pyrrole(1,4)benzodiazepine antitumor antibiotics,[14] MOA of DNA synthesis inhibitors,[15] and inhibitors of mercapto enzymes.[16] Clinical results obtained with the most effective adjuvant chemotherapeutic approaches were also reviewed.[18,19] A report detailing cancer survival statistics for patients diagnosed and treated at centers participating in the Cancer Surveillance, Epidemiology and End Results (SEER) program was published by the Department of Health, Education and Welfare (DHEW).[20]

Alkylating Agents and Nitrosoureas — A great deal of research continued to be stimulated by the clinical efficacy of compounds such as cyclophosphamide, L-phenylalanine mustard (L-PAM), *bis*-chloroethyl nitrosourea (BCNU; **1**), and close analogs. With the development of chlorozotocin (**2**) and streptozotocin (**3**) additional work has sought further decreases in toxicity and advantages in activity profile. 1-(2-Chloroethyl)-3-(β-D-glucopyranosyl)-1-nitrosourea (**4**) and **5** were synthesized and compared with **2**, BCNU, and CCNU.[21,22] The % increased life span (ILS) values at the LD_{50} dose (i.p.) in mice with L1210 leukemia were 90 (**4**), 429 (**5**), 332 (**2**), 260 (BCNU), and 364 (CCNU; **6**).

$ClCH_2CH_2–CNU$

1

CNU = $–NH–\overset{O}{\overset{\|}{C}}–\underset{}{\overset{NO}{\overset{|}{N}}}–CH_2CH_2Cl$

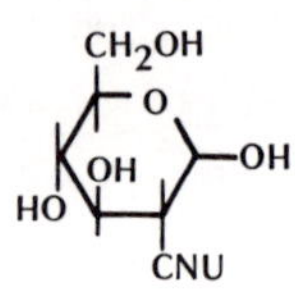

2

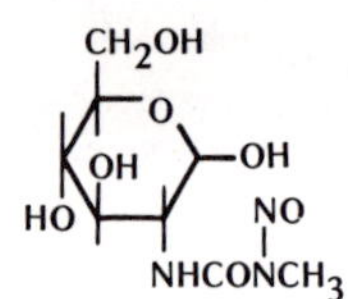

3

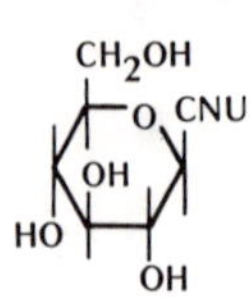

4

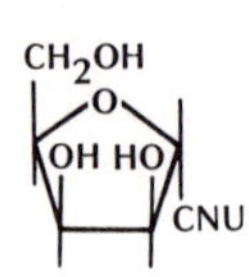

5

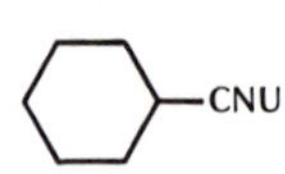

6

When compared with BCNU and CCNU, the selective reduction of myelosuppression by **4** and **2** was attributed to the glucose functionality and not the increased water solubility. Support for this hypothesis was obtained by studying the water soluble nitrosourea 7, which was active against

ISBN 0-12-040513-X

L1210 leukemia (492% ILS), but was also a potent myelotoxin.[23] The mechanism of nitrosourea action remained unclear, as antineoplastic activity did not correlate with carbamoylating

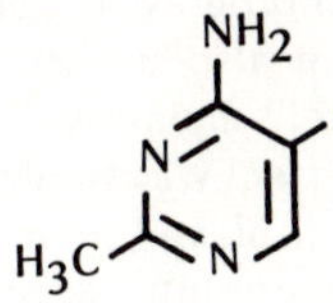

7

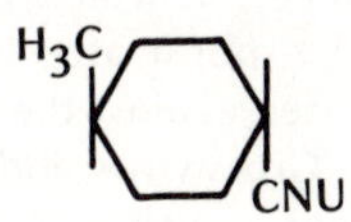

8

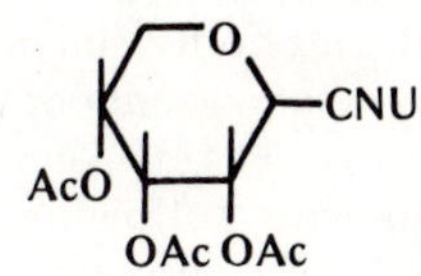

9

activity, alkylating activity or LD_{10} in mice; however, stability appeared inversely proportional to alkylating activity.

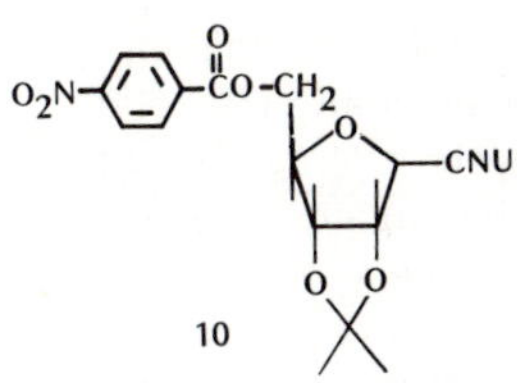

10

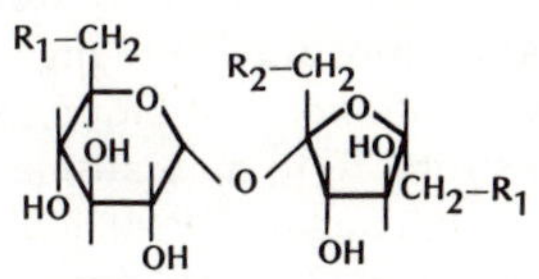

	R_1	R_2
11;	$NHCON(NO)CH_3$	OH
12;	$NHCON(NO)CH_3$	$NHCON(NO)CH_3$

Ribose-containing nitrosoureas **9** and **10** displayed activity against Friend leukemia and L1210, respectively,[24,25] and clinical evaluation of **10** has begun because of its superior therapeutic index (TI ~ 4). Based on reports that the blood-brain barrier prevented access of sucrose to normal brain tissue, but not brain tumors, 6,6′-dideoxy-6,6′ di(3-methyl-3-nitrosoureido)sucrose (**11**) and 1′,6,6′-trideoxy-1′,6,6′-tri(3-methyl-3-nitrosoureido)sucrose (**12**) were synthesized and tested in mice at doses of 200 mg/kg against both L1210 leukemia [treated/control (T/C) = 137 and 137, respectively] and ependymoblastoma brain tumor (T/C = 148 and 133, respectively).[26] A series of substituted cyclohexyl-CNU derivatives were prepared to investigate the known greater activity of the *trans* configuration of MeCCNU (**8**) versus the *cis*.[27] The compounds were active in L1210 leukemia with little differentiation between *cis* and *trans,* however, against Lewis lung carcinoma[28] it became clear that maximum activity was observed when substituents were at the 4-position of the cyclohexyl and *trans* to the CNU. A structural modification of BCNU, CNU-$(CH_2)_n$-OH (n = 2-4), designed to give a water-soluble alkylating agent, resulted in activity similar to BCNU against Walker carcinosarcoma.[29] A quantitative structure activity relationship (SAR) correlation equation based on lipophilic-hydrophilic balance (R_m) and L1210 activity was obtained for dialkanolamine dialkanesulfonic esters (**13**).[30] The homo-aza-steroidal ester (ASE; **14**) of *p-bis*-(2-chloroethyl)aminophenylacetic acid was active against L1210 and P388 leukemias, while the parent compound, phenestrin, was inactive. This provided the first example of a steroid alkylating agent active in the L1210 system.[31]

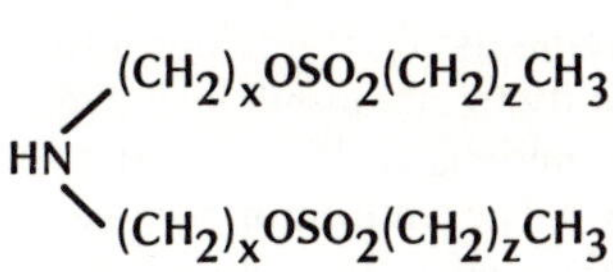

13

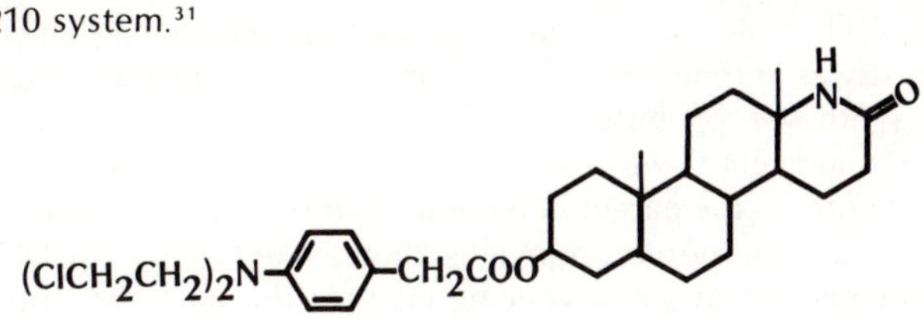

14

A series of Mannich bases were prepared with and without N-mustard groups and their SAR studied in a variety of tumor systems.[32] Bases with the N-mustard as the amine were particularly active against myeloid leukemia LAJ-1 and Walker 256. Two reports detailed progress toward a chemoimmunotherapeutic approach to cancer, in which an alkylating agent also served as a hapten, thus producing both a cell-mediated response after binding to tumor cells and providing a means for using a cytotoxic antibody generated against the hapten.[33,34] This effect was similar to the observation that EL4 leukemia and Gross-virus induced leukemia displayed new immunogenic properties following treatment with 5-(3,3-dimethyl-1-triazeno)imidazole-4-carboxamide (DIC).[35] The absolute configuration of (+)-cyclophosphamide was obtained by x-ray diffraction and will allow determination of the absolute configuration at the phosphorus of all chiral metabolites of cyclophosphamide.[36]

Natural Products and Semi-synthetics — Screening of compounds from fermentation and other natural sources continued to provide the greatest number of new antineoplastic agents. Two antibiotics structurally related to bleomycin, tallysomycin A and B, were identified as having antitumor activity comparable to bleomycin.[37] Antitumor activity (5 mg/kg, i.v.) against an S180 solid tumor in mice was described for a new antitumor antibiotic, sporamycin.[38] A group of fermentation-derived ansamycins, similar in structure to maytansine and active against a broad range of tumor systems, displayed strongest activity against P388 leukemia in mice at daily doses as low as 0.8-25 μg/kg (i.p.).[39] The SAR of septicidin (**15**) and close analogs was investigated by varying the fatty acid, glycine and amino sugar groups attached to the adenine unit. Activity against murine P388 leukemia was observed if the fatty acid contained 12-16 carbons, the amino acid was gycine or β-alanine, and CH_3 or CH_2OH replaced $CHOHCH_2OH$ in the sugar. Septacidin's ability to inhibit nucleic acid syntheses was assumed not to be due to direct attack on DNA because of a negative Ames test.[40] Analogs of sparsomycin (**16**) were compared with the parent compound and found to require the sulfoxide moiety and a D-configuration at the chiral carbon atom for activity against P388 leukemia.[41] However, conflicting with the above data was a report

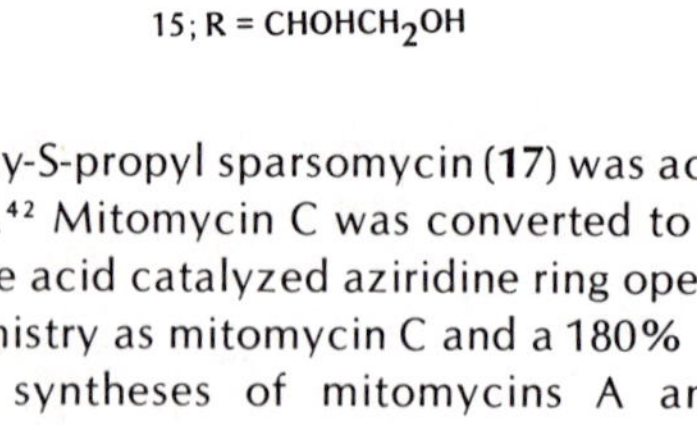

15; R = $CHOHCH_2OH$

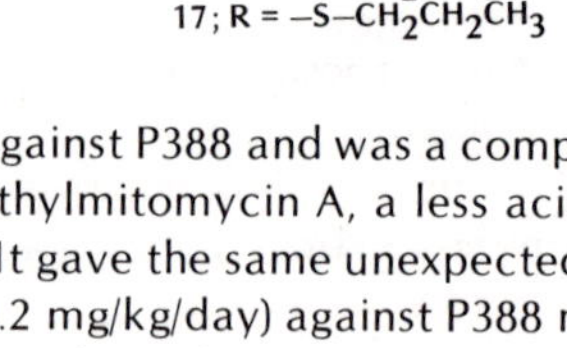

16; R = $-\overset{O}{\overset{\|}{S}}-CH_2SCH_3$
17; R = $-S-CH_2CH_2CH_3$

that S-deoxy-S-propyl sparsomycin (**17**) was active against P388 and was a competitive inhibitor of puromycin.[42] Mitomycin C was converted to N-methylmitomycin A, a less acid-sensitive analog, to study the acid catalyzed aziridine ring opening. It gave the same unexpected *cis*-aminoalcohol stereochemistry as mitomycin C and a 180% T/C (3.2 mg/kg/day) against P388 murine leukemia.[43] The total syntheses of mitomycins A and C and porfiromycin were also reported.[44,45] 2-Deaminoactinomycin D was found by a variety of physical measurements to intercalate into DNA as efficiently as the parent compound, but had only 1/100 the ability to inhibit nucleic acid synthesis. The 2-amino group, originally thought necessary for DNA binding, was proposed as slowing displacement by an advancing enzyme during transcription.[46] The antitumor protein, neocarzinostatin, was reported readily purified over earlier isolates and found 2x as inhibitory for human leukemia (CCRF-CEM) cells and 40x for Sarcina lutea.[47] A new quassinoid glycoside, bruceoside-A, was identified and tested against P388 leukemia (156% T/C at 6 mg/kg/day).[48]

Synthetic efforts in the terpene area have focused attention on vernolepin and vernomenin, and a number of synthetic routes to them and their analogs were reported.[49-54] The mechanism for inhibition of nucleic acid synthesis by the sesquiterpenes helenalin and tenulin was studied and proposed as a Michael-type addition of sulfhydryl groups of key regulatory enzymes.[55,56] The synthesis and activity of analogs of podophyllotoxin, an inhibitor of the microtubule system, were investigated to study the dependence of the *trans*-fused ring system on activity, a necessary feature of the parent compound.[57-59] A semisynthetic podophyllotoxin, 4'-demethyl-epipodophyllotoxin 9-(4,6-0-ethylidene-β-D-glucopyranoside), was tried against small cell anaplastic carcinoma (SCAC), and gave a 50% overall response rate after oral dosing, thereby, making it one of the most active single agents against SCAC.[60] In the area of alkaloid research the SAR of vinca alkaloids was studied by correlating LD_{50} data and anti-P388 activity with partition coefficients, pKa, and binding to tubulin.[61] The SAR of 4'-dehydrated vinca alkaloids revealed that a combination of 3',4' double bond and 4-deacetylation in vincristine resulted in a significant increase in TI against B-16 melanoma.[62] In a study of ergot alkaloids, two prolactin inhibitors, Deprenon and ergocryptine, proved to be highly effective against DMBA-induced rat mammary carcinomas.[63] The antitumor SAR of cephalotaxine esters was investigated, and particularly active were methyl (-)-cephalotaxyl itaconate and fumarate. However, there was a lack of correlation between activity and structure of α,β-unsaturated esters, which were 50-100 times less active than the naturally occurring esters.[64] New syntheses were reported for the alkaloids, trilobine, isotrilobine, obaberine,[65] camptothecin,[66] and ellipticine.[67,68]

Anthracyclines — Adriamycin (ADR) has continued to show dramatic clinical efficacy along with serious toxicity. In spite of the drawbacks, its success against solid tumors has led to a great deal of research centered around the anthracycline nucleus. The design, synthesis and SAR of daunorubicin (DNR), ADR and their new analogs have been carefully reviewed.[7] Labelled DNR and ADR have in the past been prepared by catalytic tritium exchange, which yielded products that readily exchanged during drug distribution studies. This problem was circumvented by synthesis of [14-^{14}C]DNR and [14-^{14}C]ADR using ^{14}C-diazomethane.[69] 4-Demethoxy DNR (i.v.) compared favorably with DNR and ADR (i.v.) against Gross leukemia and S180 tumor bearing mice, however, when given orally (2.55 mg/kg), it was effective (50% reduction in tumor growth and increase in survival time), where ADR and DNR were either ineffective or effective at large multiples of the optimal dose.[70] The importance of stereochemistry at C-9 was demonstrated when 9-deacetyl DNR displayed a 2-fold greater TI over 9-epi-deacetyl DNR against P388 lymphocytic leukemia in mice.[71] Studies on prevention and reversal of ADR associated cardiotoxicity showed that coenzyme Q reduced tachycardia, ECG and histological changes induced in long-term ADR treated rabbits.[72] In a clinical investigation, treatment with digoxin and diuretics reversed ADR-associated cardiac failure.[73] Carminomycin, the 4-demethyl analog of DNR developed in the USSR, has been reviewed and reported not to possess the cardiac toxicity associated with DAR.[74] Recent screening has resulted in a large number of ε-pyrromycinone (**18**) and 1-ε-deoxypyrromycinone (**19**) analogs with potent L1210 activity.[75-77] Only marginal anti-leukemia activity was observed when deoxy sugar glycosides (**20**) of **19** were synthesized.[78]

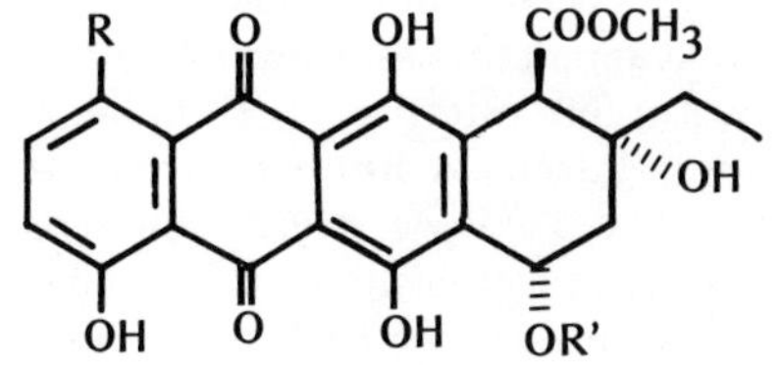

18; R = OH, R' = H
19; R = H; R' = H
20; R = H; R' = deoxysugar

Nucleoside Analogs — Ara-CDP-dipalmitin, after conversion to ara-CMP and phosphatidyl inositol,[79] increased the life of L5187Y leukemia-bearing mice (173% at 50 mg/kg i.p.). Both N⁴-behenoyl-1-β-D-arabinocytosine and N⁴-stearoyl-1-β-D-arabinocytosine were more active *in vivo* than 1-β-D-arabinocytosine, apparently because the N⁴ substituents protected against degradation by cytidine deaminase.[80] New syntheses were reported for ftorafur [1-(2-tetrahydrofuryl)-5-fluorouracil],[81,82] and no differences were seen in biological activities of the R and S isomers. Tumor regression was seen in a Phase I study of advanced gastrointestinal cancer following treatment with ftorafur and mitomycin C or MeCCNU.[83] The chemistry and biology of 5-azacytidine were reviewed.[84] Additional work with 5,6-dihydro-5-azacytidine, the stable analog of 5-azacytidine, demonstrated more efficacy than the parent against cerebral L1210 and had a better TI.[85] Several sulfur-substituted analogs of the α and β anomers of 2′-deoxy-6-thioguanosine had substantial antileukemia activity in mice,[86] but none was as potent as the parent compound.

Metal Complexes — With the clinical utility of *cis*-platinum diamminodichloride (PDD) repeatedly reinforced,[87,88] work has continued toward establishing the MOA of this compound and the growing number of cytotoxic, heavy metal complexes. PDD was found to be synergistic with cyclophosphamide in L1210 leukemia[89] and with 2,2′-anhydro-1-β-D-arabinofuranosyl-5-fluorocytosine in L1210 and P388 systems resistant to 5-FU or MTX.[90] A series of *cis*-dichlorobis(1-methyl-imidazole-2-thiol)Pt(II) and Pd(II) compounds were complexed with nucleosides to determine the binding properties of the metals. IR and NMR were used to show Pt and Pd bound to N^7 in guanosine and adenosine and N^6 in cytidine.[91] Acetylacetonate-1,5-cyclooctadienerhodium(I) (AC) and *cis*-dichlorotetrakisdimethylsulfoxide ruthenium(II) (CR) compared favorably with PDD *in vivo* against Ehrlich ascites carcinoma, however, only AC and PDD were effective in L1210.[92] Cyclic and polymeric amino phosphazenes have been reacted with K_2PtCl_4, resulting in water-soluble complexes with cytostatic activity in mouse P388 leukemia and Ehrlich ascites tumor regression systems.[93] Partition coefficients for rhodium(II) carboxylates were correlated with activity in mice bearing the Ehrlich ascites tumor. The data showed increases in lipophilicity gave increases in %ILS and TI, until steric factors or too little water solubility lessened the effects.[94] Evidence has been obtained for cytotoxic copper and rhodium complexes reacting with enzymes containing essential -SH groups.[95,96] Concentrations of rhodium carboxylates that will inhibit -SH enzymes have been correlated with maximal survival times of mice bearing Ehrlich ascites tumors.[97]

Miscellaneous Agents — Anti-L1210 leukemia activity was correlated with a lipophilic-hydrophilic balance for a series of 4′-(9-acridinylamino)alkanesulfonanilides.[98,99] Acridines substituted in the 3-position with lipophilic groups were found more active when further substituted with hydrophilic groups. *In vivo* reduction of nitro derivatives of 4′-(9-acridinylamino)methanesulfonanilide (AMSA) had been postulated to explain the activity of these weakly basic compounds, however, 3- and 4-aza analogs of AMSA had similar base strength and were equally active.[100] Joining two acridine rings at the 9-amino position by a varying number of methylene units yielded a series of *bis*-intercalating diacridines, shown to have an inverse correlation between %ILS (P-388) and agglutination involving S180 cells treated with Con-A.[101] The SAR of a group of N-protected amino acids converted to their vinyl, 1,2-dihaloethyl and cyanomethyl esters was reported; particularly active against Ehrlich ascites carcinoma were the esters of N-carbobenzoxy-L-phenylalanine, glycine, and leucine.[102,103] 1,8-Di-N-*bis*-(*n*-butyloxycarbonylaminomethyl)-L-citrulline was shown to be orally effective against rats implanted with AH 41C ascites hepatoma (i.v.).[104] In a study concerned with homocysteine metabolism in neoplastic tissue, arachidonoyl homocysteine thiolactone (HCT) amide decreased growth, and oleoyl HCT amide increased growth of A-10 mammary adenocarcinoma.[105] 1-Formylpyridine thiosemicarbazone has been shown to have the E-configuration,[106] and in a series of 5,6-dihydro-8(7H)-quinoline thiosemicarbazones, investigation of structural requirements revealed that the E-isomers were slightly more active than the Z-isomers against P388 leukemia.[107] 4-Methyl-5-amino-1-formylisoquinoline thiosemicarbazone (i.p.) significantly increased survival time in mice bearing S180, L1210 and P388 leukemia, B16 melanoma or Lewis lung carcinoma.[108] Analogs of **21** and **22**, structurally similar to mitomycins and pyrrolizidine alkaloids, were found effective against P388 *in vivo*.[109,110] 5,5-*Bis*(4-chlorophenyl)-1,3-dichlorohydantoin was the most active (190% T/C) of a group of hydantoins tested against P388 leukemia.[111]

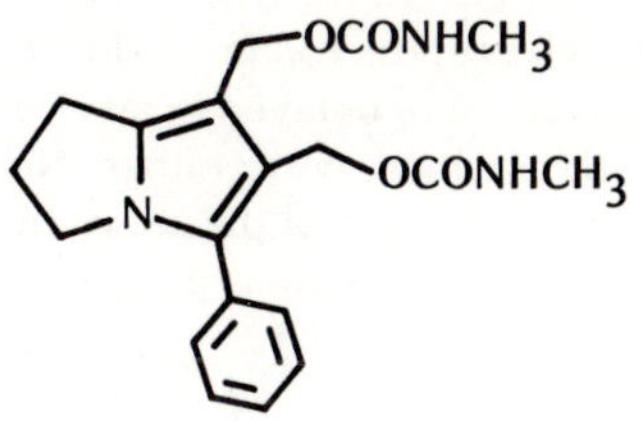

21

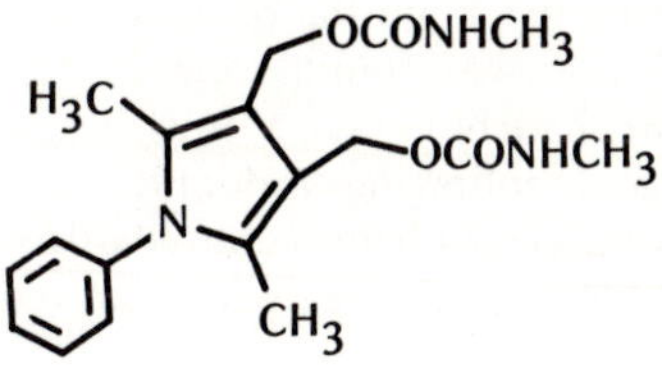

22

Immunotherapeutics — No new significant immunotherapeutic agents have been reported, but the approach has been accepted as clinically useful, and BCG, MER, *C. parvum*, and levamisole usage continued to grow. The general subject was comprehensively reviewed,[3,112] as well as the specific topics, MER-BCG,[113] levamisole,[12] and clinical trials of immunotherapy in man.[114] The mechanism of macrophage activation by BCG was studied with respect to lysosomal enzymes and the presence of intracellular free radical species.[115] A vaccine of BCG plus x-irradiated L10 hepatocarcinoma cells eliminated a disseminated tumor burden in guinea pigs.[116] This approach has been extended to the clinic where good results against acute lymphoid leukemia have been observed after chemotherapy followed by active immunotherapy with BCG.[117] *C. parvum* (i.v.) was found more effective than BCG in reducing incidence of regional lymph node metastases after surgery of adenocarcinoma in rats.[118] The mechanism of *C. parvum* antimetastatic activity has been explained as mediation by macrophages with T-cell cooperation[119] and a T-cell independent activation.[120] Various combinations of *C. parvum* given s.c., i.v. and i.p. increased survival of Fischer 344 rats bearing 13762 adenocarcinoma.[121] Pulmonary, peritoneal, and splenic macrophages from these animals were cytotoxic toward target 13762 tumor cells *in vitro*. An objective response was seen in human ovarian cancer with *C. parvum* and a program of Cytoxan, adriamycin, and 5-FU, where conventional therapy had failed.[122] Levamisole was reported to inhibit s.c. malignant neurinoma growth in 80% of treated rats.[123] Skin tests, E-rosettes, and cAMP levels have been measured in patients with malignant melanoma and squamous cell cancer of the head and neck, and improved values correlated with responders to levamisole therapy.[124]

Drug Delivery — There has been a persistent effort in increasing selectivity of antitumor agents by altering physical, chemical and biochemical parameters.[125-127] Emulsions[128,129] have been applied to delivery of agents to lymphatics, and liposomes have been used to enhance the action of nitrogen mustard,[130] specific tumor cell antibody[131] and a variety of cytotoxic agents.[127] The proposed lisosomal membrane alteration of target cells has been extended to Amphotericin B (AMP B), which is known to alter membrane permeability.[132,133] AMP B has enhanced BCNU uptake into tumor cells and stimulated host response to killed cells.[134] Objective clinical responses were observed when AMP B was used during combination chemotherapy.[135,136] Macromolecular species such as BSA, IgG, poly amino acids,[137] and Con A[138] have been used as carriers of antitumor agents to increase specificity and TI. MTX covalently coupled to tumor associated antibodies (ab) was shown to be more effective against C3H murine ovarian carcinoma thanthe agent alone or a simple mixture of ab and MTX.[139] Specificity has also been sought by incorporating alkylating groups on hydantoin,[140] pyrimidine[141] and isoquinoline[142] pharmacophores.

Anticarcinogens — Published reports concerning compounds inhibiting tumors induced by carcinogens have continued to grow. Dithiocarbamates such as disulfiram (**23**) and diethyldithocarbamic acid prevented 1,2-dimethyl hydrazine (DMH)-induced large bowel tumors in mice.[143] Selenium supplementation of diet decreased colon cancer induction in rats by DMH.[144] Similarly, incidence of rat intestinal and bladder tumors induced by bracken fern was decreased by addition to the diet of BHA, PVP, calcium chloride, and disulfiram.[145] The most studied class of compounds in this area has been the retinoids, thought to act via control of epithelial cell growth. Retinyl methyl ether was found superior to natural retinyl acetate for inhibition of DMBA-induced mammary cancer in rats.[146] Invasive cancer was prevented or delayed in rats treated with 13-*cis*-retinoic acid following induction of preneoplastic lesions with either N-methyl-N-nitrosourea or N-butyl-N-(4-hydroxybutyl)nitrosamine.[147-149] Systemic use of the aromatic retinoid, Ro 10-9359, (**24**) successfully treated DMBA-induced skin papillomas in Swiss mice.[150]

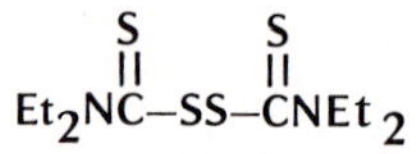

23

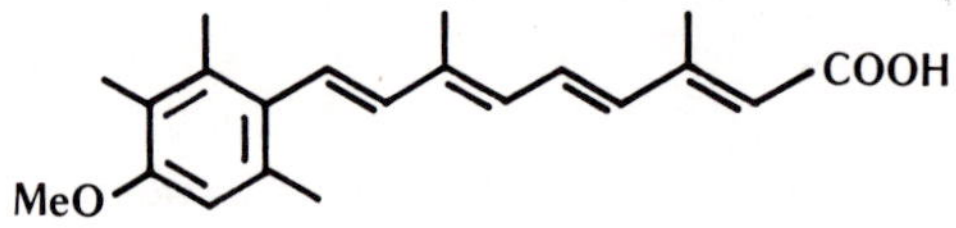

24

REFERENCES

1. F.F. Becker, Ed., "Cancer: A Comprehensive Treatise," Vol. 5, Plenum Press, New York, 1977.
2. R.L. Clark and R.W. Cumley, Eds., "The Yearbook of Cancer," Yearbook Medical Publishers, Chicago, 1977, p. 277.
3. E.M. Hersh, G.M. Mavligit, J.U. Gutterman and S.P. Richman, "Cancer: A Comprehensive Treatise," Vol. 6, F.F. Becker, Ed., Plenum Press, 1977, p. 425.
4. W.A. Woods, Adv. Pharmacol. Chemother.,**14,** 143 (1977).
5. H.F. Oettgen, New Engl. J. Med., **297,** 484 (1977).
6. S.A. Rosenberg and W.A. Terry, Advan. Cancer Res., **25,** 323 (1977).
7. F. Arcamone, J. Nature Prod., **40,** 45 (1977).
8. M.E. Wall and M.C. Wani, Ann. Rev. Pharmacol. Toxicol., **17,** 117 (1977).
9 G.A. Cordell and N.R. Farnsworth, J. Natur. Prod. **40,** 1 (1977).
10. W. Sadee and C.G. Wong, Clinical Pharmacokinetics, **2,** 437 (1977).
11. W.A. Bleyer, Cancer Treat. Rev. **4,** 87 (1977).
12. W.K. Amery, F. Spreafico, A.F. Rojas, E. Denissen and M.A. Chirigos, Cancer Treat. Rev., **4,** 167 (1977).
13. H. Umezawa, J. Natur. Prod., **40,** 67 (1977).
14. L.H. Hurley, J. Antibiotics, **30,** 349 (1977).
15. N.R. Cozzarelli, Ann. Rev. Biochem., **46,** 641 (1977).
16. E. Fujita and Y. Nagao, Bio-Org. Chem., **6,** 287 (1977).
17. M.T. Shaw and R.D. Stebbins, "Cancer: A Comprehensive Treatise," Vol. 5, F.F. Becker, E., Plenum Press, New York, 1977, p. 163.
18. L.W. Keiser and R.L. Capizzi, "Cancer: A Comprehensive Treatise," Vol. 5, F.F. Becker, Ed., Plenum Press, New York, 1977, p. 163.
19. R.L. Capizzi, L.W. Keiser and A.C. Sartorelli, Semin. Oncol., **4,** 227 (1977).
20. L.M. Axtell, A.J. Asire and M.H. Myers, Eds., "Cancer Patient Survival Report Number 5," DHEW Publication No. (NIH) 77-992, U.S. Government Printing Office, Washington, D.C. (1976).
21. L.C. Panasci, D. Green. R. Nagourney, P. Fox and P.S. Schein, Cancer Res., **37,** 2615 (1977).
22 .P.A. Fox, L.C. Panasci and P.S. Schein, Cancer Res., **37,** 783 (1977).
23. R.A. Nagourney, P. Fox and P.S. Schein, Cancer Res., **38,** 65 (1978).
24. N. Larnicol, Y. Augery, C. Jasmin, J.L. Montero and J.L. Imbach, Biomedicine, **26,** 176 (1977).
25. J.L. Montero, A. Moruzzi, J. Oiry and J.L. Imbach, Eur. J. Med. Chem., **12,** 397 (1977).
26. R.G. Almquist and E.J. Reist, J. Med. Chem., **20,** 1246 (1977).
27. T.P. Johnston, G.S. McCaleb, S.D. Clayton, J.L. Frey, C.A. Krauth and J.A. Montgomery, J. Med. Chem., **20,** 279 (1977).

28. J.A. Montgomery, G.S. McCaleb, T.P. Johnston, J.G. Mayo and W.R. Laster, J. Med. Chem., **20,** 291 (1977).
29. H.H. Fiebib, G. Eisenbrand, W.J. Zeller and W.T. Deutsch, Eur. J. Cancer, **13,** 937 (1977).
30. B.F. Cain and W.A. Denny, J.Med. Chem., **20,** 515 (1977).
31. G.L. Wampler and P. Catsoulacos, Cancer Treat. Rep., **61,** 37 (1977).
32. W. Werner, W. Jungstand, W. Gutsche and K. Wohlrabe, Pharmazie, **32,** 431 (1977).
33. A.H. Soloway, J.E. Wright, V. Subramanyam and J.J. Gozzo, J. Med. Chem., **20,** 1357 (1977).
34. J.E. Wright, M.J. Hayes, V. Subramanyam and A.H. Soloway, J. Med. Chem., **20,** 1700 (1977).
35. A. Nicolin, M. Cavalli, A. Missiroli and A. Goldin, Eur. J. Cancer, **13,** 235 (1977).
36. I.L. Karle, J.M., Karle, W. Egan, G. Zon and J.A. Brandt, J. Amer. Chem. Soc., **99,** 4803 (1977).
37. M. Konishi, K. Saito, K. Nuhata, T. Tsuno, K. Asama, H. Tsukiura, T. Naito and H. Kawaguchi, J. Antibiot., **30,** 789 (1977).
38. K. Komiyama, K. Sugimoto, H. Takeshima and H. Umezawa, J. Antibiot., **30,** 202 (1977).
39. E. Higashide, M. Asi, K. Ootsu, S. Tanida, Y. Kozai, T. Hasegawa, T. Kishi, Y. Sugino and M. Yoneda, Nature, **270,** 721 (1977).
40. E.M. Acton, K.J. Ryan and A.E. Luetzow, J. Med. Chem., **20,** 1362 (1977).
41. L.L. Chie-Chang and R.J. Dubois, J. Med. Chem., **20,** 337 (1977).
42. R. Vince, J. Brownell and C.K. Lee, Biochem. Biophys. Res. Commun., **75,** 563 (1977).
43. L. Cheng and W.A. Remers, J. Med. Chem., **20,** 767 (1977).
44. T. Fukuyama, F. Nakatsubo, A.J. Cocuzza and Y. Kishi, Tetrahedron Lett., 4295 (1977).
45. F. Naktasubo, T. Fukuyama, A.J. Cocuzza and Y. Kishi, J. Amer. Chem. Soc., **99,** 8115 (1977).
46. C.W. Mosher, K.F. Kuhlmann, D.G. Kleid and D.W. Henry, J. Med. Chem., **20,** 1055 (1977).
47. T.S.A. Samy, J.M. Hu, J.L. Meienhofer, H. Lazarus and R.K. Johnson, J. Natl. Cancer Inst., **58,** 1765 (1977).
48. K.H. Lee, Y, Imakura and H.C. Huang, J. Chem. Soc. Chem. Commun., 69 (1977).
49. P.A. Grieco, M. Nishizawa, T. Oguri, S.D. Burke and N. Marinovic, J. Amer. Chem. Soc., **99,** 5773 (1977).
50. S. Danishefsky, P.F. Schuda, T. Kitahara and S.J. Etheredge, J. Amer. Chem. Soc., **99,** 6066 (1977).
51. P.A. Grieco, J.A. Noguez and Y. Masaki, J. Org. Chem., **42,** 495 (1977).
52. F. Zutterman, P. deClercq and M. Vandewalle, Tetrahedron Lett., 3191 (1977).
53. P.A. Grieco, J.A. Noguez, Y. Masaki, K. Hiroi and M. Nishizawa, J. Med. Chem., **20,** 71 (1977).
54. M. Isobe, H. Iio, T. Kawai and T. Goto, Tetrahedron Lett., 703 (1977).
55. K.H. Lee, Science, **196,** 533 (1977).
56. I.H. Hall, K.H. Lee, E.C. Mar and C.O. Starnes, J.Med. Chem., **20,** 333 (1977).
57. W.J. Gensler, C.D. Murphy and M.H. Trammell, J. Med. Chem., **20,** 635 (1977)
58. V.N. Aiyar and F.C. Chang, J. Org. Chem., **42,** 246 (1977).
59. S.D. Jolad, R.M. Wiedhopf, and J.R. Cole, J. Pharm. Sci., **66,** 892 (1977).
60. M. Hansen, F. Hirsch, P. Dombernowsky and H.H. Hansen, Cancer, **40,** 633 (1977).
61. R.J. Owellen, D.W. Donigan, C.A. Hartke and F.Q. Hains, Biochem. Pharmacol., **26,** 1213 (1977).
62. J.C. Miller, G.E. Gutowski, G.A. Poore and G.B. Boder, J. Med. Chem., **20,** 409 (1977).
63. M.N. Teller, C.C. Stodk, L. Hellman, I.M. Mountain, M. Bowie, B.J. Rosenberg, R.M. Boyer and J.M. Budinger, Cancer Res., **37,** 3932 (1977).
64. K.L. Mikolajczak, C.R. Smith and D. Weisleder, J. Med. Chem., **20,** 328 (1977).
65. Y. Inubushi, Y. Ito, Y Masaki and T. Ibuka, Chem. Pharm. Bull., **25,** 1636 (1977).
66. J. Quick, Tetrahedron Lett., 327 (1977).
67. A.H. Jackson, P.R. Jenkins and P.V.R. Shannon, J. Chem. Soc., 1698 (1977).
68. A.P. Kozikowski and N.M. Hasan, J. Org. Chem., **42,** 2039 (1977).
69. S. Penco, G. Vicario, F. Angelucci and F. Arcamone, J. Antibiot., **30,** 773 (1977).
70. A. DiMarco, A.M. Casazza and G. Pratesi, Cancer Chemother. Rep., **61,** 893 (1977).
71. S. Penco, F. Angelucci, A. Vigevani, E. Arlandini and F. Arcamone, J. Antibiot., **30,** 764 (1977).
72. C. Bertazzoli and M. Ghione, Pharmacol. Res. Commun., **9,** 235 (1977).
73. S.A.D. Al Ismail, D.H. Parry and J.A. Whittaker, Brit. J. Med., 815 (1977).
74. S.T. Crooke, J. Med., **8,** 295 (1977).
75. D.E. Nettleton, W.T. Brander, J.A. Bush, A.B. Coon, J.E. Moseley, R.W. Myllymaki, F.A. O'Herron, R.H. Schreiber and A.L. Vulcano, J. Antibiot., **30,** 525 (1977).
76. I. Kitamura, N. Shibamoto, T. Oki, T. Inui, H. Naganawa, M. Ishizuka, T. Masuda, T. Takeuchi and H. Umezawa J. Antibiot., **30,** 616 (1977).
77. T. Oki, N. Shibamoto, Y. Matsuzawa, T. Ogaswara, A. Yoshimoto, I. Kitamura, T. Inui, H. Naganawa, T. Takeuchi and H. Umezawa, J. Antibiot., **30,** 683 (1977).
78. H.S. El Khadem, D.L. Swartz and R.C. Cermak, J. Med. Chem., **20,** 957 (1977).
79. C.R.H. Raetz, M.Y. Chu, S.P. Srivastava and J.G. Turcotte, Science, **196,** 303, (1977).
80. M. Aoshima, S. Tsukagoshi, Y. Sakurai, J. Oh, T. Ishida and H. Kobayashi, Cancer Res., **37,** 2481 (1977).
81. T. Kametani, K. Kigasawa, M. Hiiagi, K. Wakisaka, O. Kusama, K. Kawasaki and H. Sugi, J. Heterocyc. Chem., **14,** 473 (1977).

82. M. Yasumoto, A. Moriyama, N. Unemi, S. Hahimoto and T. Suzue, J. Med. Chem., **20**, 1592 (1977).
83. T. Buroker, L. Baker, J. Correa, L.A. Schwartz and V.K. Vaitkevicius, Cancer Treat. Rep., **61**, 463 (1977).
84. D.D. von Hoff and M. Slavik, Adv. Pharmacol. Chemother., **14**, 285 (1977).
85. J.A. Beisler, M.M. Abbasi, J.A. Kelley and J.S. Driscoll, J. Med. Chem., **20**, 806 (1977).
86. A.P. Marinez, W.W. Lee and D.W. Henry, J. Med. Chem., **20**, 341 (1977).
87. R.E. Wittes, E. Cvitkovic, J. Shah, F.P. Gerold and E.W. Strong, Cancer Treat. Rep., **61**, 359 (1977).
88. A. Yagoda, Cancer Res., **37**, 2775 (1977).
89. M. Rozencweig, D.D. von Hoff, M. Slavik and F.M. Muggia, Ann. Internal Med., **86**, 803 (1977).
90. J.H. Burchenal, T. O'Toole, K. Kalaher and J. Chisholm, Cancer Res., **37**, 4908 (1977).
91. J. Dehand and J. Jordanov, J. Chem. Soc., 1588 (1977).
92. T. Giraldi, G. Sava, G. Bertoli, G. Mestroni and G. Zassinovich, Cancer Res., **37**, 2662 (1977).
93. H.R. Allcock, R.W. Allen and J.P. O'Brien, J. Amer. Chem. Soc., **99**, 3984 (1977).
94. R.A. Howard, E. Sherwood, A. Erck, A.P. Kimball and J.L. Bear, J. Med. Chem., **20**, 943 (1977).
95. D.T. Minkel and D.H. Petering, Cancer Res., **38**, 227 (1977).
96. D.T. Minkel, L.A. Saryan and D.H. Petering, Cancer Res., **38**, 124 (1977).
97. R.A. Howard, T.G. Spring and J.L. Bear, Cancer Res., **36**, 4402 (1976).
98. B.F. Cain, G.J. Atwell and W.A. Denny, J. Med. Chem., **20**, 987 (1977).
99. G.J. Atwell, B.F. Cain and W.A. Denny, J. Med. Chem., **20**, 1128 (1977).
100. W.A. Denny, G.J. Atwell and B.F. Cain, J. Med. Chem., **20**, 1242 (1977).
101. R.M. Fico, T.K. Chen and E.S. Canellakis, Science, **198**, 53 (1977).
102. L.J. Loeffler, Z. Sajadi and I.H. Hall, J. Med. Chem., **20**, 1578 (1977).
103. L.J. Loeffler, Z. Sajadi and I.H. Hall, J. Med. Chem., **20**, 1584 (1977).
104. H. Fujita, T. Sakurai, H. Ichimura, H. Sato and S. Toyoshima, Cancer Treat. Rep., **61**, 1577 (1977).
105. K.S. McCully and P. Clopath, Chemotherapy, **23**, 44 (1977).
106. I. Antonini, F. Claudi, P. Franchetti, M. Grifantini and S. Martelli, J. Med. Chem., **20**, 447 (1977).
107. T.L. Lemke, T.W. Shek, L.A. Cates and L.K. Smith, J. Med. Chem., **20**, 1351 (1977).
108. K.C. Agrawal, J.B. Schenkman, H. Denk, P.D. Mooney, E.C. Moore, I. Wodinsky and A.C. Sartorelli, Cancer Res., **37**, 1692 (1977).
109. W.K. Anderson and P.F. Corey, J. Med. Chem., **20**, 812 (1977).
110. W.K. Anderson and P.F. Corey, J. Med. Chem., **20**, 1691 (1977).
111. T.R. Rodgers, M.P. LaMontagne, A. Markovac and A.B. Ash, J. Med. Chem., **20**, 591 (1977).
112. C.M. Haskell, Ann. Rev. Pharmacol. Toxicol., **17**, 179 (1977).
113. S.M. Mikulski and F.M. Muggia, Cancer Treat Rev., **4**, 103 (1977).
114. S.E. Salmon, Cancer Res., **37**, 1245 (1977).
115. J.B. Weinberg and J.B. Hibbs, Clin. Res., **25**, 163A (1977).
116. M.G. Hanna and L.C. Peters, Cancer Res., **38**, 204 (1977).
117. G. Mathe, F. Vassal, L. Schwarzenberg, M. Delgado, R. Weiner, M.A. Gil, J. Pena-Angula, D. Belpomme, P. Pouillart, D. Machover, J.L. Misset, J.L. Pico, C. Jasmin, M. Hayat, M. Schneider, A. Cattan, J.L. Amiel, M. Musset and C. Rosenfeld, Cancer Immunol. Immunother., **2**, 225 (1977).
118. J.A. Greager and R.W. Baldwin, Cancer Res., **38**, 69 (1977).
119. P.D. Jones and J.E. Castro, Brit. J. Cancer, **35**, 519 (1977).
120. M.F. Woodruff and N.L. Warner, J. Natl. Cancer Inst., **58**, 111 (1977).
121. V.V. Likhite, Cancer Immunol. Immunother., **2**, 173 (1977).
122. B. Rao, H.J. Wanebo, M. Ochoa, J.L. Lewis, and H.F. Oettgen, Cancer, **39**, 514 (1977).
123. S. Aleksic, F. Drnovski, A. Bloom, H. Rappaport, and J. Ransohoff, J. Natl. Cancer Inst., **59**, 1565 (1977).
124. S.A. Wilkins and Z.L. Olkowski, Cancer, **39**, 487 (1977).
125. P.J. Cox and P.B. Farmer, Cancer Treat. Rev., **4**, 47 (1977).
126. P.J. Cox and P.B. Farmer, Cancer Treat. Rev., **4**, 119 (1977).
127. G. Gregoriadis, Nature, **265**, 407 (1977).
128. M. Hashida, Y. Takahashi, S. Muranishi and H. Sezaki, J. Pharmacokin. Biopharm., **5**, 241 (1977).
129. M. Hashida, M. Egawa, S. Muranishi and H. Sezaki, J. Pharmacokin. Biopharm., **5**, 225 (1977).
130. R.J. Rutman, N.G. Avadhani and C. Ritter, Biochem. Pharmacol. **26**, 85 (1977).
131. G. Gregoriadis, D.E. Neerunjun and R. Hunt, Life Sci., **21**, 357 (1977).
132. F.J. Schiffman and D.T. Vistica, Lancet, 141 (1977).
133. I. Klein and F.J. Schiffman, Clin. Res., **25**, 408A (1977).
134. G. Medoff, F. Valeriote, J. Ryan and S. Tolen, J. Natl. Cancer Inst., **58**, 949 (1977).
135. S.D. Reich, Ann. Internal. Med., **86**, 656 (1977).
136. C.A. Presant, C. Klahr and R. Santala, Ann. Internal. Med., **86**, 47 (197).
137. M. Szekerke and J.S. Driscoll, Eur. J. Cancer, **13**, 529 (1977).
138. T. Kitao and K. Hattori, Nature, **265**, 81 (1977).
139. S. Burstein and R. Knapp, J. Med. Chem., **20**, 950 (1977).
140. J. Plowman, D.B. Lakings, E.S. Ownes and R.H. Adamson, Pharmacology, **15**, 359 (1977).

141. K.H. Lee, Y.S. Wu and I.H. Hall, J. Med. Chem., **20,** 911 (1977).
142. C.N. Filer, F.E. Granchelli, A.H. Soloway and J.L. Neumeyer, J. Med. Chem., **20,** 1504 (1977).
143. L.W. Wattenberg, L.K. Lam, A.V. Fladmoc, and P. Borchert, Cancer, **40,** 2432 (1977).
144. M.M. Jacobs, Cancer, **40,** 2557 (1977).
145. A.M. Pamukcu, S. Yalciner and G.T. Bryan, Cancer, **40,** 2450 (1977).
146. C.J. Grubbs, R.C. Moon, M.B. Sporn and D.L. Newton, Cancer Res., **37,** 599 (1977).
147. J.M. Smith, M.L. Wenk and S. Springer, Cancer Res., **37,** 2930 (1977).
148. J.M. Smith, M.L. Wenk and S. Springer, Science, **195,** 487 (1977).
149. C.J. Grubbs, R.C. Moon, R.A. Squire, G.M. Farrow, S.F. Stinson, D.G. Goodman, C.C. Brown and M.B. Sporn, Science, **198,** 743 (1977).
150. A. Matter and W. Bollag, Eur. J. Cancer, **13,** 831 (1977).

Chapter 14. Antiparasitic Agents

M. H. Fisher and C. C. Wang, Merck Sharp & Dohme Research Laboratories
Rahway, New Jersey

General - Chapters were published on drugs for intestinal parasitism[1] and current treatment of protozoan and helminth parasites.[2]

Malaria - Reviews appeared on antimalarial drugs.[3,4] A screening method was described using owl monkeys bearing human parasites.[5] Further evaluation of phenanthrene methanols showed WR 122,455 (1) to be effective against chloroquine-resistant *Plasmodium berghei* in mice[6] and chloroquine-resistant *Plasmodium falciparum* in man.[7] Activity differences among analogs of (1) were correlated with their conformation.[8] The active conformation of each structure was such that it allowed the formation of a hydrogen bond between the hydroxyl and protonated amine functions.

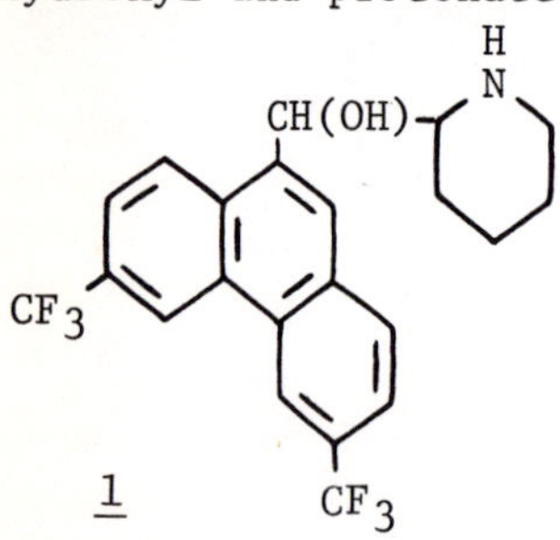

1

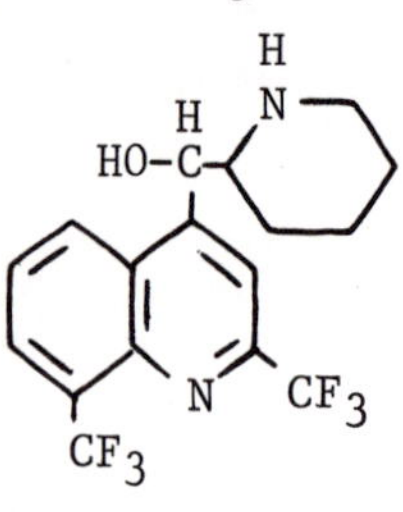

2

The DNA binding of quinolinemethanols was studied.[9] Mefloquine (2), a potent antimalarial found clinically effective against chloroquine-resistant *P. falciparum*,[10] bound weakly compared to compounds such as quinacrine, ethidium or daunorubicin. The finding questions the role of DNA binding for the antimalarial activities of quinoline methanolamines. Similar doubts cast previously on the mode of antimalarial action of chloroquine and related compounds have led to the hypothesis[11] that these compounds possess just the right combination of lipid solubility and doubly protonated form to be concentrated into the trophozoite phagosomes of the parasites. As a result, the pH in the phagosomes increases, probably beyond the optimum range for the acid proteases which are responsible for digesting host hemoglobin. The net outcome is an acute amino acid deprivation of the parasites. Quinolinemethanolamines could act *via* a similar mechanism. But their inhibition of haemozoin clumping,[12] which follows exposure of the parasites to chloroquine or its active analogs,[13] suggests that the two classes of compounds do not act in exactly the same way. Primaquine, an 8-aminoquinoline antimalarial drug, was recently re-evaluated in rhesus monkeys.[14] It was found that the *d*-isomer had a therapeutic index at least twice that of the *dl*-isomer due to the much lower toxicity of the former. The finding may represent a separation between toxicity and antimalarial activity.

Smith *et al.*[15] noted that among many compounds tested, L-serine was the only methyl group donor for *Plasmodium knowlesi* in rhesus monkey erythrocytes. The observation agreed with a previous report by Platzer[16] that 10-formyltetrahydrofolate synthetase and 5,10-methylenetetrahydrofolate dehydrogenase were apparently absent in *P. lophurae*, whereas serine hydroxymethyl transferase was present in abundance in the cytosolic fraction of the parasite.[17]

ISBN 0-12-040513-X

The methyl group from serine was about evenly distributed between methionine and thymidylate in *P. knowlesi*.[18] p-Aminobenzoate, dihydrofolate and tetrahydrofolate stimulated the incorporation, whereas pyrimethamine and 5-fluoroorotic acid inhibited it,[15] as one would expect. It will be interesting to see if specific inhibitors of plasmodial serine hydroxymethyl transferase can be found and if they will demonstrate *in vivo* antimalarial activity.

A quantitative structure-activity relationship of antimalarial activity and bacterial dihydrofolate reductase inhibition by quinazolines and 5-substituted benzyl-2,4-diaminopyrimidines was formulated.[19] Two fermentation products, erythromycin[20] and aplasmomycin,[21] a boron containing ionophore,[22] were active against *P. berghei* in mice.

Helminthiasis - Reviews were published on drugs used in the treatment of helminthiasis,[23,24,25] the control of parasites by drugs,[26] anticestodal and antinematodal drugs[27] and anthelmintics from laboratory animals to the target species.[28]

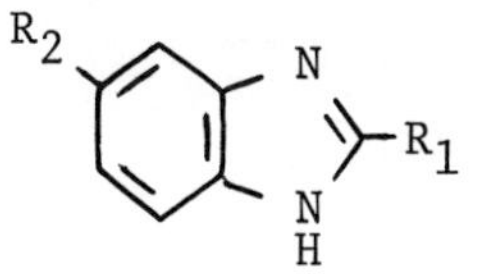

R_1

3, $-NHCOOCH_3$
4, $-NHCOOCH_3$
5, $-NHCOOCH_3$
6, $-NHCOOCH_3$
7, 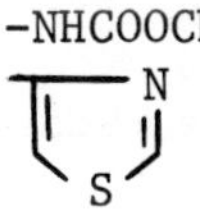
8, $-NHCOOCH_3$

R_2

3, $-O-CH_2CH_2CH_3$
4, $-S(\rightarrow O)-C_6H_5$
5, $-S-CH_2CH_2CH_3$
6, $-S-C_6H_5$
7, $-NHCOOCH(CH_3)_2$
8, $-C(=O)-C_6H_5$

Many efficacy studies were reported on the newer benzimidazole anthelmintics, oxibendazole (3), oxfendazole (4), albendazole (5), and fenbendazole (6), in papers presented at an international conference.[29] The compounds were generally effective against most important nematodes of sheep and cattle at oral doses of 2.5 to 10 mg/kg. Other studies further confirmed these observations for oxibendazole,[30] oxfendazole[31,32,33] and albendazole.[34,35,36,37] At higher doses albendazole eliminated adult *Fasciola hepatica* from sheep[38] and *Paragonimus kellicotti* from cats.[39] Cambendazole (7) was shown to be effective against *Dicrocoelium dendriticum*[40] and fenbendazole against *Moniezia expansa* infections.[41] Fenbendazole and mebendazole (8) were active against developing but not against mature *Trichinella spiralis* infections in mice.[42]

The existence of cross-resistance in *H. contortus* and *T. colubriformis* to all the benzimidazole anthelmintics has been well documented.[43] Because of the capability of thiabendazole in inhibiting embryonation of nematode eggs at very low concentrations,[44] suggestions were made by Le Jambre[45] and Coles and Simpkin[46] almost simultaneously that the ovicidal activity of benzimidazoles may be used to indicate cross-resistance among nematode eggs. Results presented in these two papers indicated that eggs from benzimidazole-resistant nematodes were also resistant to the ovicidal action of benzimidazoles. A test such as this could be used as a screen for detecting resistance to benzimidazoles.

Among other established anthelmintics, oxantel[47] was shown to be active against *Trichuris trichiura* in man and levamisole resinate[48] was active against *Dirofilaria immitis* microfilaria and partially effective against adult worms in dogs.

Newly described anthelmintic structures included 2-tolylazo-2-thiazoline (9),[49] dihydroquinoxalino[2,3-b]quinoxalines (10),[50] and isoxazoles, (11) and (12).[51] Ethyl-6-ethoxybenzothiazole-2-carbamate (13), a benzimidazole isostere, was a broadly effective anthelmintic in horses, pigs, chickens and sheep but was less potent than analogous benzimidazoles.[52] Methyl 6-(phenylsulfinyl)imidazo[1,2-a]pyridine-2-carbamate (14) was shown to be orally active against a broad range of helminths in sheep and cattle at 2.5 mg/kg and in swine and dogs at higher doses.[53]

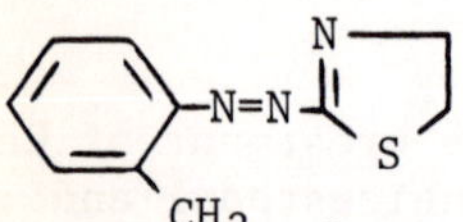
9

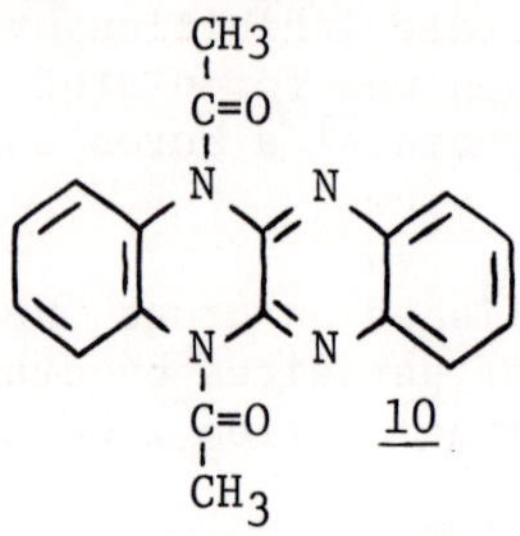
10

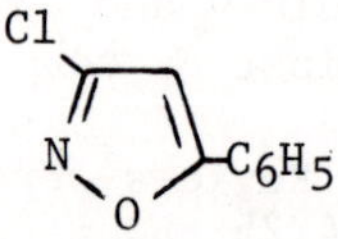
11

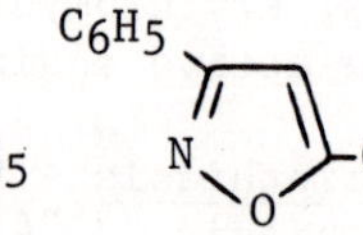
12

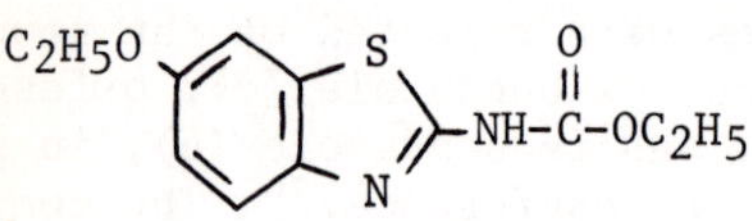
13

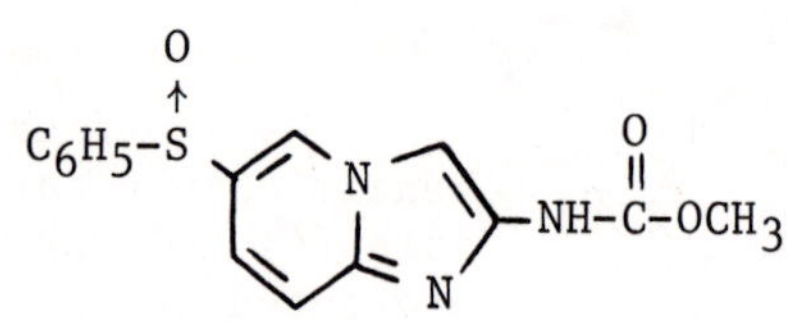
14

New tapeworm agents included praziquantel (EMBAY 8440, Droncit) (15), active against schistosomes and cestodes[54] in mice, rats[55] and dogs[56] by oral or parenteral administration. Uredofos (RH-565, diuredosan) (16), was shown to be effective against tapeworms, hookworms and whipworms in dogs.[57,58,59] Butamisole (17) was active against hookworms and whipworms in dogs but poorly effective against ascarid and tapeworm infections.[60] Nitroscanate (Lopatol) (18) was active against most nematodes and cestodes of dogs but inactive against whipworms.[61]

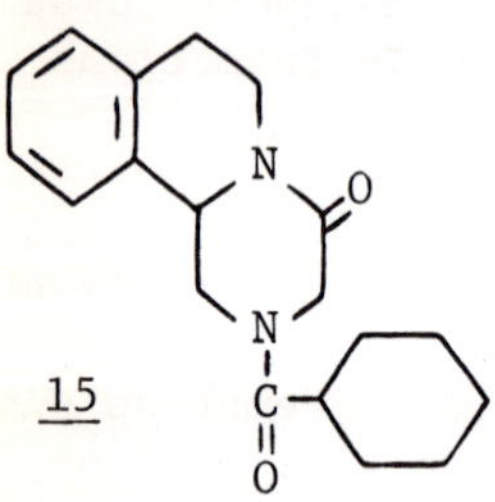
15

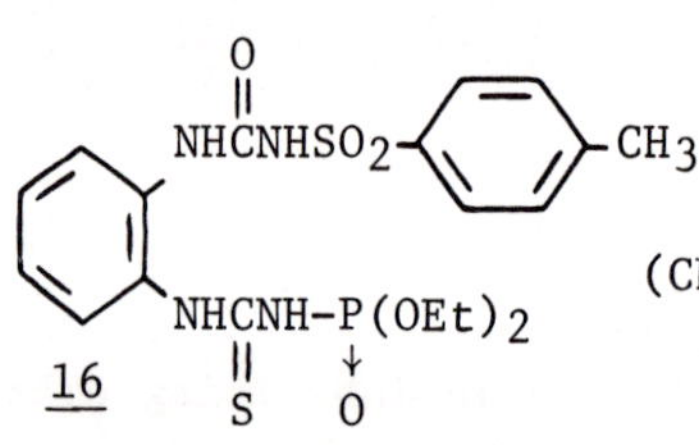
16

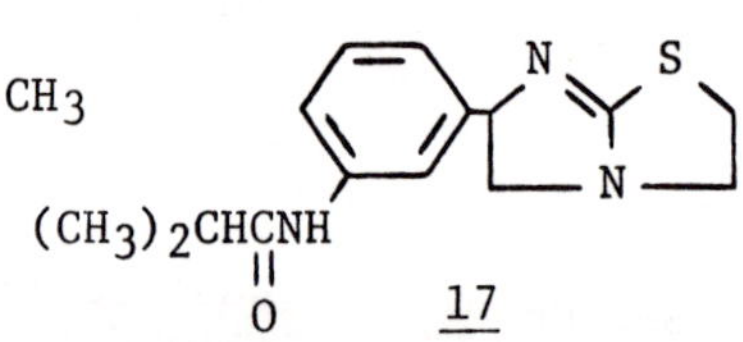
17

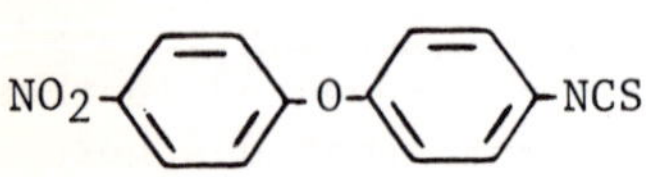
18

New drugs for the treatment of *Fasciola hepatica* in sheep and cattle included a benzenedisulfonamide (19)[62,63,64] active against mature flukes at 3.75 mg/kg, immature flukes at 10-15 mg/kg and possessing a wide margin of safety. Acemidophen (20), an analog of diamphenethide, showed expected superior activity against immature flukes.[65] Carbonyldicyanide phenylhydrazones exemplified by (21) were active but toxic.[66] 4-Isothiocyanato-4'-nitrodiphenylamine (C.9333-GO/CC_1P 4540) (22) was active against human hookworm infections.[67,68]

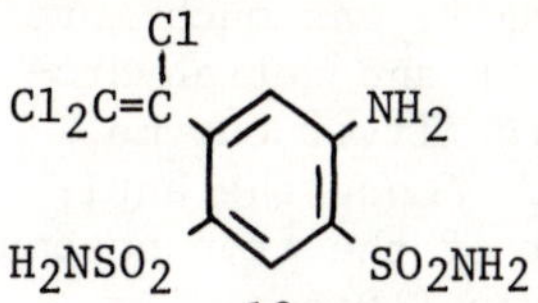

19

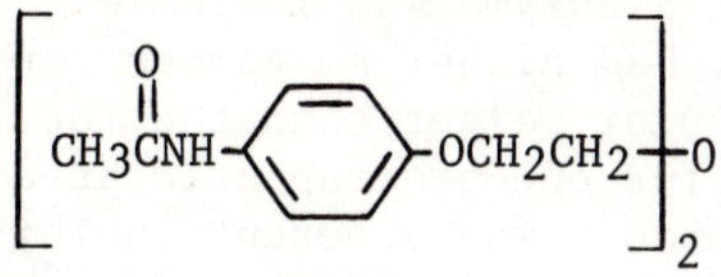

20

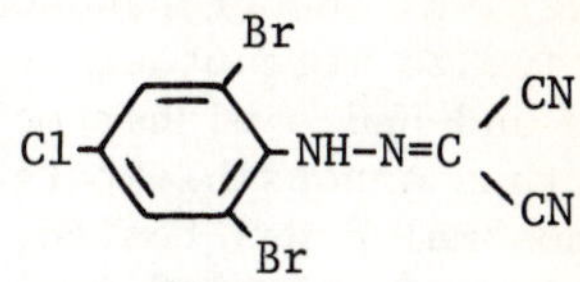

21

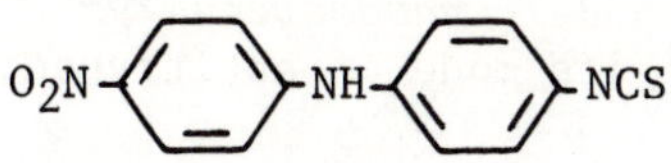

22

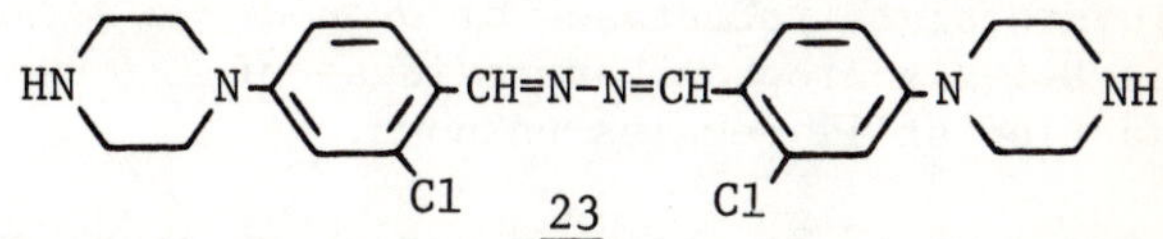

23

Schistosomiasis - Reviews were published on the chemotherapy of *Schistosoma mansoni*[69] and the chemistry of schistosomicides.[70] A series of papers[71,72,73,74,75] described the excellent activity of praziquantel, (15), against all species of schistosomes in mice, hamsters, monkeys and baboons by oral or parenteral administration. Studies on the antischistosomal drug 4-isothiocyanato-4'-nitrodiphenylamine (22) and its isocyanate analog[76] demonstrated that the latter compound was mutagenic and lacked activity against schistosomes. Several antischistosomal drugs including furapranidium, hycanthone, oxamniquine and metrifonate were shown to be mutagenic.[77,78] New structural types with reported antischistosomal activity were the benzalazine (23),[79] 5-(2,4,5-trichlorophenyl)hydantoin (24)[80] and N-acyl derivatives of N^4-(N-alkylglycyl)sulfanilamides (25).[81]

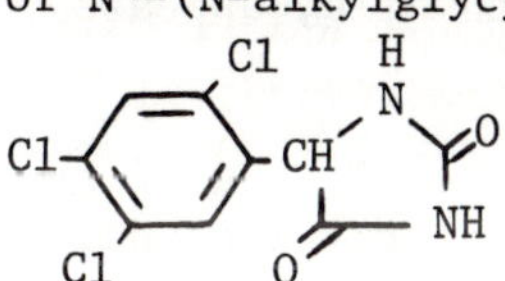

24

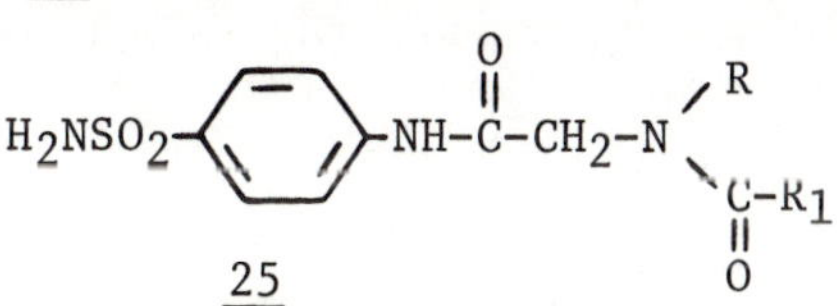

25

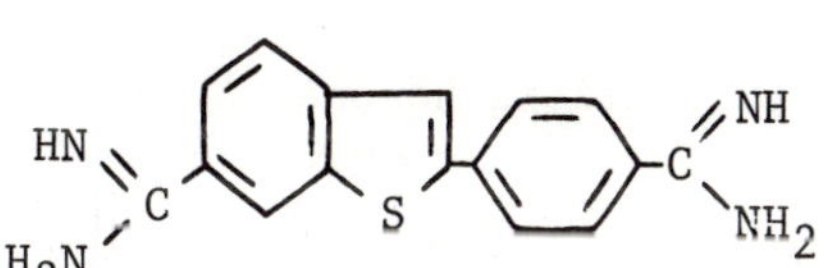

26

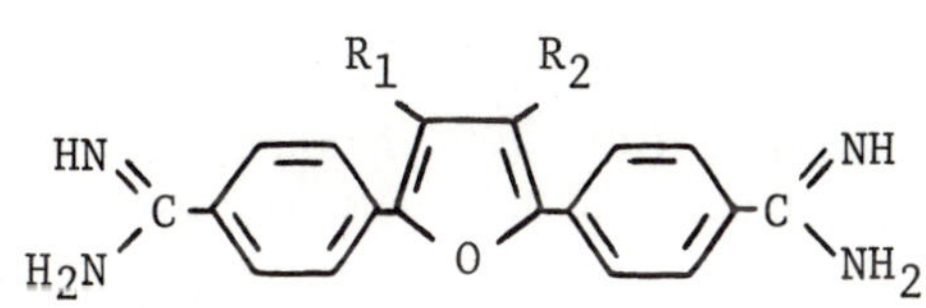

27

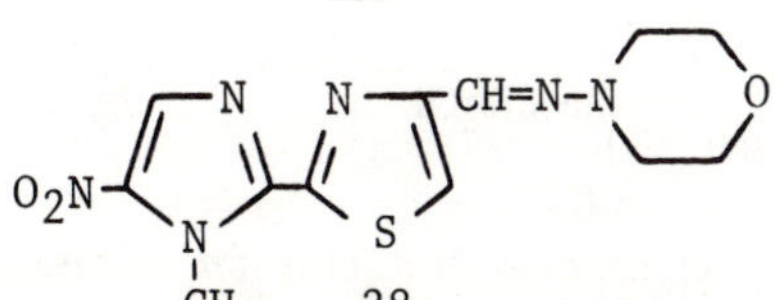

28

Trypanosomiasis - A review of the biochemistry of *Trypanosoma cruzi* was published.[82] A session was organized to discuss the relevance of trypanosome biochemistry to control.[83] A novel approach to drug screening was proposed using African trypanosomes in the presence of SHAM or glycerol.[84] A mouse model was used to try to uncover new trypanosomiasis leads.[85] No entirely new antitrypanosomal structures were described. Variations of older types included the bisamidines 98/202 (26)[86] and (27)[87] and nitro heterocycles, the most potent of which was the nitroimidazole (28).[88]

Thymidylate synthetase activities were detected in *Crithidia fasciculata, Crithidia oncopelti,* the bloodstream forms of *Trypanosoma brucei, T. congolense* and *T. lewisi* and the blood, intracellular and culture forms of

T. cruzi.[89] The trypanosomatid enzyme was inhibited by Mg^{++}, was much more sensitive to mercaptoethanol, had higher Km values for dUMP and tetrahydrofolate and had a higher molecular weight than the fetal rat liver enzyme. It is thus a possible target for chemotherapeutic attack. Among the antitrypanosomal drugs tested, suramin was a potent inhibitor of the trypanosomatid enzyme ($ID_{50} \approx 1.8 \times 10^{-6}M$) but not the mammalian enzyme ($ID_{50} \approx 1.1 \times 10^{-3}M$). However, since suramin also inhibits, at similar concentrations, the dihydrofolate reductases of *Onchocerca volvulus* and *T. rhodesiense*[90] and the L-α-glycerophosphate oxidase of *T. brucei*,[91] its mode of antitrypanosomal action still remains unknown.

Cross *et al.*[92] observed extensive breakdown of L-threonine to equimolar amounts of glycine and acetate during growth of *T. brucei* in culture. The pathway, which involves L-threonine dehydrogenase and aminoacetone synthetase and subsequent hydrolysis of acetyl-CoA, is most active in cultured trypanosomes but is also present in bloodstream forms.[93] The acetyl-CoA generated from threonine was apparently utilized by the parasite as a preferred source of carbon for lipid synthesis.[94] Antabuse was a strong inhibitor of threonine catabolism, probably due to its strong inhibition of L-threonine dehydrogenase ($ID_{50} = 5.2 \times 10^{-6}M$).[92,93] It also blocked the growth of *T. brucei* in culture,[92] and inhibited O_2 uptake and motility of bloodstream *T. brucei*.[95] The drug was, however, unable to cure trypanosome infection in mice[92] which was attributed to probable inactivation or sequestering of the drug by blood cells.[95] The catabolism of threonine in trypanosomes, meanwhile, appears to be an attractive target for chemotherapy.

The successful *in vitro* cultivation of animal-infective *T. brucei* by Hirumi *et al.*[96] has opened the opportunity of evaluating new trypanocidal drugs *in vitro*.

Trichomoniasis - The only new drugs described were variations of nitroimidazoles, *e.g.*, HOE316 (29),[97] ornidazole (30),[98] pirinidazole (HOE088) (31)[99] and chloronizole (32).[100] A study was made of the antitrichomonal activity of nitropyridines and nitroimidazopyridines.[101]

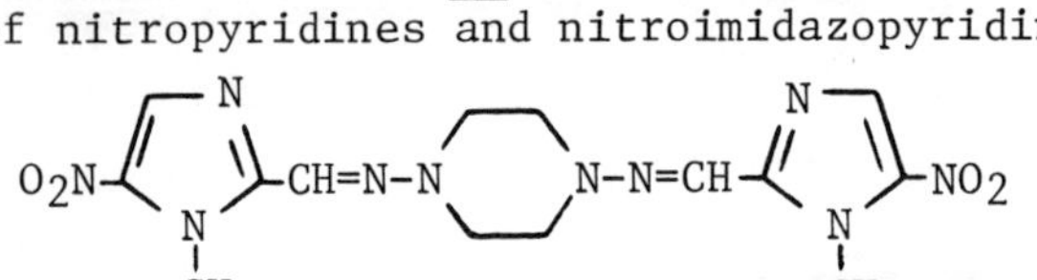
29

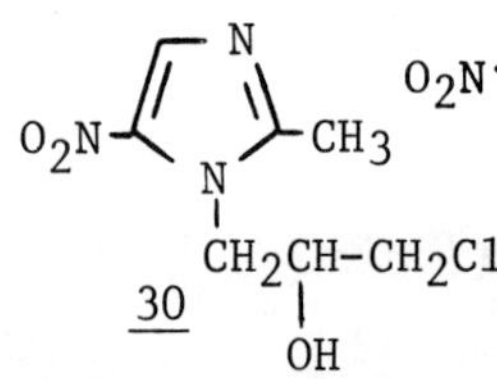
30

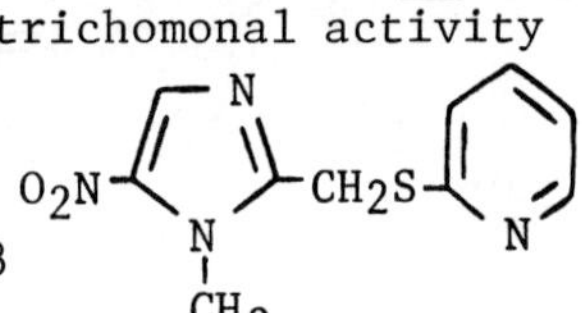
31

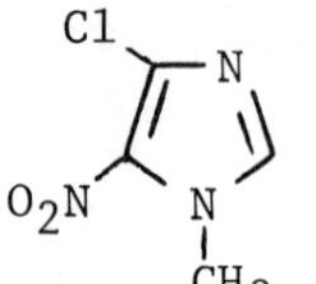
32

Leishmaniasis - The nutritional requirements for the *in vitro* cultivation of *Leishmania donovani* and *Leishmania braziliensis* were described.[102] A number of antiparasitic agents were tested against *Leishmania mexicana* in tissue culture. Those which showed good activity were also active in mice.[103] Mycobacillin, a polypeptide antifungal, was active against *L. donovani*, presumably by disruption of the membrane.[104]

Amebiasis - Further studies were carried out on nitroimidazoles,[98] nitrobenzofurans,[105] nitropyridines and nitroimidazopyridines[101] and 4-alkylaminoquinolines and 4-alkylaminoquinaldines.[106,107]

Babesiosis - A comprehensive review of ovine babesiosis was published[108] covering most aspects of biology and chemotherapy. The first isolation of babesia in sheep in Great Britain was reported.[109] A potential *in vitro* screen was described, measuring the inhibition of hypoxanthine incorporation into *Babesia rodhaini*.[110]

Toxoplasmosis - Treatment of *Toxoplasma gondii* infected cats with 2-sulfamoyl-4,4'-diaminodiphenylsulfone and sulfadiazine reduced oocyst shedding but did not eliminate infection. Clindamycin appeared to have superior efficacy.[111] Robenidene and sulfamonomethoxine were effective in chicks, mice, rats and rabbits.[112]

Cultivation of *T. gondii* in human fibroblast tissue cultures enabled the isolation of temperature-sensitive and drug-resistant mutants of the parasite by Pfefferkorn and Pfefferkorn.[113,114] An adenine-arabinoside resistant mutant was found deficient in adenosine kinase which could be the first successful step to convert the drug to its active form.[115] It was apparent that the parasite can grow without adenosine kinase. *T. gondii* was able to grow in Lesch-Nyhan cells and incorporate hypoxanthine or guanine from the culture medium.[116] The evidence suggests that the parasite depends mainly on the hypoxanthine-guanine phosphoribosyl transferase pathway for its purine supply.

Similar observations were made on pyrimidine metabolism by Pfefferkorn and Pfefferkorn.[117] Uracil was not significantly incorporated into the nucleic acids of human fibroblast cells but was extensively incorporated into the intracellular parasite. There was little or no uridine kinase but high levels of uridine and deoxyuridine phosphorylases and uracil phosphoribosyl transferases in the parasite.[118] A single-step mutant resistant to 5-fluorodeoxyuridine[119] was lacking the enzyme uracil phosphoribosyl transferase.[118] Apparently, uridine, deoxyuridine and 5-fluorodeoxyuridine all enter the parasite by the phosphorylase-phosphoribosyl transferase pathway. That the parasite could grow without uracil phosphoribosyl transferase suggests its ability to synthesize pyrimidines *de novo*.

Coccidiosis - Studies were reported distinguishing coccidiostatic from coccidiocidal effects,[120,121] isolation of oocysts,[122] and purification of schizonts,[123] sporocysts and sporozoites[124] and the development of resistance.[125,126,127,128] Arprinocid (MK-302) (33)[129,130] had excellent activity against several virulent field isolates of coccidia at 60 to 70 ppm. New 1-benzyl (34)[131] and 1-phenyl (35)[132] derivatives of 6-azauracil were reported to have high anticoccidial activity. Polyether ionophore antibiotics with reported anticoccidial activity included sephamycin,[133] salinomycin,[134,135] etheromycin[136] and glucopyranosylmonensin.[137]

Several types of riboflavin antagonists showed excellent anticoccidial activity.[138,139] The most potent compound in the group was 5-deazariboflavin (36). 1-Substituted-4(1H)-pyridinone hydrazones (37) were found to have broad anticoccidial activity. ^{13}C NMR spectroscopy and computer-assisted molecular modeling compared the conformation of (37) with robenedine (38).[140,141] Although the calculations did not permit an unambiguous assignment of bioactive conformations, structural similarities were apparent in the low energy conformers of both compounds. The cross-resistance of (37) with (38) could be explained on this basis. Dithiosemicarbazones[142] showed activity against several *Eimeria* species whereas oxadiazoles, triazoles,[143] and 5-nitronicotinamide[144] and flutamide[145] were active only against *Eimeria tenella*.

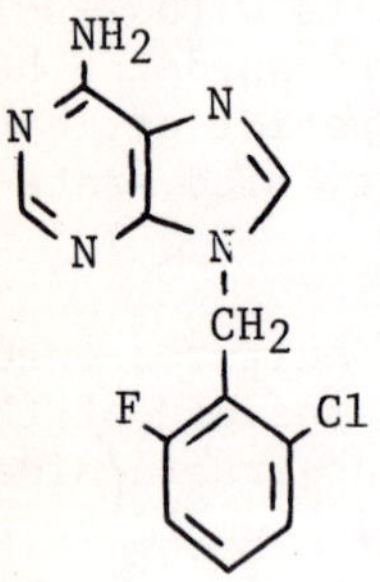

33

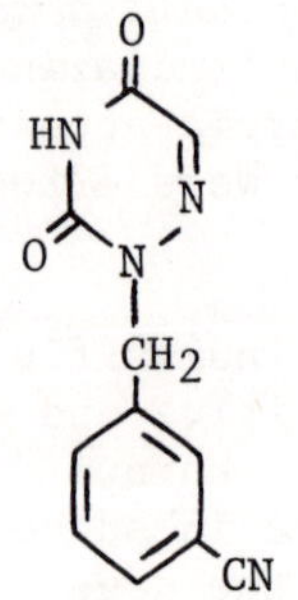

34

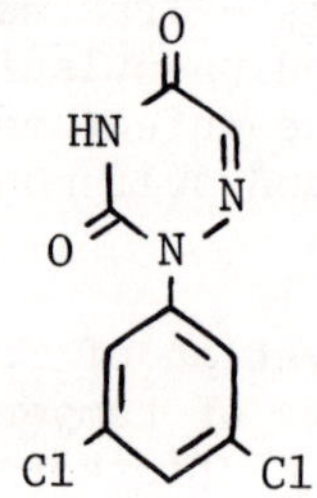

35

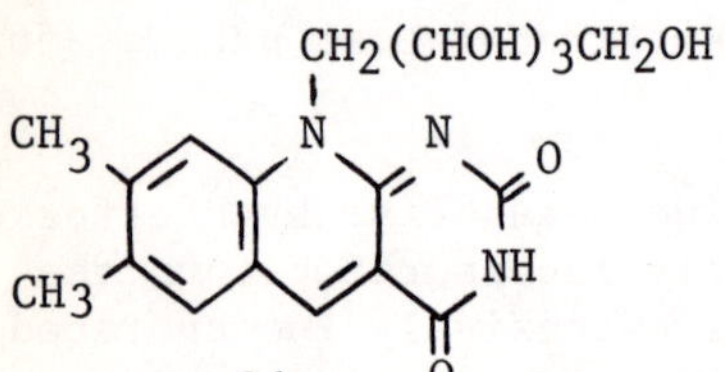

36

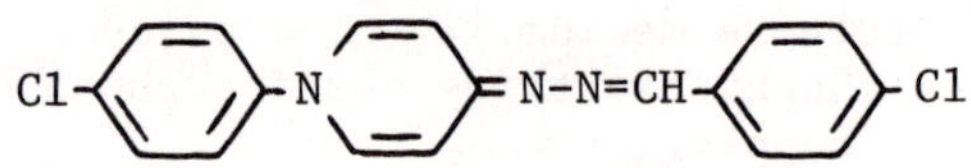

37

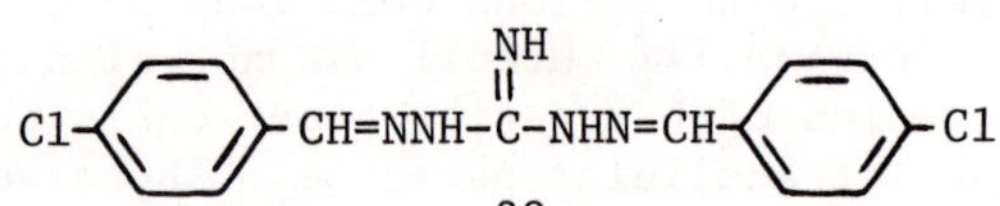

38

REFERENCES

1. B.H. Kean and D.W. Hostans, Drugs Choice 1976-1977, W. Modell, Ed., Mosby, St. Louis, p. 356.
2. M.J. Miller, *Prog.Drug.Res.*, *20*, 433 (1976).
3. A.I. White, *Textb.Org.Med.Pharm.Chem.*, 7th Ed., Lippincott, Philadelphia 1977, p. 247.
4. L.E. Cluff, Drugs Choice 1976-1977, W. Modell, Ed., Mosby, St. Louis, p. 160.
5. W.E. Rothe, *Bol.Of.Sanit.Panam.*, *81*, 338 (1976).
6. W. Peters and M. Porter, *Ann.Trop.Med.Parasitol.*, *70*, 271 (1976).
7. J. Rinehart, J. Arnold and C.J. Canfield, *An.J.Trop.Med.Hyg.*, *25*, 769 (1976).
8. G.H. Loew and R. Sahakian, *J.Med.Chem.*, *20*, 103 (1977).
9. M.W. Davidson, B.G. Griggs, D.W. Boykin and D.W. Wilson, *J.Med.Chem.*, *20*, 1117 (1977).
10. G.M. Trenholme, R.L. Williams, R.E. Desjourdin, H. Frischer, P.E. Carson, K.H. Rieckmann and C.J. Canfield, *Science*, *190*, 792 (1975).
11. C.A. Homewood, D.C. Warhurst, W. Peters and V.C. Baggaley, *Nature*, Lond., *235*, 50 (1972).
12. D.C. Warhurst and S.C. Thomas, *Biochem.Pharmacol.*, *24*, 2047 (1975).
13. D.C. Warhurst and V.C. Baggaley, *Trans.Roy.Soc.Trop.Med.Hyg.*, *66*, 5 (1972).
14. L.H. Schmidt, S. Alexander, L. Allen and J. Rasco, *Antimicrobial Agents and Chemotherapy*, *12*, 51 (1977).
15. C.C. Smith, G.J. McCormick and C.J. Canfield, *Exptl.Parasitol.*, *40*, 432 (1976).
16. E.G. Platzer, *Trans.N.Y.Acad.Sci.*, *34*, 200 (1972).
17. E.G. Platzer, *Life Science*, *20*, 1417 (1977).
18. C.C. Smith, G.J. McCormick and C.J. Canfield, *Exptl.Parasitol.*, *40*, 432 (1976).
19. C. Hansch, J.Y. Fukunaga, P.Y.C. Jow and J.B. Hynes, *J.Med.Chem.*, *20*, 96 (1977).
20. D.C. Warhurst, B.L. Robinson and W. Peters, *Ann.Trop.Med.Parasitol.*, *70*, 253 (1976).
21. Y. Okami, T. Okazaki, T. Kitahara and H. Umezawa, *J.Antibiot.*, *29*, 1019 (1976).
22. H. Nakamura, Y. Iitaka, T. Kitahara, T. Okazaki and Y. Okami, *ibid.*, *30*, 714 (1977).
23. M. Katz, *Drugs*, *13*, 124 (1977).
24. J.H. Thompson, *Ess.Pharmacol.* 2nd Ed., 1977, Harper & Row, Hagerstown, p. 512.
25. I.M. Rolls, *Pharmacol. Basis Ther.* 5th Ed., 1975, L.S. Goodman and A. Gilman Ed., Macmillan, New York, p. 1018.
26. W.C. Campbell, *Proc.Helminthol.Soc.Wash.*, *44*, 17 (1977).
27. E.I. Robertson, *Vet.Pharmacol.Ther.* 4th Ed., 1977, Iowa State Univ. Press, p. 994, 1052.
28. V.J. Theodorides, *Chemother.Infect.Dis.*, 71 (1976).
29. Abstracts of papers presented at the 8th Int. Conf. World Assoc. Adv. Vet. Parasitol., Sydney, July 11-15, 1977.
30. J.W. Crowley, A.C. Todd, D.H. Bliss and T.J. Kennedy, *Am.J.Vet.Sci.*, *37*, 1285 (1976).
31. R.M. Corwin, *ibid.*, *38*, 465 (1977).
32. N.F. Baker and R.A. Fisk, *ibid.*, *38*, 1315 (1977).

33. N.E. Downey, *Vet.Rec.*, *99*, 267 (1976).
34. V.J. Theodorides, T. Nawalinski and J. Chang, *Am.J.Vet.Res.*, *37*, 1515 (1976).
35. V.J. Theodorides, T. Nawalinski and J. Murphy, *ibid.*, *37*, 1517 (1976).
36. H. Herlich, *ibid.*, *38*, 1247 (1977).
37. G.W. Berz and J.V. Ernst, *ibid.*, *38*, 1425 (1977).
38. R.A. Knight and M.L. Colglazier, *ibid.*, *38*, 807 (1977).
39. J.P. Dubey, P.C. Stromberg and M.J. Toussant, *Experientia*, *33*, 1154 (1977).
40. J. Foix, *Rev.Med.Vet.*, *128*, 1111 (1977).
41. D.G. McBeath, M.J. Best and N.K. Preston, *Vet.Rec.*, *101*, 408 (1977).
42. S.S.E. Fernando and D.A. Denham, *J.Parasitol.*, *62*, 874 (1976).
43. J.D. Kelly, C.A. Hall, H.V. Whitlock, H.G. Thompson, N.J. Campbell and I.C.A. Martin, *Res.Vet.Sci.*, *22*, 161 (1977).
44. J.R. Egerton, *Texas Reports on Biology and Medicine*, *27* (Suppl. 2), 561 (1969).
45. L.F. LeJambre, *Vet.Parasitol.*, *2*, 385 (1976).
46. G.C. Coles and K.G. Simpkin, *Res.Vet.Sci.*, *22*, 386 (1977).
47. E.G. Garcia, *J.Med.Genet.*, *25*, 914 (1976).
48. R.E. Bradley and B.T. Alford, *Med.Vet.Pract.*, *58*, 518 (1977).
49. M.T. Wu, F.S. Waksmunski, D.R. Hoff, M.H. Fisher, J.R. Egerton and A.A. Patchett, *J.Pharm.Sci.*, *66*, 1150 (1977).
50. M.H. Fisher and A. Lusi, *ibid.*, *66*, 1349 (1977).
51. J.B. Carr, H.G. Durham and D.K. Hass, *J.Med.Chem.*, *20*, 934 (1977).
52. E. Panitz, *J.Helminth.*, *51*, 23 (1977).
53. R.J. Bochis, R.A. Dybas, J.R. Egerton, P. Eskola, P. Kulsa, B.O. Linn, E.P. Meitzner, J. Milkowski, H. Mrozik, L.E. Olen, D.A. Ostlind, L.H. Peterson, R.L. Tolman, A.F. Wagner and F.S. Waksmunski, Abs. 174th ACS Meeting, Chicago, 1977, MEDI-046.
54. J. Seubert, R. Pohlke and F. Loebich, *Experientia*, *33*, 1036 (1977).
55. H. Thomas and R. Gönnert, *Z.Parasiterk.*, *52*, 117 (1977).
56. M.A. Gemmell, P.D. Johnstone and G. Oudemans, *Res.Vet.Sci.*, *23*, 121 (1977).
57. E.L. Roberson, *Am.J.Vet.Med.*, *37*, 1483 (1976).
58. E.L. Roberson and A.L. Ager, *ibid.*, *37*, 1479 (1976).
59. K.S. Todd and R.L. Yates, *ibid.*, *37*, 1329 (1976).
60. N.C. Ronald and R.R. Bell, *Southwest Vet.*, *29*, 217 (1976).
61. J.C. Boray, Proc. 54th Ann. Conf. Aust. Vet. Assoc., Perth, 1977, p. 123.
62. D.A. Ostlind, W.C. Campbell, R.F. Riek, P. Baylis, S. Cifelli, R.K. Hartman, R.K. Lang, R.W. Butler, H. Mrozik, R.J. Bochis, P. Eskola, A. Matzuk, F.S. Waksmunski, L.E. Olen, G. Schwartzkopf, A. Grodski, B.O. Linn, A. Lusi, M.T. Wu, C.H. Shunk, L.H. Peterson, J.D. Milkowski, D.R. Hoff, P. Kulsa and R.E. Harmon, *Brit.Vet.J.*, *133*, 211 (1977).
63. H. Mrozik, R.J. Bochis, P. Eskola, A. Matzuk, F.W. Waksmunski, L.E. Olen, G. Schwartzkopf, A. Grodski, B.O. Linn, A. Lusi, M.T. Wu, C.H. Shunk, L.H. Peterson, J.D. Milkowski, D.R. Hoff, P. Kulsa, D.A. Ostlind, W.C. Campbell, R.F. Riek and R.E. Harmon, Abs. 173rd ACS Meeting, New Orleans, 1977, MEDI-15.
64. H. Mrozik, R.J. Bochis, P. Eskola, A. Matzuk, F.S. Waksmunski, L.E. Olen, L.H. Peterson, J.D. Milkowski, D.R. Hoff, P. Kulsa, D.A. Ostlind, W.C. Campbell, R.F. Riek and R.E. Harmon, *J.Med.Chem.*, *20*, 1226 (1977).
65. A. Visnaukas, N.V. Demidov and Z. Barckute, *Tr.Vses.Inst.Gel'mintol.*, *21*, 217 (1974).
66. G.R. Brown, G.C. Coles and A. Hayes, *Eur.J.Med.Chem.*, *12*, 361 (1977).
67. A.B. Vaidya, N.A. Mankowi, T. Paul and U.K. Sheth, *Brit.J.Pharmacol.*, *4*, 463 (1977).
68. J.C. Doshi, A.B. Vaidya, H.G. Sen, N.A. Mankodi, C.N. Nair and R.S. Grewal, *Am.J.Trop.Med.Hyg.*, *26*, 636 (1977).
69. N. Katz, *Adv.Pharmacol.Chemotherap.*, *14*, 1 (1977).
70. H.A. Shoeb, *Egypt J.Bilharz*, *3*, 11 (1977).
71. P. Andrews, *Parasitology*, *75*, 17 (1977).
72. R. Gönnert and P. Andrews, *Zeitsch. fur Parasit.*, *52*, 129 (1977).
73. J. Pellegrino, F.F. Lima-Costa, M.A. Carlos and R.T. Mello, *ibid.*, *52*, 151 (1977).
74. G. Webbe and C. James, *ibid.*, *52*, 169 (1977).
75. C. James, G. Webbe and G.S. Nelson, *ibid.*, *52*, 179 (1977).
76. A.W. Coulter, E. Bueding and R.P. Batzinger, *J.Med.Chem.*, *20*, 981 (1977).
77. T.M. Ong, D.F. Callen, S.L. Huang, R.P. Batzinger and E. Bueding, *Mutat.Res.*, *48*, 37 (1977).
78. R.P. Batzinger and E. Bueding, *J.Pharmacol.Exp.Ther.*, *200*, 1 (1977).
79. J. Hildebrandt, G. Ascher, H. Reinshagen and H. Mieth, *Tropenmed.Parasit.*, *28*, 51 (1977).
80. L.M. Werbel, E.F. Elslager, P.J. Islip and M.D. Closier, *J.Med.Chem.*, *20*, 1569 (1977).
81. H. Horstmann, S. Schütz, R. Behnisch, R. Gönnert and P. Andrews, *Eur.J.Med.Chem.*, *12*, 387 (1977).
82. W.E. Gutteridge, *Sci.Bull.Pan.Amer.Health Org.*, *318*, 135 (1976).
83. L.G. Goodwin, *Trans.Roy.Soc.Trop.Med.Hyg.*, *71*, 1 (1977).
84. A.H. Fairlamb, F.R. Opperdoes and P. Borst, *Nature*, *265*, 270 (1977).
85. K.E. Kinnamon, E.A. Steck, W.L. Hanson and W.L. Chapman, *J.Med.Chem.*, *20*, 741 (1977).
86. W. Roether and H. Seidenath, *Tropenmed.Parasit.*, *27*, 238 (1976).
87. B.P. Das and D.W. Boykin, *J.Med.Chem.*, *20*, 531 (1977).
88. M.C. Neville and J.P. Verge, *ibid.*, 946 (1977).
89. K. Al Chalabi and W.E. Gutteridge, *Biochim.Biophys.Acta.*, *481*, 71 (1977).
90. J.J. Jaffe, J.J. McCormack Jr. and E. Maymarian, *Biochem.Pharmacol.*, *21*, 719 (1972).
91. A.H. Fairlamb and I.B.R. Bowman, *Exptl.Parasitol.*, *43*, 353 (1977).
92. G.A.M. Cross, R.A. Klein and D.J. Linstead, *Parasitology*, *71*, 311 (1975).
93. D.J. Linstead, R.A. Klein and G.A.M. Cross, *J.Gen.Microbiol.*, *101*, 243 (1977).
94. R.A. Klein and D.J. Linstead, *Biochem.Soc.Trans.*, *4*, 48 (1976).
95. P. Borst, *Trans.Roy.Soc.Trop.Med.Hyg.*, *71*, 3 (1977).
96. H. Hirumi, J.J. Doyle and K. Hirumi, *Science*, *196*, 992 (1977).
97. W. Roether, H. Seidenath and E. Winkelmann, *Arzneium.Forsch.*, *27*, 968 (1977).
98. M. Skold, H. Gnorpe and L. Hillstrom, *Brit.J.Ven.Dis.*, *53*, 44 (1977).
99. W. Roether and E. Winkelmann, Proc. 9th Int. Cong. Chemother., London 1975, Plenum, N.Y., p. 45.
100. G. Dillemann, *Ann.Pharm.*, *34*, 17 (1976).
101. E. Winkelmann, W. Roether, M. Hartung and W.H. Wagner, *Arzneim.Forsch.*, *27*, 82 (1977).

102. R.F. Steiger and E. Steiger, *J.Protozool.*, *24*, 437 (1977).
103. W. Peterson, Proc. 2nd Int. Symp. Biochem. Parasit., 1976, H. Van den Bossche Ed., North-Holland, Amsterday, p. 523.
104. T.K. Chattopadhyay, S.N. Chatak, A.N. Bhaduri and D.K. Ghost, *J.Antibiot.*, *30*, 262 (1977).
105. R. Cavier and J. Cenac, *Ann.Pharm.*, *34*, 139 (1976).
106. S. Renault, J. Renault and R. Cavier, *Eur.J.Med.Chem.*, *7*, 555 (1970).
107. S. Renault, J. Renault and R. Cavier, *ibid.*, *7*, 561 (1976).
108. R.S. Aragon, *Vet.Bull.*, *46*, 903 (1976).
109. J.F. Reid, J. Armour, F.W. Jennings and G.M. Urquhardt, *Vet.Rec.*, *99*, 419 (1976).
110. A.D. Irwin and E.R. Young, *Nature*, *269*, 407 (1977).
111. J.P. Dubey and R.A. Yeary, *Can.Vet.J.*, *18*, 51 (1977).
112. A. Sokolov, *Russ.Vet.Bull.*, *47*, 1520 (1977).
113. E.R. Pfefferkorn and L.C. Pfefferkorn, *Exptl.Parasitol.*, *39*, 365 (1976).
114. E.R. Pfefferkorn and L.C. Pfefferkorn, *J.Parasitol.*, *62*, 993 (1976).
115. E.R. Pfefferkorn and L.C. Pfefferkorn, *Exptl.Parasitol.* (in press).
116. E.R. Pfefferkorn and L.C. Pfefferkorn, *ibid.*, *41*, 95 (1977).
117. E.R. Pfefferkorn and L.C. Pfefferkorn, *J.Protozool.*, *24*, 449 (1977).
118. E.R. Pfefferkorn, *Exptl.Parasitol.*, *44*, 26 (1978).
119. E.R. Pfefferkorn and L.C. Pfefferkorn, *Exptl.Parasitol.*, *42*, 44 (1977).
120. J.F. Ryley and R.G. Wilson, *Parasitology*, *73*, 287 (1976).
121. R.G. Wilson, *ibid.*, *3*, 283 (1976).
122. J.F. Ryley, R. Meade, J. Hazelhurst and T.E. Robinson, *ibid.*, *73*, 344 (1976).
123. M.A. Fernando and J. Pasternak, *Parasitology*, *74*, 19 (1977).
124. R.L. Stotish, P.M. Simashkevitch and C.C. Wang, *J.Parasitol.*, *63*, 1124 (1977).
125. H.D. Chapman, *Parasitology*, *73*, 265 (1976).
126. H.D. Chapman, *ibid.*, 275 (1976).
127. T.K. Jeffers, *Z.Parasitenkd.*, *50*, 251 (1976).
128. R.M. Weppelman, J.A. Battaglia and C.C. Wang, *Exp.Parasitol.*, *42*, 56 (1977).
129. B.M. Miller, E.C. McManus, G. Olson, K.D. Schleim, A.A. VanIderstine, D.W. Graham, J.E. Brown and E.F. Rogers, *Poult.Sci.*, *56*, 2039 (1977).
130. T. Tamas, G. Olson, E.C. McManus and B.M. Miller, *Poult.Sci.*, *56*, 1761 (1977).
131. B.L. Mylari, M.W. Miller, H.L. Howes, S.K. Figdar, J.E. Lynch and R.C. Koch, *J.Med.Chem.*, *20*, 475 (1977).
132. M.W. Miller, B.L. Mylari, H.L. Howes, J.E. Lynch, M.J. Lynch and R.L. Koch, Abs. 173rd ACS Meeting, New Orleans 1977, MEDI-8.
133. J.G. Meingassner, J. Hildebrandt, R. Leskova and H. Mieth, *Poult.Sci.*, *56*, 1281 (1977).
134. H.D. Danforth, M.D. Ruff, W.M. Reid and R.L. Miller, *ibid.*, *56*, 926 (1977).
135. H.D. Danforth, M.D. Ruff, W.M. Reid and J. Johnson, *ibid.*, *56*, 933 (1977).
136. M. Mitani, T. Umetsu, T. Yamanishi and N. Otake, *J.Antibiot.*, *30*, 239 (1977).
137. S. Omura, C. Kitao, H. Tanaka, R. Oiwa, Y. Takahashi, A. Nakagawa, M. Shimada and Y. Iwai, *ibid.*, *39*, 876 (1976).
138. D.W. Graham, J.E. Brown, R.D. Brown, W.T. Ashton and E.F. Rogers, Abs. 173rd ACS Meeting, New Orleans 1977, MEDI-9.
139. D.W. Graham, J.E. Brown, W.T. Ashton, R.D. Brown and E.F. Rogers, *Experientia*, *33*, 1274 (1977).
140. A.W. Douglas, M.H. Fisher, J.J. Fishinger, P. Gund, E.E. Harris, G. Olson, A.A. Patchett and W.V. Ruyle, Abs. 173rd ACS Meeting, New Orleans 1977, MEDI-10.
141. A.W. Douglas, M.H. Fisher, J.J. Fishinger, P. Gund, E.E. Harris, G. Olson, A.A. Patchett and W.V. Ruyle, *J.Med.Chem.*, *20*, 939 (1977).
142. E. Winkelmann, W. Wagner and H. Wirth, *Arzneim.Forsch.*, *27*, 950 (1977).
143. M. Mano, T. Seo, T. Matsuno and K. Imai, *Chem.Pharm.Bull.*, *24*, 2871 (1976).
144. Y. Morisawa, M. Kataoka, N. Kitano and T. Matsuzawa, *J.Med.Chem.*, *20*, 129 (1977).
145. E. Panitz and C.A. Stahl, *Proc.Helminth.Soc.Wash.*, *44*, 102 (1977).

Chapter 15. Antiviral Agents

C. E. Hoffmann, Pharmaceuticals Division, Biochemicals Department
E. I. du Pont de Nemours & Co., Inc., Wilmington, Delaware

Introduction - A sign of the advances in antiviral chemotherapy is the large number and variety of review articles published on the subject. Clinical applications for available antiviral agents are covered in reports by Becker,[1] Diana and Pancic,[2] Kaufman,[3] Pradalies and Leynadier,[4] Waldman,[5] James,[6] and Hermans.[7] The review by Maugh[8] discusses the history and present status of antiviral agents in the U.S.A. More generalized reviews on the trends in antiviral research are covered in reviews by Becker,[9] Galabov,[10] Meyer and colleagues,[11] and Hoffmann.[12] The papers presented at two symposia, "Antivirals with Clinical Potential" and the "Third Conference on Antiviral Substances," have been published[13,14] and provide a broad overview of both interferon and its inducers and compounds with antiviral activity.

Antiviral agents are currently available for clinical use against herpes- and influenza-caused infections. This has resulted in a series of papers related to clinical treatment of the disease. Reports by Rawls[15] and Dostal, *et al.*[16] cover the treatment of herpesvirus infections, with others covering the treatment of herpes skin infections[17] and herpes-caused encephalitis.[18] Testing and model systems for herpesvirus studies have also appeared with descriptions of test methods for herpes keratitis[19] and for intranasal testing.[20] A study of the polypeptides and antigens of herpesvirus has been used as a guide for studies of chemotherapy and epidemiology of herpes infections.[21] The chemoprophylaxis and prevention of respiratory diseases are discussed in articles by Jackson and Stanley[22] and Batten.[23] Douglas,[24] Knight,[25] and Dolin[26] report on influenza as a disease and cover methods for its control. More specifically, Couch[27] provides an assessment of amantadine's use for influenza and Hoffman and Dixon[28] review the problem of influenza in hospitals and methods for control.

The control of herpesvirus disease remains a major target of virus chemotherapy with many studies aimed at this and other DNA viruses. A comparison of the activities of the better known antiherpes compounds in tissue culture and *in vivo* was reported by Collins and Bauer,[29] in the hairless mouse model by Harris and Boyd,[30] and in hamsters by Renis.[31] The utility of nucleoside analogs for treatment of non-neoplastic diseases was discussed by Calabresi, *et al.*[32] while Fox discussed the pharmacology and chemistry of inhibitors of herpes replication.[33]

Adenine Arabinoside (Ara-A, Vidarabine) - A breakthrough in the treatment of herpes simplex encephalitis with the use of Ara-A (1) was reported by Whitley and colleagues in a collaborative NIAID study.[34] In 28 clinical biopsy-proved cases, i.v. administration reduced mortality from 70 to 28%, and if started early enough, prevented subsequent debilitating neurological sequela. Treatment started after severe neurological damage had occurred could prevent death, but could not reverse the damage. Another clinical

ISBN 0-12-040513-X

study on six patients with severe herpesvirus infections showed a clinical response and cure of the infection by a 15 mg/kg/day i.v. treatment.[35] In double-blind and open studies of the treatment of IDU refractory herpetic keratitis, Ara-A treatment provided clinical improvement and appeared useful for the treatment of this disease.[36] Other clinical studies have reported a degree of efficacy on herpes zoster in immunosuppressed[37] patients. In two cases of severe chickenpox and one of *Purpura fulminans*, rapid cure was reported from i.v. Ara-A treatment.[38] No effect on the human cellular immune mechanism was seen from treatment with this compound, an important consideration in an infection where host defense is of such importance.[39] Although these studies are encouraging, the insolubility of Ara-A, its requirement for i.v. administration, and its rapid *in vivo* deamination to the less active ara-hypoxanthine (Ara-Hx) pose severe problems for widespread use and have resulted in continuing research to provide a better agent.

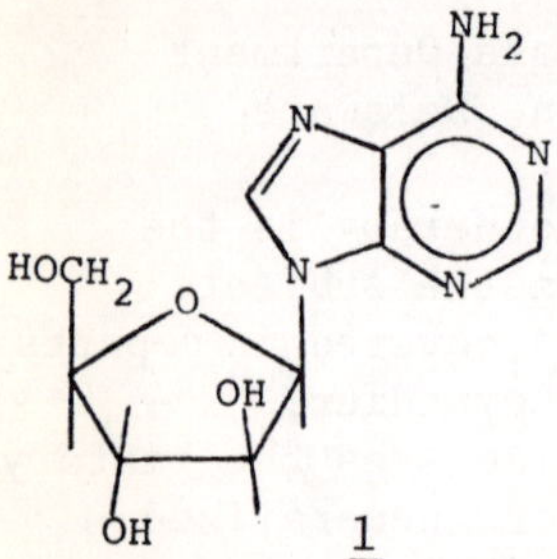

1

One promising compound is adenine arabinoside monophosphate (Ara-AMP) which is more soluble and has been shown to build high intra-ocular levels in rabbits dosed i.v. with small amounts of the compound.[40] Other studies have shown that Ara-A and Ara-AMP ointment were able to prevent fatal herpesvirus encephalitis when used as an ointment and neither caused skin irritation.[41] Treatment of established herpetic keratitis in rabbits indicated that Ara-AMP was superior to Ara-A and low doses of Ara-Hx or Ara-HxMP.[42] Due to the higher solubility of Ara-AMP, greater doses could be administered. A comparison study in mice infected with three different herpesvirus hominis infections showed Ara-AMP to be superior to Ara-A which was superior to phosphonoacetic acid.[43] Almost the reverse was observed in the treatment of genital herpesvirus hominis infections in mice where PAA ointment was effective whereas neither Ara-A nor Ara-AMP ointment provided protection.[44] Several studies have been carried out comparing the relative activities of Ara-A and Ara-Hx,[45,46,47] with Ara-A found to be ten times or more active than Ara-Hx. In the presence of coformycin, an adenine deaminase inhibitor, Ara-A in tissue culture was 35-70 times more potent than Ara-Hx.[48] In order to establish the role of antibody in control of herpesvirus infections, Ara-A was tested in mouse herpes encephalitis infections with and without rabbit immune globulin. The combination produced greater efficacy than either treatment alone, suggesting that severe infections may require a combination therapy for control.[49]

Cytosine Arabinoside (Cytarabine, Ara-C) - In spite of its higher toxicity and immunosuppressive action,[50] there is continued interest in its clinical application. In an open study it was reported that intravenous doses of cytarabine (2) reduced the shedding of type 1 and 2 herpesvirus to 4 days in 15 of 17 patients whereas without treatment, shedding would be expected to continue for several weeks.[51] An uncontrolled study of cytarabine in 61 patients with herpes zoster suggested a beneficial effect, but a randomized double-blind study in 30 patients provided no evidence of a benefit. In fact, the blister healing time was greater for the treated group.[52]

Another open study on herpes zoster in patients with malignancies reported 9 of 10 to be benefited by single daily i.v. doses of cytarabine.[53] Studies on the use of cytarabine against herpes encephalitis in children and infants indicated a beneficial effect if given early enough;[54,55] however, it would appear that vidarabine is a better agent. Neither cytarabine nor IDU were effective in treatment of cytomegalovirus infections of newborn mice indicating that they would be of little value in treatment of this disease in human neonates.[56] In an effort to bypass some of the toxicity of these agents yet retain antiviral efficacy, albumin conjugates of IDU and Ara-C were made and tested in ectromelia-infected mice.[57] Less toxicity and more activity was observed than with the free compounds.

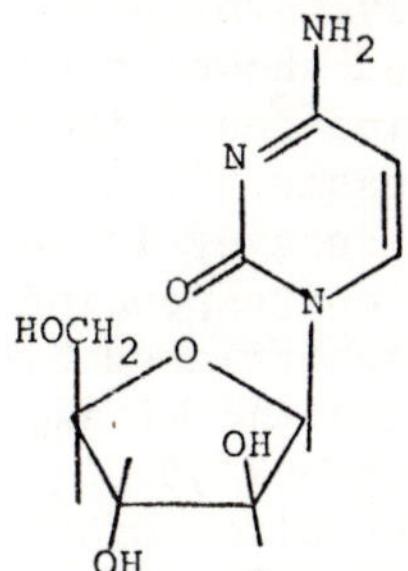

2

Idoxuridine (IDU - 5-Iodo-2'-deoxyuridine) - Idoxuridine (3) was used successfully in the treatment of recurrent genital herpes when applied topically in a solution of dimethyl sulfoxide.[58] Twenty percent idoxuridine gave the best response, although 5% solutions were better than placebo. Recurrence rates were not affected by these treatments. A similar effect was seen with this combination for the treatment of zoster lesions.[59] A study of 6-azauridine and IDU showed about a 50% response on relapsing genital herpes for either alone, but an 82% response for a combination of the two.[60] The present status of idoxuridine for herpes infections is discussed by Stuart-Harris[61] and Grupper.[62]

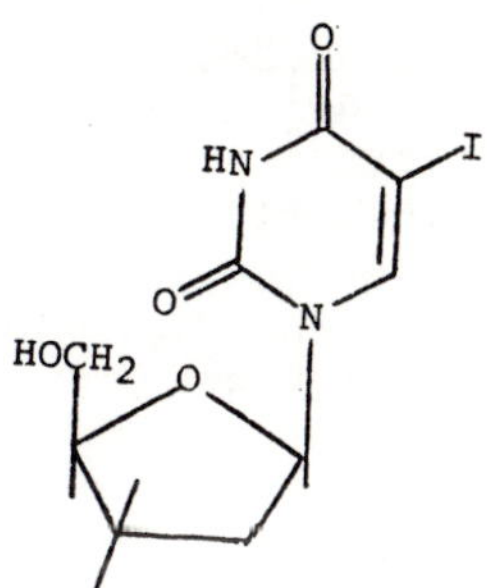

3

Other Purine and Pyrimidine Analogs - In continuing effort to obtain increased activity and safety, a large number of purine and pyrimidine analogs have been tested in laboratory systems. Among these are 5,6-dihydro-5-azathymidine with prophylactic and therapeutic activity against herpes infections in mice,[63] 5-iodo-2'-deoxycytidine (IDC) with therapeutic activity equal or better than IDU against herpetic keratitis in rabbits and man,[64] and 5-trifluoromethyl-2'-deoxyuridine, which was well tolerated and showed a dose-dependent protection of mice infected intracerebrally with type 1 herpesvirus, but was inactive against encephalitis in mice due to EMC, an RNA virus.[65] A combination of 2-deoxy-D-glucose and 3-deazauridine provided a synergistic effect against Japanese B encephalitis in tissue culture with no increased cytotoxicity, again suggesting combinations of agents for virus chemotherapy.[66] Continued studies with 3-deazaguanine (4) and its nucleoside and nucleotide suggested broad-spectrum activity with nine RNA viruses and seven DNA viruses sensitive in tissue culture. *In vivo* activity was demonstrated against influenza A and B and parainfluenza virus infections[67] as well as against Friend leukemia

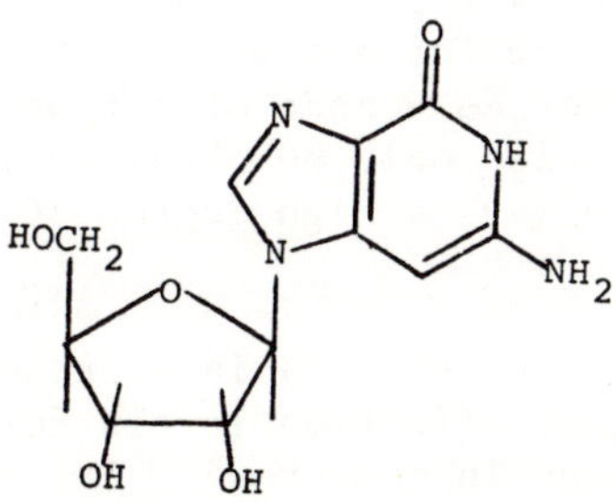

4

splenomegaly in mice. More basic studies have attempted to determine the mechanism of action for a number of active analogs. Arabinosylthymine (Ara-T), which has selective activity against herpesvirus, was shown to be phosphorylated and activated only by a virus-induced pyrimidine deoxyribonucleoside kinase and was not a substrate for normal cell kinases.[68] A similar effect was demonstrated in the case of 5-halogenated deoxycytidine analogs which were 10-100 times less toxic to cells than the corresponding 5-halogenated uridine analogs. The former could only be phosphorylated by a virus-induced kinase whereas normal cells contained an activating kinase for the latter compounds.[69,70] A new thymidine analog, 5'-amino-2',5-dideoxy-5-iodouridine (AIU), has been shown to be a potent inhibitor of herpesvirus, but has essentially no cellular toxicity.[71] It appears to selectively block an intracellular event during virus replication, an event occurring 4-6 hours after infection, and has no effect on infected or uninfected cell RNA synthesis, although blocking DNA synthesis in infected, but not uninfected, cells.

Ribavirin (Virazole - 1-β-D-Ribofuranosyl-1,2,4-triazole-3-carboxamide) - Oral doses (600 mg/day) (5) showed no demonstrable effect in volunteers challenged with influenza A virus[72] and a marginal effect on volunteers challenged with influenza B.[73] Dosage at 1000 mg/day resulted in a reduction in signs and symptoms in volunteers infected with the Victoria strain of influenza A, but had no effect on antibody response or virus shedding.[74]

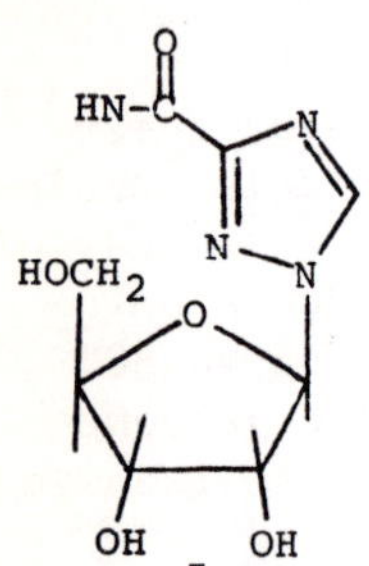

5

In ferrets, 100 mg/kg/day, but not lower doses, caused a marked reduction in symptoms from influenza A challenge infection. However, this was also accompanied by an immunosuppressive effect.[75] Activity by aerosol or i.p. administration to mice infected with influenza A and parainfluenza has been reported.[76,77]

Mode-of-action studies show that virus RNA synthesis is inhibited by ribavirin and this can be reversed by guanosine or xanthosine.[78] Additional studies with cell-free influenza virus ribonucleic acid polymerase showed that the inhibition is not by ribavirin but by its 5'-triphosphate, indicating the necessity for cellular phosphorylation for activity.[79] A general effect of the compound on cellular processes as a mode of action is suggested by the fact that no resistance to ribavirin could be obtained in herpesvirus after 10 passages, whereas idoxuridine gave a high degree of resistance under similar passage.[80]

Phosphonoacetic Acid (PAA) - Disodium phosphonoacetic acid (6) in a cream base proved to be too irritating at effective levels for use in treating herpesvirus lesions in monkeys.[81] It, but none of its analogs, was active against Marek's disease virus replication in tissue culture. However, it was ineffective against the disease in chickens.[82] PAA produced a significant effect when applied topically on superficial herpetic keratitis of rabbits against both IDU-sensitive and

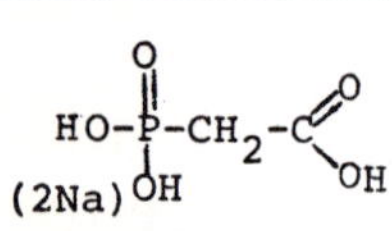

6

-resistant strains.[83] Mode-of-action studies indicate it is active on Marek's disease herpesvirus and on the virus-induced DNA polymerase where it acts by binding with the pyrophosphate site of the enzyme.[84] Herpes-virus mutants resistant to PAA can be produced and the DNA polymerase isolated from these mutants, although of the same molecular weight, are also resistant.[85,86] A review of the data on PAA to 1977 discussed some possible problems with PAA, the development of resistance, and the chance that the agent would be sequestered like pyrophosphate causing long-term complications.[87]

<u>Amantadine HCl (1-Adamantanamine HCl)</u> - Until 1976, FDA clearance for amantadine HCl (7) was for the prophylaxis of influenza A2 (Asian) infection only. In 1976 this was broadened to include use for the prevention and symptomatic management of infections caused by influenza A viruses. A report of the VIII Influenza Workshop[88] covered much of the work to 1975. More recent reports assess the use of amantadine HCl for influenza.[89,90] Double-blind controlled studies showed that amantadine HCl was effective in reducing the incidence of 1973 and 1974 influenza A outbreaks, but did not provide activity against influenza B occurring at the same time.[91] In another study, illness due to an influenza A outbreak was significantly reduced in students treated prophylactically. However, during a post-treatment period with influenza still present, an accelerated rate of illness occurred in the previously protected group, indicating treatment should be continued until the outbreak is over.[92] A study of students with natural influenza A infection indicated that the therapeutic use of amantadine HCl resulted in an accelerated physiologic improvement with a significant increase in helium-oxygen flow rate.[93] Influenza A/New Jersey/8/76 (Hsw1N1) was found to be inhibited by amantadine HCl in tissue culture, *in ovo*, and in mice,[94] and amantadine HCl was also inhibitory to the formation of virus-induced polypeptides in tissue culture.[95] High doses of amantadine HCl given orally to ferrets produced no activity against influenza A infection and caused toxic effects. In contrast, low doses, 6 mg/kg, provided as an aerosol, were consistently effective and without side effects.[96] Aerosols of amantadine, rimantadine (8) and ribavirin have also been effective for treatment of influenza A infections in mice.[97] Studies on the formation of amantadine- and rimantadine-resistant variants of influenza suggest this is due to a selection of resistant particles from a nonhomogeneous population and not due to a mutagenic effect.[98] More recent studies on the mode of action of these compounds suggest a possible effect on virus-associated RNA-dependent RNA polymerase which occurs at an early phase of infection.[99,100]

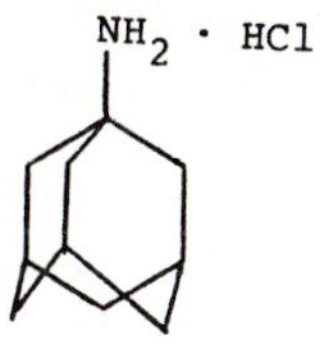

7

<u>Rimantadine HCl (α-Methyl-1-adamantanemethylamine HCl)</u> - In the USSR, rimantadine HCl (8) (available as Remantadini) is used as an antiviral chemotherapeutic agent due to good therapeutic activity and good tolerance. Although many studies have been carried out in the USSR, most of the literature on these studies is not available in the U.S. Available reports of clinical studies have shown that prolonged administration of the drug is safe, well tolerated,[101] and also effective and well tolerated against

influenza A infections, including the influenza A/Victoria/3/76 type.[102,103,104] Aerosol administration of the compound to mice infected with influenza A virus significantly increased survival rates.[105,106] A combination of rimantadine and ribavirin provided a synergistic effect[107] in both tissue culture and mouse infections with influenza A. Rimantadine was highly active against the 1976 influenza A/New Jersey isolate in a chick embryo test[108] and other studies in tissue culture[109,110] suggest that rimantadine has a direct effect on influenza virus RNA-dependent RNA polymerase and that this is the mode of action of the compound.

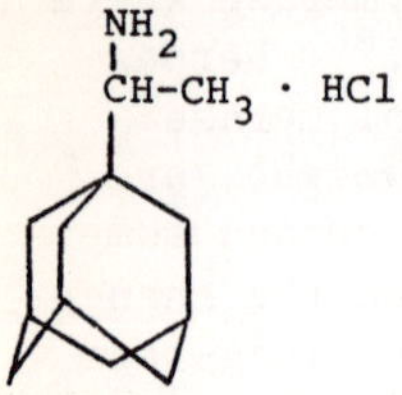

8

Tromantadine HCl (Viru-Merz) - Continued studies abroad with tromantadine HCl (9) indicate clinical efficacy against primary and recurring herpesvirus infections in man.[111,112] Used as an ointment it was reported to provide an excellent response in acute and chronic eye trachoma infections with little evidence of irritation[113] Low toxicity and minor irritation was reported from topical and systemic applications. Tissue culture studies indicate it is active at the stage of virus penetration or uncoating rather than at an inhibition of nucleic acid synthesis.[114]

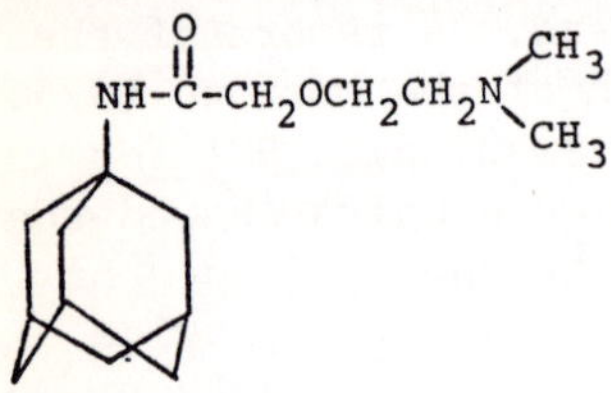

9

Isoprinosine (Paracetamidobenzoic Acid Salt of Inosine Dimethylaminoisopropanol) - This agent continues to be controversial. In a study to determine its effect on the immune system, it was found to have a direct effect on the proliferation of lymphocytes, but with an action different from other immunopotentiating agents such as levamisole.[115] Results from a clinical study in Brazil indicated activity against herpes simplex and herpes zoster infections.[116] However, in 1977 the FDA terminated the IND on isoprinosine due to a lack of evidence of efficacy.[117]

Vitamin C (Ascorbic Acid) - Additional trials have failed to provide substantive evidence of activity of vitamin C against the common cold. A co-twin study of 44 school-aged twins showed no significant overall effect of ascorbic acid, although treated girls in the youngest groups had shorter and less severe illnesses.[118] The study was double-blind, but several of the mothers reported tasting the capsules and thus knew who was receiving ascorbic acid. In order to check on earlier positive studies, a double-blind trial of vitamin C was performed in 868 Navajo school children. No effect was observed, and it was concluded that vitamin C was not an effective prophylactic or therapeutic agent.[119] Overall, an analysis of the clinical studies indicate a lack of significant effect of vitamin C on the common cold.[120]

Arildone {Win 38,020 [4-(6-((2-chloro-4-methoxy))phenoxyhexyl)-3,5-heptonedione]} - Arildone (10) was the most active of a series of β-diketones against a number of both RNA and DNA virus strains[121] with activity shown both in tissue culture and in animal studies. It is reported to be effective topically against herpesvirus types 1 and 2 in the rabbit eye and guinea pig skin.[122]

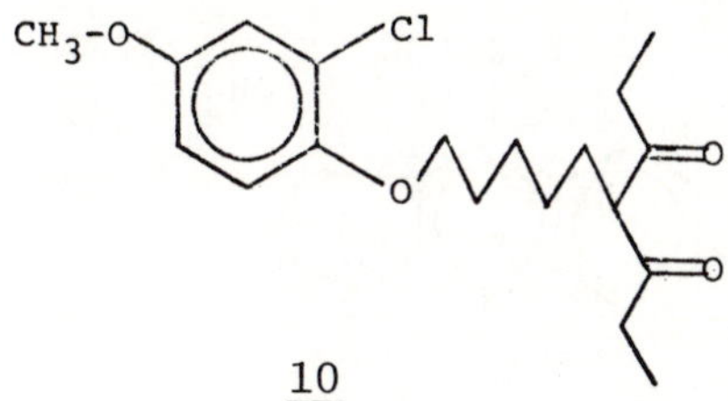

10

Bonapthon (6-Bromonaphthaquinone) - A study showed bonapthon to reduce pneumonia and improve symptoms in mice infected with influenza virus when given orally and to have a beneficial effect on herpetic keratitis in rabbits when applied as an ointment.[123] In contrast, other laboratory studies showed no activity and some toxicity,[124] the lack of activity being confirmed in a clinical trial with influenza.[103]

Other Compounds Tested Clinically - A number of compounds, including an interferon inducer, have been tested by intranasal administration to volunteers infected with rhinoviruses. A new antiviral agent, 1-phenyl-3-(4-phenyl-2-thiazolyl)guanidine was ineffective in moderating clinical illness due to rhinovirus type 44 challenge.[125] Three unrelated compounds with antirhinovirus activity in tissue culture - SKF-40491 {4-(8-amino-7-chloro-5-methyl-5H-as-triazino[5,6-b]indol-3-yl)amino-2-methyl-2-butanol}; GL R9-338 (3-α-naphthyl-5-diethylcarbamoyl-1,2,4-oxadiazole); and RP 19326 (2,6-diphenyl-3-methyl-2,3-dihydroimidazo[2,1-b]thiazole) were given intranasally to volunteers infected with rhinovirus types 3 or 9. All caused a reduction in mean viral titer from nasal washing and RP 19326 also provided a slight reduction in symptoms.[126] The lack of a striking response was thought due to inability to maintain adequate concentrations of compound. A similar study was carried out with an interferon inducer, CP 20961 (N,N-dioctadecyl-N',N'-bis(2-hydroxyethyl)propanediamine), which was found to induce interferon, and if timing and number of doses were correct, also reduce clinical symptoms of a rhinovirus challenge.[127] In such challenge studies the timing can be carefully controlled which is not the case in natural infections.

Compounds with *In Vivo* Antiviral Activity - D-Glucosamine, an inhibitor of the glycosylation of the viral coat, decreased tumor growth due to Rous sarcoma virus in chicks and quails and increased survival of mice infected with influenza when administered by i.p. injection, but provided essentially no protection to mice when administered intranasally.[128] A new compound, AMCT (11), was active on influenza A virus strains in tissue culture and in experimental mouse infections, but was inactive on influenza B. Timing experiments indicated it acts at a very early stage of virus growth (penetration or uncoating). These results are similar to those observed with amantadine HCl.[129]

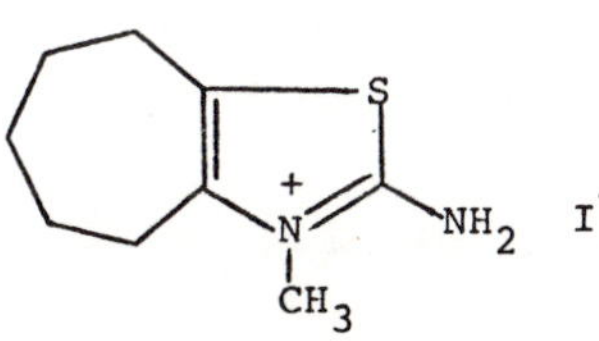

11

Interferon Inducers - The two most active analogs (12) of a series of bis-basic substituted polycyclic aromatic compounds have provided significant amounts of interferon in mice and afforded protection against infection with both RNA and DNA viruses.[130,131] BL 3849A (13) has a similar effect and is also active in mice against RNA and DNA viruses by oral administration.[132] CMA (10-carboxymethyl-9-acridanone Na salt) protected

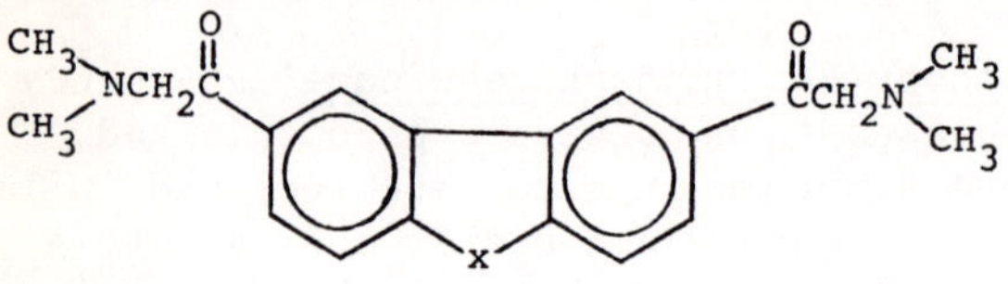

x = O or S · 2HCl · $2H_2O$

12

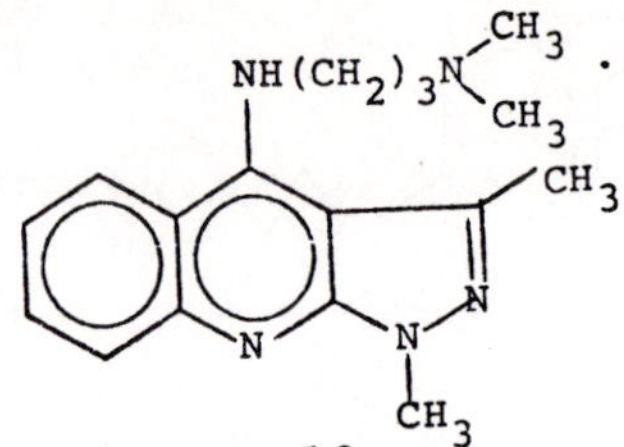

· 2HCl

13

mice infected with a variety of viruses and produced an interferon-like substance in mouse cell culture and mice.[133]

Conclusion - Antiviral chemotherapy has come of age. Broadened and more effective applications of available and new agents will require a continuing effort by researchers on methods for best treating virus diseases and on bringing this to the attention of physicians and public health authorities.

References

1. Y. Becker in "Antiviral Drugs - Monographs in Virology," Vol. 11, S. Karger, N.Y., 1976.
2. G. D. Diana and F. Pancic, Angew. Chem. Int. Ed. Engl., 15 (2), 410 (1976).
3. H. E. Kaufman, Int. J. of Dermatol., 16, 464 (1977).
4. A. Pradalier and F. Leynadier, Gaz. Med. Fr., 82 (32), 3795 (1975).
5. R. H. Waldman and J. D. Lee, Compr. Ther. 3 (7), 10 (1977).
6. D. G. James, Practitioner, 217 (1300), 603 (1976).
7. P. E. Hermans, Mayo Clin. Proc., 52 (11), 683 (1977).
8. T. H. Maugh, II, Science (Wash.), 192 (4235), 128 (1976).
9. Y. Becker, Isr. J. Med. Sci., 11 (11), 1135 (1975).
10. A. S. Galabov, Forsch., 26 (2), 169 (1976).
11. F.-P. Meyer, H. Walther and L. Domner, Biol. Rundsch. 13 (6), 358 (1975).
12. C. E. Hoffmann, Ann. Rep. Med. Chem. 11, 128 (1976).
13. T. C. Merigan, J. Inf. Dis., 133, A1 (1976).
14. E. C. Herrmann, Jr., Ed., Ann. N.Y. Acad. of Sci. 284, 1 (1977).
15. W. E. Rawls, JAMA, 235 (13), 1365 (1976).
16. V. Dostal, D. Fanta and R. J. Reiss-Gutfreund, Wein Klin Wochenschr. 89 (22), 741 (1977).
17. E. B. Smith, JAMA, 235 (16), 1731 (1976).
18. M. Longson, J. Antimicrob. Chemo. 3 (Suppl. A), 115 (1977).
19. M. G. Falcon and B. R. Jones, *ibid*, 3 (Suppl. A), 83 (1977).
20. E. DeClercq and M. Luczak, J. Inf. Dis., 133, A226 (1976).
21. D. H. Watson and R. W. Honess, J. Antimicrob. Chemo. 3, (Suppl. A), 33 (1977).
22. G. G. Jackson and E. D. Stanley, JAMA, 235 (25), 2739 (1976).
23. J. Batten, Postgrad. Med. J. 52, 571 (1976).
24. R. G. Douglas, Jr., Hosp. Pract. 11 (12), 43 (1976).
25. V. Knight, Dis.-M. XX (11), Year Book Medical Publishers, Inc., Chicago, Ill. (1976).
26. R. Dolin, Amer. Family Physician 14, 72 (1976).
27. R. B. Couch, J. Inf. Dis. 7 (9), 4 (1977).
28. P. C. Hoffman and R. E. Dixon, Ann. Intern. Med. 87 (6), 725 (1977).
29. P. Collins and D. J. Bauer, J. Antimicrob. Chemo. 3 (Suppl. A), 73 (1977).
30. S. R. B. Harris and M. R. Boyd, *ibid*, 3 (Suppl. A), 91 (1977).
31. H. E. Renis, Antimicrob. Ag. Chemother. 11 (4), 701 (1977).
32. P. Calabresi, C. H. Doolittle, III, G. H. Heppner, and C. J. McDonald, Ann. N.Y. Acad. Sci., 255, 190 (1975).
33. B. W. Fox, J. Antimicrob. Chemo. 3 (Suppl. A), 23 (1977).
34. R. J. Whitley, S.-J. Soong, R. Dolin, G. J. Galasso, L. T. Ch'ien, C. A. Alford and Coll. Study Group, New Eng. J. Med. 297, 289 (1977).

35. M. D. Aronson, C. F. Phillips, D. W. Gump. R. J. Albertini and A. Phillips, JAMA, 235 (13), 1339 (1976).
36. D. Pavan-Langston and R. A. Buchanan, Trans. Am. Acad. Ophthalmol. Otolaryngol., 81 (5), 813 (1976).
37. R. J. Whitley, S.-J. Soong, R. Dolin, G. J. Galasso, L. T. Ch'ien, C. A. Alford and the Coll. Study Group, New Eng. J. Med. 297 (6), 1193 (1976).
38. B. Juel-Jensen, J. Antimicrob. Chemo. 2, 261 (1976).
39. R. W. Steele, I. A. Capa, M. M. Vincent, S. A. Hensen and R. E. Keeney, Antimicrob. Ag. Chemother. 7 (2), 203 (1975).
40. D. Pavan-Langston, R. D. North, Jr., P. A. Geary, and A. Kinkel, Arch. Ophthalmol. 94 (9), 1585 (1976).
41. R. J. Klein and A. E. Friedman-Kien, Antimicrob. Ag. Chemother. 12 (5), 577 (1977).
42. H. E. Kaufman and E. D. Varnall, *ibid*, 10 (6), 885 (1976).
43. E. R. Kern, J. T. Richards, J. C. Overall, Jr., and L. A. Glasgow, *ibid*, 13 (1), 53 (1978).
44. E. R. Kern, J. T. Richards, J. C. Overall, Jr., and L. A. Glasgow, J. Inf. Dis. 135 (4), 567 (1977).
45. B. B. Williams, E. J. Bailey and A. M. Lerner, J. Lab. Clin. Med. 89 (4), 687 (1977).
46. Y. J. Bryson and J. D. Connor, Antimicrob. Ag. Chemother. 9 (3), 540 (1976).
47. C. Shipman, Jr., S. H. Smith, R. H. Carlson and J. C. Drach, *ibid*, 9 (1), 120 (1976).
48. P. M. Schwartz, C. Shipman, Jr., and J. C. Drach, *ibid*, 10 (1), 64 (1976).
49. C. T. Cho, K. K. Feng and N. Brahmacupta, J. Inf. Dis. 133 (2), 157 (1976).
50. P. Peller, O. Goetz and M. Rath, Infection 4 (3), 130 (1976).
51. B. Juel-Jensen, J. Antimicrob. Chemo. 3 (Suppl. A), 125 (1977).
52. C. E. Orfanos, A. Weese, U. Runne, J. Kratka and G. Goerz, Dtsch. Med. Wochenschr. 102 (9), 312 (1977).
53. S. Kernbaum, Br. Med. J. 1 (6003), 224 (1976).
54. B. Wolman and M. Longson, Acta Paediatr. Scan. 66 (2), 243 (1977).
55. B. Lagerkvist and H. Ekelund, Scand. J. Infect. Dis. 7 (2), 81 (1975).
56. D. K. Kelsey, E. R. Kern, J. C. Overall, Jr., and L. A. Glasgow, Antimicrob. Ag. Chemother. 9 (3), 458 (1976).
57. P. G. Balboni, A. Minia, M. P. Grossi and G. Barbanti-Brodano, Nature 264, 181 (1976).
58. J. D. Parker, J. Antimicrob. Chem. 3 (Suppl. A), 131 (1977).
59. T. Nasemann, Hautarzt 27 (9), 463 (1976).
60. R. M. Bikbulatov and V. N. Grebenyuk, Vopr. Virusol. (2), 228 (1977).
61. C. Stuart-Harris, J. Antimicrob. Chemo. 2 (2), 112 (1976).
62. C. Grupper, Z. Hautkr. 52 (8), 483 (1977).
63. G. E. Underwood and S. D. Weed, Antimicrob. Ag. Chemother. 11 (4), 765 (1977).
64. G. Takenaka, Nichidai Igaku Zasshi 35 (4), 427 (1976).
65. D. W. Clough and J. R. Parkhurst, Antimicrob. Ag. Chemother. 11 (2), 307 (1977).
66. D. R. Woodman and J. C. Williams, *ibid*, 11 (3), 475 (1977).
67. L. B. Allen, J. H. Huffman, P. D. Cook, R. B. Meyer, Jr., R. K. Robins and R. W. Sidwell, *ibid*, 12 (1), 114 (1977).
68. J. F. Aswell, G. P. Allen, A. T. Jamieson, D. E. Campbell and G. A. Gentry, *ibid*, 12 (2), 243 (1977).
69. I. Schildkraut, G. M. Cooper and S. Greer, Mol. Pharmacol. 11, 153 (1975).
70. M. J. Dobersen, M. Jerkofsky, and S. Greer, J. Virol. 20 (2), 478 (1976).
71. Y. C. Cheng, B. Goz, J. P. Neenin, D. C. Ward and W. H. Prusoff, *ibid*, 15 1284 (1975).
72. A. Cohen, Y. Togo, R. Khakoo, R. Waldman and M. Sigel, J. Inf. Dis. 133, A114 (1976).
73. Y. Togo and E. A. McCracken, *ibid*, 133, A109 (1976).
74. C. R. Magnussen, R. G. Douglas, Jr., R. F. Betts, F. K. Roth and M. P. Meagher, Antimicr. Ag. Chemother. 12 (4), 493 (1977).
75. R. J. Fenton and C. W. Potter, J. Antimicrob. Chem. 3, 263 (1977).
76. R. F. Berendt, J. S. Walker, J. W. Dominik and E. L. Stephen, Antimicrob. Ag. & Chemother. 11 (6), 1069 (1977).
77. E. W. Larson, E. L. Stephen and J. S. Walker, *ibid*, 10 (4), 770 (1976).
78. C. Scholtissek, Arch. Virol. 50 (4), 349 (1976).
79. B. Eriksson, E. Helgstrand, N. G. Johansson, A. Larsson, A. Misiorny, J. O. Noren, L. Philipson, K. Stenberg, G. Stening, S. Stridh and B. Oberg, Antimicrob. Ag. Chemo. 11 (6), 946 (1977)
80. L. B. Allen and C. M. Fingal, *ibid*, 12 (1), 120 (1977).
81. A. E. Palmer, W. T. London and J. L. Sever, *ibid*, 12 (3), 510 (1977).
82. L. F. Lee, K. Nazerian, S. S. Leinbach, J. M. Reno and J. A. Boezi, J. Natl. Cancer Inst. 56 (4), 823 (1976).
83. R. F. Meyer, E. D. Varnell and H. E. Kaufman, Antimicrob. Ag. Chemo. 9 (2), 308 (1976).
84. S. S. Leinbach, J. M. Reno, L. F. Lee, A. F. Isbell and J. A. Boezi, Biochemistry (Wash.), 15 (2), 426 (1976).

85. Y. Becker, Y. Asher, Y. Cohen, E. Weinberg-Zahlering and I. Shlomai, Antimicrob. Ag. Chemo. 11 (5), 919 (1977).
86. B. Fridlander, N. Chejanovsky and Y. Becker, *ibid*, 13 (1), 124 (1978).
87. J. May, S. M. Brown, A. T. Jamieson, F. J. Rixon, H. Moss, D. A. Dargan and J. H. Subak-Sharpe, *ibid*, 3, 63 (1977).
88. R. B. Couch and G. G. Jackson, J. Inf. Dis. 134 (5), 516 (1976).
89. R. B. Couch, *ibid*, Sept. (1977).
90. A. Chanin, JAMA, 236 (18), 2050 (1976).
91. A. W. Galbraith, J. Antimicrob. Chemo. 1 (Suppl.), 81 (1975).
92. R. L. Muldoon, E. D. Stanley and G. G. Jackson, Amer. Rev. Resp. Dis. 113, 487 (1976).
93. J. W. Little, W. J. Hall, R. G. Douglas, Jr., R. W. Hyde and D. M. Speers, Ann. Inter. Med. 85, 177 (1976).
94. R. R. Grunert and C. E. Hoffmann, J. Inf. Dis. 136 (2), 297 (1977).
95. J. S. Oxford and G. C. Schild, FEMS Microb. Letters 1, 223 (1977).
96. R. J. Fenton, C. Bessell, C. R. Spilling and C. W. Potter, J. Antimicrob. Chemother. 3, 463 (1977).
97. J. S. Walker, E. L. Stephen and R. O. Spertzel, J. Inf. Dis. 133, A140 (1976).
98. V. I. Ilyenko, Vopr. Virusol. (2), 199 (1975).
99. V. A. Kalninya and M. K. Indulen, Acta. Virol. 20, 343 (1976).
100. J. H. Skehel, A. J. Hay and J. A. Armstrong, J. gen. Virol. 38, 97 (1977).
101. V. Mazhinskaya and R. Antipova Khimi, Khimio. Grippai, Mater. Vses. Simp. 1st, 92 (1972).
102. V. F. Krylov, A. A. Alekseeva, T. Ia. Liarskaia, T. G. Poliakova and L. M. Kupriashina, Vopr. Virusol. (2), 186 (1976).
103. N. P. Obrosova-Serova, L. M. Kupryashina, G. V. Shtunderendo, G. S. Churkin, E. A. Severin, and G. A. Galegov, *ibid*, (3), 295 (1977).
104. A. Denys, S. Szram, W. T. Kaczewski, H. Niedzielska, J. Bochenska, M. Kulawczyk, L. Szymanski and E. Zujewski, Acta. Microbiol. Polonica Ser. A V(22), 219 (1973).
105. J. B. Arensman, J. W. Dominik and D. E. Hilmas, Antimicrob. Ag. Chemo 12 (1), 40 (1977).
106. J. S. Walker, E. L. Stephen and R. O. Spertzel, J. Inf. Dis. 133, A140 (1976).
107. G. Galegov, N. Pushkarskaya, N. Obrosova-Serova and V. Zhdanov, Experientia 33 (7), 905 (1977).
108. N. L. Pushkarskaya, V. K. Blinova, R. Ya. Podchernyaeva, N. P. Obrosova-Serova, G. A. Galegov, D. K. L'vov and V. M. Zhdanov, Vopr. Virusol (3), 369 (1977).
109. G. Galegov, A. Yatsna, G. Linitskaya and N. Pushkarskaya, Biochemistry 41, 2 (1976).
110. V. A. Kalninya and M. K. Indulen, Acta virol. 20, 343 (1976).
111. P. M. Ahumada, Ther. Ggw. 116 (1), 100 (1977).
112. D. Fanta, Wien Med. Wschr. 126, 315 (1976).
113. M. M. Hassan, Rev. Int. Trach. 53 (3-4), 105 (1976).
114. Wien. Klin. Wochenschr. 85 (37), 614 (1973). (Authors not stated.)
115. J. W. Hadden, E. M. Hadden and R. G. Coffey, Infect. & Immun. 13 (2), 1382 (1976).
116. R. D. Azulay and E. Azulay, Rev. Bras. Med. 32 (2), 105 (1975).
117. Scrip, p. 16, Sept. 1977.
118. J. Z. Miller, W. E. Nance, J. A. Norton, R. L. Wolen, R. S. Griffith and R. J. Rose, JAMA 237 (3), 248 (1977).
119. J. L. Conlehan, S. Eberhard, L. Kapner, F. Taylor, K. Rogers, and P. Garry, New Eng. J. Med. 295, 973 (1976).
120. Editorial, Brit. Med. J. 1 (6010), 606 (1976).
121. G. D. Diana, J. Med. Chem. 20 (6), 757 (1977).
122. F. Pancic, B. Steinberg, G. Diana, W. Gorman, and P. Came, 17th Intersci. Conf. Antimicrob. Ag. Chemo., New York (Oct. 12-14), 1977 Abst. #289.
123. I. S. Nikolaeva, S. N. Kutchak, N. S. Bogdanova and G. N. Pershin, Farmakol. Toksikol. (Moscow) 3, 336 (1976).
124. N. Gustman, I. Zastavnii, L. Manakhova and I. Balandin, Vopr. Virusol (6), 738 (1975).
125. Y. Togo, F. E. Durr and D. A. Laurenzana, Med. Microbiol. Immunol. 163 (1), 37 (1977).
126. S. E. Reed, J. W. Craig and D. A. J. Tyrrell, J. of Inf. Dis. 133, A128 (1976).
127. E. D. Stanley, G. G. Jackson, V. A. Dirda and M. Rubenis, *ibid*, 133, A121 (1976).
128. F. Floc'h and G. H. Werner, Arch. Virol. 52, 169 (1976).
129. K. Shinkai and T. Nishimura, Ann. Rep. Sankyo Res. Lab. 28, 93 (1976).
130. W. L. Albrecht, J. Med. Chem. 20 (3), 364 (1977).
131. A. A. Carr, *ibid*, 19 (9), 1142 (1976).
132. E. R. Kern, J. R. Hamilton, J. C. Overall, Jr., and L. A. Glasgow, Antimicrob. Ag. Chemo. 10 (4), 691 (1976).
133. M. J. Kramer, R. Cleeland and E. Grunberg, *ibid*, 9 (2), 233 (1976).

Chapter 16. Structure-Activity Relationships of "Non-Classical" β-Lactam Antibiotics

L. D. Cama and B. G. Christensen
Merck Sharp & Dohme Research Laboratories, Rahway, New Jersey 07065

Introduction - Although examples of semi-synthetic penicillins 1 (R = COOH) and cephalosporins 2 (R = COOH) have been known for over twenty years, the thousands of semi-synthetic analogs which have been prepared by medicinal chemists are almost exclusively the C6(7)-amide type. The only other common variants are those produced at the C-3 methylene of cephalosporins by nucleophilic displacement of the naturally-occurring acetoxyl function. These simple derivatives or "classical" β-lactam antibiotics have been the subject of many reviews[1] and will not be considered here. Instead, attention will be directed to a discussion of the biological activities of those derivatives in which the bicyclic nucleus itself is altered either by the addition of a substituent[2] or by the synthesis[3,4] or isolation of a new nucleus itself. This report will attempt to highlight the unusual structural features of these "non-classical" analogs and detail the effects of these features on biological activity.

S-1 Substituents - It has long been supposed that oxidation of penicillins and cephalosporins to the sulfoxide or sulfone results in a marked loss of antibacterial activity.[1] In contrast to the penicillin sulfoxides and the S-cephalosporin sulfoxides, R-sulfoxides of various cephalosporins when compared to the parents show variable changes in biological activity.[5] However R-sulfoxides of cephalosporins are usually more active than the S-isomer *in vitro* and 7-phenylacetamidodeacetoxycephalosporanic acid R-sulfoxide has even higher antibacterial activity than the unoxidized parent.

Carboxyl Variations - Early attempts to modify the C-3(4) carboxyl groups of penicillins and cephalosporins were largely discouraging.[1] The homopenicillins and cephalosporins 1b[6] and 2b[7] were obtained from 1a and 2a. The cephem aldehyde, 2g,[8] has been prepared from the 4-hydroxymethyl precursor *via* a Moffatt oxidation. The aldehyde was then converted to 2h-m. None of these derivatives are active at <25 μg/ml. All modifications, 1a,b and 2a-f were less active analogs, supporting the contention that an acidic function at C-3(4) is essential for activity. The importance of the position of the carboxyl function is indicated by the lack of bioactivity in 1b and 2b. It is of interest to note that the homopenicillins are powerful inducers of penicillinase formation. Replacement of the carboxyl function with a phosphonate[9] results in a less active compound than the analogous cephalosporin.

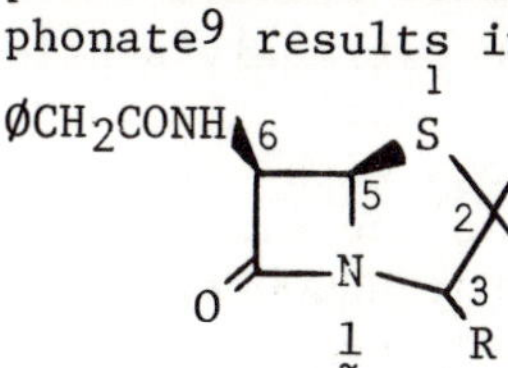

1

1a, R = $-COCHN_2$
1b, R = $-CH_2CO_2H$

One of the more interesting modifications of the penicillin molecule has been the conversion of the C-3 carboxyl group to that of a tetrazole. Two examples of 3-(5-tetrazolyl) penams have been reported to date. CP-35,587,[10] the better documented of the two analogs, is more potent than amoxicillin against *Klebsiella pneumoniae*, *Enterobacter*, *Serratia marcescens*, *Citrobacter*, *Providentia* and *Salmonella typhimurium*. Although less

ISBN 0-12-040513-X

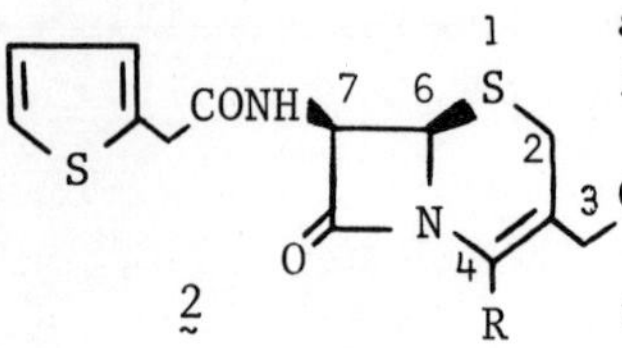

2

2a, R = $-COCHN_2$
2b, R = $-CH_2CO_2H$
2c, R = $-COCH_2Cl$
2d, R = $-COCH_2OAc$
2e, R = $-COCH_2OMe$
2f, R = $-CH_2OH$
2g, R = -CHO
2h, R = 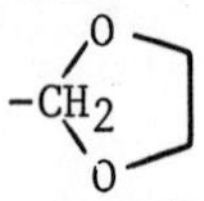
2i, R = -CH=NOH
2j, R = -CH=NOMe
2k, R = $-CH{=}NNHCONH_2$
2l, R = $-CH{=}NOCH_2CO_2H$
2m, R = 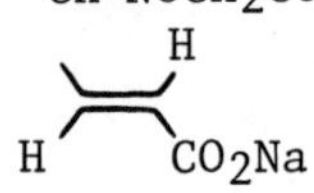

active than amoxicillin against other strains, CP-35,587 nevertheless is highly potent (1.56-12 μg/ml). The extension of spectrum is presumably due to the stability of β-lactamase conferred upon the compound by the tetrazolyl functionality. The extrapolation of the *in vitro* activities to *in vivo* efficacy in protecting mice against experimental infections has also been demonstrated. CP-38,118 is also stable to penicillinase and the extension of its spectrum to include anti-pseudomonal activity is claimed.[11] Thus, the substitution of a 3-(5-tetrazolyl) function for a carboxyl in the penicillin series seems compatible with retention of bioactivity while conferring increased β-lactamase stability to the penam nucleus.

C-5(6) Substituents - The bridgehead position has not been substituted extensively in penicillins or cephalosporins. Only one example in each case is known. Penicillin V has been substituted at C-5 by an α-phenyl group.[12] The compound shows only 1/1000 the activity of the parent compound. An α-methoxy group has been substituted at the C-6 position of cephalothin.[13] Again, the compound has a very low order of activity. The low activity of the 6α-methoxy cephalosporin derivative is not easily understood since 7α-methoxy cephalothin has excellent activity.[14]

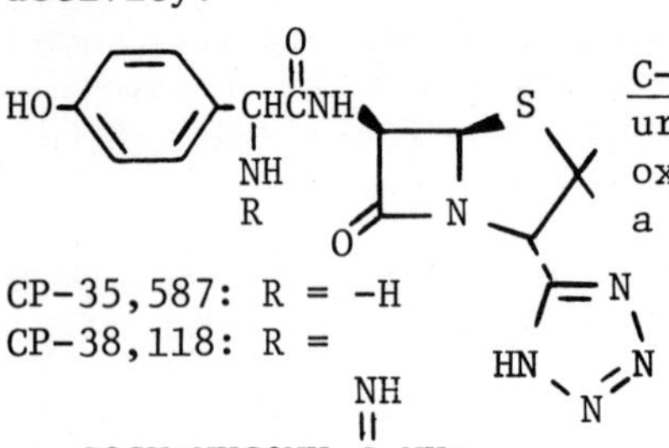

CP-35,587: R = -H
CP-38,118: R = $-COCH_2NHCONH-C(=NH)-NH_2$

C-6(7) Substituents - The discovery of the naturally-occurring cephamycin[15] family of 7α-methoxycephalosporins has stimulated the synthesis of a large number of C-6(7) substituents in the penicillin and cephalosporin series. The primary interest in this class derives from their stability to β-lactamase. Substitution at C-7 in the cephalosporin series uniformly increases stability to these enzymes. Under conditions where >96% of cephalothin is destroyed by the β-lactamase from *E. coli* MB 2885, the following C-7 substituted analogs of cephalothin were destroyed to the indicated extent:[14]

TABLE I

7-Substituent	-H	$-OCH_3$	$-OCH_2CH_3$	$-SCH_3$	$-CH_2OH$
% Destruction	>96%	16%	0%	20%	0%

Disruption of the azetidinone by β-lactamase appears to be extremely sensitive to steric bulk in the 7α position. On the other hand, while the introduction of a 7α-methoxy group produces cephalosporin analogs with high antibacterial potency, there is a rapid decrease in activity as the size of the ether group is increased. Other groups, such as CHO, $COCH_3$, NHCOOEt, CH_3 and -CH(Ø)OH, are also devoid of useful activity and indeed these groups and even the 6α-methoxy group on penicillin does not lead to useful compounds. Thus, the utility of the 7α-methoxy group is due to its unique ability to confer stability of the cephalosporin molecule to β-lactamase while retaining full antibacterial activity. It has long been clear that since the 7α-methoxycephalosporin class of β-lactam antibiotics possesses the attributes of the cephalosporins combined with β-lactamase stability, a family of new clinically useful antibacterials should result. Cefoxitin,[16] 3, is the most studied of this type. Cefoxitin, when compared to a classical cephalosporin, *e.g.*, cephalothin 2 (R = COOH), shows comparable safety, pharmacokinetics,[17] and inhibition of the cephalosporin sensitive organisms.[18] However, because of its β-lactamase stability,[19] 3 is also active against many cephalosporin-resistant gram-negative bacteria including the anaerobic organism, *Bacteroides fragilis*.[20]

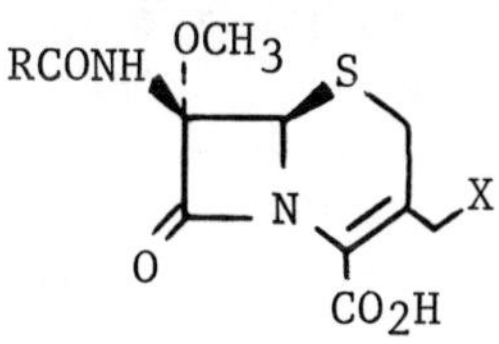

	R	X
3,	C_4H_3S-CH_2-	-OC(=O)-NH_2
4,	$NCCH_2$-SCH_2-	-SHet.
5,	CF_3S-CH_2-	-SHet.
6,	C_4H_3S-CH(NH-C(=O)-NH_2)-	-SHet.

C_4H_3S =

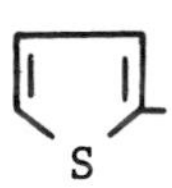

Het. =

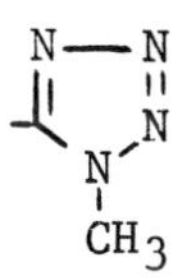

Three other 7α-methoxycephalosporins have received considerable attention. They are 4 (CS-1170),[21] 5 (SKF 73678)[22] and 6 (SQ 14,359).[23] They share similar pharmacokinetics to cefoxitin and enhanced *in vitro* potency.

C-6(7) Side Chains Other than Those Derived from C-6(7) Amino Function - A number of penicillins and cephalosporins having side chains other than those derived from the C-6(7) amino group have been prepared.

Simple groups (Cl, Br, OH, CH_3) on penicillins[24] or cephalosporins[25] give compounds devoid of activity. The details of the activity of penicillin and cephalosporin analogs in which the nitrogen of the amide side chain has been replaced by O, CH_2 or S,[26] are not available but all show some antibacterial activity. Thus, though a β-amide is necessary for good activity, any carbonyl function isosteric with the amide seems to contribute positively toward antibiotic activity.

The 1-hydroxyethyl side chain is of considerable interest when it occurs on the C-6α position of the very active naturally-occurring thienamycin.[61] This side chain has been substituted on penicillins and cephalosporins at the C-6(7) α and β positions. The compounds obtained were markedly lower in activity than those with the amide side chain. Surprisingly, the C-6 β (1-hydroxyethyl) penicillin is slightly more active than the α isomer.[27]

β-Amidino Penicillins - These remarkable examples of non-amide side chain β-lactams have been reviewed recently[28] and will not be commented on further. Mecillinam (FL1060) 7 is used clinically.

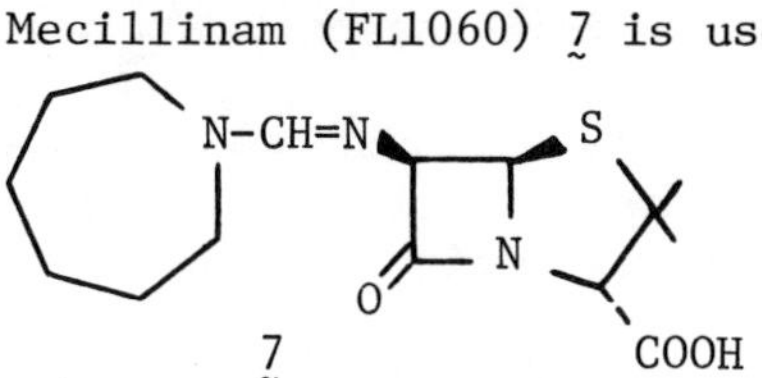

7

Substitution of the β-Lactam Carbonyl Oxygen - Compounds 8 and 9 in which the β-lactam carbonyl oxygen is replaced by a sulfur have been reported.[29] These compounds have from 1/20 to 1/1000 the activity of the parent compounds. This may be a reflection of the larger bond order and decreased reactivity of the 4-7 (5-8) C-N bond.

Nuclear Analogs of Cephalosporins - In 1971, Lowe and co-workers[30] described 10, a compound in which the sulfur atom of a cephalosporin was replaced by carbon. Compound 10 was inactive because it lacked the Δ^3 double bond necessary for activity in the cephalosporin system. The first nuclear analogs which had all the features of cephalothin (2, R = COOH) except that the sulfur atom was replaced by oxygen[31] and carbon[32] were prepared by total synthesis. Compounds 11a (R^1 = thienylacetyl; R^2 = H; R^3 = OAc; X = O) and 11b (R^1 = thienylacetyl; R^2 = H; R^3 = OAc; X = CH_2) were found to parallel cephalothin in their antibiotic spectrum with the oxygen analog 11a about twice as active and the carbon analog 11b 1/2 as active as cephalothin. This was the first demonstration of the fact that the sulfur atom was not essential for antibiotic activity in the cephalosporins. This has been followed by the total synthesis of oxa and carba derivatives of cefamandole, 11c (R^1 = mandelyl; R^2 = H; R^3 = 5-thiomethyltetrazolyl; X = O), 11d (R^1 = mandelyl; R^2 = H; R^3 = 5-thio-1-methyltetrazolyl; X = CH_2), and the 1-carba derivatives of cefoxitin,[33] 11e (R^1 = thienylacetyl; R^2 = OCH_3; R^3 = $OCONH_2$; X = CH_2). The activity of these compounds again compares favorably with the corresponding cephalosporin derivative.

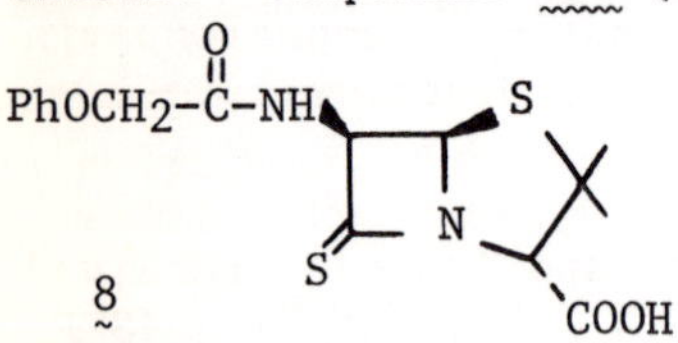

8

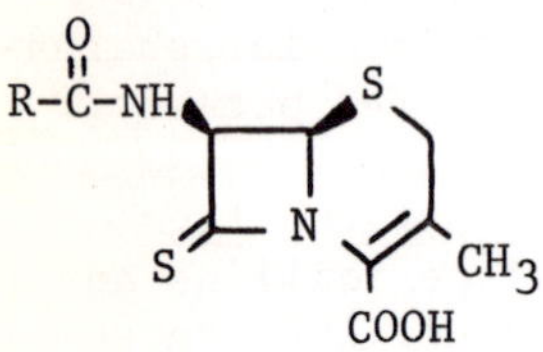

9a, R = $PhOCH_2$
b, R = $PhCH_2$

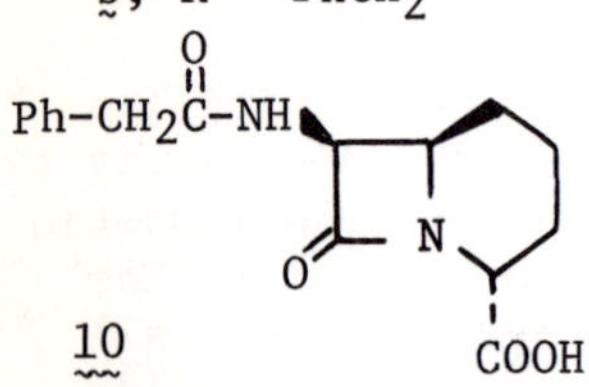

10

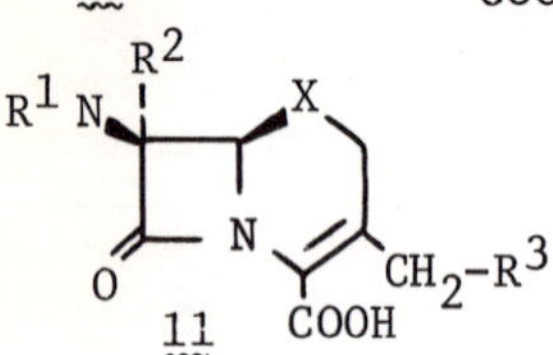

11

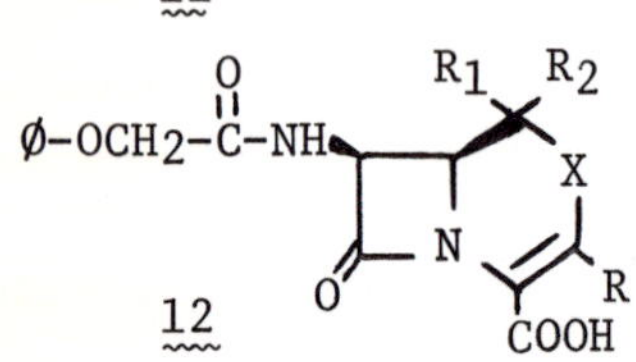

12

	R	R^1	R^2	X
a,	H	H	H	O
b,	CH_3	H	H	O
c,	$CH_2Ø$	H	H	O
d,	$CH_2CH_2Ø$	H	H	O
e,	CH_3	CH_3	H	O
f,	CH_3	H	CH_3	O
g,	CH_3	- O -		O
h,	H	H	H	$N-CH_3$
i,	H	H	H	$N-\overset{O}{\overset{\|\|}{C}}-OC_2H_5$

O-2-Isocephems - Compounds 12a to 12d, obtained *via* total synthesis by Doyle and co-workers,[34] show activity which is somewhat better than or comparable to the corresponding cephalosporins. 12e and 12f, in which the 1-CH_2 group is substituted by an α-methyl or β-methyl, have also been synthesized.[35] These are reported to have antibacterial activity but the details are not reported. A very interesting compound, 12g, in which the 1-CH_2 is replaced by a carbonyl has also been made.[36] This lactone acid, 12g, is unstable and the instability is due to opening of the highly strained and reactive β-lactam carbonyl (whose IR frequency appears at 1800 cm^{-1}) and not due to hydrolysis of the lactone functionality. 12g appears to be too unstable to be a useful antibiotic.

N-2-Isocephems - Doyle and co-workers have also reported the synthesis of N-2-isocephems, 12h and 12i.[37] Compound 12h is relatively unstable and also has a low order of antibiotic activity. However, 12i is more stable and is active as an antibiotic but the details of the activity have not been reported.

2-Isocephems - Two groups have reported the synthesis of 2-isocephem compounds, 13. Compounds 13 are reported as quite active.[38,39] The activity of 13a has been compared with the corresponding cephalosporin.[39] Its gram-positive activity is poorer but it shows better gram-negative activity. The 7α-methyl-2-isocephem, 13e, has been reported by Lowe,[40] which like the 7α-methyl cephalosporins,[41] also shows very low antibacterial activity. Thus a 7α-methyl group is detrimental to activity in both nuclei. Transposition of the hetero atom to position 2 gives rise to compounds whose antibiotic activity shows some difference in their gram-positive and gram-negative spectra, but the change in spectrum or overall activity is not drastically different from the corresponding cephalosporins. This finding is commensurate with the small changes in the reactivity of the β-lactam caused by shifting of the hetero atom or replacement of the sulfur by oxygen.

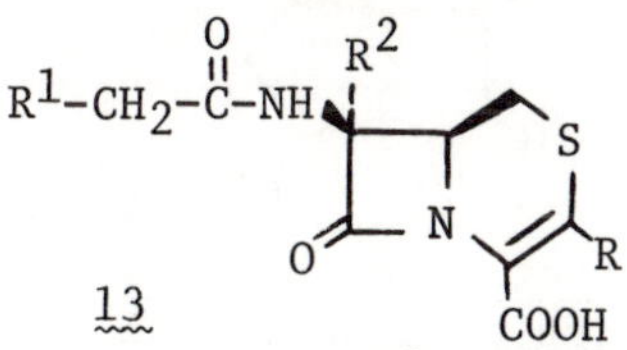

13

	R	R^1	R^2
a,	H	2-thienyl	H
b,	H	ØO-	H
c,	CH_3	ØO-	H
d,	CH_2OAc	ØO-	I
e,	H	C_6H_5	CH_3

Compounds with 3 Hetero Atoms in the 6-Membered Ring of Cephalosporins - A number of compounds of this type have recently been reported. They lack Δ^3 double bond and show very little or no activity.[42,43]

1-Oxapenams - Penicillins in which the sulfur atom of a penicillin nucleus is substituted by the smaller oxygen atom have been reported.[44,45] The compounds 14a, b, and c are considerably less active than the corresponding penicillins. This is surprising since fusion of the β-lactam ring to the oxazolidine ring should give a more strained, more reactive β-lactam than the β-lactam of a penicillin. The C-3 epimer of 14c is unstable.[45]

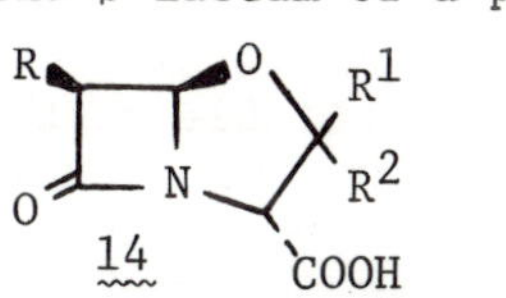

14

a, R = $C_6H_5CH_2\overset{O}{\overset{\|}{C}}$-NH; $R^1 = R^2 = H$

b, R = $C_6H_5OCH_2\overset{O}{\overset{\|}{C}}$-NH; $R^1 = R^2 = H$

c, R = $C_6H_5OCH_2\overset{O}{\overset{\|}{C}}$-NH; $R^1 = R^2 = CH_3$

N-2-Isopenam - Though the 1-aza penicillin nucleus has not been reported, the 2-aza-penicillin 15 has been reported recently.[46] This compound (mixture of C-3 epimers) is unstable in aqueous solution but shows low antibacterial activity against *B. subtilis, S. aureus* and *Shigella paradysenteriae*. The IR of the benzyl ester of 15 shows a β-lactam absorption at 1795 cm^{-1} indicating a highly strained β-lactam which should be more reactive. This is reflected in the instability of 15 but not in its bioactivity.

Carbapenam - A nuclear analog of penicillin in which the sulfur is replaced by carbon has been reported.[47] Compound 16 is reported as unstable.

2-Penem Nucleus - Woodward and co-workers[48] have reported the synthesis of 17. These have antibacterial activity but the details are not available. The β-lactam carbonyl of the *t*-butyl ester of 17 (R = H) appears at 1805 cm^{-1} indicating a highly strained, reactive β-lactam. Whether this implies that it is relatively unstable or has very high antibiotic activity is not reported.

1-Oxa-2-Penem Nucleus - The oxygen analog of the penem nucleus, 17, has been recently synthesized.[49] 18 is unstable as the ester. The free acid has not been reported. In the case of the saturated nuclear analogs of penicillins, replacement of the ring sulfur by smaller atoms seems to give unstable compounds. In spite of the more strained β-lactams in these systems, the antibiotic activity is lower, contrary to expectation. It would appear that a certain amount of chemical stability is essential for good activity. Analogs of the penicillin nuclei which have a double bond in the 5-membered ring are extremely interesting. Though compound 18 is probably unstable, compound 17 and thienamycin and its epimers are relatively stable and thienamycin shows excellent antibiotic activity.

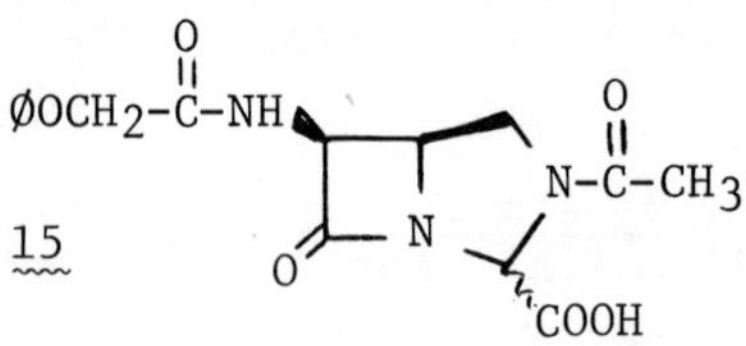

15

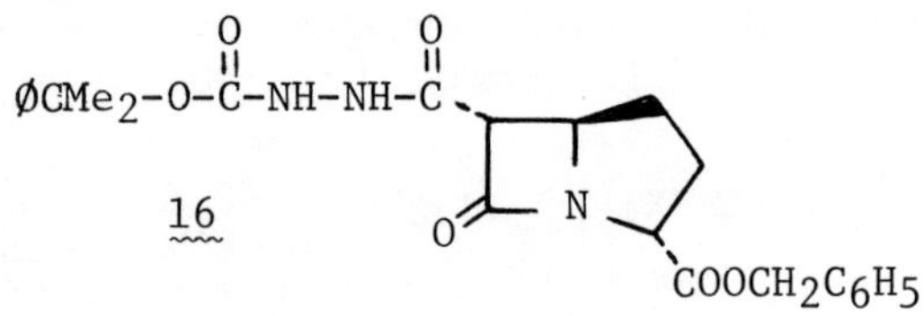

16

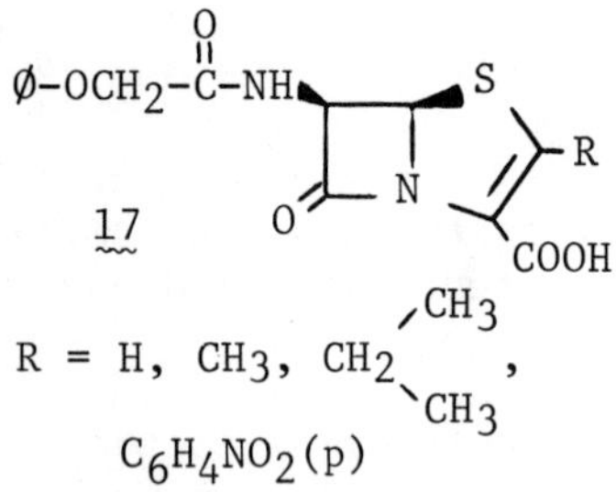

17

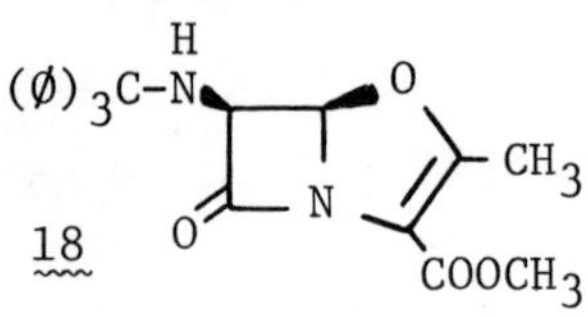

18

New, Naturally-Occurring β-Lactam Antibiotics - Nocardicin A and B - The first of a series of structurally remarkable β-lactam antibiotics was reported by the Fujisawa group. Nocardicin A and B[50] have been assigned structures 19 and 20 respectively. These new antibiotics were isolated from *Nocardia uniformis* subsp. *tsuyamaniasis*[51] and were surprisingly active when one recalls the lack of potency[52] exhibited by 21. It should be noted that these workers ascribe the name 3-aminonocardicinic acid (3-ANA) to the nucleus, 22, by analogy to the penicillanic and cephalosporanic acid nomenclature. Nocardicin A is stable to the action of several β-lactamases (except from *Proteus vulgaris*), but demonstrates poor gram-positive activity (MIC's of 50 and 800 against *B. subtilis* and *S. aureus*, respectively). However, some quite low MIC's against gram-negative organisms have been observed, *e.g.*, *Sh. sonnei*, 12.5; *Sal. typhimurium*, 25; *A. lwoffi*, 3.13; *Pr. mirabilis*, 1.56; *Pr. vulgaris*, 1.56; *Pr. rettgeri*, 3.13; *Pr. inconstans*, 12.5; *Ps. aeruginosa*, 12.5; *N. gonorrhoeae*, 1.56 and *N. meningitidis*, 1.56. Other gram-negative MIC's ranged from 100-800 μg/ml. In addition to its novel structure, perhaps the other most surprising feature is the unexpectedly high *in vivo* activity which is observed. This enhanced potency may be related to the observed increase in *in vitro* bactericidal activity in the presence of rabbit polymorphonuclear leukocytes.[53] Nocardicin A is more effective than carbenicillin in some gram-negative animal infections.[54] No cross resistance is seen between Nocardicin A and other β-lactam antibiotics and higher serum levels than carbenicillin are observed.[55]

Clavulanic Acid - Clavulanic acid 23[56] is the second in a structurally remarkable series of naturally-occurring β-lactam antibiotics of novel structure isolated during the last few years. Its antibacterial activity has been characterized as "weak," but it is a potent β-lactamase inhibitor.[57] Levels of 1-10 μg/ml, when added to penicillinase-labile penicillins, *e.g.*, ampicillin or amoxicillin, can protect the antibiotics and extend their spectrum to include resistant strains of *Staphylococcus, Klebsiella, Proteus* and *E. coli*.[58] I_{50}s (μg/ml) of 0.06, .03, .03 and .08 are reported for β-lactamases isolated from these organisms. Table II shows the *in vitro* protection afforded by clavulanic acid to ampicillin in the presence of these β-lactamases. Clavulanic acid is a progressive and irreversible inhibitor of these enzymes. 25a-c were prepared by total synthesis and reported as moderate inhibitors, while 25d is a potent inhibitor.

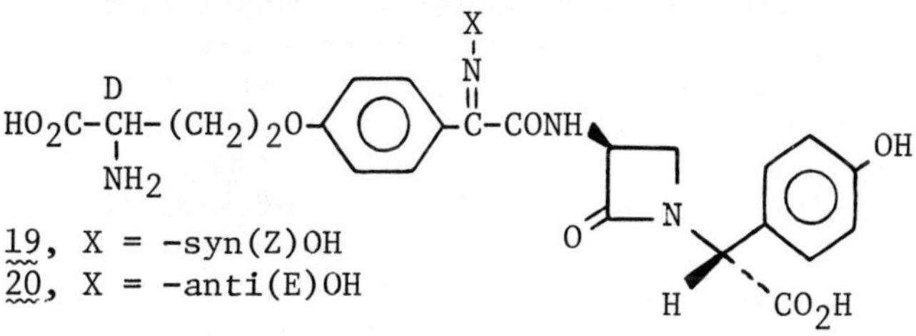

19, X = -syn(Z)OH
20, X = -anti(E)OH

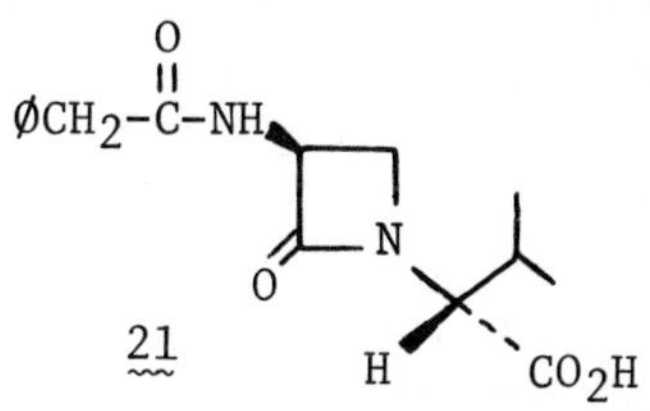

21

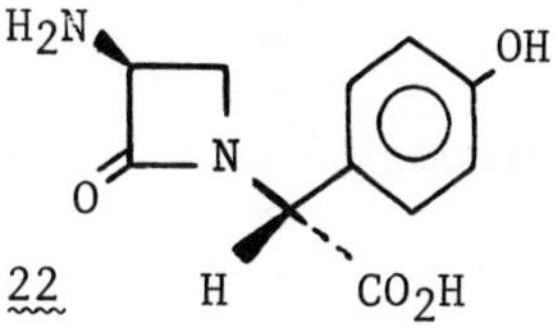

22

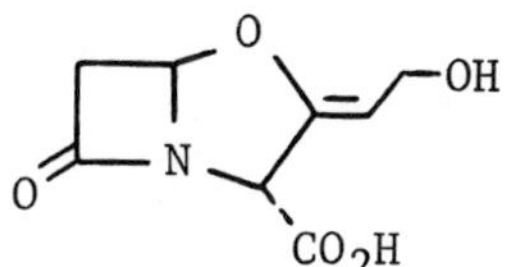

23

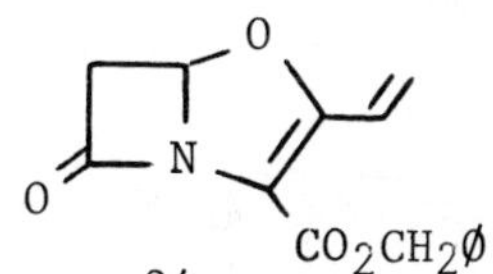

24

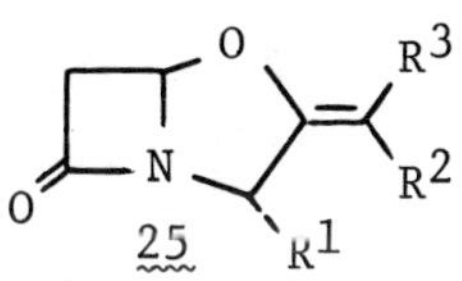

25

a, R^1 = H; R^2 = $COOCH_3$; R^3 = H
b, R^1 = H; R^2 = H; R^3 = $COOCH_3$
c, R^1 = H, R^2 = $COOCH_3$; R^3 = Cl
d, R^1 = COONa; R^2 = H; R^3 = Ø

The mode of action of clavulanic acid is similar to other β-lactam antibiotics since it binds to the same enzyme site as benzylpenicillin.[59] Clavulanic acid has been converted to the novel 1-oxapenem system 24,[60] but no bioactivities are reported.

Thienamycin - Thienamycin[61] (26) is the final and perhaps most remarkable of the naturally-occurring β-lactam antibiotics of novel structure found during the past few years. Although its properties are only described in abstracts,[62] it appears to be the most potent and broadest spectrum β-lactam anti-

TABLE II

	MIC (μg/ml)			
	S. aureus	*K. aerogenes*	*Pr. mirabilis*	*E. coli*
Na Clavulanate alone	15	31	62-125	31
Ampicillin alone	500	250	>2000	>2000
Ampicillin + 5 μg/ml Na Clavulanate	.02	.1	8	4

biotic reported. MIC's and, with few exceptions, MBC's of ≤10 μg/ml were reported for both gram-positive and gram-negative bacteria including *Pseudomonas, Serratia* and anaerobic *Bacteroides* species. 26 is fully effective against β-lactamase-producing strains at the same levels. Presumably the 2-carbon chain of the 6α-hydroxyethyl side chain provides β-lactamase stability while the hydroxyl can hydrogen bond to the same site as the amide side chain of classical β-lactams. Thienamycin is not absorbed orally, but is effective s.c. at levels of 0.005-0.2 mg/kg for gram-positive infections and 2-10 mg/kg for gram-negative ones. Against *Ps. aeruginosa*, thienamycin is active at levels one-quarter those for gentamicin. Thienamycin also binds to the same protein-binding site as benzylpenicillin.[59] Several "epi" thienamycins have been reported.[64] 27, 28 and 29 are "powerful" inhibitors of β-lactamases and "potent" antibacterials.[63] 27 (also known as MM13902) is more potent than 28 (MM 4550) inhibiting a wide range of bacteria at concentrations less than 5 μg/ml. 30-33 have also been isolated.[65] All are cell-wall biosynthesis inhibitors, but while some have equal or greater activity against the *Enterobacteriaceae* than thienamycin, none are as active against other organisms and up to a ten-fold difference is observed. Wide variation in β-lactamase stability is also observed.

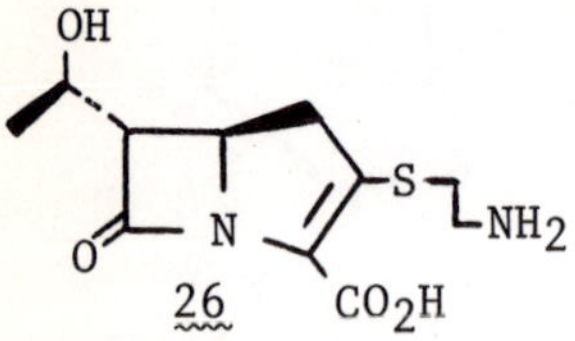

26

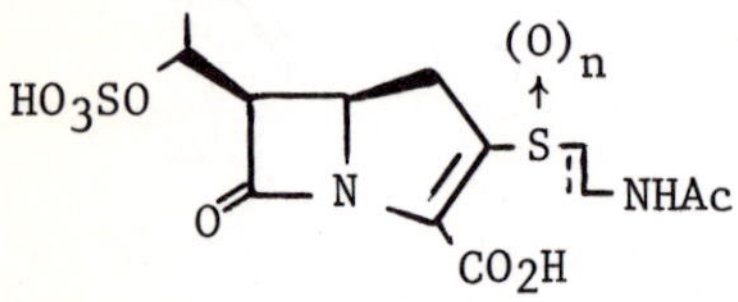

27, n = 0 (side chain unsaturated)
28, n = 1 (side chain unsaturated)
29, n = 0 (side chain saturated)

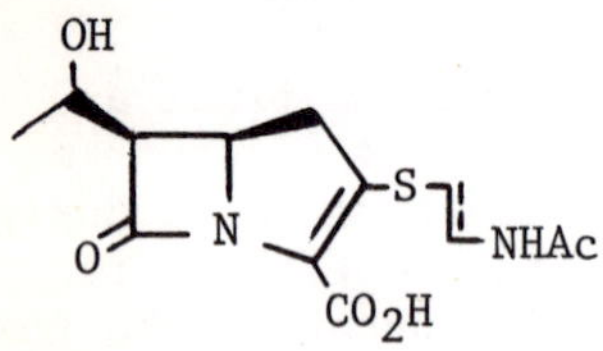

30 (side chain saturated)
31 (side chain unsaturated)

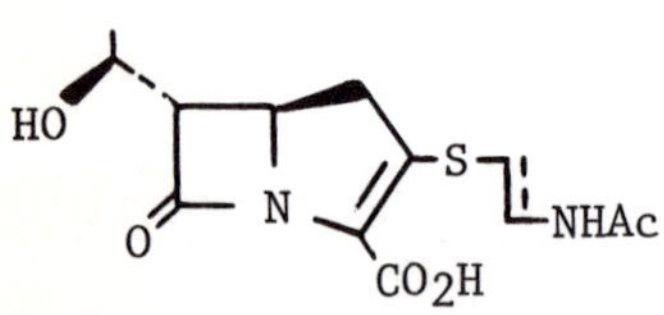

32 (side chain saturated)
33 (side chain unsaturated)

Conclusion - The previous efforts of medicinal chemists to vary the C-6(7) β-amide side chains of penicillins and cephalosporins, as well as the C-3 position of cephalosporins remains an important part of medicinal chemical lore and have provided many different clinically useful antibiotics. The exact medical position of the "non-classical" β-lactam antibiotics remains unknown, for only two of these new-generation antibiotics, cefoxitin and mecillinam have been approved in any country. One conclusion, however, has become abundantly clear. Virtually all of the "classical" structure-activity relationships of β-lactam antibiotics,[34,66] must be revised. The S-1 sulfur atom may be modified (α-sulfoxide) or replaced (by oxygen or methylene) with full retention of activity. Similarly, the carboxyl group may be replaced by an isosteric acidic function (tetrazolyl) with not only retention of activity but with the added feature of β-lactamase stability. Cephalosporanic acids may be substituted with a methoxyl function conferring β-lactamase stability upon the molecule. The penicillin and cephalosporanic acid nuclei, previously considered essential for activity, may be replaced by other bicyclic nuclei (thienamycin) and by a monocyclic nucleus (Nocardicin A). Finally, the C-6(7) amide side chain may be absent while retaining full or even enhanced potency (thienamycin). Indeed when these new structural features, all of which are consistent with full biological activity, are considered, the only essential common feature remains the azetidinone ring system itself.

REFERENCES

1. K.E. Price, M.L. Sassiver and A. Lewis, J.A. Webbe, and J.L. Ott in "Structure-Activity Relationships Among the Semi-synthetic Antibiotics," D. Perlman, Ed., Academic Press, New York, N.Y., 1977, pp. 1-84, 87-160 and 161-238.
2. J.C. Jaszberenyi and T.E. Gunda in "Progress in Medicinal Chemistry," Vol. 12, G.P. Ellis and G.B. West, Ed., North-Holland Publishing Co., New York, N.Y., 1975, pp. 395-477.
3. B.G. Christensen and R.W. Ratcliffe in *Ann.Repts.Med.Chem.*, Vol. II, F.H. Clarke, Ed., Academic Press, New

York, N.Y., 1976, pp. 271-280.
4. K. Heusler in "Cephalosporins and Penicillins," E.H. Flynn, Ed., Academic Press, New York, N.Y., 1972, pp. 255-279.
5. J.J. deKoning, A.F. Marx, M.M. Post, P.M. Smid and J. Verivey in "Recent Advances in the Chemistry of β-Lactam Antibiotics," J. Elks, Ed., The Chemical Society, London, England, 1977, pp. 161-6.
6. E.M. Kleiner, L.B. Senzavina and A.S. Khokklov, *Khim.Geterot.Soedienii*, 2, 70-5 (1966).
7. T. Jen, B. Dienel, J. Frazee and J. Weisbach, *J.Med.Chem.*, *15*, 1172 (1972).
8. P.J. Beeby, *ibid.*, 20, 173 (1977).
9. N.G. Steinberg, R.W. Ratcliffe, B.G. Christensen, Abstracts, 5th International Congress of Heterocyclic Chemistry, Ljublana, Yugoslavia, 58 (1975).
10. A.R. English, J.A. Retsema and J.E. Lynch, *Antimicrob.Ag.Chemother.*, *10*, 132 (1976).
11. A.R. English, J.A. Retsema and J.E. Lynch, Abstracts, 16th Interscience Conf. on Antimicrobial Agents and Chemotherapy, Chicago, Ill., 225 (1976).
12. H. Vanderhaeghe and J. Thomis, *J.Med.Chem.*, *18*, 486 (1975).
13. B.G. Christensen, K. Hoogsteen, F. Plavac and R.W. Ratcliffe, "Recent Advances in the Chemistry of β-Lactam Antibiotics," J. Elks, Ed. Special Publication No. 28, The Chemical Society, 1977, p. 269.
14. E.O. Stapley, D.R. Daoust, D. Hendlin, A.K. Miller, S.B. Zimmerman, J. Birnbaum, L.D. Cama and B.G. Christensen in Proc. 2nd Tokyo Symposium on Microbial Drug-Resistance, Tokyo, Japan (1977).
15. R. Nagarajan, L.D. Boeck, M. Gorman, P.I. Hamill, C.E. Higgins, M.M. Hoehn, W.M. Stork and J.G. Whitney, *J.Am.Chem.Soc.*, *93*, 2308 (1971); E.O. Stapley, M. Jackson, S. Hernandez, S.B. Zimmerman, S.A. Currie, S. Mochales, J.M. Mahn, H.B. Woodruff and D. Hendlin, *Antimicrob.Ag.Chemother.*, *2*, 122 (1972).
16. H. Wallick and D. Hendlin, *Antimicrob.Ag.Chemother.*, *5*, 25 (1974).
17. J. Kosmidis, J.M.T. Hamilton-Miller, J.N.G. Gilchrist, D.W. Kerry and M. Brumfitt, *Brit.Med.J.*, *3*, 653 (1973).
18. R.C. Moelloring, M. Dray and L.J. Kunz, *Antimicrob.Ag.Chemother.*, *6*, 320 (1974).
19. H.R. Onishi, D.R. Daoust, S.D. Zimmerman, D. Hendlin and E.O. Stapley, *ibid.*, *5*, 38 (1974).
20. F.P. Talley, N.V. Jacobus, J.G. Bartlett and S.L. Gorbach, *ibid.*, *7*, 1128 (1975).
21. H. Nakao, H. Yanagisawa, B. Shimizu, M. Kaneko, M. Nagano and S. Sugawara, *J.Antibiotics*, *29*, 534 (1976).
22. R.M. DeMarinis, J.V. Uri and J.A. Weisbach, *ibid.*, 973 (1976).
23. H.H. Gadebusch, G.J. Miraglia and H.I. Basch, Abstracts, 17th Interscience Conf. on Antimicrob. Ag. Chemother., New York, N.Y., 415 (1977).
24. J.C. Jaszberenyi and T.E. Gunda, "Progress in Medicinal Chemistry," G.P. Ellis and G.B. West, Ed., American Elsevier Publishing Co., Inc., N.Y., p. 395.
25. J.S. Weiring and H. Wynberg, *J.Org.Chem.*, *41*, 1574 (1976).
26. a) Y.S. Lo and J.C. Sheehan, *J.Am.Chem.Soc.*, *94*, 8253 (1972); b) J.C. Sheehan and Y.S. Lo, *J.Org.Chem.*, *38*, 3227 (1973); c) J.C. Sheehan, T.J. Commons and Y.S. Lo, *ibid.*, *42*, 2274 (1977); d) J.C. Sheehan, Y.S. Lo and D.R. Ponzi, *ibid.*, *42*, 1012 (1977).
27. F. DiNinno, T.R. Beattie and B.G. Christensen, *J.Org.Chem.*, *42*, 2960 (1977).
28. F.J. Lund in "Recent Advances in the Chemistry of β-Lactam Antibiotics," J. Elks, Ed., The Chemical Society, London, England, 1977, pp. 25-45.
29. P.W. Wojtkowski, J.E. Dolfini, O. Kocy, C.M. Cimarusti, *J.Am.Chem.Soc.*, *97*, 5628 (1975).
30. D.M. Brunwin, G. Lowe and J. Parker, *J.Chem.Soc.* Chem. Comm., 865 (1971), *J.Chem.Soc.* (C) 3757 (1971).
31. L.D. Cama and B.G. Christensen, *J.Am.Chem.Soc.*, *96*, 7582 (1974).
32. R.N. Guthikonda, L.D. Cama and B.G. Christensen, *ibid.*, *96*, 7584 (1974).
33. R.A. Firestone, J.L. Fahey, N.S. Maciejewicz, G.S. Patel and B.G. Christensen, *J.Med.Chem.*, *20*, 551 (1977).
34. T.W. Doyle, B. Belleau, B. Luh, T.T. Conway, M. Menard, J.L. Douglas, D.T. Chu, G. Lim, L.R. Morris, P. Rivest and M. Casey, *Can.J.Chem.*, *55*, 484 (1977).
35. T.W. Doyle, B. Luh and A. Martel, *ibid.*, *55*, 2700 (1977).
36. T.W. Doyle, A. Martel and B. Luh, *ibid.*, *55*, 2708 (1977).
37. T.W. Doyle, B. Luh, D.T. Chu and B. Belleau, *ibid.*, *55*, 2719 (1977).
38. T.W. Doyle, J.L. Douglas, B. Belleau, J. Meunier and B. Luh, *ibid.*, *55*, 2873 (1977).
39. D.B. Bryan, R.F. Hall, K.G. Holden, W.F. Huffman and J.G. Gleason, *J.Am.Chem.Soc.*, *99*, 3453 (1977).
40. D.M. Brunwin and G. Lowe, *J.Chem.Soc.*, Perkin I, 1321 (1973).
41. E.H.W. Bohme, H.E. Applegate, B. Toeplitz, J.E. Dolfini and J.Z. Gougoutas, *J.Am.Chem.Soc.*, *93*, 4326 (1971).
42. J. Finkelstein, K.G. Holden, R. Sneed and C.D. Perchonock, *Tetrahedron Lett.*, 1855 (1977).
43. M.J. Pearson, *J.Chem.Soc.*, Perkin I, 189 (1977).
44. L.D. Cama, R.A. Firestone and B.G. Christensen, Abstracts, 10th ACS Middle Atlantic Regional Meeting, Philadelphia, Pennsylvania, 1976.
45. R.A. Alexander and R. Southgate, *J.Chem.Soc.*, Chem. Comm., 405 (1977).
46. W.F. Huffman, K.G. Holden, T.F. Buckley, III, J.G. Gleason and L. Wu, *J.Am.Chem.Soc.*, *99*, 2353 (1977).
47. G. Lowe and D.D. Ridley, *J.Chem.Soc.* Chem. Comm., 328 (1973), *J.Chem.Soc.*, Perkin I, 2024 (1973).
48. R.B. Woodward, "Recent Advances in the Chemistry of β-Lactam Antibiotics," J. Elks, Ed., Special Publication No. 28, The Chemical Society, Lond, 1977, p. 167.
49. A.J. Eglington, *J.Chem.Soc.*, Chem. Comm., 720 (1977).
50. M. Hashimoto, T. Komori and T. Kamiya, *J.Antibiotics*, *29*, 890 (1976).
51. H. Aoki, H. Sakai, M. Kohsaka, T. Konomi, J. Hosada, Y. Kubachi, E. Iguchi and H. Imanaka, *ibid.*, *29*, 492 (1976); M. Kurita, K. Jomon, Y. Konori, N. Miyairi, H. Aoki, S. Kuge, T. Kamiya and H. Imanaka, *ibid.*, *24*, 1243 (1976).
52. E. Kaczka and K. Folkers in "The Chemistry of Penicillin," H.J. Clarke, J.R. Johnson and R. Robinson, Eds., Princeton Univ. Press. Princeton, N.J., 1949, 256.
53. M. Nishida, Y. Mine, S. Nonoyama and H. Kojo, *J.Antibiotics*, *30*, 917 (1977).
54. Y. Mine, S. Nonoyama, H. Kojo, S. Fukuda and M. Nishida, *ibid.*, *30*, 932 (1977).
55. Y. Mine, S. Nonoyama, H. Kojo, S. Fukuda and M. Nishida, *ibid.*, *30*, 938 (1977).
56. T.J. Howarth, A.G. Brown and T.J. Kind, *J.Chem.Soc.*, Chem. Comm., 266 (1976).
57. P.A. Hunter and C. Reading, Abstracts, 16th Interscience Conf. Antimicrob. Ag. Chemother., Chicago, Ill., 211 (1976).
58. C. Reading and M. Cole, Antimicrob. Ag. Chemother., *11*, 852 (1977).
59. B.G. Spratt, V. Jobamputra and W. Zimmerman, *ibid.*, *12*, 406 (1977).
60. D.F. Corbett, T.J. Howarth and I. Stirling, *J.Chem.Soc.*, Chem. Comm., 808 (1977).

61. G. Albers-Schönberg, B.H. Arison, O.D. Hensens, J. Hirshfield, K. Hoogsteen, E.A. Kaczka, R.E. Rhodes, J.S. Kahan, F.M. Kahan, R.W. Ratcliffe, E. Walton, L.J. Ruswinkle, R.B. Morin and B.G. Christensen, *J.Am.Chem. Soc.*, in press.
62. J.S. Kahan, F.M. Kahan, R. Goegelman, S.A. Currie, M. Jackson, E.O. Stapley, T.W. Miller, A.K. Miller, D. Hendlin, S. Mochales, S. Hernandez and H.B. Woodruff, Abstracts, 16th Interscience Conf. Antimicrob. Ag. Chemother., Chicago, Ill. (1976). Abstract 227; H. Kropp, J.S. Kahan, F.M. Kahan, J. Sundelof, D. Darland and J. Birnbaum, *ibid.*, Abstract 228; G. Albers-Schönberg, B.H. Arison, E. Kaczka, F.M. Kahan, J.S. Kahan, B. Lago, W.M. Maiese, R.E. Rhodes, J.L. Smith, *ibid.*, Abstract 229.
63. A.G. Brown, D. Butterworth, M. Cole, G. Hanscomb, J.D. Hood, C. Reading and G.M. Rolinson, *J.Antibiotics, 29,* 668 (1976); D.F. Corbett, A.J. Eglington and T.J. Howarth, *J.Chem.Soc.*, Chem. Comm., 953 (1977).
64. P.J. Cassidy, E.O. Stapley, R. Goegelman, T.W. Miller, B.H. Arison, G. Albers-Schönberg, S.B. Zimmerman and J. Birnbaum, Abstracts, 17th Interscience Conf. Antimicrob. Ag. Chemother., New York, N.Y., 1977, Abstract 81.
65. E.O. Stapley, P. Cassidy, S.A. Currie, D. Daoust, R. Goegelman, S. Hernandez, M. Jackson, J.M. Mata, A.K. Miller, R.L. Monaghan, J.B. Tunac, S.B. Zimmerman, D. Hendlin, *ibid.*, Abstract 80.
66. K. Heusler, Medicinal Chemistry Special Contributions - Milan, 1972, P. Pratesi, Ed., Butterworths, London, p. 13.

Section IV - Metabolic Diseases and Endocrine Function

Editor: Hans-Jürgen Hess, Pfizer Inc., Groton, Connecticut

Chapter 17. Chronic Complications of Diabetes

Dushan Dvornik, Ayerst Research Laboratories, Montreal, Canada

Introduction - Before the discovery of insulin, the greatest threat to the diabetic patient was sudden death from coma caused by acidosis. From 1894 - 1915, 64% of all diabetic patients died in coma.[1] After insulin became generally available, diabetic coma as cause of death fell to 8.3% between 1922 - 1936, and to 1% between 1950 - 1968.[2] However, diabetic coma has been more than supplanted by the composite category of cardio-renal disease, which now accounts for about 80% of total deaths of diabetics.[3] The effects of long-term diabetes were thus unmasked, and, by 1950, it was evident that, whilst prolonging life, insulin treatment cannot prevent the appearance of disabling complications of chronic diabetes,[4] such as retinopathy, nephropathy, neuropathy, cataracts and generalized atherosclerosis.

Diabetic Microangiopathy - One of the most striking features of diabetes is the slow and progressive development of vascular abnormalities, particularly in the small blood vessels.[5] Diabetic retinopathy and nephropathy are, thus, rarely found at the onset of the disease.[6,7] The slow, progressive development of vascular changes during the years of incompletely normalized metabolism suggests that diabetic angiopathy is secondary to the metabolic abnormality(ies) characterizing diabetes mellitus.[5] According to McMillan,[8] the development of diabetic microangiopathy proceeds through several stages: at the onset, blood flow is disturbed in several body areas, and dilatation of small veins increases slowly until, in established diabetes, it becomes irreversible. Later, periodic arteriolar vasoconstriction sets in. As diabetes becomes long-standing, sclerosis of the vessels of the entire microcirculation develops which, finally, results in progressive decompensation of the microcirculation.

The following categories of alterations appear to contribute to diabetic angiopathy: (1) Basement membrane thickening, although the role remains unclear; however, hydroxylysine-linked glucosylgalactose units in basement membranes appear to be greatly increased in diabetes.[9,13] (2) Functional alterations, e.g. impaired phagocytosis,[14] abnormal lymphocytes,[15] and increased levels of lysosomal enzymes,[16] may affect the microcirculation by altering passage of blood, vascular tone and removal of basement membranes. (3) Altered cell metabolism, e.g. increased activity of the polyol pathway (see below).[17] (4) Altered blood flow characteristics, e.g. enhanced erythrocyte aggregation, increased plasma viscosity,[18] and increased resistance to blood flow.[8] (5) Increased sensitivity of platelets to aggregation correlating with elevated levels of von Willebrand's factor,[19] possibly due to excess of growth hormone (GH). (6)

ISBN 0-12-040513-X

Impaired oxygen transport, e.g. by $HbAI_c$, a minor variant of hemoglobin with greater avidity for oxygen than normal hemoglobin; $HbAI_c$ is about twice as abundant in insulin-treated diabetics as in control subjects and accounts for about 10% of total erythrocyte hemoglobin.[20,21] Increased erythrocyte 2,3-diphosphoglycerate, directly related to plasma phosphate, can compensate for impaired oxygen release by decreasing the oxygen affinity of HbA.[22,23] (7) Altered hormone production, e.g. of GH,[24] whose levels are 3-4 times higher in juvenile diabetics than in normal subjects.[5] The significance of increased glucagon levels in diabetic hyperglycemia is still controversial.[25] In addition to increasing glucose output by the liver, glucagon stimulates the formation of "acute phase" proteins,[26] thus possibly contributing to altered blood viscosity.

The pattern of deterioration of the microcirculation in diabetes is, however, not satisfactorily explained by any single category of these alterations. The slow progression of diabetic microangiopathy favors a mixture of adaptation and degeneration in response to several strains placed upon the microcirculation by the diabetic state.[8]

Diabetic Retinopathy is present in 60-80% of long-term diabetics. Five to 10% of diabetics surviving 20 years from the time of diagnosis will be blind, mostly from retinopathy, which ranks as leading cause of blindness in Great Britain[28] and the U.S.[29] In 1970, in the U.S., 8.5/100,000 persons were reported to be blind from diabetic retinopathy.[30] The prevalence of retinopathy increases with the duration of diabetes. Retinopathy is conventionally divided into a simple or non-proliferative, and a proliferative category. Non-proliferative retinopathy is characterized by alterations occurring in the original retinal vessels, e.g. microaneurisms, hemorrhages, exudates, and changes in retinal veins. Changes superimposed on the simple variety constitute proliferative retinopathy, e.g. new vessel development, vitreous hemorrhage and fibrous tissue proliferation, leading to traction retinal detachment. Proliferative retinopathy has a poor prognosis for retention of vision and, after five years, 43% of juvenile-onset and 60% of adult-onset diabetics become blind.[31] Proliferative retinopathy is associated with other long-term vascular complications, such as nephropathy and coronary heart disease. The development of retinopathy is accelerated by high blood pressure and low intraocular pressure.[32] The cause of diabetic retinopathy is unclear, and the mechanism of the early breakdown of the blood-retinal barrier is unknown. Several mechanisms have been proposed to explain the development of capillary occlusions, e.g. increased platelet aggregation,[19] decreased fibrinolytic activity,[33] increased plasma viscosity,[18] elevated $HbAI_c$,[20] and increased microvascular protein passage and deposition in the walls of the arterioles.[34] Since the introduction of hypophysectomy for diabetic retinopathy, in 1953, attention has been placed on GH as a causal factor in the development of diabetic angiopathy;[5] however, GH levels were not higher in juvenile diabetics with proliferative retinopathy than in those with minimal, or no retinopathy.[35] The question requires further study.

Diabetic Nephropathy - The kidneys of the diabetic patient are a target for structural damage which mainly involves the small blood vessels, i.e.

the glomerular capillaries and the associated arterioles, leading successively to proteinuria, impaired renal function and hypertension. There is a close correlation between the diabetic microvascular changes in the kidney and in the retina; however, while retinopathy is readily detected by ophthalmoscopy, renal involvement may cause few immediate clinical features until well advanced.[36] The earliest clinical feature of nephropathy is symptomless proteinuria. The time-interval between the detection of proteinuria and the deterioration of renal function varies considerably. In a recent retrospective analysis,[37] nephropathy accounted for 53% of deaths among juvenile diabetics; the mean duration of diabetes to the onset of proteinuria was 17.3 years and the duration of life after the onset of proteinuria was 4.8 years. The first symptom of nephropathy usually consists of peripheral edema, probably worsened by vasomotor defects caused by peripheral neuropathy; finally symptoms characteristic of renal failure develop, with fluid retention as one of the major problems.[38] In man, diabetic nephropathy is irreversible: once the clinical signs of nephropathy become evident, the natural course is inexorably progressive to death. In the later stages, the rate of progression is accelerated by the appearance and progression of other complications of diabetes, such as retinopathy, neuropathy and cardiovascular disease.[37] The factors causing diabetic nephropathy and those determining its progression are still unknown, and there is no convincing evidence that poor glucose control causes diabetic nephropathy or in any way alters its course.[39]

Diabetic Neuropathy of varying degree probably afflicts the majority of people with recognized diabetes mellitus. Clinically manifest problems which accrue from diabetic neuropathy are evident in over 50% of the American diabetic population.[40] The varying underlying pathogenic mechanisms and the resulting diversity of clinical manifestations suggest that, in diabetes, there are neuropathies - rather than a single entity of neuropathy. The spectrum of involvement is wide, with virtually every organ system at risk.[41] Ellenberg has broadly divided the manifestations of diabetic neuropathy into peripheral and visceral, and their subdivisions.[41] While peripheral neuropathy is the most common form, visceral neuropathy is also highly significant and may affect every part of the gastrointestinal tract, the genitourinary tract,[42,43] sexual function,[44] as well as the autonomic[45] and, possibly, the central nervous system.[46] Possible explanations for the development of diabetic neuropathy are based on theories of either microangiopathy and occlusive vascular disease, on abnormalities of metabolism, or on both.[47] Recent investigations suggest that chronic metabolic disturbances[48] are an underlying factor in nerve affection.[41] The most prominent lesion of the peripheral nerve fibers affected by diabetic neuropathy is segmental demyelination.[49] Since the myelin sheath is formed by spiral folding of Schwann cell membranes, diabetic neuropathy may, in fact, result from a metabolic defect of the Schwann cell.[49] The characteristic decrease in conduction-velocities of peripheral motor and sensory nerves may be due to segmental demyelination. Recently, it has been postulated that Schwann cell loss and abnormalities may be caused by increased aldose reductase activity resulting in intracellular accumulation of sorbitol (see below).[17] An interesting relationship between impaired motor-nerve-conduction-velocity and decreased myoinositol concentration has been found in the nerves of streptozotocin-diabetic rats.[48] Furthermore, decreased myoinositol and increased sorbitol levels have been found in cerebrospinal fluid of patients with diabetic polyneuropathy.[50]

Diabetes and Cataract - Although it is generally believed that diabetes causes cataracts, there is no scientific study supporting this view.[51] Nevertheless, in contrast to the lack of data on a correlation between diabetes and prevalence of cataracts, several hospital surveys indicate that diabetics undergo cataract extraction 5 to 9 times more frequently than non-diabetics.[51,52,53] It thus appears that the rate of cataract development in the diabetic is increased, thus resulting in cataract extraction at an earlier age.[54] In Britain, approximately one diabetic becomes blind from cataract for every three becoming blind from retinopathy;[55] in Canada, the proportion is one to four.[56] Recent evidence implicates aldose reductase as the key factor in the initiation of diabetic cataract (see below.)[53]

Role of Aldose Reductase - The clinical expression and the development of diabetic complications depend mainly on the duration of diabetes; current means of therapy are therefore, at best, only partly effective. It is pertinent that the tissues (lens, nerve, retina, kidney, blood vessels and islet cells) afflicted by diabetic manifestations do not require insulin for uptake of glucose. These tissues are thus exposed to any circulating levels of glucose without a protective barrier.[17] Recent experimental evidence suggests that the metabolic disposition of excess glucose in some of these tissues proceeds via the polyol pathway, and that the polyol produced initiates the changes leading to the development of diabetic complications. The polyol pathway consists of two enzymes: aldose reductase (AR), catalyzing the NADPH-dependent reduction of glucose and other aldoses to the corresponding polyol, and polyol dehydrogenase, catalyzing NAD-dependent oxidation of sorbitol to fructose.

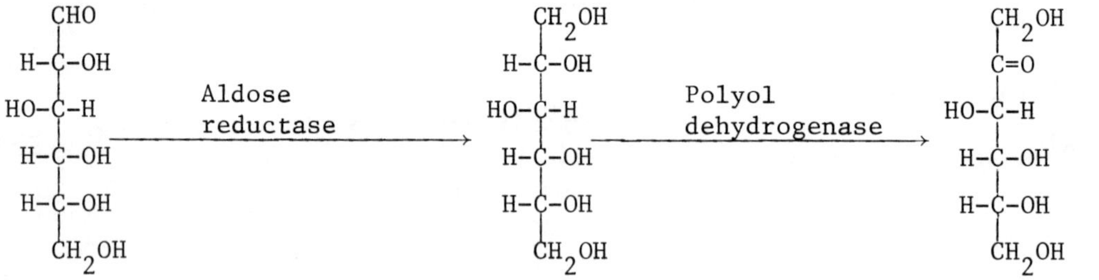

D-glucose Sorbitol D-fructose

The polyol pathway was first identified in seminal vesicles,[57] and later in lens[58] and other tissues.[59,60,61] The physiological function of the polyol pathway in these tissues remains unknown. The possible role of AR in the development of diabetic complications is based largely on the role of AR in the initiation of sugar cataracts.

The lens is uniquely vulnerable to diabetic conditions for the following reasons:[51] (1) since glucose uptake does not depend on insulin,[62] the lens is exposed to ambient glucose concentrations; (2) metabolism of glucose via the glycolytic pathway is controlled by hexokinase,[63] whose activity is low, but avidity for glucose is high:[64] hexokinase is thus easily saturated, making any excess glucose available to AR;[58,62,65] (3) as affinity of AR for glucose is low,[66] appreciable AR activity is attained only at high intracellular concentrations of glucose, as in diabetes; (4) sorbitol is not efficiently metabolized, e.g. by polyol dehydrogenase,[67] and does not readily diffuse through cell membranes, hence accumulates. The resulting increased osmotic pressure within the lens causes water uptake and lens swelling leading to loss of transparency, i.e. cataract. These events form the basis of Kinoshita's osmotic hypothesis,[68] which attributes the association between increased polyol levels and cataractogenesis[58,65] to the osmotic effects of increased polyol levels in a lens exposed to high sugar concentrations.[69] The concept has been substantiated by biochemical studies in vitro[51] and in laboratory animals by the use of AR inhibitors.[70,72] The identification of sorbitol in the lens of the human diabetic, whether cataractous or not, suggests that the sequence of events postulated by the osmotic hypothesis also occurs in man.[73]

The intriguing question is whether the consequences of increased AR activity in hyperglycemia also play a role in the development of other diabetic complications. In neuropathy, the case for the osmotic hypothesis is supported by the presence of AR in Schwann cells of peripheral nerves,[74] and the finding that, both in diabetic[75,76] and galactosemic rats,[77,78] polyol accumulates in the sciatic nerve, and that the accumulation was prevented by an AR inhibitor.[71] Furthermore, the defect in motor-nerve-conduction-velocity, occurring in both human[79] and experimental diabetes,[80] is controlled with insulin, and occurrence of a similar defect in galactosemic rats was delayed by an AR inhibitor.[80] Osmotic damage resulting from sorbitol accumulation has been suggested to be responsible for diabetic capillary disease in the retina.[81] AR has been found in the retina,[60] and sorbitol was found to accumulate in the retina of diabetic rats, albeit at low levels.[82] In addition, tissue cultures of mural cells from human retinal capillaries contain AR and accumulate sorbitol when incubated in high glucose medium.[83] Except for the localization of AR in the papilla of the kidney,[60] no information is available on the possible role of AR in nephropathy. Thus, the presently available evidence supports the postulate that AR is involved in the initiation of diabetic cataracts and, possibly, diabetic neuropathy.

AR Inhibitors - If AR is indeed responsible for initiating the development of some diabetic complications, then inhibition of AR may represent a pharmacological approach to their delay and, possibly, prevention. The approach is attractive because AR appears to play an important role only in a non-physiological state, such as created by high blood glucose levels. The first compounds reported to inhibit AR in vitro were medium-chain aliphatic fatty acids (C_6-C_8)[66] and, later, tetramethyleneglutaric acid (1), which was used to corroborate the osmotic hypothesis in vitro.[70]

Alrestatin (AY-22,284) (2), an orally active AR inhibitor, decreased polyol accumulation in lens and sciatic nerve of galactosemic and diabetic rats,[71] and suppressed cataract formation when administered either orally,[71] or topically.[84] AR inhibitory activity in vitro has also been reported for a series of flavonoids,[85,86] and the most potent compound, quercitrin (3), delayed the appearance of cataracts in the diabetic degu,[87] a South American rodent prone to rapid cataract development. AR inhibitors are thus useful to further elucidate the role of AR in the development of chronic diabetic complications.

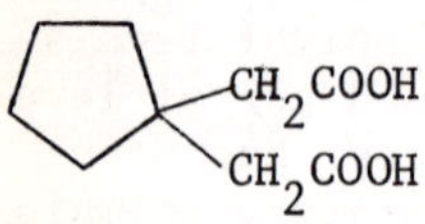

1

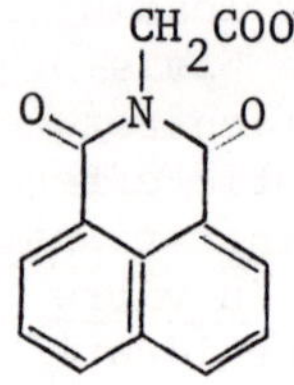

2

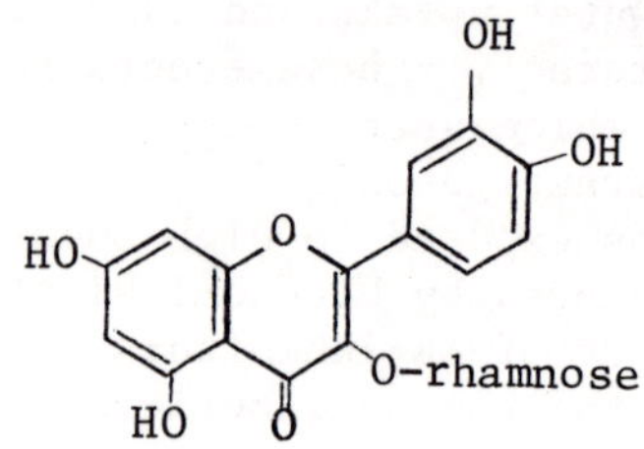

3

References

1. E.P. Joslin, in "The Treatment of Diabetes Mellitus," Lea and Febiger, Philadelphia, 1916, p.54.
2. H.H. Marks and L.P. Krall, in "Joslin's Diabetes Mellitus," 11th Ed., A. Marble, P. White, R.F. Bradley and L.P. Krall, Eds., Lea and Febiger, Philadelphia, 1971, p.2.
3. H. Keen, Postgrad. Med.J. 52, 445 (1976).
4. A. Marble, Diabetologia 12, 193 (1976).
5. K. Lundbaek, Diabetes 25 (Suppl.2), 845 (1976).
6. P. White, Diabetes 5, 445 (1956).
7. R. Østerby, Acta Med.Scand. 574 (Suppl.), 1 (1975).
8. D.E. McMillan, Diabetes 24, 944 (1975).
9. R.G. Spiro, Diabetes 25 (Suppl.2), 909 (1976).
10. N.A. Kefalides, J.Clin.Invest. 53, 403 (1974).
11. T. Sato, H. Munakata, K. Yoshinaga and Z. Yosizawa, Clin.Chim.Acta 61, 145 (1975).
12. N.G. Westberg, Diabetes 25 (Suppl.2), 920 (1976).
13. R.G. Spiro, Diabetologia 12, 1 (1976).
14. J.D. Bagdade, R.K. Root and R.J. Bulger, Diabetes 23, 9 (1974).
15. Z. Skrabalo, in "Vascular and Neurological changes in Early Diabetes," R.A. Camerini-Davalos and H.S. Cole, Eds., Academic Press, New York, 1973, p.311.
16. F. Belfiore, E. Napoli and L. Lovecchio, Diabetes 21, 1168 (1972).
17. K.H. Gabbay, Ann.Rev.Med. 26, 521 (1975).
18. D.E. McMillan, Diabetes 25 (Suppl.2), 858 (1976).
19. J.A. Colwell, P.V. Halushka, K. Sarji, J. Levine, J. Sagel and R.M.G. Nair, Diabetes 25 (Suppl.2), 826 (1976).

20. S. Rahbar, O. Blumenfeld and H.M. Ranney, Biochem.Biophys.Res.Comm. 36, 838 (1969).
21. H.F. Bunn, K.H. Gabbay and P.M. Gallop, Science 200, 21 (1978) and ref. cited.
22. H.F. Bunn and R.W. Briehl, J.Clin.Invest. 49, 1088 (1970).
23. J. Ditzel, Diabetes 25 (Suppl.2), 832 (1976).
24. K. Lundbaek, V.A. Jensen, T.S. Olsen, H. Orskov, N.J. Christensen, K. Johansen, A.P. Hansen and R. Østerby, Lancet 2, 131 (1970).
25. R. Levine, New Engl.J.Med. 294, 494 (1976).
26. L.L. Miller, Diabetes 25 (Suppl.2), 865 (1976).
27. M. Amherdt, V. Harris, A.E. Renold, L. Orci and P.H. Unger, J.Clin. Invest. 54, 188 (1974).
28. E.M. Kohner and N.W. Oakley, Metabolism 24, 1085 (1975).
29. P.H. Morse and T.G. Duncan, New Eng.J. Med. 292, 87 (1976).
30. H.A. Kahn and R. Hiller, Am.J.Opthalmol. 78,58 (1974).
31. P.F. Palmberg, Diabetes 26, 703 (1977).
32. B. Becker, Am.J.Opthalmol. 71, 1 (1971).
33. L. Almer and M. Pandolfi, Diabetes 25 (Suppl.2), 807 (1976).
34. H. Parving, Diabetes 25 (Suppl.2), 884 (1976).
35. P.M. Holland, M.B. Landers, 3rd. H.E. Lebovitz and M.L. Wolbarscht, Am.J.Opthalmol. 82, 612 (1976).
36. J.T. Ireland, Brit.J.Clin.Pract. 30, 149 (1976).
37. M.J. Kussman, H.H. Goldstein and R.E. Gleason, J.Am.Med.Assoc. 236, 1886 (1976).
38. P.J. Watkins, V. Parsons and M. Bevick, Clin.Nephrology 7, 243 (1977).
39. Leading article, Brit.Med.J. 3, 5 (1975).
40. A.M. Lawrence and C. Abraira, Ann.Clin.Lab.Sci. 6, 78 (1976).
41. M. Ellenberg, Metabolism 25, 1627 (1976).
42. J.T. Andersen and W. Bradley, Urology 7, 442 (1976).
43. A.C. Buck, P.I. Reed, Y.K. Siddiq, G.D. Chisholm and T. Russell Fraser, Diabetologia 12, 251 (1976).
44. R.C. Kolodny, C.B. Kahn, H.H. Goldstein and D.M. Barnett, Diabetes 23, 306 (1973).
45. I.W. Campbell, Brit.J.Clin.Pract. 30, 153 (1976).
46. R.N. De Jong, Postgrad.Med. 61, 101 (1977).
47. B.C. O'Malley, W.R. Timperley, J.D. Ward, N.R. Porter and F.E. Preston, Lancet 2, 1274 (1975).
48. A.I. Winegrad and D.A. Greene, New Engl.J.Med. 295, 1416 (1976).
49. P.K. Thomas and R.G. Lascelles, Lancet 1, 1355 (1965).
50. C. Servo, L. Berstrom and R. Fogelholm, Acta Med.Scand. 202, 301 (1977).
51. J.H. Kinoshita, S.D. Varma and H.N. Fukui, Jap.J.Opthalmol. 20, 399 (1976).
52. A. Pirie, Isr.J.Med.Sci. 8, 1550 (1972).
53. J.H. Kinoshita, Invest.Opthalmol. 13, 713 (1974).
54. F.I. Caird, M. Hutchinson and A. Pirie, Br.J.Prev.Soc.Med. 19, 80 (1965).
55. British Diabetes Assoc., London, 1970.
56. A.E. MacDonald, Can.Med.Assoc.J. 92, 264 (1965).
57. L.G. Hers, Biochim.Biophys. Acta 22, 202 (1956).
58. R. Van Heyningen, Nature 184, 194 (1959).

59. S. Hayman, M.F. Lous, L.O. Merola and J.H. Kinoshita, Biochim.Biophys. Acta 128, 474 (1966).
60. K.H. Gabbay, Isr.J.Med.Sci. 8, 1626 (1972).
61. A.I. Winegrad, A.D. Morrison and R.S. Clements, Jr., in "Diabetes," N.J. Malaisse, J. Pirart and J. Valance-Owen, Eds., Excerpta Medica, Amsterdam, 1974, p.387, and ref. cited.
62. F.I. Caird, A. Pirie and T.G. Ramsell, in "Diabetes and the Eye," Blackwell Sci.Publ., Oxford, 1969, p.140, and ref.cited.
63. J.H. Kinoshita, Invest. Ophthalmol. 4, 619 (1965).
64. P.K. Pottinger, Biochem.J. 104, 663 (1967).
65. R. van Heyningen, Exp.Eye.Res. 1, 396 (1962).
66. S. Hayman and J.H. Kinoshita, J.Biol.Chem. 240, 877 (1965).
67. J.G. Collins and C.N. Corder, Invest.Opthalmol. 16, 242 (1977).
68. J.H. Kinoshita, Invest.Opthalmol. 4, 786 (1965).
69. J.H. Kinoshita, L.O. Merola and S. Hayman, J.Biol.Chem. 240, 310 (1965).
70. J.H. Kinoshita, D. Dvornik, M. Kraml and K.H. Gabbay, Biochim.Biophys. Acta 158,472 (1968).
71. D. Dvornik, N. Simard-Duquesne, M. Kraml, K. Sestanj, K.H. Gabbay, J.H. Kinoshita and L.O. Merola, Science 182, 1146 (1973).
72. S.D. Varma, A. Mizuno and J.H. Kinoshita, Science 195, 205 (1977).
73. A. Pirie and R. van Heyningen, Exp.Eye Res. 3, 124 (1964).
74. K.H. Gabbay, New Engl.J.Med. 288, 831 (1973).
75. K.H. Gabbay, L.O. Merola and R.A. Field, Science 151, 209 (1966).
76. M.A. Stewart, W.R. Sherman and S. Anthony, Biochem.Biophys.Res.Comm. 22, 488 (1966).
77. K.H. Gabbay and J.P. O'Sullivan, Diabetes 17, 239 (1968).
78. M.A. Stewart, W.R. Sherman, M.M. Kurien, G.I. Moonswammy and M. Wisgerhof, J. Neurochem. 14, 1057 (1967).
79. G. Gregersen, Diabetologia 4, 273 (1968).
80. K.H. Gabbay, in "Vascular and Neurological Changes in Early Diabetes", R.A. Camerini-Davalos and H.S. Cole, Eds., Academic Press, New York, N.Y., 1973, p.417.
81. P. Beaumont, F.C. Hollows, P.J. Schofield, J.F. Williams and W. Steinbeck, Lancet 1, 579 (1971).
82. J.C. Hutton, P.J. Schofield, J.F. Williams and F.C. Hollows, Austral. J.Exp.Biol.Med.Sci. 52, 361 (1974).
83. S.M. Buzney, R.N. Frank, S.D. Varma, T. Tamshima and K.H. Gabbay, Invest.Opthalmol.Visual Sci. 16, 392 (1977).
84. S.D. Varma and J.H. Kinoshita, Documenta Opthalmol. Proc.Series 8, 305 (1976).
85. S.D. Varma, I. Mikuni and J.H. Kinoshita, Science 188, 1215 (1975).
86. S.D. Varma and J.H. Kinoshita, Biochem.Pharmacol. 25, 2505 (1976).
87. S.D. Varma, A. Mizuno and J.H. Kinoshita, Science 195, 205 (1977).

Chapter 18. Newer Agents for the Treatment of Arthritis

Joseph G. Lombardino, Pfizer Central Research, Groton, CT. 06340

Introduction — Many compounds are in use or under study for the control of the painful symptoms of arthritis and other inflammatory diseases of the musculoskeletal system. The literature on non-steroidal antiinflammatory (NSAI) drugs has increased dramatically since Wong[1] last surveyed the field for this series in 1975. In addition to the NSAI agents, several immunoregulatory drugs, last reviewed by Chang,[2] have been shown to control immune-mediated inflammation and, although still in the experimental phase of clinical trials, such agents offer the possibility of achieving more than palliative control of the symptoms of arthritis. Among the various anti-arthritic agents, the NSAI drugs are by far the largest and most important class. More than 120 such compounds have been assigned a generic name, suggesting that many have progressed beyond initial testing in animals. Several such agents have recently been marketed with claims for rheumatoid arthritis (RA), osteoarthritis (OA) and acute inflammatory conditions of connective tissue. The present review will focus on the literature of 1975-1977, with emphasis on the newer, more potent compounds of both the NSAI and immunoregulatory type. Several recent reviews and texts are available which discuss the drugs used in the treatment of arthritis[3-8] and their possible mechanisms of action.[9-14] Reviews of the inflammatory process,[15-16] the rheumatic diseases,[17-22] including the rheumatism literature[19] for the years 1973-1974, and a compilation of papers from an international meeting on inflammation,[23] have also appeared.

Mechanisms of Action — Some new insights have been gained concerning the mechanisms by which NSAI agents control inflammation. The ability of these agents to influence the biosynthesis of prostaglandins (PG), reviewed more recently by Vane and Lewis,[24] is viewed as a basic mode of action of these drugs.[25] Support was obtained for a role for PG in RA when elevated PG levels were found in articular tissue from arthritis patients,[26,27] and by the detection of a human lymphocyte factor which stimulates PG production in rheumatoid synovial cells.[28] Furthermore, NSAI drugs inhibit PG production by synovial cells in organ culture[29,30] and PG levels are reduced in synovial fluid of arthritic patients dosed orally with NSAI agents.[31] The PG inhibitory potency of NSAI agents *in vitro* is dependent on both the tissue source and the way the prostaglandin biosynthetase system is handled.[32] As a result, studies with NSAI agents have shown either good correlations[29,33,34] or poor correlations[35-39] between *in vitro* inhibition of PG synthesis and *in vivo* antiinflammatory activity. It is not unexpected that *in vitro* activity should fail to correlate with *in vivo* activity when one considers that complex metabolic and pharmacokinetic factors may be superimposed on the *in vivo* situation.

Whereas steroids block both PG and collagenase production by RA synovial cells, indomethacin inhibits PGE_2 production but stimulates collagenase production.[40] This finding may explain in part why NSAI drugs relieve inflammation but do not prevent tissue damage in arthritic patients. A further difference between steroids and NSAI agents is that the former inhibit the release of arachidonic acid from cell membranes[41] whereas the latter inhibit the cyclooxygenase step in PG production.

ISBN 0-12-040513-X

Evidence exists suggesting that inhibition of PG synthesis does not entirely explain the antiinflammatory activity of NSAI drugs.[42-45] Information on a possible role of the endoperoxide PGG_2 in inflammation has been obtained from studies with MK-447.[46] This compound has significant antiinflammatory activity in the rat but does not inhibit the PG cyclooxygenase. It does, however, suppress PGG_2 levels suggesting that PGG_2 or some substance derived from PGG_2, rather than PGE or PGF, may trigger the inflammatory response.[46] An understanding of the role of the thromboxanes in inflammation[47] may offer new therapeutic approaches for agents with more specific actions, especially in view of the compounds (e.g. dipyridamole, N-0164, L-8027) already reported[48-50] to preferentially inhibit thromboxane production. Other

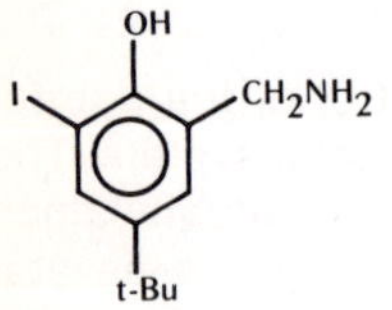

MK-447

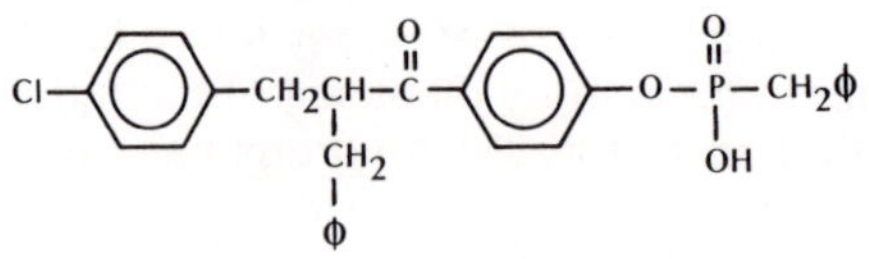

N-0164

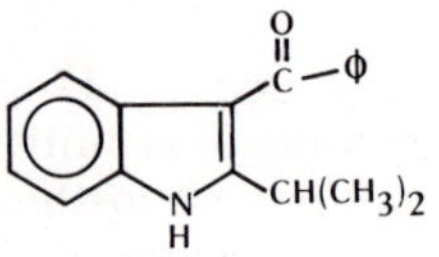

L-8027

effects observed with NSAI agents which may contribute to their mechanism of action include: inhibition of neutrophil chemotaxis,[51] reduced leukocyte migration,[52] effects on lysosomal enzyme release,[53-55] impairment of phagocytosis,[56] inhibition of superoxide anion production in macrophages,[57] stabilization of cell membranes[58] and inhibition of the production of vasodilator mediators.[59]

The mechanism of action of immunoregulatory agents of both the suppressive and stimulatory type, and the basis for their use in the treatment of RA, have been discussed by Chang[2] and Maini.[22]

Methodology — Various, now generally standard, animal models of inflammation have been reviewed.[60,61] The most commonly used test for the identification and characterization of antiinflammatory agents is the rat foot edema (RFE) test in which an edema is provoked in the paw of a rat by injection of carrageenan. This test has a PG mediated phase of the inflammatory response which is less intense in essential fatty acid deficient rats,[62] presumably due to deficient levels of arachidonic acid. Another widely used model, the rat adjuvant arthritis (RAA) test, produces a more chronic type of inflammation. In this model there is evidence for an immune-mediated inflammatory component involving a critical role for T-cells.[63,64] Modifications of this procedure permit the detection of immunological agents,[65,66] analgesics,[67] as well as NSAI drugs.[68] Morphological studies suggest a similarity between the lesions in the RAA model and human RA.[69,70] Considerable effort is being directed toward the development of other models of chronic inflammation.[71] In this regard, ovalbumin,[72] carrageenan,[73] bovine serum albumin,[74] Fab_2,[75] or an extract of *Erysipelothrix rhusiopathiae*[76] have been utilized to provoke synovitis in rabbits. Although evaluation of compounds in the rabbit synovitis model is relatively time consuming, its similarity to human RA will likely encourage its use.

A detailed discussion of the immunologically-based models is beyond the scope of this review. *In vitro* methods for measuring cell-mediated immunity[77] and models of lymphokine production,[78] and of autoimmune diseases,[79] are available. Reviews on lymphocyte function[80] and the role of lymphocytes in clinical disorders[81] provide a useful background for models suitable for measuring drug effects on the immune response.

Compounds Under Investigation

Immunoregulatory Agents — There has been an explosive increase in the literature on the use of levamisole (LVS, **1**) in several inflammatory diseases. A valuable entry to the more than 400 publications on this drug is provided by a review of the literature through late 1976.[82] LVS has achieved particular attention for the treatment of RA (reviewed through 1976 by Trabert *et al.*[83]), with mostly positive effects observed but some negative results and often severe side effects also reported.[82-86] Double-blind clinical trials of LVS in RA confirm the results achieved in most open clinical trials — i.e. when LVS is administered against a background of NSAI drugs, clinical symptoms of RA improve in many patients after three months of therapy.[87] However, immunological parameters do not necessarily correlate with clinical improvement, and side-effects, in particular agranulocytosis, can be serious, occurring in up to 20% of patients.[88]

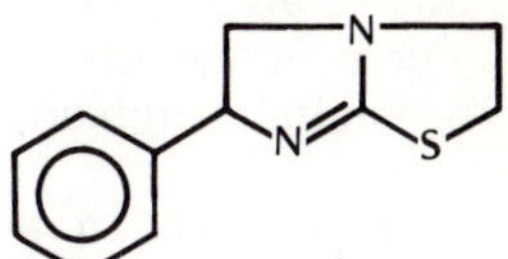

1

Several mechanisms of action, mainly involving T-cell function, have been proposed to explain the beneficial effect of LVS.[82] Enhanced phagocytosis[89,90] and chemotaxis[91,92] have been observed *in vitro*, but the clinical relevance of some of these *in vitro* effects, which have sometimes been observed with concentrations as high as 1 mM, is not certain. Variable results are obtained with levamisole in the RAA model,[93,94] and in the autoimmune disease model of NZB/W mice.[95,96] Delayed hypersensitivity in rats is enhanced by LVS.[97]

Other immunostimulatory compounds include Wy-13,876 (**2**), which increases T-lymphocytes and rosette formation in rats and inhibits tumor growth in mice.[98] The anthranilic acid derivative, **3**, promotes lymphocyte blastogenesis and antibody production in rats and suppresses both RAA and the autoimmune disease of NZB/W mice.[99]

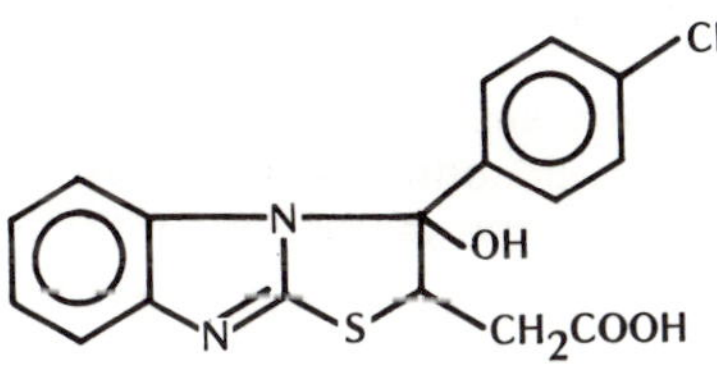

2

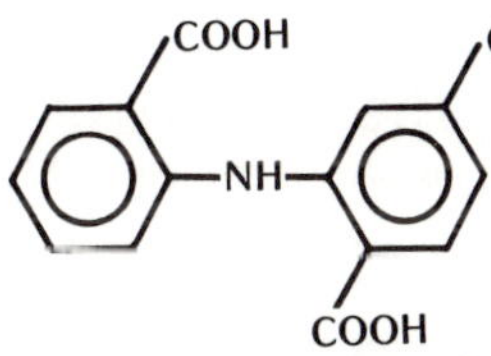

3

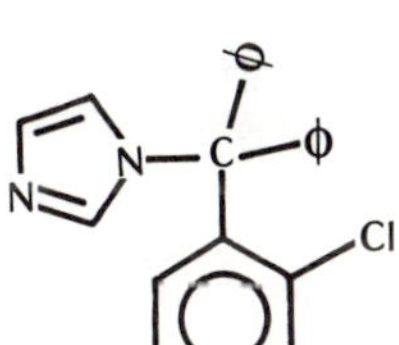

4

Among the immunosuppressive agents receiving attention are two imidazole derivatives, clotrimazole (**4**) and niridazole (**5**), the pyridine derivative oxisuran (**6**), and frentizole (**7**).

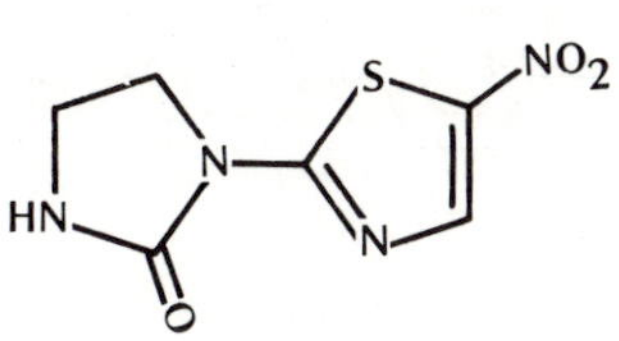

5

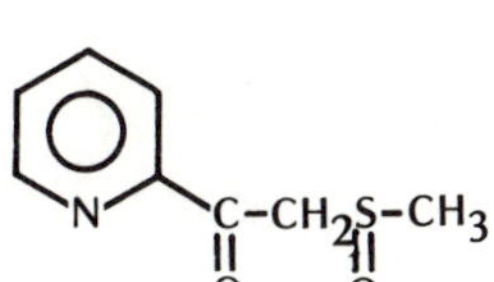

6

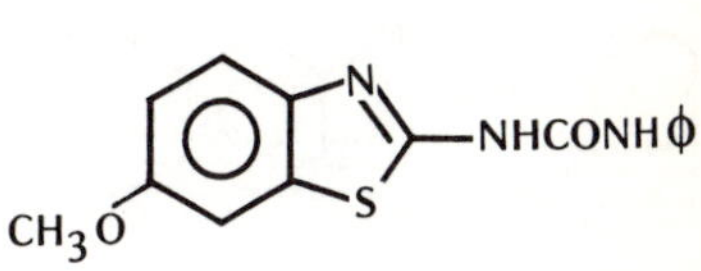

7

Clotrimazole (**4**), an antifungal agent, was reported to produce rapid improvement in 10 RA patients.[100] Data from animal studies[101] and another clinical trial in RA patients[102] suggest that stimulation of the adrenal glands, with an ensuing elevation of serum cortisol levels, is responsible for the activity of clotrimazole. Niridazole (**5**), a human anthelmintic drug, has modest antiinflammatory properties[103] and is a suppressor of cellular hypersensitivity,[104,105] perhaps due to an active metabolite formed *in vivo*.[106] The drug suppresses experimental allergic encephalomyelitis in rats[107] and mice[108] but is carcinogenic in rodents.[109,110] In man, niridazole inhibits the mixed lymphocyte reaction.[111]

Oxisuran (**6**) has been reported to be a differential inhibitor of cell-mediated hypersensitivity.[112] Recent data suggest that this compound acts by stimulating the pituitary adrenal system, producing elevated levels of circulating steroids.[113] Indeed, the effects of oxisuran have been duplicated in mice by administration of corticosterone.[113]

The immunosuppressive urea derivative frentizole (**7**) inhibits murine lymph node cells and suppresses macrophage phagocytosis.[114] The compound was found to either increase or decrease survival time of mice infected with various bacterial, viral or fungal organisms,[115] suggesting a differential drug effect on the immune response to these organisms.

NSAI Agents — These agents are conveniently grouped into acidic compounds of the arylcarboxylic or enolic type and non-acidic compounds.

A. *Arylcarboxylic Acids* — Carboxylic acids form the largest structural class of NSAI drugs. Indomethacin and the more recently marketed drugs, naproxen, ibuprofen, fenoprofen and tolmetin, have been thoroughly reviewed elsewhere[3-9,116] and will not be discussed here. Approximately 70 other carboxylic acids have been reported to have significant antiinflammatory activity in animal models and some in man. Some of these compounds, such as ketoprofen, alclofenac and flurbiprofen have been discussed in earlier reviews in this series (e.g. Wong[1]). This review will focus on a discussion of the newer agents. The relative antiinflammatory potencies of several NSAI drugs have been published.[117-120] All of the NSAI agents have a similar profile of activity which includes anti-edema, antipyretic and analgesic effects. None of the NSAI agents are clinically clearly superior to high doses of aspirin but some are less toxic and are used in patients who are not controlled by aspirin. All of these agents, like aspirin, have gastrointestinal side-effects but the search for a more potent and safer drug continues.

Among benzoic acid derivatives reported to exhibit antiinflammatory activity, fendosal (HP-129, **8**), possesses prolonged analgesic effects.[121] Tolfenamic acid (**9**), 600 mg/d, controls the symptoms of RA[122,123] and is reported to cause only minor gastrointestinal effects.[124] Diflunisal (**10**), an aspirin derivative, differs from the latter drug principally by a longer half-life and greater potency.[125,126]

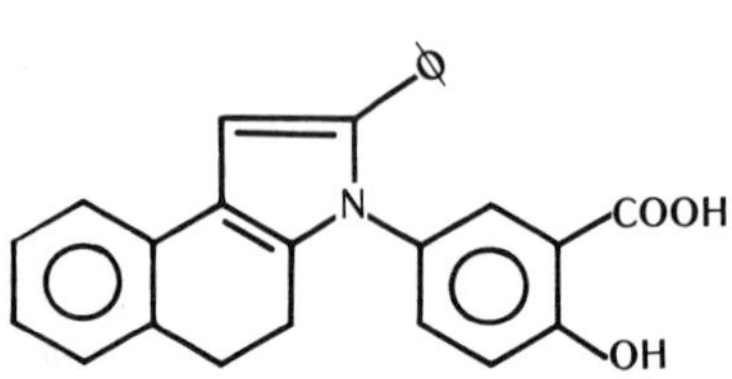

8

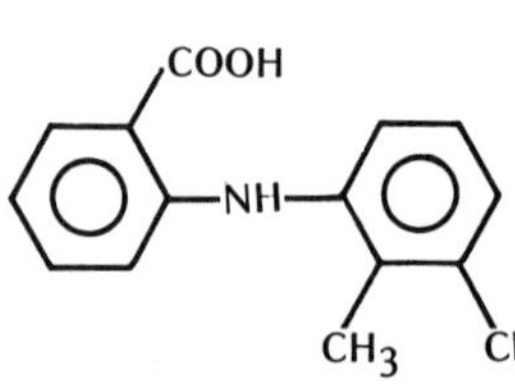

9

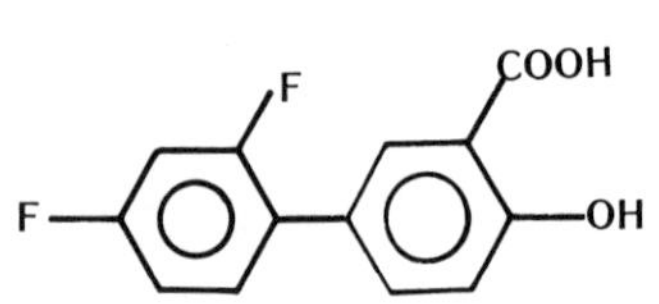

10

Acetic acid derivatives are well represented among the NSAI agents. Sulindac (**11**), an indene derivative of indomethacin, is effective in OA[127,128] and in RA[129] at daily doses of 300-400 mg. In several models of inflammation the sulfide metabolite derived from **11** is more potent than sulindac itself,[130] indicating the sulfide to be the active species *in vivo.* Mucosal injury[131] and intestinal blood loss[132] are reported to be less severe with sulindac than with aspirin.

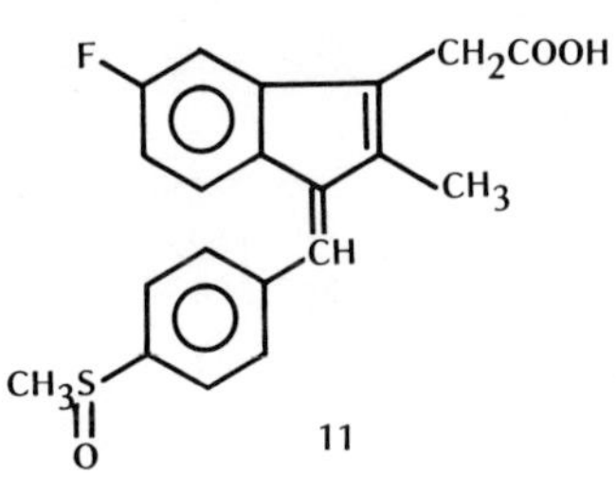

11

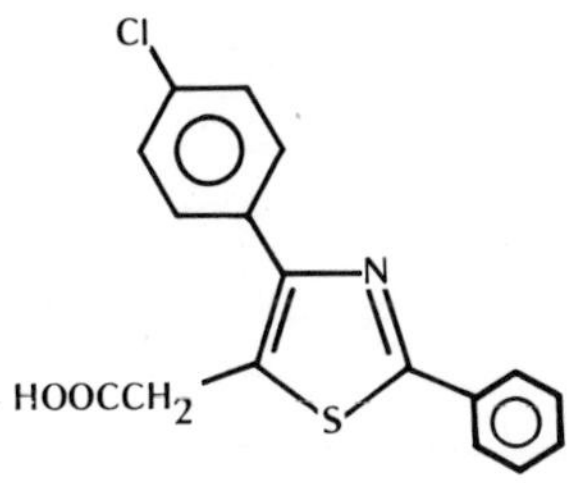

12

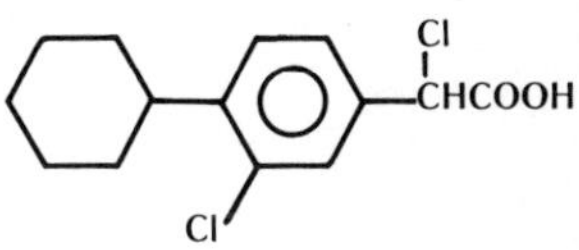

13

Fentiazac (BR-700, **12**) is more potent than ibuprofen in the RFE test,[134] is an effective analgesic in rodents, suppresses RAA,[133] and reduces mononuclear cell migration into granulomas *in vivo.*[135] Fenclorac (WHR-539, **13**) is one-third as potent as indomethacin as an inhibitor of the RFE test (ED_{50} 7.9 mg/kg),[137] but is more potent than indomethacin as an inhibitor of PG synthesis.[136] The half-life of this compound in man is 3 hr.[138]

Etodolic acid (AY-24,236, **14**) is equipotent with phenylbutazone in the RFE test,[140] and is a potent inhibitor of RAA.[139] Similarly, tianafac (**15**) is as active as phenylbutazone in the RFE test, but is less ulcerogenic.[141,142] A series of abstracts report the pharmacology and antiarthritic efficacy (300 mg/d) of clopirac (BRL-13,856, **16**).[143]

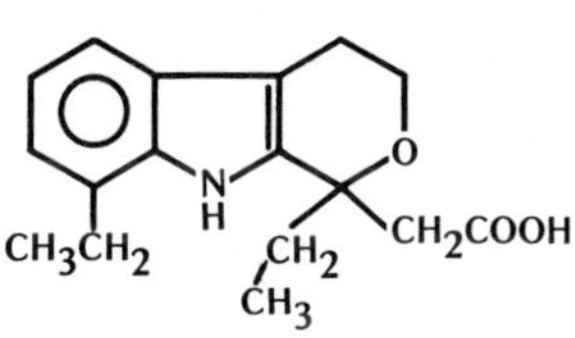

14

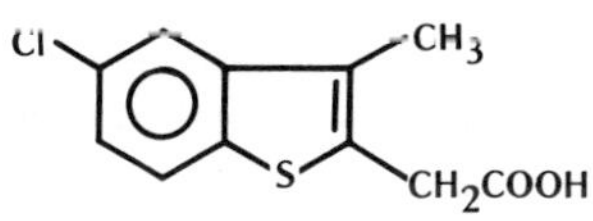

15

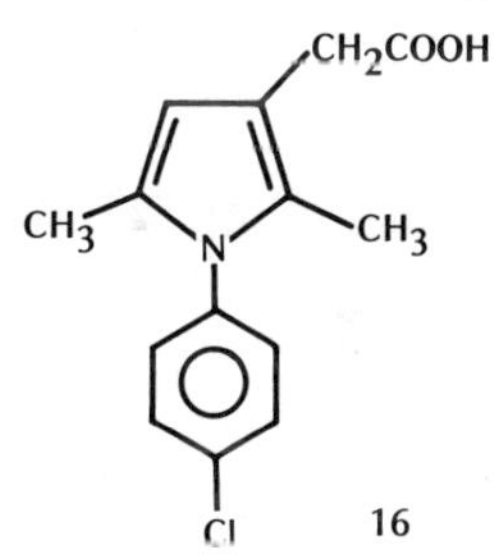

16

Clometacine (RU-3959, **17**), a positional isomer of indomethacin, is much less potent than indomethacin.[144] DD-3314 (**18**) is more than twice as active as indomethacin in the RFE test.[145] A basic derivative of fentiazac, the thiazole acetic acid **19**, was reported to be more potent than phenylbutazone in the RFE test.[146]

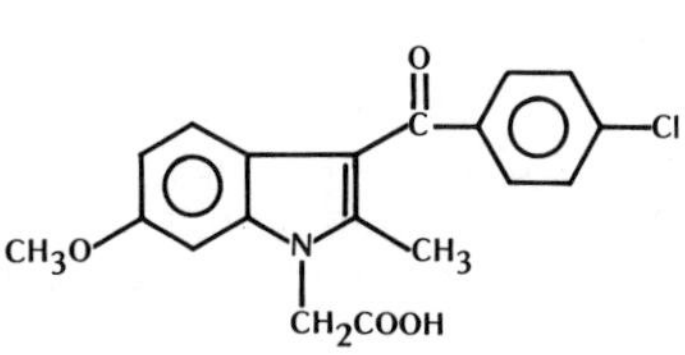

17

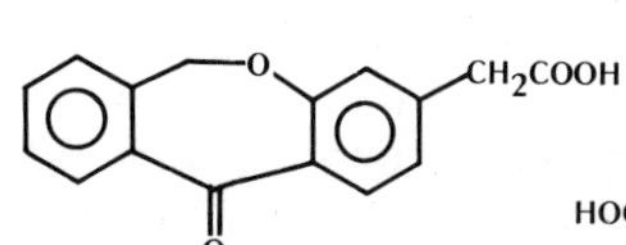

18

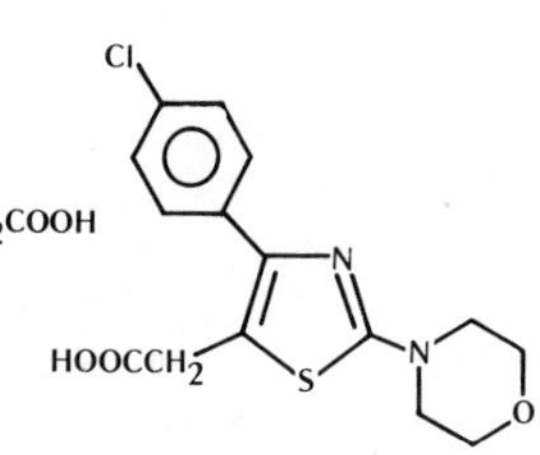

19

Many propionic acid derivatives related to ibuprofen have been shown to control inflammation. Benoxaprofen (**20**) is 5 times more potent than phenylbutazone in the RFE test.[147] The compound exhibits only weak PG synthetase inhibiting properties[148] and has a long half-life (37 hr) in man.[149] The isoindole derivative indoprofen (K-4277, **21**) is 19 times more potent than phenylbutazone[150] and has a half-life of 3 hr in man.[151,152] The drug causes less fecal blood loss than aspirin.[153] In the treatment of OA[154] it is comparable (600 mg/d) to ibuprofen (900 mg/d).

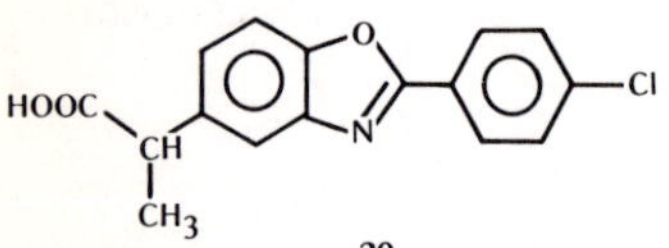

20

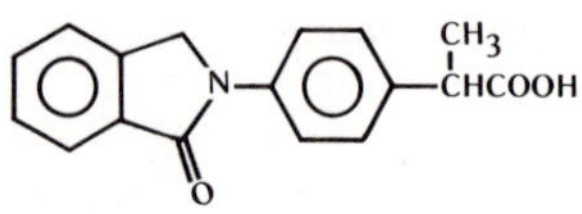

21

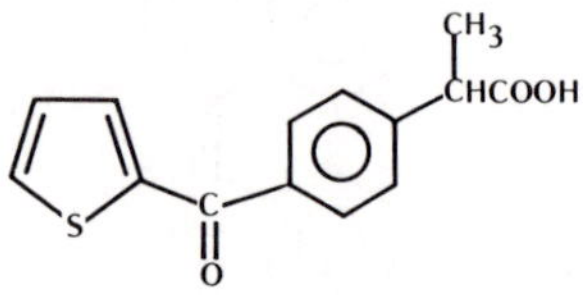

22

Several publications summarize the pharmacological and toxicological properties of suprofen (R-25,061, **22**), a potent antiinflammatory acid (e.g. in RAA, ED_{50} = 6 mg/kg).[155,156]

Other heterocyclic propionic acids include carprofen (Ro-5720, **23**), tiaprofenic acid (RU-15,060, **24**) and R-803 (**25**). Carprofen (**23**) is as potent as indomethacin in the RFE test but less potent in the RAA test.[157] In rodents, relatively low doses of carprofen have been reported to produce gastric ulcers.[157,158] Co-administration with aspirin results in lower peak plasma levels of carprofen.[159] The d-isomer of carprofen is more potent than the l-isomer both in the RAA test and as a PG synthetase inhibitor.[160] Early clinical evidence suggests that carprofen (300 mg/d) is effective in RA.[161] The pharmacokinetics of tiaprofenic acid (**24**) in man and animals have been reported and two metabolites identified.[162] The compound appears to be as potent as indomethacin in RA.[163,164] The benzofuran propionic acid R-803 (**25**) has an ED_{50} of 10 mg/kg in the RFE test and inhibits ultraviolet-induced erythema in guinea pigs and granuloma formation in rats.[165] Gastrointestinal bleeding in man following administration of 1200 mg of R-803 is reported to be less than with 3600 mg of aspirin.[166]

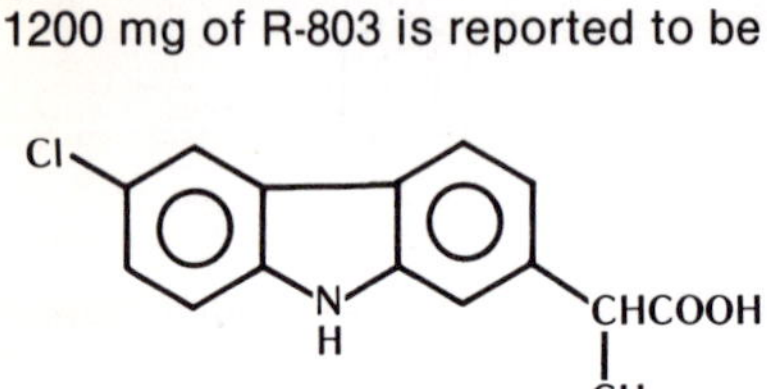

23

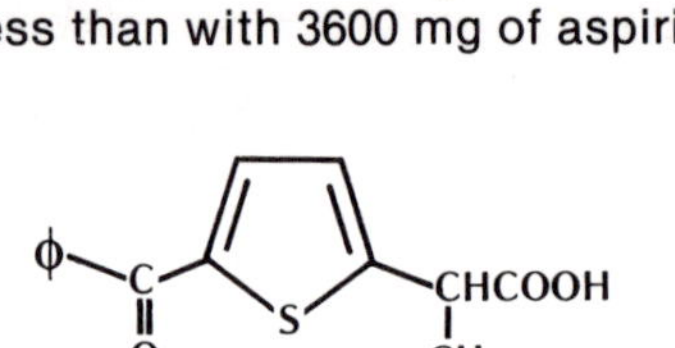

24

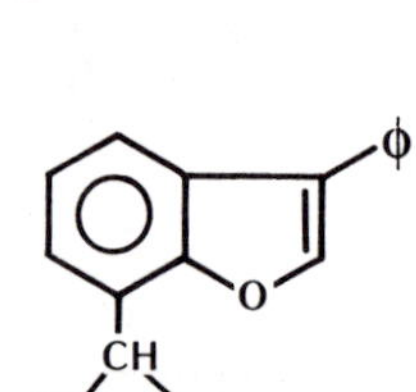

25

B. *Enolic Acids* — Several antiinflammatory agents are acidic but are not carboxylic acids. Phenylbutazone has been known for some time to be an effective NSAI agent and this has encouraged further research around this structure. A series of 26 publications has appeared on feprazone (DA-2370, **26**)[167] discussing the pharmacology, toxicology and clinical results with this compound. Clinical trials indicate 300-800 mg/d of feprazone to be effective in controlling the symptoms of inflammation in RA[168-170] and OA.[171] Gastrointestinal effects were milder, but other side-effects (rash, headache, etc.) resembled those seen with phenylbutazone.[172] The half-life in man is shorter (39 hr) than that of phenylbutazone (72 hr).[173] Trimethazone (**27**), 1000 mg/d, was as effective as phenylbutazone, 600 mg/d, in a trial in RA and was better tolerated.[174]

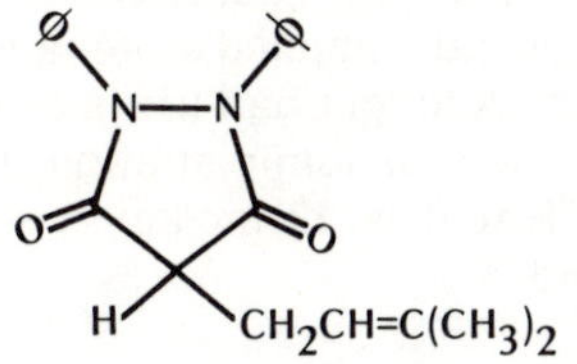

26

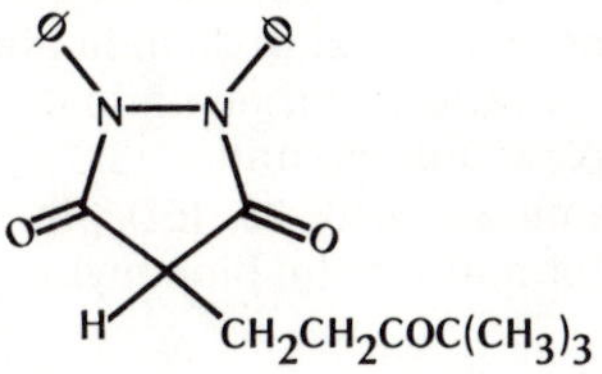

27

The potent antiinflammatory properties and long biological half-life of piroxicam (CP-16,171, **28**) have been reviewed.[175] Oral ED_{50} values in the RFE test (2 mg/kg) and in RAA (0.5 mg/kg),[176] and a long half-life in several species, including man (48 hr), are reflected clinically where the compound dosed at 20 mg once-a-day is found effective in RA and OA.[177,178,180] In contrast to other NSAI agents, concomitant salicylate administration does not affect the plasma kinetics of piroxicam.[180] Piroxicam is a potent (IC_{50} 0.2 μM) inhibitor of prostaglandin synthesis in cultures of MC5-5 cells.[179] The related compound isoxicam (W 8495, **29**), which is less potent in the RFE test (ED_{50} 50 mg/kg),[181] is reported to exhibit reduced gastric irritating effects in rodents.[181-183] Structure-activity relationships determined for a number of analogs indicate a crucial role of the 5-substituent of bucolome (**30**) for antiinflammatory activity.[184,185]

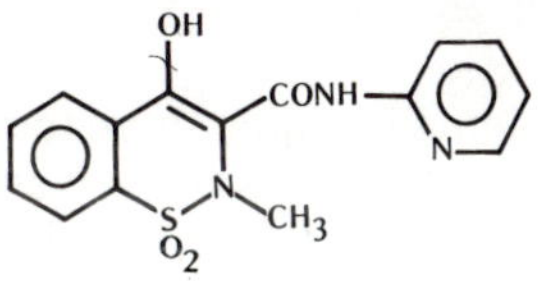

28

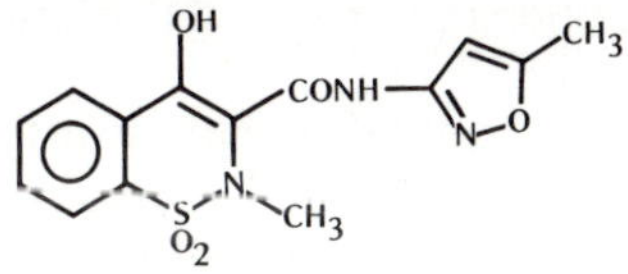

29

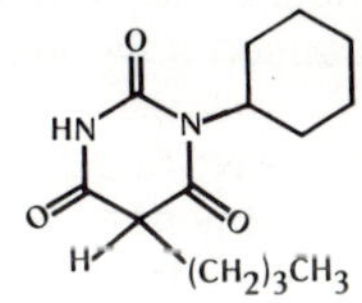

30

C. *Non-Acidic Compounds* — Non-acidic NSAI drugs, reviewed recently by Shen,[186] comprise a much smaller class of drugs, especially when one considers that several such compounds are merely pro-drugs (esters, hydroxamic acids, etc.) of the corresponding carboxylic acids. Meseclazone (W 2395, **31**) is active in the RFE test (ED_{50} 41 mg/kg) and the RAA model[187,188] and is less ulcerogenic than phenylbutazone in rats. The active species, however, is the hydrolysis product 5-chlorosalicylic acid.[189,190] The hydroxamic acids ibuproxam[191] (**32**) and indoxamic acid[192] (**33**) are related to ibuprofen and indomethacin, respectively. Rapid conversion of **32** to ibuprofen has been demonstrated in man.[193]

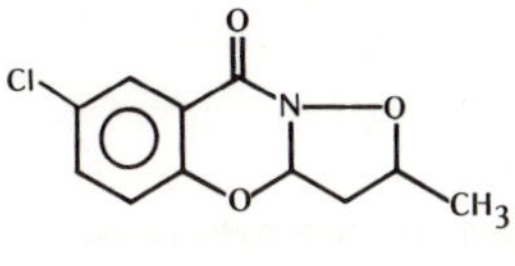

31

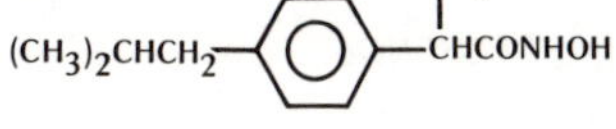

32

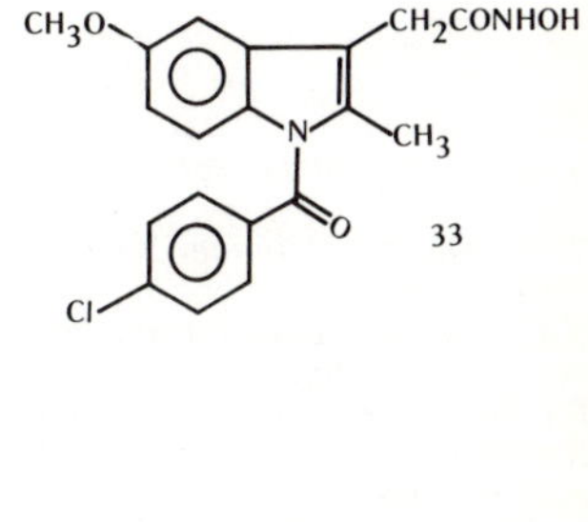

33

Etofenamate (**34**) is an ester pro-drug of flufenamic acid that rapidly penetrates skin after topical application. The pharmacology and toxicology of etofenamate are reported in a series of publications.[194] Clinical trials indicate that topically applied etofenamate produces beneficial effects in a variety of rheumatic diseases.[194] A longer half-life is observed for the parent drug after topical administration (3.3 hr) than after oral administration (1.6 hr). The activity of diphenpyramide (Z-876, **35**) (ED_{50} in the RFE test is 13 mg/kg) is reported to be mediated by its major metabolite, biphenylacetic acid.[195]

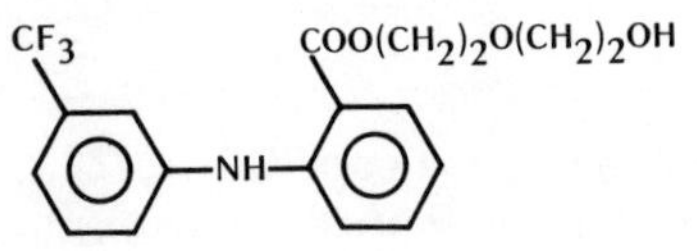

34

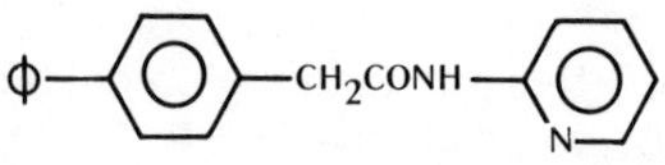

35

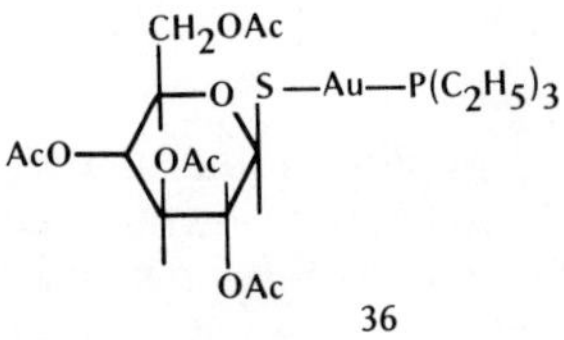

36

Auranofin (SKF D-39162, **36**), a gold derivative, has demonstrated activity following oral administration to either animals (RAA model)[196] or man (RA),[197] and serum IgG levels were observed to fall during therapy in man.

A series of publications review the present place of penicillamine in therapeutics.[199] In a recent double-blind multicenter trial, improvement was seen in a majority of RA patients but the drug caused adverse reactions in nearly 50% of patients.[198]

Conclusion — NSAI agents are of definite benefit to arthritic patients in aiding them to maintain a reasonably normal life by controlling the symptoms of inflammation. Although aspirin at high doses is often an effective antiinflammatory drug, toxic side-effects can limit its use. Individual variability in absorption and excretion leads to wide differences in serum concentrations after administration of a fixed dose of aspirin. Several of the newer NSAI drugs are more potent than aspirin on a dose basis and offer needed improved toleration. A longer half-life of some of the newer agents offers the convenience of less frequent dosing and provides more constant plasma drug levels with more uniform control of the symptoms of inflammation.

The immunoregulatory agents are at an earlier stage of development and those in clinical trials generally exhibit limiting side-effects. However, this class of compounds, rather than primarily alleviating symptoms, as the NSAI drugs do, offer the possibility of arresting the arthritic disease process and thereby halting progressive joint destruction. The trend in current drug research is toward the development of well-tolerated and safe drugs which will arrest or reverse the arthritic disease process.

REFERENCES

1. *S. Wong in "Annual Reports in Medicinal Chemistry, Vol. 10", Ed. R.V. Heinzelman, Academic Press, N. Y., 1975, p. 172.*
2. *Y.-H. Chang in "Annual Reports in Medicinal Chemistry, Vol. II", Ed. F.H. Clarke, Academic Press, N.Y., 1976, p. 138.*
3. *J.A. Mills, New Eng. J. Med.,* **290,** *781 and 1002 (1974).*
4. *W.L. Norton and M.A.P. Meisinger, Inflammation,* **2,** *37 (1977).*
5. *R.L. Roe, Med. Clinics North America,* **61,** *405 (1977).*
6. *R.L. Kaye and R.E. Pemberton, Arch. Int. Med.,* **136,** *1023 (1976).*
7. *E.C. Huskisson, Sem. Arth. Rheum.,* **7,** *1 (1977).*
8. *E. Arrigoni-Martelli, "Inflammation and Antiinflammatories", Halsted Press, New York, 1977.*

9. C.J. Smyth and J.F. Bravo, Drugs, **10,** 394 (1975).
10. N.J. Gilmore, Ann. of Allergy, **37,** 420 (1976).
11. K. Brune, M. Glatt and P. Graf, Gen. Pharmacol., **7,** 27 (1976).
12. J.-P. Famaey, P.M. Brooks and W.C. Dick, Sem. Arth. Rheum., **5,** 63 (1975).
13. S.H. Ferreira and J.R. Vane, Ann. Rev. Pharmacol., **14,** 57 (1974).
14. I. Bonta, J. Thompson and K. Brune, "Inflammation: Mechanisms and Their Impact on Therapy," Birkhauser-Verlag, Basel, 1977.
15. J.C. Houck, J. Invest. Dermatol., **67,** 124 (1976).
16. P. Davies and R.J. Bonney, "Annual Reports in Medicinal Chemistry, Vol. 12," Ed. R.V. Heinzelman, Academic Press, N.Y., 1977, p. 152.
17. M. Shearn, Ed., Med. Clinics North America, **61,** Number 2, March 1977.
18. E.C. Huskisson and G.P. Velo, Eds., "Inflammatory Arthropathies", Excerpta Medica, Amsterdam, 1976.
19. Twenty-second Rheumatism Review, Arthritis Rheumatism, **19,** (6) Supplement (1976), pp. 1104-1116.
20. W.W. Buchanan and W.C. Dick, "Recent Advances in Rheumatology," Parts 1 and 2, Churchill Livingstone, London, 1976.
21. J.L. Gordon and B.L. Hazleman, Eds., "Rheumatoid Arthritis — Cellular Pathology and Pharmacology," North-Holland Publishing Co., Amsterdam, 1977.
22. R.N. Maini, "Immunology of the Rheumatic Diseases", The Williams and Wilkins Co., Baltimore, 1977.
23. J.P. Giroud, D.A. Willoughby and C.P. Velo, Eds., "Future Trends in Inflammation II," Birkhauser-Verlag, Basel, 1975.
24. a. J.R. Vane, J. Allergy Clin. Immunol., **58,** 691 (1976).
    b. G.P. Lewis, J. Reticuloendothel. Soc., **22,** 389 (1977).
25. H.J. Robinson and J.R. Vane, "Prostaglandin Synthetase Inhibitors," Raven Press, New York, 1974.
26. D.R. Robinson, M.B. McGuire and L. Levine, Ann. N.Y. Acad. Sci., **256,** 318 (1975).
27. G. Husby, A.D. Bankhurst and R.C. Williams, Jr., Arth. Rheum., **20,** 785 (1977).
28. J.M. Dayer, D.R. Robinson and S.M. Krane, J. Exp. Med., **145,** 1399 (1977).
29. F.G. Kantrowitz, L. Levine and D.R. Robinson, Arth. Rheum., **18,** 407 (1975).
30. D. Crook, A.J. Collins, P.A. Bacon and R. Chan, Ann. Rheum. Dis., **35,** 327 (1976).
31. S. Bombardieri, O. diMunno, C. Patrono, B.D. Grossi, G. Ciabattoni and G.P. Pasero, Scand. J. Rheumatol., **4,** Suppl. 8, 26 (1975).
32. M. Ali, W.H. Barnett, A.J. Stoessl and J.W. McDonald, Clin. Res., **24,** 669A (1976).
33. P. Carminate and L.J. Lerner, Proc. Soc. Exp. Biol. Med., **148,** 455 (1975).
34. R. Ziel and P. Krupp, Int. J. Clin. Pharmacol., **12,** 186 (1975).
35. J.W. Horodniak, E.D. Matz, D.T. Walz, B.M. Sutton, C.E. Berkoff, J.E. Zarembo and A.D. Bender, Res. Commun. Chem. Pathol. Pharmacol., **11,** 533 (1975).
36. C. Deby, M. Descamps, F. Binon and Z.M. Bacq, Biochem. Pharmacol., **24,** 1089 (1975).
37. M.J.H. Smith, A.W. Ford-Hutchinson and P.N.C. Elliott, J. Pharm. Pharmacol., **27,** 473 (1975).
38. R. Ceserani, M. Ferrari, G. Goldaniga, E. Moro, A. Buttinoni, Life Sciences, **21,** 223 (1977).
39. R.J. Taylor, Jr. and J.J. Salata, Biochem. Pharmacol., **25,** 2479 (1976).
40. J.M. Dayer, S.M. Krane, R.G.G. Russell and D.R. Robinson, Proc. Nat. Acad. Sci., **73,** 945 (1976).
41. S.C.L. Hong and L. Levine, Proc. Natl. Acad. Sci., **73,** 1730 (1976).
42. M.J.H. Smith, Agents Actions, **5,** 315 (1975)
43. I.L. Bonta, H. Bult, J.E. Vincent and F.J. Zijlstra, J. Pharm. Pharmac., **29,** 1 (1977).
44. C.H. Cashin, W. Dawson and E.A. Kitchen, J. Pharm. Pharmac., **29,** 330 (1977).
45. R. Deraedt, S. Jouquey, J. Benzoni and M. Peterfalvi, Arch. Int. Pharmacodyn., **224,** 30 (1976).
46. F.A. Kuehl, Jr., J.L. Humes, R.W. Egan, E.A. Ham, G.C. Beveridge, and C.G. Van Arman, Nature, **265,** 170 (1977).
47. I.M. Goldstein, C.L. Malmsten, H.B. Kaplan, H. Jindahl, B. Samuelsson and G. Weissman, Clin. Res. **25,** 518A (1977).
48. K.E. Eakins and P.S. Kulkarni, Brit. J. Pharmacol., **60,** 135 (1977).
49. S. Moncada, S. Bunting, K. Mullane, P. Thorogood and J.R. Vane, Prostaglandins, **13,** 611 (1977).
50. R.J. Gryglewski, Arch. Pharmacol., **29,** 585 (1977).
51. I. Rivkin, G.V. Foschi and C.H. Rosen, Proc. Soc. Exp. Biol. Med., **153,** 236 (1976).
52. J.R. Walker, M.J.H. Smith and A.W. Ford-Hutchinson, Agents Actions, **6,** 602 (1976).
53. R.J. Smith, C. Sabin, H. Gilchrist and S. Williams, Biochem. Pharmacol., **25,** 2171 (1976).
54. P.S. Ringrose, M.A. Parr and M. McLaren, Biochem. Pharmacol., **24,** 607 (1975).
55. R.J. Smith, J. Pharm. Exp. Ther., **200,** 647 (1977).
56. I. Spilberg, A. Gallacher, B. Mandell and D. Rosenberg, Agents Actions, **7,** 153 (1977).
57. Y. Oyanagui, Biochem. Pharmacol., **25,** 1473 (1976).
58. Y. Mizushima, Y. Ishii and S. Masumoto, Biochem. Pharmacol., **24,** 1589 (1975).
59. T.J. Williams and M.J. Peck, Nature, **270,** 530 (1977).
60. R.C. Imrie, Lab. Animal Sci., **26,** 345 (1976).
61. S.R. Naik and U.K. Sheth, J. Postgrad. Med., **22,** 5 (1976).
62. I.L. Bonta and H. Bult, Life Sciences, **16,** 805 (1975).

63. *J.W. Hollingsworth, D.S. Greenberg and M. Dawson, Proc. Soc. Exper. Biol. Med.,* **152,** *183 (1976).*
64. *K. Kayashima, T. Koga and K. Onoue, J. Immunol.,* **117,** *1878 (1976).*
65. *Y.-H. Chang, J. Pharm. Exp. Therap.,* **201,** *1 (1977).*
66. *Y.-H. Chang, Arth.Rheum.,* **20,** *1135 (1977).*
67. *A.W. Pircio, C.T. Fedele and M.E. Bierwagen, Europ. J. Pharmacol.,* **31,** *207 (1975).*
68. *J. Wax, D.K. Tessman, C.V. Winder and M.D. Stephens, J. Pharm. Exp. Therap.,* **192,** *166 (1975).*
69. *W. Mohr and A. Wild, Z. Rheumatol.,* **35,** *301 (1976).*
70. *W. Mohr and A. Wild, Arzneim.-Forsch.,* **26,** *1860 (1976).*
71. *N.M. Hadler, Arth. Rheum.,* **19,** *256 (1976).*
72. *A. Fox and L.E. Glynn, Ann. Rheum. Dis.,* **34,** *431 (1975).*
73. *D.J. Carmichael, G.C. Gillard, D.A. Lowther, C.J. Handley and V.B. Santer, Arth. Rheum.,* **20,** *834 (1977).*
74. *M.B. Goldlust, L.C. Rich and T.W. Harrity, Arth. Rheum.,* **20,** *937 (1977).*
75. *K. Fehr, M. Velvart, A. Boni, H. Watanabe, M.A. Spycher and J.R. Ruttner, Ann. Rheum. Dis.,* **35,** *85 (1976).*
76. *T.G. White, J.L. Puls and P. Hargrave, Clin. Immunol. Immunopath.,* **3,** *531 (1975).*
77. *B.R. Bloom, Advances in Immunology,* **14,** *101 (1971).*
78. *S. Cohen, Amer. J. Pathol.,* **88,** *502 (1977).*
79. *M.E. Gershwin and A.D. Steinberg, Sem. Arth. Rheum.,* **6,** *125 (1976).*
80. *C.W. Parker, New Eng. J. Med.,* **295,** *1180 (1976).*
81. *T.B. Tomasi, Jr. and J.D. Stobo, Disease-a-Month,* **23** *(5), 3 (1977).*
82. *J. Symoens and M. Rosenthal, J. Reticuloendothel. Soc.,* **21,** *175 (1977).*
83. *U. Trabert, M. Rosenthal and W. Muller, Schweiz. med. Wschr.,* **106,** *1293 (1976).*
84. *Y. Dinai and M. Pras, Lancet,* **2,** *556 (1975).*
85. *M. Lequesne and J. Floquet, Nouv. Press. Med.,* **5,** *358 (1976).*
86. *J. Sany, G. Morlock, J. Clot and H. Serre, Revue Rhumatisme,* **44,** *143 (1977).*
87. *Abstracts of the XIVth International Congress of Rheumatology, San Francisco, June 1977, abstracts 1073, 1087, 1093 and 1099.*
88. *M. Rosenthal, Y. Breysse, P. Franchimont, K.L. Schmidt, E. Veys, A. St. J. Dixon, E.C. Huskisson, Y. Schuermans, T.L. Vischer, P.A.J. Janssen, J. Brugmans, W. K. Amery, J. DeCrepe, J. Symoens and A.L. Macnair, Lancet,* **1,** *904 (1977).*
89. *M.S. Al-Ibrahim, R.S. Holzman and H.S. Lawrence, J. Infect. Dis.,* **135,** *517 (1977).*
90. *L. Molin and O. Stendahl, Scand. J. Haematol.,* **19,** *93 (1977).*
91. *A.R. Rabson, D.A. Whiting, R. Anderson, A. Glover and H.J. Koornhof, J. Infect. Dis.,* **135,** *113 (1977).*
92. *M.C. Pike and R. Snyderman, Nature,* **261,** *136 (1976).*
93. *U. Trabert, M. Rosenthal and W. Muller, J. Rheumatol.,* **3,** *166 (1976).*
94. *F. Delbarre, Biomedicine,* **27,** *97 (1977).*
95. *L.W. Klassen, D.R. Budman, G.W. Williams, A.D. Steinberg and N.L. Gerber, Science,* **195,** *787 (1977).*
96. *A. Russell, J. Rheumatol.,* **3,** *380 (1976).*
97. *E. Arrigoni-Martelli, E. Bramm, E.C. Huskisson, D.A. Willoughby and P.A. Dieppe, Agents Actions,* **6,** *613 (1976).*
98. *A.L. Fenichel, F.J. Gregory and H.E. Alburn, Brit. J. Cancer,* **33,** *329 (1976).*
99. *a. Belgian Patent 842,832 (1976).*
    b. Y. Ohsugi, S-I. Hata, M. Tanemura, T. Nakano, T. Matsuno, Y. Takagaki, Y. Nishii and M. Shindo, J. Pharm. Pharmac., **29,** *636 (1977).*
100. *R. Wyburn-Mason, Lancet,* **1,** *489 (1976).*
101. *I. Otterness and J. Niblack, Lancet,* **1,** *148 (1976).*
102. *K. Lund-Olesen, Curr. Therap. Res.,* **21,** *704 (1977).*
103. *L. Riesterer, H. Majer and R. Jaques, Experientia,* **27,** *546 (1971).*
104. *L.T. Webster, Jr., A.E. Butterworth, A.A.F. Mahmoud, E.N. Mngola and K.S. Warren, New Eng. J. Med.,* **292,** *1144 (1975).*
105. *A.A.F. Mahmoud, M.A. Mandel, K.S. Warren and L.T. Webster, Jr., J. Immunology,* **114,** *279 (1975).*
106. *J.C. Daniels, K.S. Warren and J.R. David, J. Immunology,* **115,** *1414 (1975).*
107. *P.Y. Patterson, J.M. Harvey and L.T. Webster, Jr., J. Immunology,* **118,** *2151 (1977).*
108. *C.C.A. Bernard, J. Leydon, and I.R. Mackay, Int. Arch. Allergy Appl. Immunol.,* **53,** *555 (1977).*
109. *S.D. Deodhar, V.W. Lee, T. Chiang, A.F. Mahmoud and K.S. Warren, Cancer Res.,* **36,** *3147 (1976).*
110. *O. Bulay, H. Urman, D.B. Clayson and P. Shubik, J. Natl. Cancer Inst.,* **59,** *1625 (1977).*
111. *B.M. Jones, M. Bird, P. Massey, D. Millar, J.J. Miller, S. Reeves and J.R. Salaman, Brit. Med. J.,* **2,** *792 (1977).*
112. *H.H. Freedman, A.E. Fox, J. Shavel, Jr. and G.C. Morrison, Proc. Soc. Exper. Biol. Med.,* **139,** *909 (1972).*
113. *H. van Dijk, I.A. Bakker, J. Testerink, N. Bloksma and J.M. Willers, J. Immunology,* **115,** *1587 (1975).*
114. *M.E. Scheetz, L.J. Thomas, J. Harrington, and M.R. Schinitsky, Abstracts of the Reticuloendothelial Society meeting, December, 1976. Abstract 97.*
115. *M.E. Scheetz, D.G. Carlson and M.R. Schinitsky, Infect. Immun.,* **15,** *145 (1977).*
116. *R.F. Willkens and W. M. O'Brien, Bull. Rheum. Dis.,* **24,** *770 (1974).*
117. *J.G. Lombardino, I.G. Otterness and E.H. Wiseman, Arzneim.-Forsch.,* **25,** *1629 (1975).*
118. *Von U. Jahn, Th. Wagner-Jauregg, Arzneim.-Forsch.,* **24,** *494 (1974).*

119. J. Wax, C.V. Winder, D.K. Tessman and M.D. Stephens, J. Pharm. Exper. Ther., **192**, 172 (1975).
120. Von K. Morsdorf and G. Wolf, Arzneim.-Forsch., **27**, 531 (1977).
121. S.S. Bloomfield, T.P. Barden and J. Mitchell, Clin. Pharmacol. Therap., **21**, 99 (1977).
122. A. Kajander, V. Laine and G. Gothni, Scand. J. Rheumatol., **1**, 91 (1972).
123. A. Kajander, J. Martio, O. Mutru and G. Gothoni, Scand. J. Rheumatol., **5**, 158 (1976).
124. C.K. Axelsson, L.V. Christiansen, A. Johansen and P.E. Poulsen, Scand. J. Rheumatol., **6**, 23 (1977).
125. S.L. Steelman, G.O. Breault, D. Tocco, G.H. Bresselaar, K.F. Tempero, P.M. Lutterbeck, C.V. Perrier, F.W. Gribnau and M. Hinselman, Clin. Pharm. Therap., **17**, 245 (1975).
126. D.A. Willoughby, V. Wright and P. Turner, eds., Brit. J. Clin. Pharmacol., **4**, Suppl. 1, 1977.
127. P.A. Dieppe, H.C. Burry, R. Grahame and T. Perera, Rheum. Rehabil., **15**, 112 (1976).
128. J. Calabro, S.Y. Andelman, J.R. Caldwell, R.C. Gerber, D. Hamaty, H. Kaplan, B.A. Maltz, J.L. Parsons, P. Saville, H.C. Tretbar and J.R. Ward, Clin. Pharm. Therap., **22**, 358 (1977).
129. P.M.G. Reynolds, A.R. Rhymer, M.M. MacLeod and W.W. Buchanan, Curr. Med. Res. Opinion, **4**, 485 (1977).
130. D.E. Duggan, K.F. Hooke, E.A. Risley, T.Y. Shen and C.G. Van Arman, J. Pharm. Exp. Ther., **201**, 8 (1977).
131. P.G. Bianchi, M. Petrillo, E. Caruso and M. Fumagalli, Lancet, **1**, 1152 (1977).
132. A. Cohen, Clin. Pharm. Therap., **20**, 238 (1976).
133. J.E. Davies, D.N. Kellett and J.C. Pennington, Arch. Int. Pharmacodyn., **221**, 274 (1976).
134. G. D'Atri, E. Galimberti, S. Cerutti and A. Forlani, Boll. Chim. Farm., **114**, 107 (1975).
135. E. Galimberti, S. Cerutti, A. Forlani and G. d'Atri, Arzneim.-Forsch., **26**, 392 (1976).
136. R.L. Procaccini, R.D. Smyth, N.H. Reavey-Cantwell, Biochem. Pharmacol., **26**, 1051 (1977).
137. G.W. Nuss, R.D. Smyth, C.H. Breder, M.J. Hitchings, G.N. Mir and N.H. Reavey-Cantwell, Agents Actions, **6**, 735 (1976).
138. A.F. DeLong, R.D. Smyth, A. Polk, R.K. Nayak, G. Martin, G.H. Douglas and N.H. Reavey-Cantwell, Drug Metab. Disposition **5**, 122 (1977).
139. C.A. Demerson, L.G. Humber and A.H. Philipp, J. Med. Chem., **19**, 391 (1976).
140. R.R. Martel and J. Klicius, Can. J. Physiol. Pharmacol., **54**, 245 (1976).
141. M. Colot, M. VanDamme, M. Dirks, J. Beersaerts and R. Charlier, Arch. Int. Pharmacodyn., **208**, 328 (1974).
142. J. Damas and C. Deby, Biochem. Pharmacol., **25**, 983 (1976).
143. Scand. J. Rheum., **4**, Suppl. 8 (1975).
144. A. Allais, J. Meier, J. Mathieu, G. Nomine, M. Peterfalvi, R. Daraedt, L. Chifflot, J. Benzoni and R. Fournex, Eur. J. Med. Chem., **10**, 187 (1975).
145. W. Tsukada, M. Tsubokawa, T. Masukawa, H. Kojima and A. Kasahra, Jap. J. Pharmacol., **26**, Suppl. 124P (1976).
146. K. Hirai and H. Sugimoto, Chem. Pharm. Bull. (Tokyo), **25**, 2292 (1977).
147. D.W. Dunwell, D. Evens, T.A. Hicks, C.H. Cashin and A. Kitchen, J. Med. Chem., **18**, 53 (1975).
148. C.H. Cashin, W. Dawson and E.A. Kitchen, J. Pharm. Pharmac., **29**, 330 (1977).
149. G.L. Smith, R.A. Goulbourn, R.A.P. Burt and D.H. Chatfield, Brit. J. Clin. Pharmacol., **4**, 585 (1977).
150. A. Buttinoni, A. Cuttica, J. Franceschini, V. Mandelli, G. Orsini, N. Passerini, C. Turba and R. Tommasini, Arzneim.-Forsch., **23**, 1100 (1973).
151. I. Caruso, G. Corvi, L.M. Fucella, E. Moro, G. Sachetti, V. Tamassia, and G.P. Tosolini, Int. J. Clin. Pharmacol., **15**, 411 (1977).
152. V. Ventatridda, G. Martino, V Mandelli and A. Emanueli, Clin. Pharmacol. Therap., **17**, 284 (1974).
153. G.B. Porro, G. Corvi, L.M. Fuccella, G.C. Goldaniga and G. Valzelli, J. Intern. Med. Res., **5**, 155 (1977).
154. M. Peruzza, B. Finzi, J. Parini and A. Emanueli, Int. J. Clin. Pharmacol., **14**, 81 (1976).
155. F. DeClerk, J. Vermylen and R. Reneman, Arch. Int. Pharmacodyn., **216**, 263 (1975).
156. Eleven consecutive papers in Arzneim.-Forsch., **25**, pp. 1495-1542 (1975).
157. L.O. Randall and H. Baruth, Arch. Int. Pharmacodyn., **220**, 94 (1976).
158. W. Dairman, R. M. McLain, L.P. Juhasz and G. Roberts, Toxicol. Appl. Pharmacol., **37**, 184 (1976).
159. C.B. Coutinho, J.A. Cheripko and T. Crews, Toxicol. Appl. Pharmacol., **37**, 182 (1976).
160. Z.N. Gaut, H. Baruth, L.O. Randall, C. Ashley and J.R. Paulsrud, Prostaglandins, **10**, 59 (1975).
161. H.A. Silverman, T.G. Lawrence and J.D. Holloman, Abstracts of the XIVth International Congress of Rheumatology, San Francisco, 1977. Abstract 1163.
162. J. Pottier, D. Berlin and J.P. Raynaud, J. Pharm. Sci., **66**, 1030 (1977).
163. A.V. Camp, Scand. J. Rheumatol., **4**, Suppl. 8, 96 (1975).
164. M. Neuman, Drugs of Today, **12**, 238 (1976).
165. K.F. Swingle, R.A. Scherrer and T.J. Grant, Arch. Int. Pharmacodyn., **214**, 240 (1975).
166. A. Arsenault, E. LeBel and A. Lussier, J. Clin. Pharmacol., **16**, 473 (1976).
167. A series of 26 publications on Zepelin, DA-2370, Arzneim.-Forsch., **22**, issue 1a, pp. 171-278 (1972).
168. R.M. Collins, A.F. El-Ghobarey, L.S. Bain and B. Donovan, Clin. Trials J., **12**, 25 (1975).
169. R. Sturrock, A. Isaacs and F.D. Hart, Practitioner, **215**, 94 (1975).
170. P.J. Rooney, M. McLeod, D.M. Grennan and W.C. Dick, Curr. Med. Res. Opinion, **3**, 642 (1976).
171. L. Bain, M.P. Lynch and G.M. Bruce, Curr. Med. Res. Opinion, **4**, 665 (1977).
172. M.R. Fletcher, W. Loebl and J.T. Scott, Ann. Rheum. Dis., **34**, 190 (1975).
173. H.G. Dean, B. Donovan, C. Murray-Leslie and P. Rylett, Arzneim.-Forsch., **26**, 1700 (1976).
174. K. Pavelka, O. Vojtisek, A. Bremova, D. Kaukova and D. Handlova, Int. J. Clin. Pharmacol., **14**, 20 (1976).

175. J. Castaner and E. Arrigoni-Martelli, Drugs of the Future, **2**, 124 (1977).
176. E.H. Wiseman, Y-H. Chang and J.G. Lombardino, Arzneim.-Forsch., **26**, 1300 (1976).
177. Abstracts of papers, XIVth International Congress of Rheumatology, San Francisco, 1977; Abstracts 963-976.
178. M. Weintraub, R.F. Jacox, C.D. Angevine and E.C. Atwater, J. Rheumatology, **4**, 393 (1977).
179. T.J. Carty, Pharmacologist, **19**, 149 (1977).
180. E.H. Wiseman, Abstracts of papers, Piroxicam Symposium, XIVth International Congress of Rheumatology, San Francisco, 1977; Abstract 964.
181. G. DiPasquale, C. Rassaert, R. Richter, P. Welaj, J. Gingold and R. Singer, Agents Actions, **5**, 256 (1975).
182. G. DiPasquale, C. Rassaert, P. Welaj and L. Tripp, Agents Actions, **6**, 748 (1976).
183. G. DiPasquale and D. Mellace, Agents Actions, **7**, 481 (1977).
184. E. Mizuta, N. Suzuki, Y. Miyake, M. Nishikawa and T. Fujita, Chem. Pharm. Bull. (Japan), **23**, 5 (1975).
185. K. Kitani, Gastroenterology, **69**, 837 (1975).
186. T.-Y. Shen, Drugs Exptl. Clin. Res., **2**, 1 (1977).
187. R.D. Sofia, W. Diamantis, R. Gordon, M. Kletzkin, F.M. Berger, J. Edelson, H. Singer and J.F. Douglas, Eur. J. Pharmacol., **26**, 51 (1974).
188. D.B. Reisner, B.J. Ludwig, F.J. Stiefel, S. Gister, M. Meyer, L.S. Powell and R.D. Sofia, Arzneim.-Forsch., **27**, 760 (1977).
189. J. Edelson, J.F. Douglas, B.J. Ludwig, E.B. Schuster and S. Shahinian, J. Pharm. Sci., **64**, 1316 (1975).
190. R.D. Sofia, Agents Actions, **7**, 289 (1977).
191. G. Orzalesi, R. Selleri, O. Caldini, I. Volpato, F. Innocenti, J. Colome, A. Sacristan and G. Varez, Arzneim.-Forsch., **27**, 1006 (1977).
192. F. DeMartiis, N. Corsico, J.S. Franzone and T. Tamietto, Boll. Chim. Farm., **114**, 319 (1975).
193. G. Orzalesi, R. Selleri, O. Caldini, I. Volpato, F. Innocenti, J. Colome, A. Sacristan, G. Varez and G. Pisaturo, Arzneim.-Forsch., **27**, 1012 (1977).
194. A series of 10 consecutive publications in Arzneim.-Forsch., **27**, 1299-1364 (1977).
195. S. Caliari, L. Alfieri, G.B. Gervasi, M.P. Sangiovanni and F. Scrollini, Arzneim.-Forsch., **27**, 2086 (1977).
196. D.T. Walz, M.J. DiMartino, L.W. Chakrin, B.M. Sutton and A. Misher, J. Pharmacol. Exper. Therap., **197**, 142 (1976).
197. A.E. Finkelstein, D.T. Walz, V. Batista, M. Mizraji, F. Roisman and A. Misher, Ann. Rheum. Dis., **35**, 251 (1976).
198. Y. Shiokawa, Y. Horiuchi, M. Honma, T. Kageyama, T. Okada and T. Azuma, Arth. Rheum., **20**, 1464 (1977).
199. Proc. Royal Soc. Med., **70**, Suppl. 3 (1977).

Chapter 19. Mechanisms of Action of Glucocorticosteroids

Anthony S. Fauci, National Institute of Allergy and Infectious Diseases,

NIH, Bethesda, MD 20014

Introduction - Glucocorticosteroids display a variety of complex effects on different biologic systems and cell types. This review will focus on the mechanisms of action of these agents on inflammatory and immune responses, particularly with respect to human biology *in vivo*. Effects of glucocorticosteroids on vascular tissue, leukocyte kinetics and function, and various humoral factors involved in these responses will be considered. The structures of some typical corticosteroids are shown below.

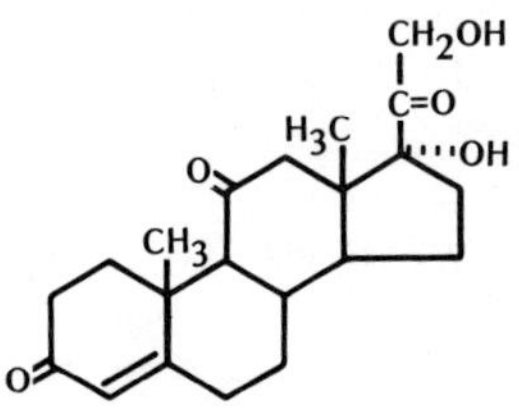

Cortisone

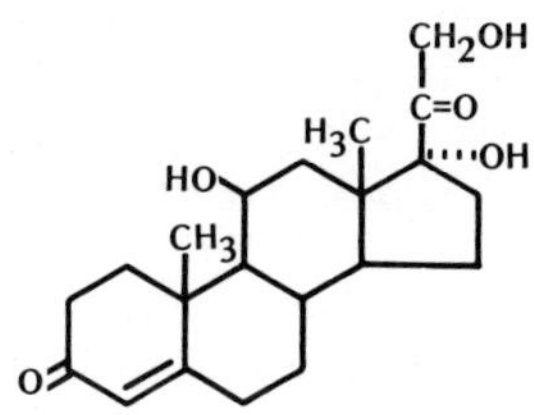

Hydrocortisone (Cortisol)

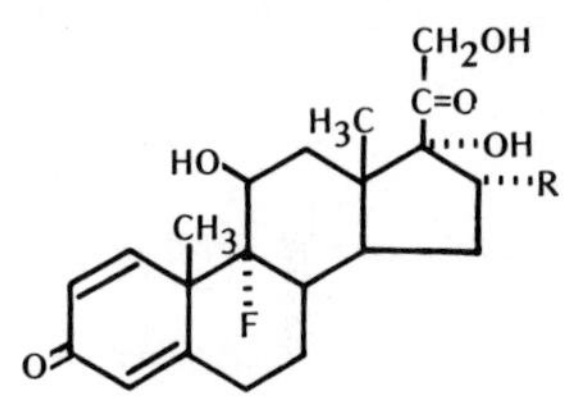

Triamcinolone (R=OH)
Dexamethasone (R=CH_3)

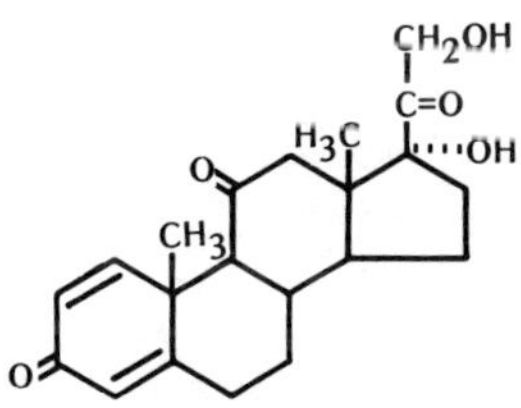

Prednisone

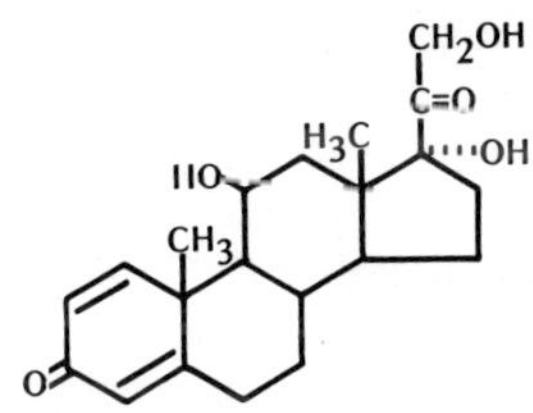

Prednisolone

Corticosteroid Receptors - The precise molecular mechanisms whereby corticosteroids exert their divergent effects are not well delineated at present. However, it has been demonstrated in a variety of models that many of the cellular and tissue effects of corticosteroids are triggered through an interaction with intracytoplasmic steroid receptors in the target cell.[1-3] The steroid-receptor complexes thus formed migrate to, and become associated with the cell nucleus. This leads to the synthesis of specific mRNA which, in turn, induces new protein synthesis. The newly synthesized protein may be an enzyme or an inhibitory protein, and it is highly likely that such a mechanism is responsible for the modulatory effect of corticosteroids on leukocytes involved in inflammatory or immune responses.[4,5]

Tissue and Vascular Effects - Inflammatory and immunologically mediated reactions are almost invariably associated with extravasation of fluid and cells from the intravascular compartment into surrounding tissues via leakage from capillaries and venules.[6]

ISBN 0-12-040513-X

Clearly, corticosteroid administration inhibits the leakage of fluids and cells into inflammatory sites.[7] Several mechanisms for this effect have been proposed, the most obvious being vasoconstriction of the capillaries.[8,9] It is not presently clear how this effect arises; however, antagonism of vasoactive substances such as histamine,[9] kinins,[10,11] or plasminogen activator[12] have been suggested to be involved.

Kinetics and Traffic of Cells - Corticosteroid administration in man has profound effects on the distribution and circulatory properties of various populations of leukocytes.[13-17] The effect is transient and related to the dose and dose-interval of administered drugs.

Approximately 4 hours following intravenous administration of 100 to 400 mg of hydrocortisone or its equivalent to man, a dramatic, but transient, lymphocytopenia and monocytopenia occur, with a return to normal counts by 24 hours.[13,16,18] The mechanism of this cell depletion from the circulation is not a result of cell death, as is the case with corticosteroid-induced lymphopenia in corticosteroid-sensitive species, such as mouse, rat and rabbit. Rather, it is caused by a redistribution of these cells out of the circulation into other body compartments, such as bone marrow.[14,15] In fact, normal human mononuclear cells are extremely resistant to corticosteroid-induced lympholysis seen in mouse and rat.

The intravascular lymphocytes most susceptible to this redistribution belong to the recirculating pool of lymphocytes which, under normal circumstances, is in constant equilibrium with the extravascular lymphocyte pool in thoracic duct, spleen, lymph nodes, and bone marrow.[14,15] Although most identifiable subpopulations of lymphocytes are affected to some degree, corticosteroid administration selectively depletes thymus-derived (T) cells more than bone marrow-derived (B) cells[13,16,18] and, within the T cell population, cells with IgM-receptors are depleted to a greater extent than cells with IgG-receptors.[19]

The eosinopenia resulting from corticosteroid administration is also thought to result from a redistribution of these cells out of the circulation into other body compartments.[20]

The precise mechanism for the redirection of cell traffic is unclear. Cells normally enter and leave the circulation by migrating through the endothelium of the microvasculature. Complementary surface configurations and interactions between the circulating cells and the endothelial cells of the vessels probably influence entrance and egress of cells to and from the intravascular compartment.[15] It is uncertain whether corticosteroids exert their effects on the circulating cells or on the vascular endothelium. However, *in vitro* alteration of the lymphocyte surface configuration results in similar changes in circulation patterns following reinfusion of these cells.[21-25] This suggests that corticosteroids alter traffic patterns of cells by affecting their surface charge or receptors, thereby interfering with lymphocyte-microvascular interactions.

Corticosteroid administration also markedly influences neutrophil kinetics. The resulting granulocytosis is a consequence of multiple effects including enhancement of neutrophil release from bone marrow reserves, prolongation of neutrophil half-life, and inhibition of neutrophil migration into inflammatory sites.[17] It is this last effect which is closely linked to the anti-inflammatory effects of corticosteroids.

Corticosteroids inhibit the adherence of neutrophils to the microvascular endothelium of an inflammatory locus.[26] In addition, it has been shown that in vivo administration of corticosteroids results in decreased in vitro adherence of neutrophils to nylon wool columns.[27] Since one of the first recognizable events in the process of neutrophil influx into inflammatory loci is adherence of neutrophils to the vascular endothelium, it appears likely that inhibition of this intial step is an important mechanism in the interruption of neutrophil migration.

Functional Capabilities of Cells. To accurately delineate the effects of corticosteroids on various functional parameters of the different classes of leukocytes one has to distinguish between effects which are attainable in vivo and effects which cannot be achieved in vivo because they require suprapharmacologic drug concentrations.

The activities of corticosteroids both in vivo and in vitro on most recognizable cell functions involved in inflammatory and immunologic reactions have been described.[1,2,17,28,29,30] These include effects on cell activation, proliferation, and differentiation; expression of cell surface markers and surface receptor function; phagocytosis, lysosomal membrane stability, antigen processing, and microbial killing; and cytotoxic functions and response to soluble mediators. All of these functions can be suppressed by sufficiently high concentrations of corticosteroids in vitro. However, relatively few of these are affected by drug concentrations that can be achieved in man in vivo.[17] In contrast, the effects of corticosteroids on cell kinetics and migration patterns are elicited readily by concentrations that are achieved in vivo.[17]

If one compares the relative corticosteroid effects on the functional capabilities of the two major circulating phagocytic cells, the neutrophil and monocyte, it is clear that the monocyte is more susceptible to drug concentrations attainable in vivo. Not only are the circulatory kinetics of the monocyte sensitive to these concentrations, but functional properties, such as phagocytosis and microbial killing, are also impared.[31] Neutrophil phagocytosis and microbial killing are more resistant to corticosteroids at comparable drug concentrations.[17]

Cellular functions of lymphocytes such as occur during autologous mixed leukocyte reactions[32] and in the expression of suppressor cell activities[33,34] are particularly sensitive to physiologic concentrations of corticosteroids.

Despite studies showing corticosteroid-induced host defense effects, a low incidence of spontaneous infections has been reported in patients receiving corticosteroids.[17]

Effects on Humoral Factors - It is difficult to separate corticosteroid effects on humoral factors involved in inflammatory and immunologic reactions from effects on cellular functions since, in most cases, the humoral factors are cellular-derived. However, certain well defined humoral mechanisms are clearly influenced by corticosteroid administration.

Although antibody production, particularly secondary responses, are resistant to the effects of corticosteroids, total immunoglobulin synthesis can be suppressed by *in vivo* administration of high doses of corticosteroids.[35] Also, high doses of corticosteroids can result in a decreased level of serum complement components.[36] This effect is probably a manifestation of both decreased production and increased catabolism. Corticosteroids also can interfere with binding of certain immunoglobulins to the Fc receptor of certain cell types,[37,38] thus interfering with related functions such as phagocytosis and cytotoxic effector capabilities. Other potentially important effects of corticosteroids on humoral factor-related phenomena *in vitro* include inhibition of the response of macrophages to various lymphokines, particularly macrophage migration inhibitory factor,[39] and the interference with the response of neutrophils to soluble chemotactic factors.[40] The latter effect may be related to corticosteroid mediated inhibition of neutrophil adherence to vascular endothelium *in vivo*.

Summary - Corticosteroids can potentially interfere with virtually every phase of inflammatory and immunologic reactivity. Generally, kinetics and circulatory patterns of leukocytes are more sensitive to corticosteroid modulation than are functional effects of cells. In addition, various classes and subclasses of leukocytes appear to differ in sensitivity to corticosteroid effects. The precise mechanisms of their effects are still unclear. However, it is likely that they relate at least in part to specific receptor interaction of corticosteroid with the involved cells.

References

1. J.D. Baxter and P.H. Forsham, Am. J. Med. 53, 573 (1972).
2. E.B. Thompson and M.E. Lippman, Metabolism, 23, 159 (1974).
3. B.L. Levinson, J.D. Baxter, G.G. Rousseau and G.M. Tomkins, Science, 175, 189 (1972).
4. C. Hallahan, D.A. Young and A. Munck, J. Biol. Chem. 248, 2922 (1973).
5. J.D. Baxter and A.W. Harris, Transplant. Proc., 7, 55 (1975).
6. R.H. Ebert and L. Grant, In: "The Inflammatory Process". Zweifach, B.W., Grant, L., McCluskey, R.T. (eds.). New York: Academic Press, 1974.
7. B.W. Zweifach, E. Shorr and M.M. Black, Ann. N.Y. Acad. Sci., 56, 626 (1953).
8. L.C. Wyman, G.P. Fulton, M.H. Shulman and L.L. Smith, Am. J. Physiol. 176, 335 (1954).

9. R.W. Schayer, Prog. Allergy, 7, 187 (1963).
10. M.J. Cline and K.L. Melmon, Science, 153, 1135 (1966).
11. R.P. Suddick, Am. J. Physiol., 211, 844 (1966).
12. J. Vassalli, J. Hamilton and E. Reich, Cell, 8, 271 (1976).
13. A.S. Fauci and D.C. Dale, J. Clin. Invest., 53, 240 (1974).
14. A.S. Fauci and D.C. Dale, Blood, 46, 235 (1975).
15. A.S. Fauci, Transplant. Proc., 7, 37 (1975).
16. A.S. Fauci and D.C. Dale, J. Clin. Invest., 55, 22 (1975).
17. A.S. Fauci, D.C. Dale and J.E. Balow, Ann. Intern. Med., 84, 304 (1976).
18. D.T.Y. Yu, P.J. Clements, H.E. Paulus, J.B. Peter, J. Levy and E.V. Barnett, J. Clin. Invest. 53, 565 (1974).
19. B.F. Haynes and A.S. Fauci, J. Clin. Invest., 61, 703 (1978).
20. D.C. Dale, R.T. Hubert and A.S. Fauci, J. Lab. Clin. Med., 87, 487 (1976).
21. B.M. Gesner and V. Ginsburg, Proc. Natl. Acad. Sci. (USA), 52, 750 (1964).
22. J. Woodruff and B.M. Gesner, Science, 161, 1976 (1968).
23. H. Jacobsson and H. Blomgren, Clin. Exp. Immunol., 13, 439 (1973).
24. M. Schlesinger and E. Israel, Cell. Immunol., 14, 66 (1974).
25. J.J. Woodruff and J.R. Woodruff, Cell. Immunol., 10, 78 (1974).
26. R.H. Ebert and W.R. Barclay, Ann. Intern. Med., 37, 506 (1952).
27. R.R. MacGregor, P.J. Spagnuolo and A.L. Lentknek, N. Engl. J. Med. 291, 642 (1974).
28. D.S. David, M.H. Grieco and P. Cushman, Jr., J. Chronic Dis., 22, 637 (1970).
29. A.E. Gabrielsen and R.A. Good, Adv. Immunol., 6, 91 (1967).
30. R.B. Zurier and G. Weissman, Med. Clin. North Am., 57, 1295 (1973).
31. J.J. Rinehart, A.L. Sagone, S.P. Balcerzak, G.A. Ackerman, and A.F. LoBuglio, N. Engl. J. Med., 292, 236 (1975).
32. D.N. Ilfeld, R.S. Krakauer, and R.M. Blaese, J. Immunol., 119, 428 (1977).
33. A.S. Fauci, K.R. Pratt, and G. Whalen, J. Immunol., 119, 598 (1977).
34. S. Gupta and R.A. Good, Cell. Immunol., 34, 10 (1977).
35. W.T. Butler and R.T. Rossen, J. Clin. Invest., 52, 2629 (1973).
36. J.R. Atkinson and M.M. Frank, J. Immunol., 111, 1061 (1973).
37. A.D. Schreiber, J. Parsons, P. McDermott and R.A. Cooper, J. Clin. Invest., 56, 1189 (1975).
38. G.W. Hunninghake and A.S. Fauci, J. Immunol, 118, 146 (1977).
39. J.E. Balow and A.S. Rosenthal, J. Exp. Med., 137, 1031 (1973).
40. J.I. Gallin, J.R. Durocher and A.P. Kaplan, J. Clin. Invest., 55, 967 (1975).

Chapter 20. Pharmacologic Regulation of Serum Lipoproteins

Charles E. Day, The Upjohn Company, Kalamazoo, MI 49001

Introduction - Serum lipoproteins interact with the arterial wall to modulate the pathologic process of atherosclerosis. Therefore, regulation of serum lipoproteins is one rational approach toward the treatment and prophylaxis of this disease. This report will review some of the recent advances made in the pharmacologic control of serum lipoproteins in experimental animals and man.

Although the basic relationships between the different classes of serum lipoproteins and atherosclerosis have been known since 1950, the relevance of this information remained largely unappreciated until quite recently. The reexamination by Miller and Miller[1] of the relationship between serum high density lipoproteins (HDL) and coronary artery disease (CAD) sparked a resurgence of interest in the serum lipoproteins and their control. Therefore, most studies concerned with the effect of drugs on lipoproteins have been reported within the past two years.

Of the four basic classes of lipoproteins in human serum, three promote and one retards the development of atherosclerosis. Very low density lipoproteins (VLDL) and low density lipoproteins (LDL) are definitely atherogenic,[2-4] and chylomicrons are probably atherogenic as well.[5] A large body of recent epidemiologic information indicates an inverse relationship between HDL cholesterol and CAD.[6-10] In view of the known relationships between serum lipoproteins and atherosclerosis, a logical framework for combating this disease is to reduce LDL and VLDL and/or increase HDL. But even when the concentrations of serum lipoproteins can presumably be favorably altered by a drug, it should not be assumed that the atherosclerotic process is influenced similarly. It is conceivable, although unlikely, that a drug could reduce serum LDL for example by causing it to deposit in arteries. Any drug that regulates lipoproteins must necessarily be tested for its effect on atherosclerosis.

Effects of Specific Drugs on Lipoproteins

Adamantyloxyphenyl Compounds - One of the first agents reported to markedly decrease LDL and VLDL, while simultaneously increasing HDL in experimental animals, is adamantyloxyphenylpiperidine (AOPP) (1). In cholesterol-cholic acid fed hypercholesterolemic rats, AOPP, at a dose of 200 mg/kg/day, reduced atherogenic lipoproteins (LDL + VLDL) to 153 mg/dl from a control level of 1804 mg/dl, while concomitantly increasing HDL from 87 to 557 mg/dl.[11] AOPP was active after a single dose orally or intravenously and decreased hepatic cholesterol concentration after prolonged administration.[12] In our laboratory all lipoprotein modifying agents are routinely evaluated in SEA Japanese quail for their effect on atherosclerosis.[13-15] AOPP was lethal at an effective lipoprotein modifying dose in this model. However, a closely related analog, adamantyloxyaniline (2),

ISBN 0-12-040513-X

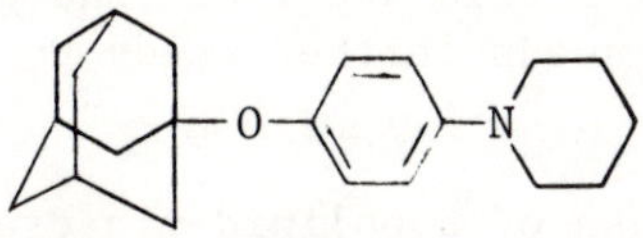

1 Adamantyloxyphenylpiperidine

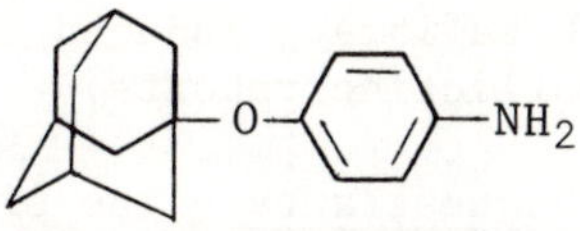

2 Adamantyloxyaniline

inhibited the development of experimental atheromas in proportion to the reduction of serum atherogenic lipoprotein levels.[16] The adamantyl compounds were discovered as a result of structure activity studies of their bicyclo-octyl analogs for which lipoprotein modifying activity was first reported.[17]

p-Aminosalicylic Acid (3) - This antituberculosis drug has been used on a very limited basis as a lipid lowering agent since it was first reported to lower serum cholesterol in 1954. A detailed study of its effect on serum lipoproteins was first published in 1976 when a reduction in VLDL, LDL, and HDL cholesterol levels of 49, 8, and 14%, respectively, was noted in patients who were mostly type II hyperlipoproteinemics.[18] Expanded studies on 30 patients consisting of both type II and type IV hyperlipoproteinemic individuals substantiated the decrease in VLDL and LDL cholesterol (46 and 6%, respectively) but failed to detect any change in HDL cholesterol.[19] In another study on 63 type II patients treated with this drug a 25% decrease in LDL cholesterol was noted.[20]

Bezafibrate (4) - This recently developed analog of clofibrate affects serum lipoproteins in much the same way as clofibrate, although at a somewhat lower dose (0.6 vs 1.5 g/day). In one study[21] bezafibrate reduced VLDL cholesterol and triglycerides in both types II and IV hyperlipoproteinemic patients. LDL cholesterol was reduced only in type II patients, and HDL cholesterol was not affected in either type II or IV individuals. Subsequent reports[22,23] by the same authors on a population of mixed hyperlipoproteinemic patients confirmed the reduction in VLDL cholesterol and triglycerides and in addition revealed that bezafibrate increased serum

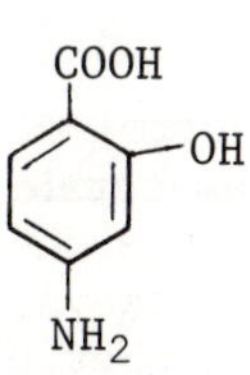

3 p-Aminosalicylic acid

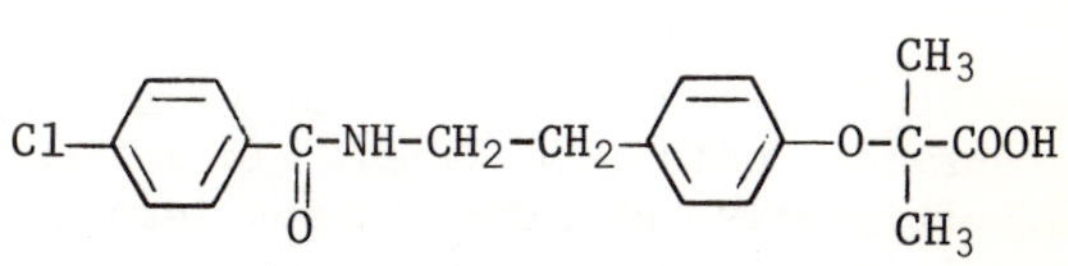

4 Bezafibrate

HDL cholesterol concentrations in the range of 20-30%. Another group of investigators[24,25] confirmed the rather marked effect of bezafibrate in reducing VLDL cholesterol and triglycerides but was not able to demonstrate an effect on HDL cholesterol. It was also noted that LDL cholesterol decreased by 15% in type II patients and increased by 16% in type IV individuals. This is consistent with an earlier finding[21] that the decrement in LDL cholesterol is proportional to the initial LDL level and that an increment in LDL may occur when initial levels are low. The question of a bezafibrate induced increment in HDL needs further study to resolve conflicting reports.

Bile Acid Sequestrants - The effect of this class of hypolipidemic drugs on serum lipoproteins and atherosclerosis was reviewed recently.[26] The clinically tested bile acid sequestrants (cholestyramine, colestipol, and polidexide) appear to be approximately equivalent in their biological effects. They reduce LDL, transiently increase VLDL, have no effect on HDL, and probably inhibit and reverse atherosclerosis. Greater LDL reduction can be achieved with sequestrants than with any other drugs presently commercially available in the U.S. Because of a reduction in cardiovascular mortality with long-term administration of colestipol,[27] sequestrants may eventually make a significant impact on controlling atherosclerosis. Two recent studies[28,29] on the effect of cholestyramine on serum lipoproteins confirm conclusions drawn from earlier studies. Reductions in LDL cholesterol of 30 to 40% were reported.

BR-931 (5) - This compound increased HDL cholesterol levels in both ethanol induced and cholesterol-cholic acid induced hyperlipidemic rats.[30,31] In cholesterol fed rabbits BR-931 increased HDL cholesterol by 53% and significantly reduced atherosclerosis in the aortic arch by 39%.[31] Like its parent compound, WY-14,643 (6), BR-931 is a potent inducer of hepatic peroxisomes.

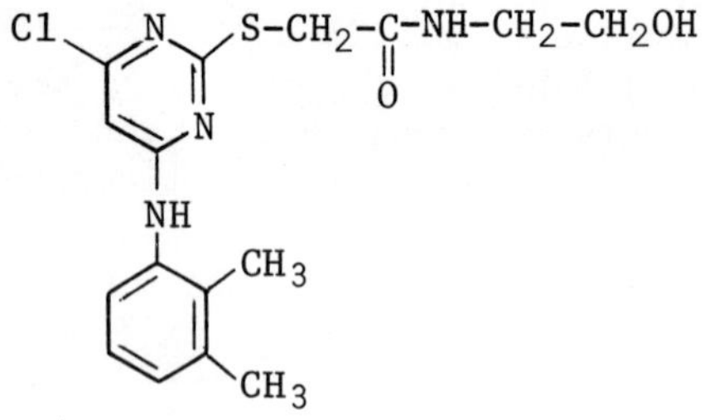

5 BR-931

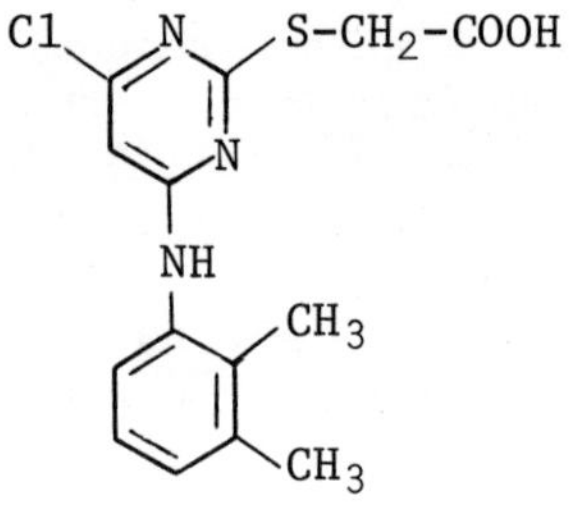

6 WY-14,643

Cetaben (7) - One of the most promising new agents for the control of atherosclerosis is cetaben. In cholesterol fed rabbits sodium cetaben significantly inhibits atherosclerosis and esterification of free cholesterol in the arterial wall.[32] In cholesterol fed cynomolgus monkeys treated with sodium cetaben at 100 mg/kg/day for 6 months, a number of beneficial effects were noted.[33] Atherosclerosis was inhibited by approximately 50% in all arterial beds examined, including coronary,

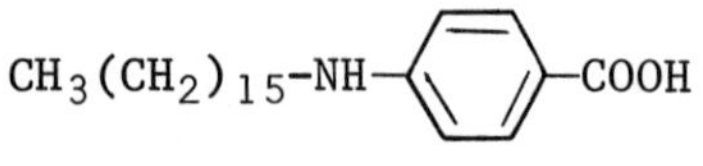

7 Cetaben

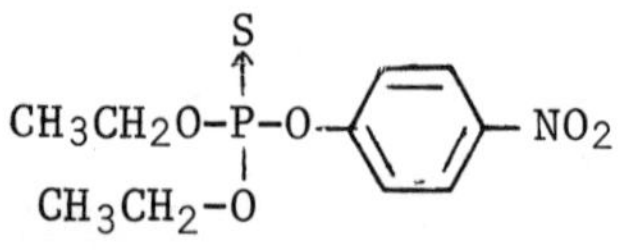

8 Parathion

carotid, and femoral arteries. Arterial cholesterol, collagen, and calcium were reduced likewise. Also, this agent reduced atherogenic LDL and VLDL concentrations in serum and increased HDL levels. Because of these numerous beneficial effects in a nonhuman primate, results of clinical testing are eagerly anticipated.

Cholinesterase Inhibitors - What may prove to be one of the most important clinical observations in the field of lipoprotein research was made by Kutty et al.[34] in 1975 on a 10 year old boy who was hospitalized after ingestion of the insecticide parathion (8). LDL levels were determined in the boy's serum drawn at 2 hour intervals for the first 12 hours after hospitalization. LDL levels dropped dramatically after only 6 hours from an initial value of 240 mg/dl to 30 mg/dl. The authors attributed the fall in LDL to the inhibition of serum cholinesterase by the parathion poisoning since this enzyme is intimately associated with LDL.[35] The same investigators have demonstrated that phospholine iodide (9) in guinea pigs[34] and

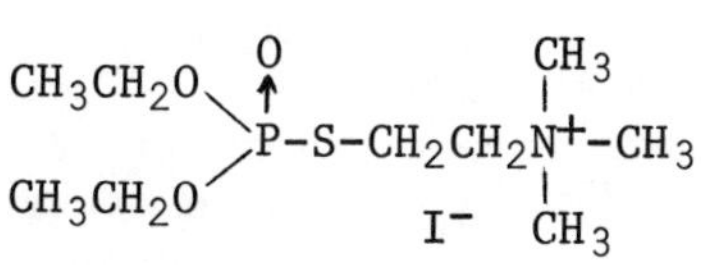

9 Phospholine iodide

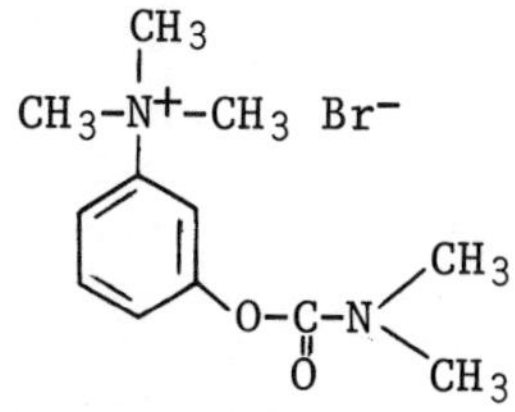

10 Neostigmine

neostigmine (10) in rats[36] cause a significant reduction in serum LDL levels that parallels the simultaneous reduction in serum cholinesterase activity. Assuming the validity of the rapid and dramatic reduction of LDL in the clinical case of parathion poisoning, much further work needs to be performed on the mechanism of this effect and the development of nontoxic drugs to mimic this activity.

Cinnarizine (11) - This antihistaminic and vasoactive agent has been used in Europe for several years to treat peripheral vascular disorders[37] and recently was tested for its effect on serum lipoproteins in a group of type II and IV hyperlipoproteinemic patients.[38] A progressive decrease in both LDL and VLDL was noted monthly through six months of treatment, at which time these lipoproteins were reduced by 35 and 78%, respectively. Even though it is vasoactive and hypolipoproteinemic, further studies will be necessary to evaluate the effect of cinnarizine on atherosclerotic disease in experimental animals or man.

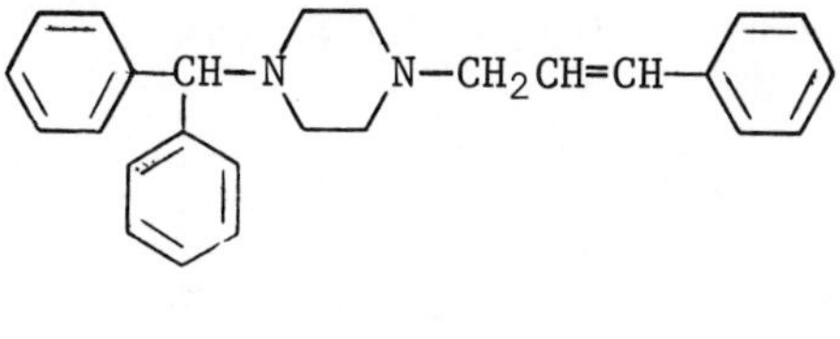

11 Cinnarizine

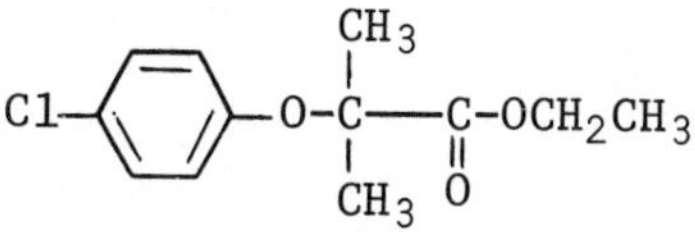

12 Clofibrate

Clofibrate (12) - Even though clofibrate is the most widely used and one of the first developed hypolipidemic agents in the world, surprisingly few studies have appeared on the effect of this drug on serum lipoproteins either in experimental animals or in man. Muller[39] reported that clofibrate in rats at 200 mg/kg/day reduced VLDL, LDL, and HDL cholesterol by 20, 22, and 41%, respectively. In another study[40] in normal rats at a dose of 120 mg/kg clofibrate reduced all lipoproteins, but with the greatest absolute reduction occurring in HDL. In normal baboons LDL cholesterol is increased by about 50% at 50 mg/kg and HDL cholesterol is decreased approximately 30% at 200 mg/kg.[41] Clinically, it has been known for several years that clofibrate exerts its greatest effect on VLDL.[42] More recently the clofibrate induced elevation in LDL was emphasized.[43] It now appears that the clofibrate induced LDL alterations from the treatment of hypertriglyceridemia are dependent on initial LDL values, with elevations occurring at initially low values and reductions effected at initially high LDL concentrations.[44] Clofibrate may induce a slight elevation in HDL cholesterol concentrations,[44-47] but at best the effect seems marginal.

Gemfibrozil (13) - Although this agent was disclosed for the first time only recently,[48,49] numerous studies have appeared concerning its effect on serum lipoproteins in man.[47,50-58] Howard[59] has recently summarized these studies, and in all clinical trials conducted with this drug there was a reduction in lipoprotein cholesterol of 58, 47, and 6% for chylomicrons, VLDL, and LDL, respectively. HDL cholesterol was increased 15%. Triglycerides were decreased in all lipoprotein fractions with reductions of 79, 43, 26, and 23% occurring in chylomicrons, VLDL, LDL, and HDL, respectively.

Like clofibrate, gemfibrozil does not appear to act via a single mechanism. It inhibits peripheral lipolysis, hepatic uptake of plasma free fatty acids, and synthesis of VLDL apoprotein.[59]

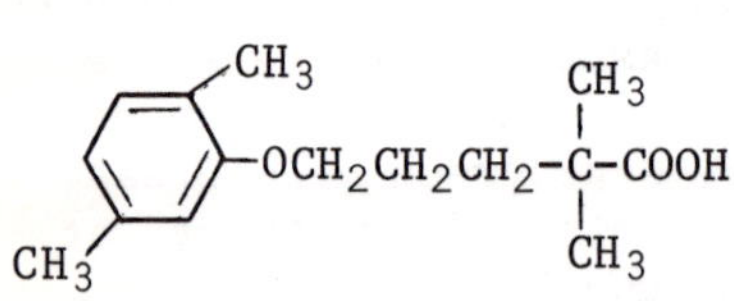

13 Gemfibrozil

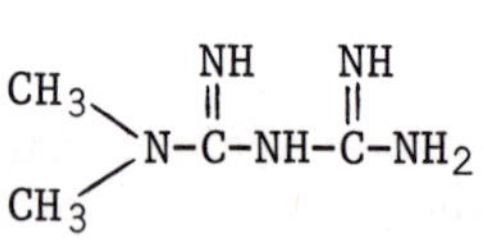

14 Metformin

Metformin (14) - Theoretically it is possible for a drug to alter the atherogenicity of a serum lipoprotein without altering its absolute concentration. The best documented example of such drug induced structural alteration in lipoproteins is metformin which inhibits the development of experimental atherosclerosis in cholesterol fed rabbits,[60] whereas other hypoglycemic agents do not.[61,62] Serum lipoproteins of cholesterol fed rabbits consist largely of cholesterol ester rich particles that float in the VLDL density range.[63,64] In a series of papers published within the past two years, Sirtori and his research group have demonstrated that metformin (a) increased the fractional catabolic rate of VLDL in hypercholesterolemic rabbits,[65] (b) altered the phospholipid composition of VLDL,[65,66] (c) reduced the interaction of VLDL with the arterial wall,[65] and (d) changed the apoprotein composition of serum lipoproteins.[66-69] Apolipoprotein E was decreased and albumin was increased in VLDL and HDL_2 by metformin in cholesterol fed rabbits. Apolipoprotein A-I levels were increased in chylomicrons, VLDL, and LDL. In man the concentrations of VLDL and intermediate density lipoprotein (IDL) were reduced in addition to the changes in apoprotein composition.[68-70]

In contrast to metformin, there is some controversy about the effect of other oral hypoglycemic agents on serum lipoproteins.[71,72] Controversy also exists about the effect of insulin on HDL in man.[72,73]

Nicotinic Acid (15) and Derivatives - In normal rats nicotinic acid decreased LDL and VLDL but had no effect on HDL cholesterol.[39] Clinically nicotinic acid has been reported to behave much like clofibrate causing a decrease in VLDL and either an increase or decrease in LDL depending on pretreatment values.[44] Xantinol nicotinate (16) has been reported to (a) decrease LDL[74] and not affect VLDL in type IIA hyperlipoproteinemia,[75] (b) decrease LDL and VLDL in type IIB,[75] (c) decrease chylomicrons and VLDL, increase LDL, and not affect HDL in type V hyperlipoproteinemia,[76] (d) decrease VLDL but not affect LDL and HDL in type IV,[77] and (e) have no effect on any lipoproteins in type IIA.[78] β-Pyridyl carbinol (17) decreased LDL approximately 30% in type IIA patients but had no effect on VLDL or HDL.[78]

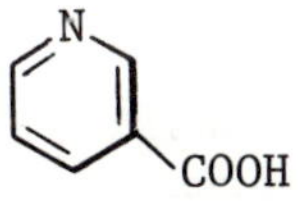

15 Nicotinic acid

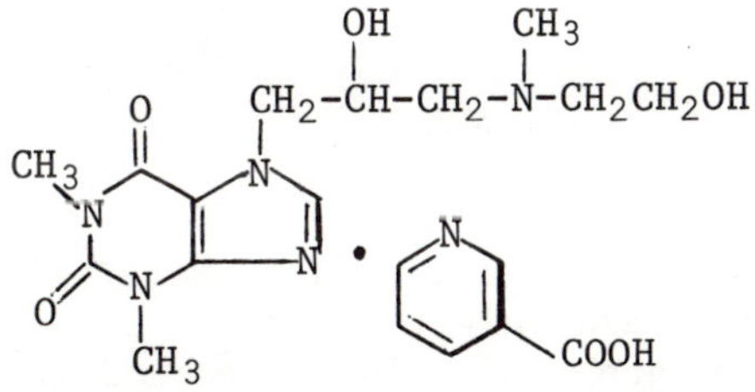

16 Xantinol nicotinate

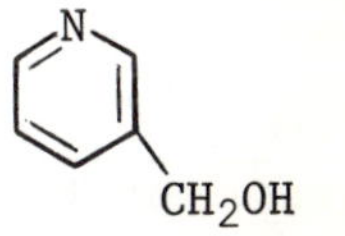

17 β-Pyridyl carbinol

Probucol (18) - Very little is known about the effect of probucol on serum lipoproteins. In a group of 30 type II patients probucol reduced both LDL and HDL cholesterol levels to a small extent but had no effect on VLDL.[79]

Procetofene (19) - This new lipoprotein modifying agent produces a more favorable effect on serum lipoproteins in man than any agent reported to date. Rossner and Oro[80,81] compared procetofene with clofibrate, bezafibrate, and gemfibrozil in type II and type IV patients and found it caused a 57% decrease in VLDL triglyceride in type IV, a 37% decrease in

LDL cholesterol in type II, and a 14% increase in HDL cholesterol in type IV. These effects of procetofene were better overall than those of any of the other drugs with which it was compared. Other investigators have also reported very favorable results with procetofene. These include a

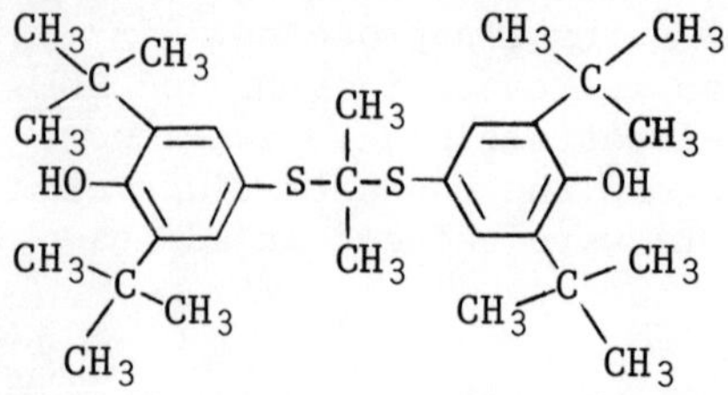

18 Probucol

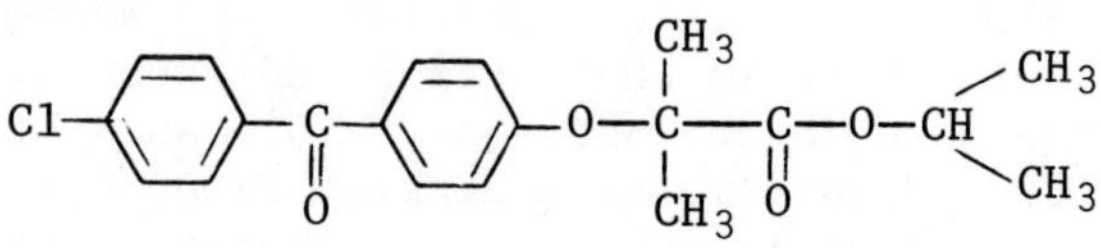

19 Procetofene

23% increase in apolipoprotein A from HDL in type II,[82] a 50 and 30% fall in VLDL and LDL cholesterol in type IIB,[83] and a 35% decrease in LDL cholesterol in type IIA.[83] In experimental animals such as hypercholesterolemic rats, procetofene markedly reduces VLDL and concomitantly increases HDL to a similar degree.[84] Based on its pronounced lipoprotein effects, this drug may retard the development of clinical atherosclerosis.

Simfibrate (20) - One would expect *a priori* that this closely related analog of clofibrate would have an identical effect on serum lipoproteins. As expected, VLDL was substantially reduced with simfibrate. Surprisingly, LDL was also reduced to a similar extent.[85,86]

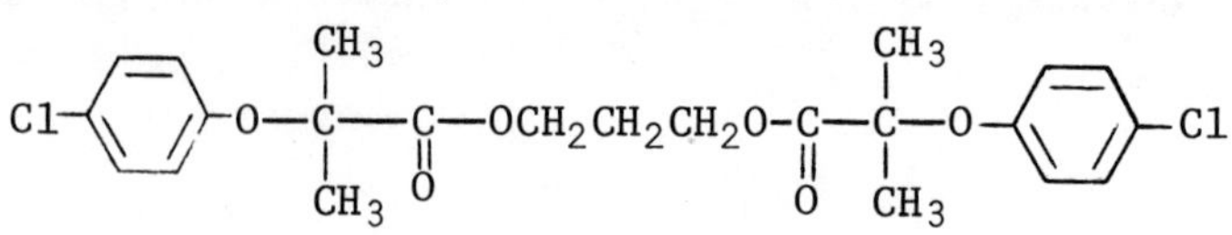

20 Simfibrate

Terbufibrol (21) - Based on preclinical data in rats[40,87] and baboons,[41] terbufibrol exerts a rather dramatic effect in the reduction of serum lipoproteins, especially LDL and VLDL. In the normal rat at a dose of 120 mg/kg/day terbufibrol caused a 32, 83, and 40% reduction in LDL, VLDL, and HDL, respectively.[40] Terbufibrol reduced also serum lipoproteins in fructose induced hypertriglyceridemic rats and in rats with hypercholesterolemia induced by thiouracil, Triton, or cholesterol feeding, apparently by inhibition of lipoprotein synthesis or release in these models.[88,89]

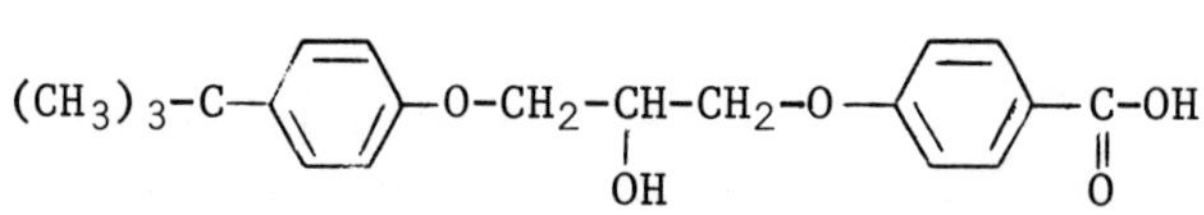

21 Terbufibrol

In the normal baboon at a dose of 200 mg/kg/day this drug reduced serum LDL and HDL by approximately 70 and 50%, respectively.[41] The effect was even greater in baboons on a high fat, high protein diet where an LDL reduction of 80% was observed at a dose of 60 mg/kg/day.

Tiadenol (22) - In type IIA hyperlipoproteinemia tiadenol reduced LDL and HDL cholesterol 23 and 36%, respectively, from basal levels after 4 months of drug therapy but had no effect on VLDL triglyceride levels.[90]

$HO-CH_2CH_2-S-(CH_2)_{10}-S-CH_2CH_2OH$

22 Tiadenol

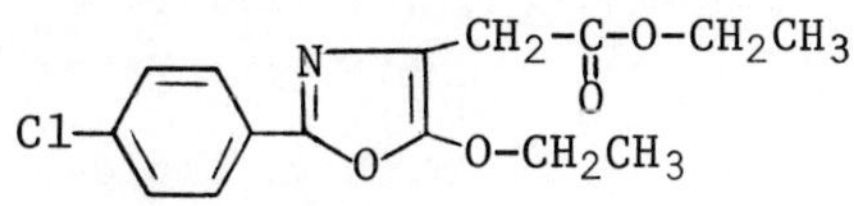

23 Y-9738

Y-9738 (23) - This newly disclosed compound effectively reduced LDL in hypercholesterolemic rats, and the 50% reduction in serum cholesterol seen in monkeys with Y-9738 treatment can be accounted for almost entirely by a reduction in LDL.[91]

Summary

A reduction of total serum cholesterol and triglycerides elicited by a drug represents only the net effect on all classes of serum lipoproteins. Since different lipoproteins may have distinctly opposite effects on atherogenesis, it is now of paramount importance to obtain information about the effect of drugs on individual lipoproteins so that some reasonable assessment can be made regarding the probability for a beneficial effect of the drug on clinical atherosclerosis. Given the present state of the art in atherosclerosis research, simple measurement of total serum cholesterol and/or triglycerides only is no longer rationally acceptable. Even when a drug appears to favorably alter lipoproteins, its effect on atherosclerosis must be verified experimentally, since an effect on lipoproteins does not necessarily assure an effect on atherosclerosis. Pharmacologic regulation of serum lipoproteins is an exciting and rapidly advancing area of research, and, as a result of intensive efforts underway in many pharmaceutical laboratories, new and better agents for controlling serum lipoproteins and atherosclerosis can be expected to be forthcoming.

REFERENCES

1. G.J. Miller and N.E. Miller, Lancet, 1, 16 (1975).
2. D.S. Fredrickson and R.I. Levy in "The Metabolic Basis of Inherited Disease," Third Edition, J.B. Stanbury, J.B. Wyngaarden, and D.S. Fredrickson, Eds., McGraw-Hill, New York, NY, 1972, p 545.
3. G. Camejo in "Low Density Lipoproteins," C.E. Day and R.S. Levy, Eds., Plenum Press, New York, NY, 1976, p 351.
4. S. Ghosh, ibid., p 371.
5. D. Zilversmit, Circ. Res., 33, 633 (1973).

6. O. Wiklund, A. Gustafson, and L. Wilhelmsen, Artery, 1, 399 (1975).
7. C.J. Glueck, R.W. Fallat, F. Millett, P. Gartside, R.C. Elston, and R.C.P. Go, Metabolism, 24, 1243 (1975).
8. G.C. Rhoads, C.L. Gulbrandsen, and A. Kagan, New Eng. J. Med., 294, 293 (1976).
9. N.E. Miller, O.H. Forde, D.S. Thelle, and O.D. Mjos, Lancet, 1, 965 (1977).
10. T. Gordon, W.P. Castelli, M.C. Hjortland, W.B. Kannel, and T.R. Dawber, Amer. J. Med., 62, 707 (1977).
11. C.E. Day, P.E. Schurr, W.E. Heyd, and D. Lednicer, Adv. Exp. Med. Biol., 67, 231 (1976).
12. P.E. Schurr and C.E. Day, Lipids, 12, 22 (1977).
13. C.E. Day and W.W. Stafford, Adv. Exp. Med. Biol., 63, 339 (1975).
14. K.P. Chapman, W.W. Stafford, and C.E. Day, Adv. Exp. Med. Biol., 67, 347 (1976).
15. C.E. Day, W.W. Stafford, and P.E. Schurr, Lab. An. Sci., 27, 817 (1977).
16. C.E. Day, W.W. Stafford, and P.E. Schurr, Prot. Biol. Fluids, 25, 519 (1977).
17. C.E. Day, P.E. Schurr, D.E. Emmert, R.E. TenBrink, and D. Lednicer, J. Med. Chem., 18, 1065 (1975).
18. B. Vessby, H. Lithell, J. Boberg, and I. Werner, Artery, 2, 70 (1976).
19. B. Vessby, H. Lithell, J. Boberg, and I. Werner, Abstracts of Sixth International Symposium on Drugs Affecting Lipid Metabolism, Philadelphia, PA, August 29-September 1, 1977, p 96.
20. P.T. Kuo, W.C. Fan, J.B. Kostis, and K. Hayase, Circulation, 53, 338 (1976).
21. A.G. Olsson, S. Rossner, G. Walldius, L.A. Carlson, and P.D. Lang, Atherosclerosis, 27, 279 (1977).
22. A.G. Olsson, S. Rossner, G. Walldius, L.A. Carlson, and P.D. Lang, Abstracts of Sixth International Symposium on Drugs Affecting Lipid Metabolism, Philadelphia, PA, August 29-September 1, 1977, p 68.
23. A.G. Olsson, L.A. Carlson, S. Rossner, G. Walldius, and P.D. Lang, Abstracts of International Conference on Atherosclerosis, Milan, Italy, November 9-12, 1977, p 270.
24. J.G. Wechsler, V. Hutt, H.U. Kloer, H. Jaeger, J. Schoenborn, and H. Ditschuneit, Abstracts of Sixth International Symposium on Drugs Affecting Lipid Metabolism, Philadelphia, PA, August 29-September 1, 1977, p 99.
25. J.G. Wechsler, V. Hutt, H.V. Kloer, J. Schoenborn, H. Jaeger, and H. Ditschuneit, Abstracts of International Conference on Atherosclerosis, Milan, Italy, November 9-12, 1977, p 272.
26. C.E. Day in "Low Density Lipoproteins," C.E. Day and R.S. Levy, Eds., Plenum Press, New York, NY, 1976, p 421.
27. A.E. Dorr, K. Gundersen, J.C. Schneider, T.W. Spencer, and W.B. Martin, J. Chronic Dis., in press.
28. A.G. Olsson and F. Dairou, Atherosclerosis, 29, 53 (1978).
29. A.G. Olsson, Pharmacotherapia, in press.
30. C.R. Sirtori, P. Gomarasca, G. d'Atri, S. Cerutti, G. Tronconi, and C. Scolastico, Abstracts of International Conference on Atherosclerosis, Milan, Italy, November 9-12, 1977, p 25.

31. C.R. Sirtori, P. Gomarasca, G. d'Atri, S. Cerutti, G. Tronconi, and C. Scolastico, Atherosclerosis, in press.
32. A.S. Katocs and S.A. Schaffer, Fed. Proc., 36, 1160 (1977).
33. W. Hollander, S. Prusty, S. Nagraj, B. Kirkpatrick, J. Paddock, and M. Colombo, Abstracts of Sixth International Symposium on Drugs Affecting Lipid Metabolism, Philadelphia, PA, August 29-September 1, 1977, p 37.
34. K.M. Kutty, J.C. Jacob, P.J. Hutton, and S.C. Peterson, Clin. Biochem., 8, 379 (1975).
35. S.H. Lawrence and P.J. Melnick, Proc. Soc. Exp. Biol. Med., 107, 998 (1961).
36. K.M. Kutty, R. Redheendran, and D. Murphy, Experientia, 33, 420 (1977).
37. H. Adriaensen, Clin. Trials J., 6, 191 (1969).
38. P. Saba, F. Galeone, F. Salvadorini, M. Guarguaglini, and J.L. Houben, Artery, 3, 250 (1977).
39. K. Muller, Abstracts of Sixth International Symposium on Drugs Affecting Lipid Metabolism, Philadelphia, PA, August 29-September 1, 1977, p 64.
40. R. Zschocke, H. Enomoto, R. Löser, and G. Hofrichter, Prot. Biol. Fluids, 25, 535 (1977).
41. A.N. Howard, G. Hofrichter, R. Zschocke, and A.V. Ginocchio, ibid., p 441.
42. D.E. Wilson and R.S. Lees, J. Clin. Invest., 51, 1051 (1972).
43. H.G. Rose, G.K. Haft, and J. Juliano, Atherosclerosis, 23, 413 (1976).
44. L.A. Carlson, A.G. Olsson, and D. Ballantyne, Atherosclerosis, 26, 603 (1977).
45. A.G. Olsson, D. Ballantyne, and L.A. Carlson, Abstracts of Sixth International Symposium on Drugs Affecting Lipid Metabolism, Philadelphia, PA, August 29-September 1, 1977, p 67.
46. S.C. Enger, J. Erikssen, V. Johnsen, A. Samuelsen, K. Herbjornsen, and E.A. Laws, Artery, 4, 28 (1978).
47. A.N. Howard and P. Ghosh, Abstracts of Sixth International Symposium on Drugs Affecting Lipid Metabolism, Philadelphia, PA, August 29-September 1, 1977, p 38.
48. P.L. Creger, G.W. Moersch, and W.A. Neuklis, Proc. Roy. Soc. Med., 69 (Suppl. 2), 3 (1976).
49. G. Rodney, P. Uhlendorf, and R.E. Maxwell, ibid., p 6.
50. A.G. Olsson, S. Rossner, G. Walldius, and L.A. Carlson, ibid., p 28.
51. B. Vessby, H. Lithell, J. Boberg, K. Hellsing, and I. Werner, ibid., p 32.
52. A. Eisalo, V. Manninen, M. Malkonen, and B. Kuhlback, ibid., p 47.
53. A. Eisalo and V. Manninen, ibid., p 49.
54. E.A. Nikkila, R. Ylikahri, and J.K. Huttunen, ibid., p 58.
55. E.D. Janus, D. Costa, I.C. Ononogbu, and B. Lewis, ibid., p 76.
56. W.F. Bremner, J.L.H.C. Third, B. Clark, C. Corstorphine, and T.D.V. Lawrie, ibid., p 83.
57. A.N. Howard and P. Ghosh, ibid., p 88.
58. B. Vessby, H. Lithell, J. Boberg, and I Werner, Abstracts of Sixth International Symposium on Drugs Affecting Lipid Metabolism, Philadelphia, PA, August 29-September 1, 1977, p 95.

59. A.N. Howard, Abstracts of International Conference on Atherosclerosis, Milan, Italy, November 9-12, 1977, p 229.
60. R. Agid and G. Marquie, C.R. Acad. Sci., Ser. D, 269, 1000 (1969).
61. J. Sterne and J. Brohon, Diabete, 21, 159 (1973).
62. R. Agid, G. Marquie, and M. Lafontan, Journ. Annu. Diabetol. Hotel-Dieu, 1975, 259.
63. C.E. Day, B. Barker, and W.W. Stafford, Comp. Biochem. Physiol., 49B, 501 (1974).
64. G. Camejo and A. Lopez, Atherosclerosis, 19, 139 (1974).
65. J. Rodriguez, A. Catapano, G.C. Ghiselli, and C.R. Sirtori, Adv. Exp. Med. Biol., 67, 169 (1976).
66. C.R. Sirtori, A. Catapano, G.C. Ghiselli, A.L. Innocenti, and J. Rodriguez, Atherosclerosis, 26, 79 (1977).
67. C.R. Sirtori, A. Catapano, G.C. Ghiselli, B. Shore, and V. Shore, Prot. Biol. Fluids, 25, 379 (1977).
68. B. Shore, C. Sirtori, A. Catapano, G.C. Ghiselli, and V. Shore, Abstracts of International Conference on Atherosclerosis, Milan, Italy, November 9-12, 1977, p 98.
69. C.R. Sirtori, G. Weber, and A. Catapano, ibid., p 97.
70. C.R. Sirtori, E. Tremoli, M. Sirtori, F. Conti, and R. Paoletti, Atherosclerosis, 26, 583 (1977).
71. H. Bar-On, D. Landau, and E. Berry, Lancet, 1, 761 (1977).
72. A. Stalenhoef, P. Demacker, J. Lutterman, and A. Van't Laar, Lancet, 1, 325 (1978).
73. E.A. Nikkila, P. Hormila, and J.K. Huttunen, Circulation, 56, III-23 (1977).
74. H. Haacke, M.R. Parwaresch, and C. Mader, Prot. Biol. Fluids, 25, 399 (1977).
75. H. Haacke, M.R. Parwaresch, and C. Mader, Med. Klin., 72, 1183 (1977).
76. H. Haacke, M.R. Parwaresch, and C. Mader, Deut. Med. Wschr., 101, 1413 (1976).
77. H. Haacke, M.R. Parwaresch, and C. Mader, Verhandl. Deut. Gesellsch. Inn. Med., 82, 829 (1976).
78. J.G. Wechsler, V. Hutt, H.U. Kloer, H. Jaeger, J. Schoenborn, and H. Ditschuneit, Abstracts of Sixth International Symposium on Drugs Affecting Lipid Metabolism, Philadelphia, PA, August 29-September 1, 1977, p 100.
79. J. LeLorier, S. DuBreuil-Quidoz, S. Lussier-Cacan, Y. Huang, and J. Davignon, Arch. Int. Med., 137, 1429 (1977).
80. S. Rossner and L. Oro, Abstracts of International Conference on Atherosclerosis, Milan, Italy, November 9-12, 1977, p 22.
81. S. Rossner and L. Oro, Abstracts of Sixth International Symposium on Drugs Affecting Lipid Metabolism, Philadelphia, PA, August 29-September 1, 1977, p 75.
82. H. Micheli, A. Gustafson, and D. Pometta, Abstracts of International Conference on Atherosclerosis, Milan, Italy, November 9-12, 1977, p 228.
83. P. Drouin, L. Mejean, D. Lambert, J.P. Sauvanet, and G. Debry, ibid., p 227.
84. E. Wulfert, ibid., p 20.

85. P. Saba, F. Galeone, F. Salvadorini, and M. Guarguaglini, ibid., p 276.
86. P. Saba, F. Galeone, F. Salvadorini, and M. Guarguaglini, Curr. Ther. Res., 22, 741 (1977).
87. H. Enomoto, Y. Yoshikuni, T. Ozaki, and R. Zschocke, Abstracts of The IVth International Symposium on Atherosclerosis, Tokyo, August 24-28, 1976, p 230.
88. R. Zschocke, H. Grill, G. Hofrichter, and H. Enomoto, ibid., p 131.
89. R. Zschocke, G. Hofrichter, A. Ginocchio, and A.N. Howard, ibid., p 176.
90. G. Baggio, G. Briani, S. Martini, R. Fellin, and G. Crepaldi, Abstracts of International Conference on Atherosclerosis, Milan, Italy, November 9-12, 1977, p 103.
91. T. Kobayakawa, K. Osuga, and H. Yasuda, Abstracts of Sixth International Symposium on Drugs Affecting Lipid Metabolism, Philadelphia, PA, August 29-September 1, 1977, p 48.

Chapter 21. Drug Metabolism

Bruce H. Migdalof, The Squibb Institute for Medical Research
New Brunswick, NJ 08903

Introduction - In this chapter selected highlights of the recent literature on drug metabolism will be presented. The material discussed will focus on compounds with pharmacological, toxicological, or biological activity, with the objective of providing information germane to medicinal chemists. It is important to point out that the state-of-the-art in this field is changing rapidly due to rapid advances in instrumentation, new methodology and the discovery of new aspects of drug disposition.[1,2]

Recent Books - There have been several books published on various aspects of drug metabolism. Drug Metabolism Concepts, the publication of an ACS symposium, discusses the enzyme systems responsible for most drug biotransformations (cytochrome P-450's, P-448's, epoxide hydrase(s), etc.), their stereospecificity and role in metabolic activation.[3] The second volume of the series on Progress in Drug Metabolism has been published.[4] An excellent volume on Interactions of Drugs of Abuse contains many excellent chapters including one by Gillette on factors affecting drug interactions.[5] Drug Interactions is the second book by the same title published in the last few years.[6,7] The third volume of The Fate of Drugs in the Organism is now available.[8] The initial volume of a new series entitled Drug Fate and Metabolism, Methods and Techniques, has also appeared.[9] Other books on more limited subjects within the field deal with pharmacokinetics in disease states,[10] metabolic activation in mutagenesis testing,[11] mass spectrometry applications,[12] and monitoring of drug levels.[13]

Methodology - One of the more active areas of methods development is the pursuit of new or improved assays for drugs and their metabolites in biological samples. This is exemplified by the increasing use of radioimmunoassay (RIA), high performance (or high pressure) liquid chromatography (HPLC), quantitative thin-layer chromatography (QTLC), and combined gas chromatography-mass spectrometry (GC/MS). GC/MS systems are often equipped with dedicated computer data systems. Chemical ionization (CI), and selected ion monitoring (SIM) procedures may provide enhanced sensitivity and specificity, and are frequently employed in the development of GC/MS assays.

A method has been reported for the simultaneous determination of d- and l-amphetamine in human plasma using gas chromatography-chemical ionization mass spectrometry (GC/CIMS) of diastereoisomer derivatives.[14] The use of stable isotope-labeled drug modifications as internal standards for the determination of drugs in biological fluids by GC/CIMS can permit quantitation in the picogram region, as shown for methadone.[15] A new technique has been reported in which ^{13}C-labeled and unlabeled drug were administered in a known ratio, and metabolites in urine were detected by a combination of gas chromatography/combustion/mass fragmentography.[16] GC/MS has been applied to studies of free organic acids extracted from human saliva.[17] Autoradiography continues to be a useful tool for studying the

ISBN 0-12-040513-X

distribution of drug-related entities and is being used increasingly in the study of feto-placental transfer.[18] QTLC continues to be a popular choice for multiple simultaneous assays,[19] and sensitivity down to 8 ng/ml of plasma has been attained for codeine phosphate, and 1 ng/ml for chlorpheniramine maleate by suitable derivatization and spectrophotometric detection.[20] The method involves nitration, reduction and diazo coupling with N-(1-naphthyl)ethylenediamine directly on thin-layer plates, and should be applicable to the analysis of other aromatic compounds.

A radioassay has been developed for the quantitation of disulfiram (1) and several of its metabolites (diethyldithiocarbamate, diethyldithiocarbamate glucuronide, inorganic sulfate and a protein bound ^{35}S fraction) from a single sample of plasma, urine, or tissue obtained after administration of disulfiram-^{35}S to laboratory animals.[21] Although the method is unusually complex, it nevertheless is a fine example of the potential for the development of specific assays for drugs and metabolites utilizing radiolabeled drugs.

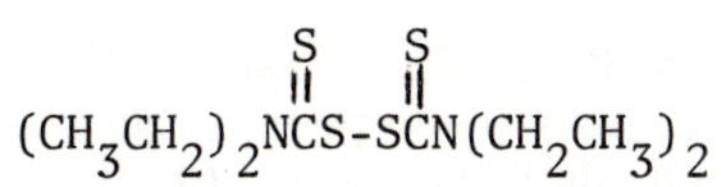

1

Hepatic Microsomal Enzymes - Research into the nature, specificity and inducibility of drug metabolizing enzymes is making steady progress. A kinetic method for the determination of multiple forms of microsomal cytochrome P-450 has been reported.[22] Further support has also been obtained for the hypothesis that drug metabolism in isolated hepatocytes correlates better with metabolism *in vivo* than does metabolism in subcellular hepatic microsomal fractions.[23] Metabolism studies in isolated rat liver parenchymal and nonparenchymal cells showed that parenchymal rat liver cells metabolized (acetylated) sulfadimidine, sulfanilamide, p-benzoic acid, and isoniazid (2), but nonparenchymal cells only metabolized isonaizid to an appreciable extent.[24] Steric factors affecting the inhibition of microsomal enzymes by imidazoles have been investigated.[25] Spectral studies suggest that cytochrome P-450 content in rat hepatic microsomes is decreased by high concentrations (≥ 0.14 M) of acetaminophen, a known hepatotoxin.[26] Two differentially inducible UDP-glucuronyl transferases present in rat liver have been separated and partially purified.[27]

An *in vitro* study of epoxide hydrase activity in human liver indicated that hydration of the 11 epoxides studied was catalyzed either by a single enzyme, or by a group of enzymes under the same regulatory control.[28] In another *in vitro* study using human liver, the intersubject variability found in the hydroxylation of a series of substrates suggests that multiple mono-oxygenases may be present in man.[29]

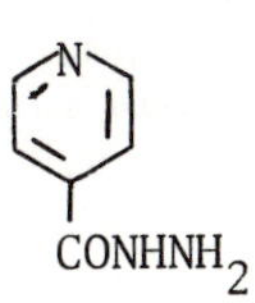

2

Extrahepatic Drug Biotransformation - Although the liver is the primary site of biotransformation of most drugs, it is not the only site in many cases. Depending upon the structure of a drug, its route of administration, and its distribution in tissues, biotransformation may occur at such extrahepatic sites as kidney, lung, skin, intestine, and blood. Recent publications on extrahepatic metabolism include a minireview on pulmonary metabolism,[30] and papers on oxidative metabolism in rat small intestine[31] and drug biotransformation in the skin.[32] The metabolism of flurazepam (3) by the small intestine was studied in man,[33] and evidence of oxidative N-dealkylation was obtained. This appears to be the first demonstration of metabolism of a benzodiazepine by human intestine *in vivo*. However, the contribution of metabolism at this site to total metabolism is not clear, since no quantitative determinations were made. The authors suggested that imiprimine might also undergo N-dealkylation in human intestine, and raised the general question as to the relative roles of the small intestines and the liver in the metabolism of drugs. Further studies are indicated.

Intestinal microflora may also be responsible for extrahepatic biotransformations, and evidence has been presented that the unusual aromatization of orally administered shikimic acid (4) to benzoic acid (6), may involve microbial formation of cyclohexane carboxylic acid (5) as an intermediate.[34] Such findings suggest that species differences in drug metabolism may sometimes be due to differences in gastro-intestinal microflora.

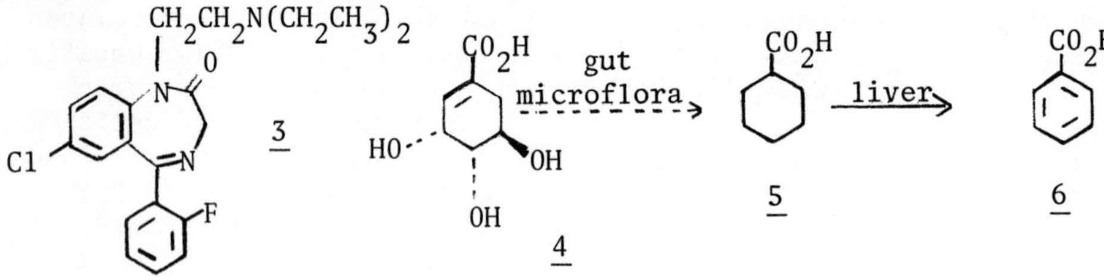

Interspecies Comparative Metabolism - Knowledge of species differences is important in evaluating the relevance of safety and efficacy data obtained in animals to man. The comparative metabolism of two arylacetic acids, 1-naphthylacetic acid (7)[35] and hydratropic acid (8) has been studied,[36] complementing earlier studies on the metabolism of phenylacetic acid (9), p-chlorophenylacetic acid (10) and indolylacetic acid (11). For these compounds qualitative and quantitative differences were observed among the species studied with regard to the percentage of the dose accounted for in urine as glucuronide, glycine, glutamine and taurine conjugates. Among the numerous papers published on the comparative metabolism of specific drugs, one, on metoclopramide (12) metabolism, is particularly noteworthy, since eight metabolites were identified from rat, dog and human urine, but only one (13) was common to all three species.[37]

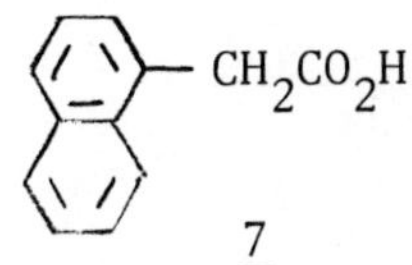

7

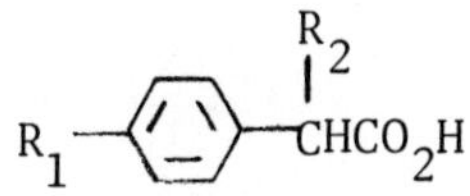

8 R_1 = H, R_2 = CH_3
9 R_1 = H, R_2 = H
10 R_1 = Cl, R_2 = H

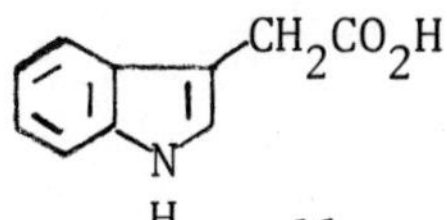

11

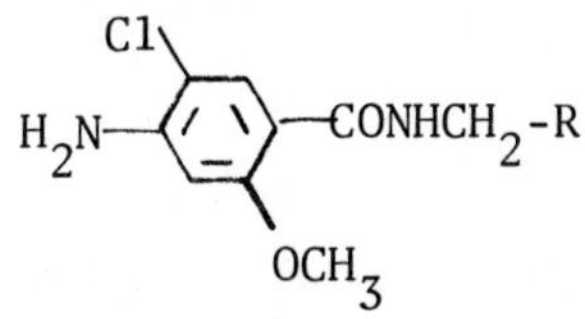

12 R = $CH_2N(C_2H_5)_2$
13 R = CO_2H

Stereoselectivity in Drug Disposition - Differences have been reported in the metabolism of R- and S-ephedrine (14),[38] R- and S-warfarin (15),[39] R- and S-methadone (16),[40] and the R/S ratio of unchanged drug excreted after oral administration of a racemic amphetamine analog (17) to rabbits varied between 1.0 to 1.7 according to dose.[41] An R/S ratio of approximately 2 was observed in rat urine after administration of 17.[42] Racemic 17 was metabolized in vitro at a different rate than either of the individual enantiomers which were metabolized at approximately the same rate.[43] Differential disposition has also been demonstrated for the two enantiomers of cocaine in rats, and may be a partial explanation for differences in pharmacological effects.[44] These observations suggest that racemates can have pharmacological and toxicological properties different from the individual enantiomers.

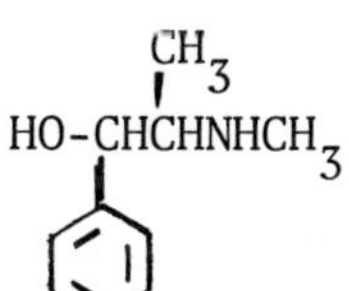

14

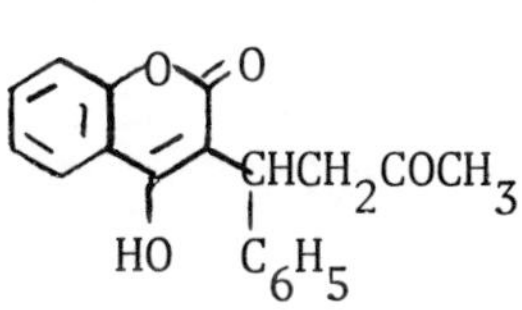

15

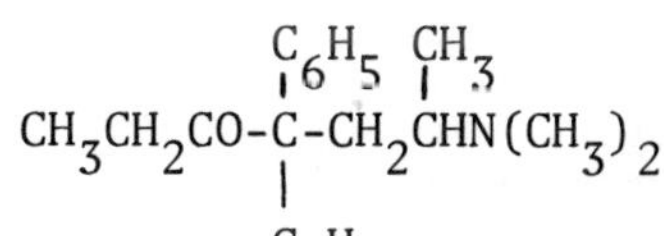

16

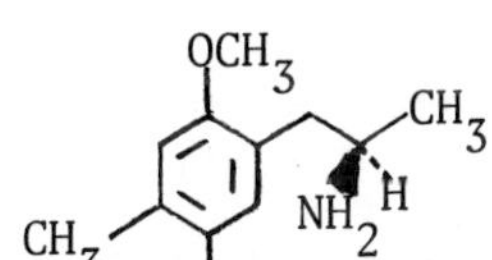

17

Biotransformation to Active Metabolites - Biotransformations may result in the formation of compounds with pharmacologic properties comparable to, or more potent than the parent compound. One such example is the antiarrhythmic drug procainamide (18), which is metabolized to an active acetyl metabolite (19).[45] The conversion of prodrugs to active substances is exemplified by sulindac (20), a nonsteroidal antiinflammatory agent which is converted in vivo to its active form 21.[46,47]

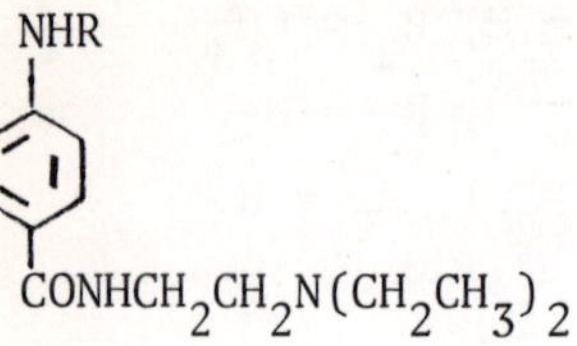

18 R = H

19 R = $\overset{O}{\overset{\|}{C}}CH_3$

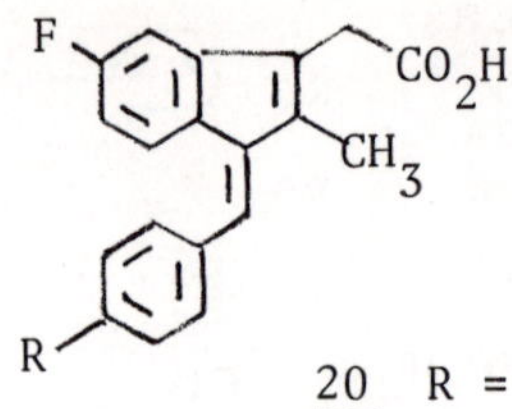

20 R = $\overset{O}{\overset{\uparrow}{S}}CH_3$

21 R = SCH_3

Highly reactive metabolites can also be produced, and such processes are being studied with increasing intensity, since they may be responsible for serious toxic effects of drugs.[11] Formation of highly reactive metabolites has been implicated as the cause of a wide array of toxic effects, from hepatic necrosis to mutagenesis and carcinogenesis, and as an explanation of the similar toxicities observed for compounds of very dissimilar structures. Reviews of the subject continue to appear in the literature.[11,48,49] Since the liver is the most common site for biotransformation, it is not surprising that hepatic necrosis, and malignant hepatic tumors are among the more frequently observed toxic manifestations when very reactive metabolites are formed. In recent years it has become increasingly apparent that the most toxic metabolites rarely survive long enough to be excreted, and studies limited to the identification of metab lites in excreta may therefore provide misleading information. It should also be mentioned that metabolic activation is an integral part of mutagenicity testing.

The teratogenicity of Δ^9-tetrahydrocannabinol (THC) (22) could be altered by stimulation and inhibition of its metabolism, and an active metabolite may be responsible.[51] *In vitro* studies of 7,12-dimethylbenz[a]-anthracene (23), a potent carcinogen have shown it to undergo bioactivation in mouse skin homogenates from mice treated with 3-methylcholanthrene.[52] A great deal of attention is currently focused on the bioactivation of the aspirin substitute, acetaminophen (24). When overdoses are ingested, a normal biotransformation pathway (conjugation with glutathione) is saturated, and a highly reactive metabolite is formed which binds irreversibly to hepatic tissue and may result in extensive hepatic necrosis.[53,54,55,56]

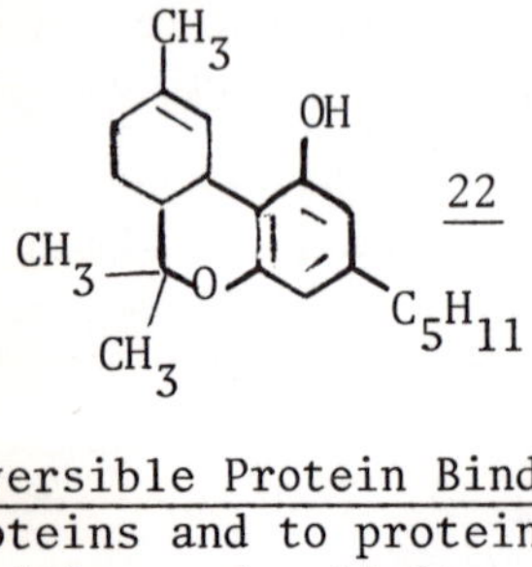

22

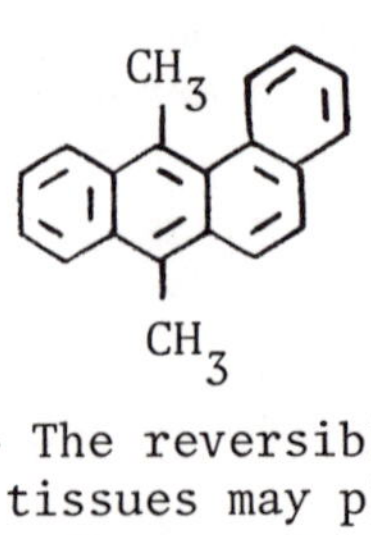

23

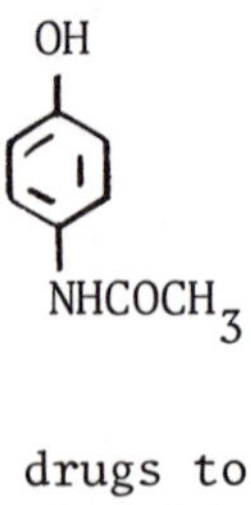

24

Reversible Protein Binding - The reversible binding of drugs to plasma proteins and to proteins in tissues may play an important role in the disposition and activity of many drugs. A comprehensive review of methods for determining protein binding has been published.[57] The effect of protein binding on pharmacokinetics and therapeutic activity of antimicrobial drugs has been reviewed.[58] Differences in the binding of some drugs to plasma proteins of neonates and adult humans has been demonstrated.[59] Species differences have been observed for the binding of warfarin to plasma proteins.[60] A *lack* of correlation between *in vitro* activity (inhibition of PG-synthetase) and *in vivo* analgesic-antiinflammatory activity (phenylquinone-induced writhing in mice, and carrageenan-induced edema in rats) for indoprofen (25) and a series of its analogs (26) was attributed to differences in plasma protein binding.[61] Evidence of non-first-order behavior for plasma levels of tolmetin (27), a new nonsteroidal antiinflammatory drug, has been reported in man and attributed to reversible tissue binding.[62]

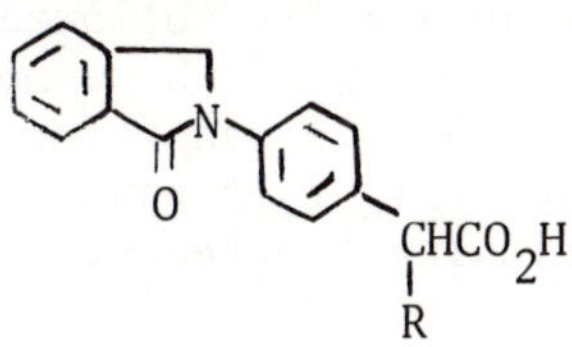

25 R = CH_3

26 R = H, ethyl, propyl or butyl

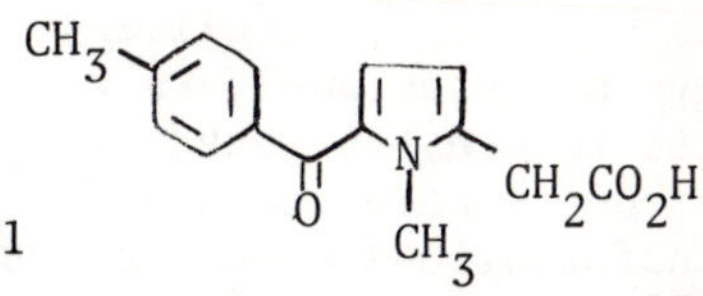

27

Pharmacokinetic-Pharmacodynamic Correlations - Pharmacokinetic evaluation of drugs and their metabolites can provide invaluable information regarding appropriate clinical dose regimens. Pharmacokinetic comparisons of analogs with similar potency in pharmacological models of human disease can assist in the selection of the compound to undergo clinical evaluation. Such studies are especially valuable when, for example, the time course of the pharmacological response can be related to that of the drug (and/or metabolites) in blood. A variety of methods are now available for obtaining serial blood microsamples from small laboratory animals and for the analysis of drug and/or metabolite concentrations in the samples.[63] Correlations of activity with blood, serum and plasma concentrations were reported for S-warfarin[64] in rats, and thioridazine (28)[65] and chlorpromazine (29)[66] in man. For chlorpromazine, an even better correlation was reported for one of its metabolites, 7-hydroxychlorpromazine (30).[67] Prolactin concentrations were found to correlate better than blood levels with clinical response following administration of thioridazine.[68] No correlation was observed between blood concentrations and antihypertensive activity of the cardioselective β-adrenergic blocking agent atenolol. (31)[69] The kinetics of the antiarrhythmic effect of procainamide showed a direct correlation with the kinetics of drug in saliva, but not in plasma.[70] This indicates that a good correlation between drug response and plasma concentrations of the drug is not always observed, but that by including metabolites in the analyses and by examining a variety of body fluids, such a correlation may be found. The effect of active drug metabolites on plasma level-response correlations has been reviewed,[71] and a pharmacokinetic model for simultaneous determination of drug levels in organs and tissues has been developed.[72]

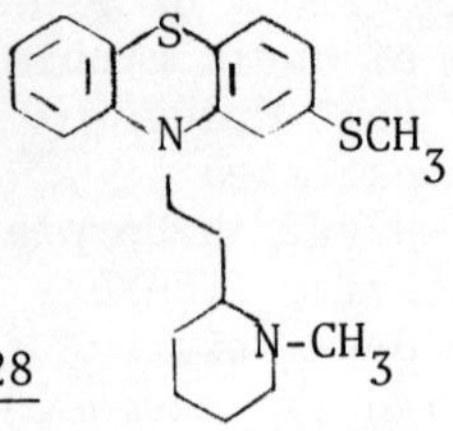

28

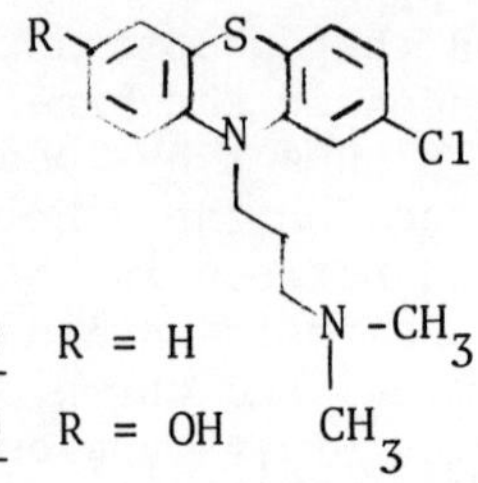

29 R = H

30 R = OH

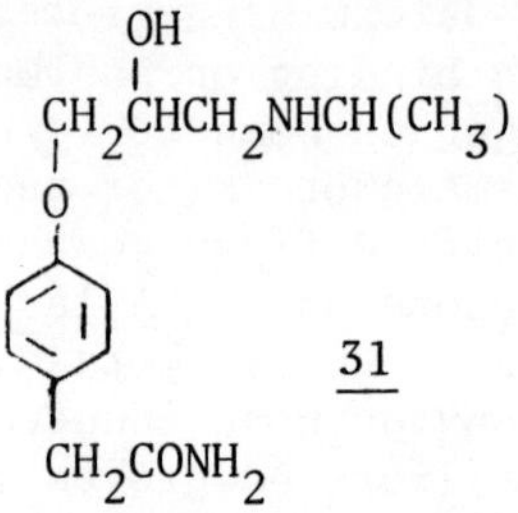

31

Novel Biotransformation Pathways and Products - The understanding of how metabolites are formed is often as important as knowing the chemical structure of the metabolites. During the past few years there have been many reports of novel metabolites, the biogenesis of which apparently followed pathways not previously known. In most cases, the structures of these metabolites were established by spectroscopic methods. Novel biotransformation products were the subject of reviews,[73,74] and several other novel biotransformations have been reported separately, including the reductive cleavage of anthracycline glycosides by cytochrome c reductase.[75] The N-methylation of benzimidazole (32) by catechol-O-methyltransferase (COMT) is the first known example of N-methylation by COMT.[76] Metabolism of clocoumarol (33), a synthetic vitamin K antagonist, by rat liver microsomes produced the new compound 34.[77] Metabolites reported for the hypnotic triazolam (35) in dogs include 36, in which the methyl carbon group is lost, presumably by an oxidation-decarboxylation pathway.[78]

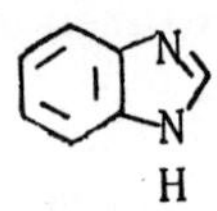

32

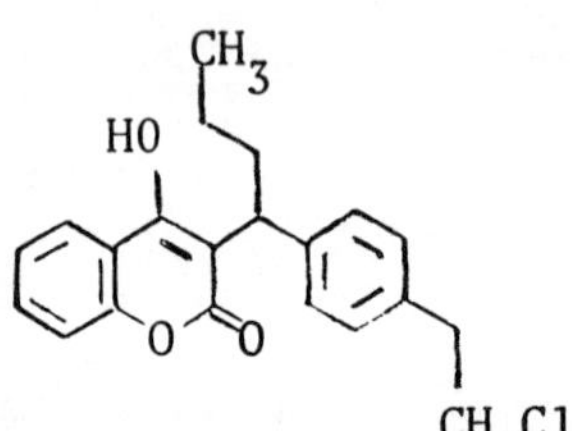

33

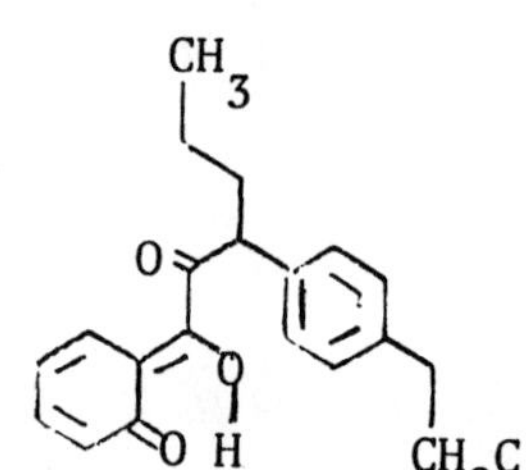

34 (cis-enol form)

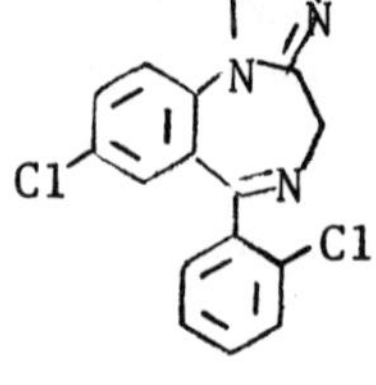

35 R = CH_3

36 R = H

REFERENCES

1. V.I. Kantemir, G. Akder and O. Tulunay, Arzneim.-Forsch. 26, 261 (1976)
2. E. Shmunes, Annals of Allergy 39, 186 (1977)
3. D.M. Jerina, ed., "Drug Metabolism Concepts", American Chemical Society, Washington, D.C., 1977
4. J.W. Bridges and L.F. Chasseaud, "Progress in Drug Metabolism", vol. 2, John Wiley & Sons, London 1977
5. E.S. Vesell and M.S. Braude, eds., "Interactions of Drugs of Abuse" (Ann. N.Y. Acad. Sci.) 281, N.Y. Acad. Sci., New York 1976
6. D.G. Grahame-Smith, ed., "Drug Interactions", Univ. Park Press, Baltimore 1977
7. P.L. Morselli, ed., "Drug Interactions", Raven Press, New York 1974
8. J. Hirz, et al., "The Fate of Drugs in the Organism: A Bibliographic Survey", vol. 3, Marcel Dekker, Inc., New York and Basel 1976
9. E.R. Garret and J.L. Hirtz, ed., "Drug Fate and Metabolism: Methods and Techniques", vol. 1, Marcel Dekker, Inc., New York 1977
10. L.Z. Benet, ed., "The Effect of Disease States on Drug Pharmacokinetics", American Pharmaceutical Association, Wash., D.C. 1976
11. F.J. de Serres, J.R. Fouts, J.R. Bend and R.M. Philpot, eds., "In Vitro Metabolic Activation in Mutagenesis Testing", North Holland Publishers, Amsterdam 1976
12. A. Frigerio and E.L. Ghisaberti, eds., "Mass Spectrometry in Drug Metabolism", Plenum Press, New York 1977
13. R.B. Stewart, L.E. Cluff and J.R. Philip, "Drug Monitoring: A Requirement for Responsible Drug Use", William & Wilkins, Baltimore 1977
14. S.B. Matin, S.H. Wan and J.B. Knight, Biomed. Mass Spectrom. 4, 118 (1977)
15. D.L. Hachey, M.J. Kreek and D.H. Mattson, J. Pharm. Sci. 66, 1579 (1977)
16. M. Sano, Y. Yotsui, H. Abe and S. Sasaki, Biomed. Mass Spectrom. 3, 1 (1976)
17. M.E. Ward, I.R. Politzer, J.L. Laseter and S.Q. Alam, Biomed. Mass Spectrom. 3, 77 (1976)
18. C. Declume and P. Bernard, Toxicology 8, 95 (1977)
19. N.T. Wad and E.J. Hanifl, J. Chromatog. 143, 214 (1977)
20. P. Haefelfinger, J. Chromatog. 124, 351 (1976)
21. M.D. Faiman, E.D. Dodd, R.J. Nolan, L. Artman and R.E. Hanzlik, Res. Comm. Chem. Pathol. & Pharmacol. 17, 481 (1977)
22. W.R. Porter, R.W. Branchflower and W.F. Trager, Biochem. Pharmacol. 26, 549 (1977)
23. R.E. Billings, R.E. McMahon, J. Ashmore and S.R. Wangle, Drug Metab. Dispos. 5, 518 (1977)
24. J. Morland and H. Olsen, Drug Metab. Dispos. 5, 511 (1977)
25. T.D. Rogerson, C.F. Wilkinson and K. Hetarski, Biochem. Pharmacol. 26, 1039 (1977)
26. R.A. Wilson and F.E. Hart, Res. Comm. Chem. Pathol. Pharmacol. 17, 605 (1977)
27. K.W. Bock, U.C. von Clausbrunch, D. Josting and H.O. Henwalder, Biochem. Pharmacol. 26, 1097 (1977)
28. J. Kapitulnik, W. Levin, A.Y.H. Lu, R. Morecki, P.M. Dansette, D.M. Jerina, and A.H. Conney, Clin. Pharmacol. Ther. 21, 158 (1977)

29. J. Kapitulnik, P.J. Poppers, and A.H. Convey, Clin. Pharmacol. Ther. 21, 166 (1977)
30. G.E.R. Hook and J.R. Bend, Life Sciences 18, 279 (1976)
31. H. Hoensch, C.H. Woo, and S.B. Raffin, Gastroenterology 70, 1063 (1976)
32. H.Y. Ando, N.F.H. Ho, and W.I. Higuchi, J. Pharm. Sci. 66, 1525 (1977)
33. W.A. Mahon, T. Inaba, and R.M. Stone, Clin. Pharmacol. Ther. 22, 228 (1977)
34. L.M. Ball, A.G. Renwick, and R.T. Williams, Xenobiotica 7, 101 (1977)
35. P.A.F. Dixon, J. Caldwell, and R.L. Smith, Xenobiotica 7, 695 (1977)
36. ibid 7, 707 (1977)
37. L. Teng, R.B. Bruce, and L.K. Dunning, J. Pharm. Sci. 66, 1615 (1977)
38. D.R. Feller and L. Malapeis, Drug Metab. Dispos. 5, 37 (1977)
39. L.R. Pohl, W.R. Porter, W.F. Trager, M.J. Fasco, and J.W. Fenton, II, Biochem. Pharmacol. 36, 109 (1977)
40. N. Gerber, R.M. Leger, P. Gordon, R.G. Smith, J. Bauer, and R.K. Lynn, J. Pharmacol. Exp. Ther. 200, 487 (1977)
41. S.B. Matin, P.S. Callery, J.S. Zweig, A. O'Brien, R. Rappoport, and N. Castignoli, Jr., J. Med. Chem. 17, 877 (1974)
42. J. Gal, J. Pharm. Sci., 66, 169 (1977)
43. N.P. McGraw, P.S. Callery, and N. Castagnoli, Jr., J. Med. Chem. 20, 185 (1977)
44. A.L. Misra and R.B. Pontani, Drug Metab. Dispos. 5, 556 (1977)
45. A.J. Atkinson, Jr., W.-K. Lee, M. Quinn, W. Kushner, M.J. Nevin, and J.M. Strong, Clin. Pharmacol. Ther. 21, 575 (1977)
46. D.E. Duggan, K.F. Hooke, E.A. Risley, T.Y. Shen, and C.G. Van Arman, J. Pharmacol. Exp. Ther. 201, 8 (1977)
47. D.E. Duggan, L.E. Hare, C.A. Ditzler, B.W. Lei, and K.C. Kwan, Clin. Pharmacol. Ther. 21, 326 (1977)
48. F. Schaffner, Vet. Pathol. 12, 145 (1975)
49. S.D. Nelson, M.R. Boyd, and J.R. Mitchell, in Drug Metabolism Concepts, D.M. Jerina, ed., ACS, Washington, D.C. 1977, pp. 155-185
50. Y. Woo, J.C. Arcos, and M.F. Argus, Biochem. Pharmacol. 26, 1535 (1977)
51. R.B. Harbison, B. Mantilla-Platt, and D.J. Lubin, J. Pharmacol. Exp. Ther. 202, 455 (1977)
52. J. DiGiovanni, T.J. Slaga, D.L. Berry, and M.R. Juchau, Drug Metab. Dispos. 5, 295 (1977)
53. M. Davis, N.G. Harrison, G. Ideo, B. Portmann, D. Labadarios, and R. Williams, Xenobiotica 6, 249 (1976)
54. M. Davis, D. Labadarios, and R.S. Williams, J. Int. Med. Res. 4, 40 (1976)
55. P.L. Madan, J. Clin. Pharmacol. 555 (1977)
56. G.J. Merrit, and P.U. Joyner, Drug Intell. Clin. Pharm. 11, 458 (1977)
57. H. Kurz, H. Trunk, and B. Weitz, Arzneim.-Forsch. 27, Nr. 8 (1977)
58. W.A. Craig and Peter Willing, Clin. Pharmacokinetics 2, 252 (1977)
59. H. Kurz, H. Michels, and H.H. Stickel, J. Clin. Pharmacol. 11, 469 (1977)
60. E.M. Sellers, M.L. Lang-Sellers, and J. Koch-Wesser, Biochem. Pharmacol. 26, 2445 (1977)
61. R. Ceserani, M. Ferrari, G. Goldaniga, E. Moro, and A. Buttinoni, Life Sciences 21, 223 (1977)

62. J.W. Ayres, D.J. Weidler, E. Sakmar, and J. Wagner, Res. Comm. Chem. Pathol. Pharmacol. 17, 583 (1977)
63. B.H. Migdalof, Drug Metab. Rev. 5, 295 (1976)
64. A. Yacobi and G. Levy, J. Pharm. Sci. 66, 1275 (1977)
65. R.G. Muusze and F.A.J. Vanderheeren, Eur. J. Clin. Pharmacol. 11, 141 (1977)
66. L. Rivera-Calimlim, H. Nasrallah, J. Strauss, and L. Lasagna, Am. J. Psychiatry 133, 64 (1976)
67. O.T. Phillipson, J.M. McKeown, J. Baker, and A.F. Healey, Brit. J. Psychiat. 131, 172 (1977)
68. G. Nikitopoulou, M. Thorner, J. Crammer, and M. Lader, Clin. Pharmacol. Ther. 21, 422 (1977)
69. A. Amery, J.-F. De Plaen, P. Lijnen, J. McAinsh, and T. Reybrouck, Clin. Pharmacol. Ther. 21, 691 (1977)
70. R.L. Galeazzi, L.Z. Benet, and L. Sheiner, Clin. Pharmacol. Ther. 20, 278 (1976)
71. A.J. Atkinson, Jr., and J.M. Strong, J. Pharmacokinetics Biopharm. 5, 95 (1977)
72. C.N. Chen and J.D. Andrade, J. Pharm. Sci. 65, 717 (1976)
73. Z.H. Disraili, P.G. Dayton, and J.R. Kiechel, Drug Metab. Dispos. 5, 411 (1977)
74. P. Jenner and B. Testa, Xenobiotica 8, 1 (1978)
75. T. Oki, T. Komiyama, H. Tone, T. Inui, T. Takeuchi, and H. Umexawa, J. Antibiotics 30, 613 (1977)
76. C.D. Arnett, P.S. Callery, and N. Zenker, Biochem. Pharmacol. 26, 377 (1977)
77. N. Thonnart, J. Med. Chem. 20, 604 (1977)
78. F.S. Eberts, Jr., Drug Metab. Dispos. 5, 547 (1977)

Section V - Topics in Biology

Editor: Christopher T. Walsh, Massachusetts Institute of Technology
Cambridge, MA 02139

Chapter 22. Molecular Aspects of Drug Metabolism

Gerald T. Miwa and Anthony Y.H. Lu, Hoffmann-La Roche Inc.
Nutley, NJ 07110

I. Introduction--The oxidation of medicinal chemicals by the cytochrome P450-containing monooxygenase system is an important initial step in determining the fate of both the chemical agent and the biological system. Metabolism can often lead to a reduction in duration of drug action through the formation of less active metabolites and the production of compounds more readily excreted into the urine by the kidneys. This process of metabolic inactivation followed by excretion is often the major pathway for terminating the action of a drug in biological systems.

Not all biotransformations catalyzed by this system are so benign, since this enzyme system can also play a central role in the formation of reactive metabolites which are either toxic, mutagenic or carcinogenic. Indeed, studies demonstrating the metabolic activation of reactive metabolites by this system have enjoyed tremendous growth in recent years[1-6]. It is now apparent that the chemistry of the metabolite(s) often determines the ultimate biological fate of an animal exposed to a chemical agent.

Although the hepatic, microsomal cytochrome P450 system metabolizes compounds at a relatively low rate (0.1 to 50 min^{-1}), it has several other features that make it uniquely suited to oxidizing nonpolar drugs. This enzyme system is able to oxidize and reduce a wide variety of structurally unrelated compounds. The membrane location and the hydrophobic nature of cytochrome P450 also favors the partitioning of nonpolar compounds from the plasma to the enzyme for metabolism[7-10]. Components of this system are located in high abundance in the liver--an organ to which about 25% of the total cardiac output is channeled. About 30% of this blood is from the hepatic artery while the remainder is supplied by the alimentary tract, pancreas and spleen via the portal vein. Thus, drugs absorbed from the gut pass directly to the liver and the cytochrome P450 enzyme system. The organism also appears to adapt to increased substrate levels through the synthesis or induction of higher amounts of these monooxygenases[11]. This feature along with adaptive increases in hepatic perfusion[12] contribute to decrease the biological half-life and duration of drug action.

This chapter is intended as an overview of the molecular aspects of drug metabolism catalyzed by this hepatic enzyme system. The recent progress in the isolation and characterization of the protein components constituting this enzyme system, the interaction between these components and the mechanism of oxygen activation are reviewed. The reader is directed to several excellent review articles which treat, in more detail, specific aspects of this system

ISBN 0-12-040513-X

such as the physical properties of its components[13-16], organization of enzyme components in the microsomal membrane[17,18], enzyme induction by chemical agents[11] and the purification and reconstitution of its components[19,20]. Three books have recently appeared treating the general properties of the microsomal cytochrome P450 drug metabolizing system and the variety of reactions catalyzed by this system[21-23]. In addition, the International Symposium on Microsomes and Drug Oxidations continues to publish its proceedings in book form[24-26].

II. Components of the Monooxygenase System--Cytochrome P450 and NADPH-cytochrome P450 reductase (or NADPH-cytochrome c reductase) are the two essential protein components of the hepatic microsomal monooxygenase system.[a] Cytochrome P450 is a b-type cytochrome with the protoporphyrin IX prosthetic group[28]. Cytochromes of the b-type are generally characterized by low-spin heme prosthetic groups octahedrally coordinated with the two z-axial positions coordinated to protein ligands[29] (Fig. 1). The two protein ligands prevent interaction of the heme iron with external ligands such as O_2, CO and CN^- and, therefore, these heme proteins are neither autoxidizable nor do they interact with the usual inhibitors of heme enzymes.

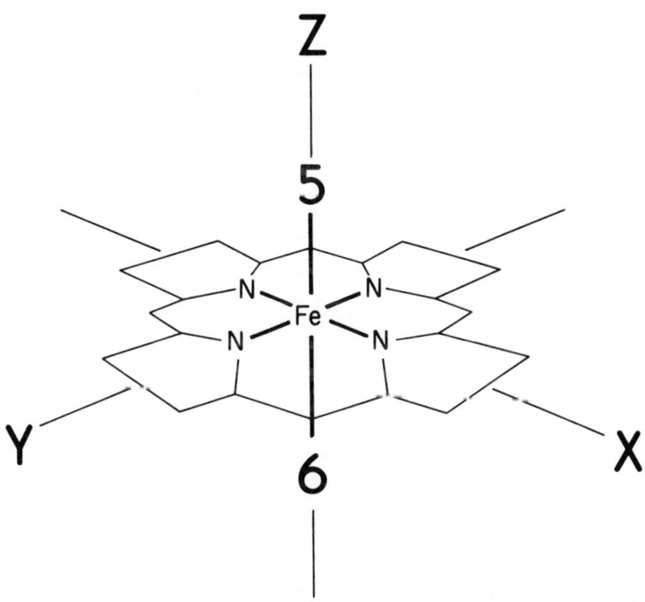

Figure 1

[a]Although cytochrome b_5 and NADH-cytochrome b_5 reductase have also been implicated in NADPH-dependent drug metabolism, these components have never been shown to be essential in reconstituting catalytic activity with purified enzyme components. A discussion of these components has therefore been omitted from the present chapter although the reader is referred to a review article on this subject[27].

Cytochrome P450 is an exceptional b-type cytochrome since it has either no protein residue[30] or an easily displaced protein residue coordinated in the sixth z-axial position[31,32]. As a result, it is readily autoxidizable[33] and combines with external ligands such as CN^- [34], CO[35], ethylisocyanide[36]. O_2 [37,38] and many drug and steroid substrates[39-41] to give complexes that can be observed by visible spectroscopy. Cytochrome P450 therefore possesses the iron and heme properties of cytochromes necessary for electron transport. Moreover, it can also bind O_2 and substrate molecules--properties that make it uniquely suited as a terminal oxidase.

The solubilization and purification of this protein from mammalian sources has permitted extensive biochemical characterization. The cytochrome exists in multiple forms with a minimum molecular weight ranging between 45,000 and 60,000 (Table 1). Multiple forms may exist in the same species of animal[42-47] and may be differentially induced by exposure of the animal to various chemical agents[11,45-48]. These different species of cytochrome P450 demonstrate different affinities or absorption maxima for ligands such as CN^-, CO and ethylisocyanide[34,47,48]. Different, but overlapping substrate specificities have also been demonstrated for these forms[45,47,49,50]. The amino acid composition has been reported for two forms of cytochrome P450 from mammalian sources [51] and, more recently, the initial amino-terminal sequence of two forms of this protein from rabbit liver microsomes has been reported[52].

The fifth z-axial position of the oxidized cytochrome is believed to be occupied by a cysteine mercaptide anion. This hypothesis, first suggested by Mason[33] is supported by several investigations. Model studies have demonstrated that a sulfhydryl ligand coordinated to the heme iron satisfactorialy explains the unusual absorption maximum at 450 nm of the reduced cytochrome-CO complex[54-58] and the characteristically low-spin EPR spectrum . Of particular interest is the recent study by Kawalek, <u>et al</u>[59] suggesting that the role of the sulfhydryl group in catalysis may be dependent on the specific form of cytochrome P450. More structural and functional studies on the purified cytochrome P450 are obviously needed to definitely establish the role of the sulfhydryl group in catalysis. Chevion, <u>et al</u>[32] have recently suggested that the sixth ligand of the oxidized cytochrome P450 may be a histidine residue.

During the course of cytochrome P450-catalyzed oxidation reducing equivalents are transferred from NADPH to the oxidized cytochrome-substrate complex by NADPH-cytochrome P450 reductase. This enzyme has been shown by various criteria to be identical with NADPH-cytochrome c reductase[53,60-62]. The enzyme contains 1 mole of FAD and 1 mole of FMN per mole of enzyme and has a molecular weight of about 79,000 [61,63,64]. The circular dichroism spectrum and amino acid composition have also been reported[65]. There is some evidence [20] for at least two forms of this enzyme in mammalian liver samples although immunological evidence suggests that only a single form exists from these sources[66,67].

In studies with the purified enzyme components and microsomal preparations, the NADPH-dependent enzyme reduces cytochrome P450 in two single electron transfer steps[68,69]. In the presence of substrate, O_2 and lipid this results in a reconstituted system capable of hydroxylating substrates without the requirement for other protein components such as cytochrome b_5 and adrenodoxin[20,70].

III. Multiple Forms of Cytochrome P450--The existence of isozymes of cytochrome P450 in liver microsomes has been suspected for many years[11,71-74]. The purification of many of these cytochrome P450 species in recent years represents a significant achievement in the area of drug metabolism. From studies with the purified enzymes, it is now clear that the species of cytochrome P450 confers the substrate specificity to the monooxygenase system[43,45,46,48,49].

Exposure of an animal to chemical agents such as phenobarbital or 3-methylcholanthrene results in the induction of cytochrome P450 species that differ in terms of the absorption maxima for the reduced cytochrome P450-carbon monoxide complex, molecular weight (Table 1) and immunological properties[76-78]. Table 1 also summarizes the metabolism of a precarcinogen, benzo[a]pyrene, and a drug substrate, benzphetamine, by various forms of cytochrome P450 in reconstituted systems containing fixed quantities of NADPH-cytochrome P450 reductase and lipid. Although all the species of cytochrome P450 catalyze the metabolism of benzo[a]pyrene and benzphetamine, the activity is markedly dependent on the particular form of cytochrome P450 examined. The activity varies over a hundred-fold range for benzo[a] pyrene hydroxylation and over a forty-fold range for benzphetamine N-demethylation. Since the isozymes of cytochrome P450 also have overlapping substrate specificities, the complex kinetics observed for substrate metabolism, patterns of inhibition[71-75] and the species, strain and sex differences, can now be explained in terms of these multiple forms in microsomal preparations.

In addition to differences in substrate specificity (Table 1), these hemeproteins also demonstrate differences in regiospecificity (different sites of oxidation on the same molecule) as has been demonstrated for testosterone[14,43,48] and benzo[a]pyrene[79,80]. These differences in catalytic properties would therefore influence the formation of potentially benign, cytotoxic or carcinogenic metabolites from drugs, polycyclic aromatic hydrocarbons and other foreign compounds.

IV. Component Organization and Interaction within the Microsomal Membrane-Cytochrome P450 is a major protein in microsomal preparations constituting up to 10% of the total, membrane-bound proteins[14]. There is a 20 to 30-fold mole excess of this protein relative to NADPH-cytochrome P450 reductase in these microsomal preparations. The spatial organization and mode(s) of interaction between these two proteins within the microsomal membrane are subjects of continued controversy. This has been comprehensively reviewed by Depierre and Dallner[17].

The surface localization of these proteins on the microsomal membrane has been investigated mainly through the use of macromolecule agents which do not penetrate the microsomal membrane. For example, the reductase flavoprotein is readily solubilized from the microsomal membrane by protease digestion[17,81] indicating that much of this protein is localized on the outer or cytoplasmic surface of the membrane. In contrast, protease treatment does not solubilize significant quantities of cytochrome P450[17,81]. Furthermore, antibodies prepared against partially purified cytochrome P420 (a degradation product of cytochrome P450 resulting from protease treatment) do not inhibit

TABLE 1

BENZO[a]PYRENE AND BENZPHETAMINE METABOLISM BY RECONSTITUTED SYSTEMS CONTAINING VARIOUS SPECIES OF CYTOCHROME P-450

Cytochrome P-450 Species[a]	Absorption maximum of reduced CO-complex (nm)	Subunit M.W.[b]	Benzo[a]-pyrene nmol products/min/nmol P-450	Benz-phetamine nmol products/min/nmol P-450	Reference
Rat (PB)	450	(44,000 (46,000 (47,000	0.2	52	15
Rat (3-MC)	447	53,000	3.9	2	15
Mouse A_2(PB)	451	50,000	0.3	5	43
Mouse C_2 (PB)	450	56,000	0.1	8	43
Rabbit LM_1	448.6	47,000	1.5	3	45
LM_2(PB)	450.8	49,000	0.6	80	
LM_{4a}(β-NF)	446.6	53,000	1.3	2	
LM_{4b}(β-NF)	447.1	.53,000	0.2	5	
LM_7	449.3	60,000	1.2	2	
LM_x(PB)	448.4	53,000	0.8	2	
Rabbit form a (TCDD)	450.5	48,000	0.4	12	50
form b (TCDD)	448	60,000	4.1	4	
form c (TCDD)	447	54,500	0.03	2	

[a]Various forms of cytochrome P-450 were purified from liver microsomes of animals treated with different inducers indicated in parentheses. PB, phenobarbital; 3-MC, 3-methylcholanthrene; β-NF, β-naphthoflavone; TCDD, 2,3,7,8-tetrachlorodibenzo-p-dioxin.

[b]Molecular weight of subunit determined by gel electrophoresis in the presence of sodium dodecyl sulfate.

microsomal benzphetamine N-demethylation[82]. These data minimally suggest that the prosthetic group of cytochrome P450 is imbedded in the microsomal membrane and is not sensitive to either proteolytic enzymes or antibodies.

On the other hand, Welton et al[83] have demonstrated the ^{125}I-radiolabelling of this enzyme by lactoperoxidase while Thomas, et al[84] have shown the inhibition of various microsomal monooxygenase reactions by antibodies prepared against highly purified, detergent solubilized, cytochrome P450 preparations. These results are consistent with the surface localization of a significant portion of these hemeproteins on the microsomal membrane.

Several studies have examined the interaction between cytochrome P450 and reductase proteins within the microsomal membrane. This has been recently reviewed by Yang[18]. Two models have been proposed for the arrangement of reductase and cytochrome P450 molecules in the membrane. A "rigid" model in which a single reductase molecule is surrounded by a cluster or sphere of the more numerous cytochrome P450 molecules[85]. Ordered regions or clusters of these enzymes form discrete electron transport complexes. Thus, translational motion of the cytochrome is not required for the electron transport between these proteins necessary for substrate oxidation.

Alternatively, a "nonrigid" model has been proposed[86] in which both the reductase and cytochrome P450 molecules are randomly distributed within the matrix of the membrane. Lateral diffusion mobility is required between reductase and cytochrome P450 for efficient electron coupling between these proteins.

V. Mechanism of the Cytochrome P450 Monooxygenase Reaction--Investigations into the mechanism of substrate oxidation by the cytochrome P450 system were initiated soon after the discovery of microsomal cytochrome P450[35,87] and the class of enzymes collectively known as oxygenases[88,89]. The monooxygenase nature of cytochrome P450-catalyzed reactions, in which one atom of molecular oxygen is transferred to the substrate, was demonstrated by Posner, et al[90] with $^{18}O_2$ experiments.

$$NADPH + SH + {}^{18}O_2 + H^+ \longrightarrow NADP^+ + S^{18}OH + H_2{}^{18}O \qquad (1)$$

Unfortunately, the microsomal enzyme system contains several enzymes such as catalase and pyrophosphatases that impeded early attempts to quantitatively elucidate the stoichiometry and mechanism of cytochrome P450-catalyzed reactions. Nevertheless, considerable knowledge about the sequence of events leading to substrate oxidation by cytochrome P450 has been obtained. This has been recently reviewed by Estabrook and Werringloer[91] and is summarized in Figure 2. Briefly, the substrate (SH) binds reversibly to the oxidized cytochrome to form a binary complex. NADPH-cytochrome P450 reductase catalyzes a one electron transfer to form a ferrous cytochrome P450-substrate complex. The reduced cytochrome can bind either CO to give a λ_{max} 450 nm absorbing species, characteristic of this protein, or to O_2 forming the ternary SH-cytochrome P450$(Fe)^{2+}$-O_2 complex. The latter species has been observed, under steady state conditions, in both microsomal[37] and purified enzyme[38] systems. A second electron equivalent is transferred from NADPH via the reductase to the ternary complex. The actual charge distribution between the cytochrome iron and O_2 are unknown in this complex and therefore a formal charge of plus one is indicated outside the brackets containing the entire complex. One possible distribution of charge within the complex giving an "active oxygen" species is also illustrated. In this case, O_2 has taken on the formal oxidation state of H_2O_2. This ternary complex, containing the "activated oxygen" then breaks down to give the hydroxylated product (SOH), water and oxidized cytochrome P450.

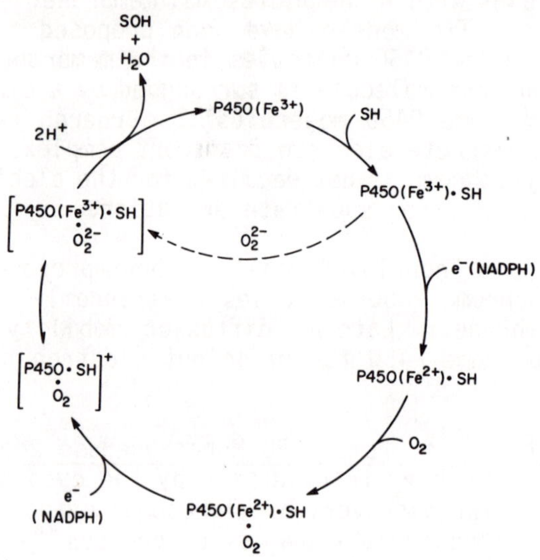

Figure 2

In recent years, the combined efforts of biochemists and organic chemists have resulted in the successful purification of various components of this multienzyme system and the elucidation of several chemical models for cytochrome P450-catalyzed reactions. Although no definitive mechanism has emerged, the arena of possible mechanisms has been considerably narrowed.

The purified and reconstituted cytochrome P450 system has been particularly useful in mechanism studies. For example, Nordblom and Coon[92] have demonstrated the 1:1:1 stoichiometry between NADPH oxidation, O_2 utilization and product(s) formation required by Equation 1 which had eluded earlier attempts with the microsomal system. In addition to the substrate hydroxylating capacity of cytochrome P450, NADPH is also oxidized by O_2 to form $NADP^+$ and H_2O_2 (Equation 2). Whether this reaction results from the autoxidation of cytochrome P450 following the second electron transfer (Equation 3) or from a reduced flavin-catalyzed formation of H_2O_2 from O_2, via free radical intermediates, by NADPH-cytochrome P450 reductase (Equation 4) or a combination of both pathways is unknown.

$$NADPH + O_2 + H^+ \longrightarrow NADP^+ + H_2O_2 \qquad (2)$$

$$P450(Fe^{++})O_2 + e^- + 2H^+ \longrightarrow P450(Fe^{+++}) + H_2O_2 \qquad (3)$$

$$FADH_2 + O_2 \longrightarrow FADH\cdot + HO_2\cdot \longrightarrow FAD + H_2O_2 \qquad (4)$$

Both reaction 1 leading to substrate hydroxylation and reaction 2 leading to H_2O_2 formation occur in microsomal[93-95] and reconstituted systems[92]. The sum of reactions 1 and 2 account for the total quantities of substrate and cofactor oxidized versus hydroxylated product(s) and H_2O_2 formed[92].

Perhaps the most plausible description of the "active oxygen" species involved in cytochrome P450-catalyzed oxidations was proposed by Hamilton[92]. By analogy to carbene and nitrene chemistry, Hamilton postulated a transition state for an electrophilic "active oxygen" species with electronic properties similar to a singlet oxygen atom. The oxygen insertion reaction catalyzed by the cytochrome P450 system of unactivated alkanes to give alcohols and of aromatic compounds to form phenols and arene oxides, finds analogy in the carbene insertion reaction between C-H bonds of alkanes to give alkylbenzenes and of aromatic compounds to form norcaradienes. This oxenoid or oxygen atom transfer mechanism is also supported by the "NIH shift" reaction[97] observed with the microsomal cytochrome P450 system. The product, 4, in which tritium

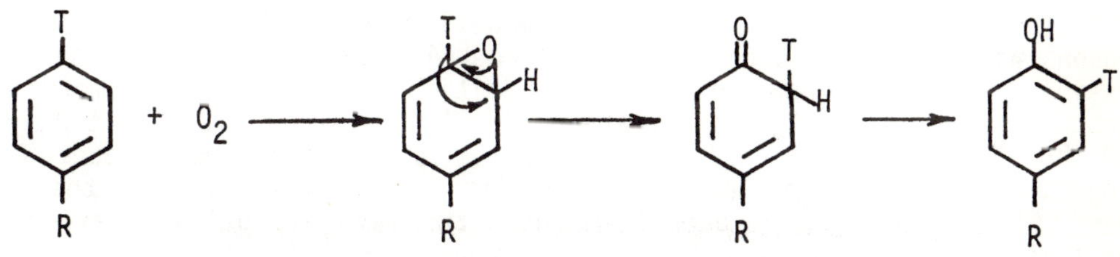

1 2 3 4

migration is observed is best explained by the epoxide intermediate, 2, formed by the electrophilic attack of an oxenoid reagent. The "NIH shift" mechanism has been recently confirmed[98] with a reconstituted system employing partially purified enzyme components.

It is generally agreed that oxidation of the substrate occurs after the second electron reduction of the ternary complex by NADPH-cytochrome P450 reductase to form $[SH\text{-}P450\text{-}O_2]^{+}$[91]. Thus, there are three possible oxenoid reagents: (1) SH-P450(Fe^{+})-O_2 complex, (2) SH-P450(Fe^{3+})-O_2^{2-} or (3) SH-P450(Fe^{5+})-O complex. Of the three, the second complex appears to be the most probable since H_2O_2[99], electrochemically generated HO_2^{-}[100], and organic hydroperoxides[101,102] can, in many cases, support substrate hydroxylation (Figure 2) in systems containing cytochrome P450 but devoid of O_2, NADPH and NADPH-cytochrome P450 reductase. The cytochrome P450-dependent oxygen insertion reaction supported by cumene hydroperoxide results in the incorporation of oxygen primarily from the peroxide[99]. Furthermore, ferrous cytochrome P450 is not involved since CO does not inhibit this reaction. Thus, the role of both inorganic and organic peroxides may be in the formation of an "active oxygen" species similar to the enzyme-peracid or enzyme-peramide intermediates postulated by Hamilton[103] for the cytochrome P450 monooxygenases.

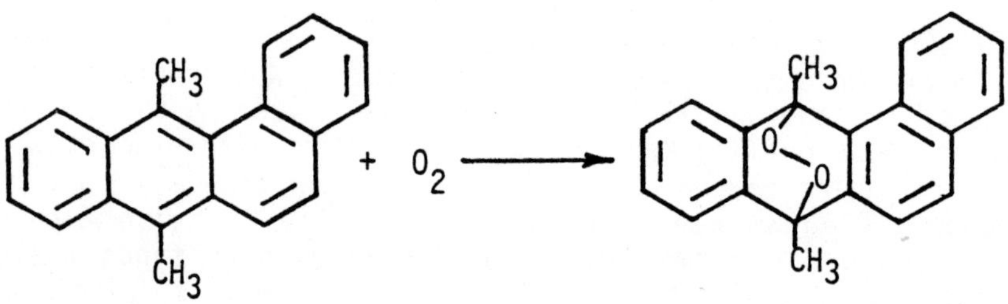

5 6

Molecular singlet oxygen has largely been ruled out for energetic reasons as an oxenoid reagent in cytochrome P450-catalyzed reactions[103]. One possible exception, however, is the addition of O_2 to 9,10-dimethyl-1,2-benzanthracene, 5, to form the transannular 1,4-peroxide, 6, reported by Chen and Tu[104]. The transannular product, 6, is the expected product from a singlet oxygen reaction with 5. Singlet O_2 originating from the Haber-Weiss[105,106] reaction has been documented and may be a possible explanation for this singlet oxygen reaction in microsomal incubations.

References

1. J.A. Miller, Cancer Res., 30, 559-576, (1970).
2. J.W. Daly, D.M. Jerina and B. Witkop, Experientia 28, 1129-1149, (1972).
3. D.M. Jerina and J.W. Daly, Science, 185, 573-582, (1974).
4. P. Sims and P.L. Grover, Adv. Cancer Res., 20, 165-274, (1974).
5. C. Heidelberger, Ann. Rev. Biochem. 44, 79-121, (1975).

6. S.D. Nelson, M.R. Boyd and J.R. Mitchell in "Drug Metabolism Concepts," D.M. Jerina, Ed., American Chemical Society, Washington, D.C., 1977, pp 155-185.
7. C.R.E. Jefcoate, J.L. Gaylor and R.L. Calabrese, Biochem, 8, 3455-3463, (1969).
8. G.M. Cohen and G.J. Mannering, Mol. Pharmacol., 9, 383-397, (1973).
9. W.J. Canady, O.A. Robinson and H.D. Colby, Biochem. Pharmacol., 23, 3075-3078, (1974).
10. A.K. Cho and G.T. Miwa, Drug Metab. Disp., 2, 477-483, (1974).
11. A.H. Conney, Pharmacol. Rev., 19, 317-366, (1967).
12. E.E. Ohnhaus and J. Th. Locher, Eur. J. Pharmacol., 31, 161-165, (1975).
13. A.Y.H. Lu, Fed. Proc., 35, 2460-2463, (1976)
14. M.J. Coon, D.A. Haugen, F.P. Guengerich, J.L. Vermilion and W.L. Dean, in "The Structural Basis of Membrane Function," Y. Hatefi and L. Djavadi-Ohaniance, Eds., Academic Press, New York, N.Y., 1976, pp. 409-427.
15. W. Levin in "Microsomes and Drug Oxidations," V. Ullrich, I. Roots, A. Hildebrandt, R.W. Estabrook, and A.H. Conney, Eds., Pergamon Press, New York, N.Y., 1977, pp 735-747.
16. A.Y.H. Lu and S.B. West, Pharmacol. Ther. Part A., 2, in press, (1977).
17. J.W. Depierre and G. Dallner, Biochim. Biophys. Acta, 415, 411-472, (1975).
18. C.S. Yang, Life Sci., 21, 1047-1058, (1977).
19. A.Y.H. Lu and W. Levin, Biochim. Biophys. Acta, 344, 205-240, (1974).
20. M.J. Coon, J.L. Vermilion, K.P. Vatsis, J.S. French, W.L. Dean and D.A. Haugen, in "Drug Metabolism Concepts," D.M. Jerina, Ed., American Chemical Society, Washington, D.C., 1977, pp 46-71.
21. "Fundamentals of Drug Metabolism and Drug Disposition," B.N. La Du, H.G., Mandel and E.L. Way, Eds., Williams & Wilkins, Baltimore, M.D., 1971.
22. "Cytochromes P450 and b_5: Structure, Function, and Interaction," D.Y. Cooper, O. Rosenthal, R. Snyder, C. Witmer, Eds., Plenum Press, New York, N.Y., 1975.
23. B. Testa and P. Jenner, in "Drug Metabolism: Chemical and Biochemical Aspects," Marcel Dekker, New York, N.Y., 1976.
24. "Microsomes and Drug Oxidations," J.R. Gillette, A.H. Conney, G.J. Cosmides, R.W. Estabrook, J.R. Fouts and G.J. Mannering, Eds., Academic Press, New York, N.Y., 1969.
25. "Microsomes and Drug Oxidations," R.W. Estabrook, J.R. Gillette and K.C. Liebman, Eds., Williams & Wilkins, Baltimore, M.D., 1972.
26. "Microsomes and Drug Oxidations," V. Ullrich, I. Roots, A. Hildebrandt, R.W. Estabrook and A.H. Conney, Eds., Pergamon Press, New York, N.Y., 1977.
27. J.B. Schenkman, I. Jansson and K.M. Robie-Suh, Life Sci., 19, 611-624, (1976).
28. M.D. Maines and M.W. Anders, Arch. Biochem. Biophys. 159, 201-205, (1973).
29. H.R. Mahler and E.H. Cordes, in "Biological Chemistry," 2nd ed., Harper and Row, New York, N.Y., 1971, p. 675.
30. B.W. Griffin, J.A. Peterson, J. Werringloer and R.W. Estabrook, Ann. N.Y. Acad, Sci., 244, 107-131, (1975).

31. J. Peisach, J.O. Stern and W.E. Blumberg, Drug Metab. Disp, 1, 45-61, (1973).
32. M. Chevion, J. Peisach and W.E. Blumberg, J. Biol. Chem., 252, 3637-3645, (1977).
33. H.S. Mason, Ann. Rev. Biochem., 34, 595-634, (1965).
34. K. Comai and J.L. Gaylor, J. Biol.Chem., 248, 4947-4955, (1973).
35. O. Garfinkel, Arch. Biochem. Biophys, 77, 493-509, (1958).
36. Y. Imai and R. Sato, Biochem. Biophys. Res. Commun., 23, 5-11, (1966).
37. R.W. Estabrook, A.G. Hildebrandt, J. Baron, K.J. Netter and K. Leibman, Biochem. Biophys. Res. Commun., 42, 132-139, (1971).
38. F.P. Guengerich, D.P. Ballou and M.J. Coon, Biochem. Biophys. Res. Commun., 70, 951-956, (1976).
39. S. Narasimhulu, D.Y. Cooper and O. Rosenthal, Life Sci., 4, 2102-2107, (1965).
40. H. Remmer, J.B. Schenkman and H. Greim, in " Microsomes and Drug Oxidations," J.R. Gillette, A.H. Conney, G.J. Cosmides, R.W. Estabrook, J.R. Fouts, and G.J. Mannering, Eds., Academic Press, New York, N.Y., 1969, pp. 371-386.
41. J.B. Schenkman, H. Remmer and R.W. Estabrook, Mol. Pharmacol., 3, 113-123, (1967).
42. D.A. Haugen, T.A. van der Hoeven and M.J. Coon, J. Biol. Chem., 250, 3567-3570, (1975).
43. M-T. Huang, S.B. West and A.Y.H. Lu, J. Biol. Chem., 251, 4659-4665, (1976).
44. R.M. Philpot and E. Arinc, Mol. Pharmacol., 12, 483-493, (1976).
45. F.P. Guengerich, J. Biol. Chem., 252, 3970-3979, (1977).
46. E.F. Johnson and U. Muller-Eberhard, J. Biol. Chem., 252, 2839-2845, (1977).
47. D.E. Ryan, P.E. Thomas and W. Levin, Mol. Pharmacol., 13, 521-532, (1977).
48. D. Ryan, A.Y.H. Lu, S.B. West and W. Levin, J. Biol. Chem., 250, 2157-2163, (1975).
49. A.Y.H. Lu, R. Kuntzman, S.B. West and A.H. Conney, Biochem. Biophys. Res. Commun., 42, 1200-1206, (1971).
50. E.F. Johnson and U. Muller-Eberhard, Biochem. Biophys. Res. Commun., 76, 644-651, (1977).
51. D.A. Haugen and M.J. Coon, J. Biol. Chem., 251, 7929-7939, (1976).
52. D.A. Haugen L.G. Armes, K.T. Yasunobu and M.J. Coon, Biochem. Biophys. Res. Commun., 77, 967-973, (1977).
53. B.S.S. Masters, E.B. Nelson, B.A. Schacter, J. Baron and E.L. Isaacson, Drug Metab. Disp., 1, 121-128, (1973).
54. J.P. Collman, T.N. Sorrell, B.M. Hoffman, J. Am. Chem. Soc., 97, 913, (1975).
55. C.K. Chang and D. Dolphin, J. Am. Chem. Soc., 98, 1607-1609, (1976).
56. H. Sakurai and M. Kito, Biochem. Pharmacol., 25, 2113-2116, (1976).
57. J.O. Stern and J. Peisach, Febs. Lett., 62, 364-368, (1976).
58. H.H. Ruf and P. Wende, J. Am. Chem. Soc., 99, 5499-5500, (1977).
59. J.C. Kawalek, W. Levin, D. Ryan and A.Y.H. Lu, Arch. Biochem. Biophys. 183, 732-741, (1977).
60. S. Orrenhius and L. Ernster, Biochem. Biophys. Res. Commun., 16, 60-65, (1964).

61. J.L. Vermilion and M.J. Coon, Biochem. Biophys. Res. Commun., 60, 1315-1322, (1974).
62. B.S.S. Masters, J. Baron, W.E. Taylor, E.L. Isaacson and J. LoSpalluto, J. Biol. Chem., 246, 4143-4150, (1971).
63. J.D. Dignam and H.W. Strobel, Biochem. Biophys. Res. Commun., 63, 845-852, (1975).
64. Y. Yasukochi and B.S.S. Masters, J. Biol. Chem, 251, 5337-5344, (1976).
65. J.A. Knapp, J.D. Dignam and H.W. Strobel, J. Biol. Chem., 252, 437-443, (1977).
66. R.I. Glazer, J.B. Schenkman and A.C. Sartorelli, Mol. Pharmacol., 7, 683-688, (1971).
67. A.F. Welton and S.D. Aust, Biochem. Pharmacol., 24, 1641-1644, (1975).
68. J.A. Peterson, R.E. White, Y. Yasukochi, M.L. Coomes, D.H. O'Keefe, R.E. Ebel, B.S.S. Masters, D.P. Ballou and M.J. Coon, J. Biol. Chem., 252, 4431-4434, (1977).
69. D.Y. Cooper, M.D. Cannon, H. Schleyer and O. Rosenthal, J. Biol. Chem., 252, 4755-4757, (1977).
70. A.Y.H. Lu, S.B. West, M. Vore, D. Ryan and W. Levin, J. Biol. Chem., 249, 6701-6709, (1974).
71. R. Kuntzman, W. Levin, G. Schilling and A. Alvares, in "Microsomes and Drug Oxidations," J.R. Gillette, A.H. Conney, G.J. Cosmides, R.W. Estabrook, J.R. Fouts and G.J. Mannering, Eds., Academic Press, New York, N.Y., 1969, pp. 349-369.
72. D.S. Hewick and J.R. Fouts, Biochem. Pharmacol., 19, 457-472, (1970).
73. T.C. Pederson and S.D. Aust, Biochem. Pharmacol., 19, 2221-2230, (1970).
74. J. Werringloer and R.W. Estabrook, Arch. Biochim. Biophys., 167, 270-286, (1975).
75. S.D. Aust and J.B. Stevens, Biochem. Pharmacol., 20, 1061-1069, (1971).
76. P.E. Thomas, A.Y.H. Lu, D. Ryan, S.B. West and W. Levin, Life Sci., 15, 1475-1483, (1974).
77. P.E. Thomas, A.Y.H. Lu, D. Ryan, S.B. West, J. Kawalek and W. Levin, J.Biol. Chem., 251, 1385-1391, (1976).
78. W.L. Dean and M.J. Coon, J. Biol. Chem., 252, 3255-3261, (1977).
79. F.J. Weibel, J.K. Selkirk, H.V. Gelboin, D.A. Haugen, T.A. van der Hoeven and M.J. Coon, Proc. Natl. Acad. Sci., 73, 3917-3920, (1975).
80. A.Y.H. Lu, W. Levin, M. Vore, A.H. Conney, D.R. Thakker, G. Holder and D.M. Jerina, in "Carcinogenesis, Vol. 1, Polynuclear Aromatic Compounds: Chemistry, Metabolism and Carcinogenesis," R.I. Freudenthal and P.W. Jones, Eds., Raven Press, New York, N.Y., 1976, pp. 115-126.
81. A. Ito and R. Sato, J. Cell. Biol., 40, 179-189, (1969).
82. A.F. Welton, F.O. O'Neal, L.C. Chaney and S.D. Aust, J. Biol. Chem., 250, 5631-5640, (1975).
83. A.F. Welton and S.D. Aust, Biochim. Biophys. Acta, 373, 197-210, (1974).
84. P.E. Thomas, A.Y.H. Lu, S.B. West, D. Ryan, G.T. Miwa and W. Levin, Mol. Pharmacol., 13, 819-831, (1977).
85. M.R. Franklin and R.W. Estabrook, Arch. Biochem. Biophys., 143, 318-329, (1971).
86. C.S. Yang, Febs. Lett., 54, 61-64, (1975).
87. M. Klingenberg, Arch. Biochem. Biophys., 75, 376-386, (1958).
88. O. Hayaishi, M. Katagani and S. Rothberg, J. Amer. Chem. Soc., 77, 5450-5451, (1955).

89. H.S. Mason, W.L. Fowlks and E. Peterson, J. Amer. Chem. Soc., 77, 2914-2915, (1955).
90. H.S. Posner, C. Mitoma, S. Rothberg and S. Udenfriend, Arch. Biochem. Biophys., 94, 280-290, (1961).
91. R.W. Estabrook and J. Werringloer, in "Drug Metabolism Concepts," D.M. Jerina, Ed., American Chemical Society, Washington, D.C., 1977, pp.1-26.
92. G.D. Nordblom and M.J. Coon, Arch. Biochem. Biophys., 180, 343-347, (1977).
93. J.R. Gillette, B.B. Brodie and B.N. La Du, J. Pharmacol. Expt. Therap., 119, 532-540, (1957).
94. R.G. Thurman, H.G. Ley and R. Scholz, Eur. J. Biochem., 25, 420-430, (1972).
95. A.G. Hildebrandt and I. Roots, Arch. Biochem. Biophys., 171, 385-397, (1975).
96. G.A. Hamilton, J. Amer. Chem. Soc., 86, 3391, (1964).
97. D.M. Jerina and J.W. Daly, in "Oxidases and Related Redox Systems, Proc. Int. Symp., 2nd," T.E. King, H.S. Mason and M. Morrison, Eds., University Park Press, Baltimore, M.D., 1973, pp. 143-161.
98. A.D. Rahimtula, P.J. O'Brien, H.E. Seifried and D.M. Jerina, Fed. Proc., 34, 623, (1975).
99. G.D. Nordblom, R.E. White and M.J. Coon, Arch. Biochem. Biophys., 175, 524-533, (1976).
100. F. Scheller, R. Renneberg, P. Mohr, G-R. Jäng and K. Ruckpaul, Febs. Lett., 71, 309-312, (1976).
101. E.G. Hrycay, J-A. Gustafsson, M. Ingelman-Sunberg and L. Ernster, Biochem. Biophys. Res. Commun., 66, 209-216, (1975).
102. E.G. Hrycay, J-A. Gustafsson, M. Ingelman-Sundberg and L. Ernster, Febs. Lett. 56, 161-165, (1975).
103. G.A. Hamilton, in "Molecular Mechanisms of Oxygen Activation," O. Hayaishi Ed., Academic Press, New York, N.Y., 1974, pp. 405-451.
104. C. Chen and M.H. Tu, Biochem. J., 160, 805-808, (1976).
105. F. Haber and J. Weiss, Proc. R. Soc., A147, 332-351, (1934).
106. E.W. Kellog and I. Fridovich, J. Biol. Chem., 250, 8812-8817, (1975).

Chapter 23. The Current Status of Iron Chelation Therapy

Robert W. Grady and Anthony Cerami, The Rockefeller University, N.Y., N.Y.

While iron deficiency is well-known and is in fact the leading cause of anemia in man,[1] the pathological accumulation of excess iron is also widespread. Iron accumulation results from hyperabsorption of dietary iron (primary hemosiderosis) or from transfusion therapy (secondary hemosiderosis). While primary hemochromatosis is a rather rare genetic disease, the thalassemia syndromes (alpha and beta) are much more common. These too are genetic disorders, the defect being an imbalance in the synthesis of the alpha and beta chains of hemoglobin respectively. Patients afflicted with either of the latter syndromes suffer from an anemia which ranges from very mild to life threatening. It is necessary to give frequent blood transfusions to those children whose anemia is severe. Worldwide, it is estimated that 3 million people show clinically significant manifestations of thalassemia. Beta-thalassemia is most common throughout the Mediterranean basin and the Middle East whereas alpha-thalassemia is prevalent in the Far East. The geographical distribution is similar to that of malaria suggesting that, as in the case of sickle cell anemia, the heterozygotes or gene carriers are somewhat protected against the malaria parasite. In some areas heterozygotes make up as much as 30% of the population.[2]

The accumulation of iron is due to the fact that man lacks a physiological means of excreting this metal. The amount of iron present in the body is regulated solely by absorption.[3] This unusual regulatory mechanism probably arose as a result of the need to conserve this essential nutrient for it is relatively difficult to obtain from the diet due to the extreme insolubility of most environmental iron. The acquisition of this element is a problem common to virtually all biological organisms. Hence the multitude of complex mechanisms for sequestration, transport and storage of iron which have been developed by microbes and plants so as to compete effectively for that which is available.[4,5]

In man, iron is stored in various tissues as either ferritin or hemosiderin. Ferritin is a protein consisting of 24 subunits arranged in the form of a shell about a core of precipitated iron oxides. That which is called hemosiderin is believed to be aggregates of ferritin which has been partially digested by lysosomes.[6] Storage of excess iron is necessary to prevent its initiation of free radical reactions within the body. In iron overload, however, <u>de novo</u> synthesis of ferritin is unable to completely protect tissues from cell damage and subsequent fibrosis. Particularly noteworthy are the progressive fibrotic changes in the liver, heart and endocrine organs of iron-overloaded patients.[7] Most untreated

ISBN 0-12-040513-X

thalassemic patients die of cardiac complications during the first or second decade while those with untreated primary hemochromatosis die in their fifties, primarily of liver failure.

The clinical management of patients with primary hemosiderosis calls for venesection at regular intervals until body stores return to normal. The removal of one unit of blood (500 ml) causes the loss of 250 mg of iron. Phlebotomy of patients with secondary hemochromatosis is obviously precluded since these patients are already anemic and in fact require blood transfusions every few weeks for the maintenance of life. Patients on chronic blood transfusion programs accumulate iron at the rate of 15 to 25 mg per day and thus would be expected to have an excess of approximately 100 g by the age of 20. Until such time as it is possible to treat the primary defect of thalassemia, therapy will most likely depend upon chronic transfusions. Accordingly, the development of an effective pharmacological means of inducing iron excretion is necessary as adjunctive therapy. During the past 20 years, several compounds have been identified as potentially useful iron-chelating drugs and are at different stages of development. Recently, the National Institutes of Health has noted the need for more efficacious drugs and has initiated a program to screen and evaluate iron chelators. Two complementary biological screening procedures are being utilized in the search for new drugs, an *in vitro* technique using Chang liver cells[8] and an *in vivo* assay employing hypertransfused rats.[9]

The compounds that have been studied to date are primarily those having functional groups found in natural products. These include hydroxamic acids and derivatives of 2,3-dihydroxybenzoic acid. These moieties possess a high affinity for ferric ions rendering compounds highly selective for this metal both *in vitro* and *in vivo*. Briefly we shall describe the current status of the iron chelators which have been identified as having potential therapeutic usefulness.

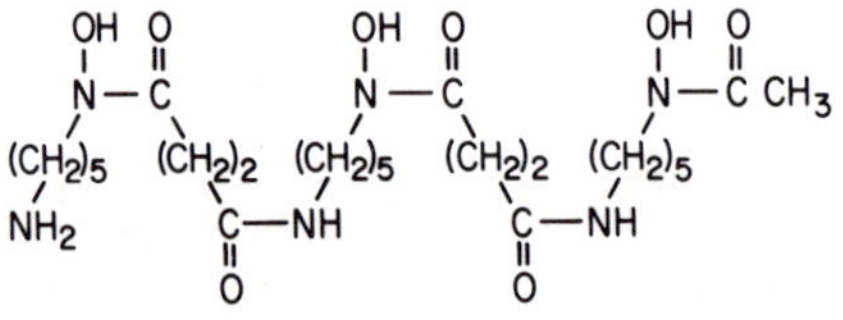

DF

Desferrioxamine - Desferrioxamine (DF) is a hexadentate iron chelator which is produced by the microbe *Streptomyces pilosus*. The three hydroxamic acid groups occupy all six sites in the octahedral coordination sphere of iron. The binding constant of this ligand is 10^{31} reflecting the very high affinity of the hydroxamate moiety for ferric ions. When evaluated in cultured Chang cells, DF is able to prevent the incorporation of iron into ferritin and can induce the mobilization of iron from preloaded ferritin.[10] Moreover, DF causes the excretion of significant amounts of iron when administered intraperitoneally to hypertransfused rats.[9] In spite of this, however, the intramuscular injection of DF into iron overloaded patients is incapable of putting them into negative iron balance. Furthermore, the injections are poorly tolerated by the patients and their parents and thus this mode of therapy has been virtually abandoned. A resurgence of interest in desferrioxamine occurred in 1974 when Barry et al.[11] reported that the persistent use of intramuscular DF-therapy over a 7-year period decreased the rate of iron accumulation in thalassemic patients. Reevaluation of DF centered on maximizing its effectiveness via alternative routes of administration. It had been observed by Smith[12] that maximum urinary excretion of iron occurred when DF was given as a slow intravenous infusion. This occurs for two reasons. First, although an iron-overloaded patient has massive amounts of iron in his body stores, most of this iron is unavailable. At any given time, there is only a small pool of iron which is accessible to low molecular weight chelators. When iron is removed from this chelatable pool, it is refilled relatively slowly from sites of iron storage. Second, the circulating half-life of DF is only 76 minutes,[13] thus a significant portion of the chelator is excreted without iron due to prior depletion of the chelatable iron pool. At the time of Smith's observation, the impracticality of administering DF as a continuous infusion precluded evaluation of this mode of therapy. Recent advances in the development of portable infusion pumps have now made this possible. While injection of a single i.m. dose of DF induces the elimination of 14 to 26 mg of iron, continuous i.v. administration of the same dose over 24 hours leads to the excretion of 74 mg of iron, close to that expected on stoichiometric grounds.[14] Similar results have been obtained upon continuous subcutaneous infusion of DF to thalassemics on an outpatient basis.[15,16] Extended clinical evaluation of this mode of administration is currently underway to determine if DF-therapy can significantly delay or, hopefully, prevent the pathological changes associated with iron overload.

Attempts to increase the size of the chelatable pool available to DF have centered upon the use of pharmacological doses of ascorbic acid. It was noted by Bothwell and his co-workers[17] that iron-overloaded patients who had concomitant scurvy showed a decreased response to DF. Administration of ascorbic acid dramatically increased the magnitude of the response. Ascorbic acid therapy has also been shown to increase urinary iron excretion in thalassemic patients treated with DF.[18,19] On the other hand, the advisability of administering DF and ascorbic acid to iron-overloaded patients has been questioned both clinically and theoretically. Apparent cardiac toxicity has been noted in several patients placed on this regimen.[20.21] Moreover, there is justifiable concern about increasing the pool of chelatable iron in the presence of excess ascorbic acid since ferric ascorbate is well known as an initiator of free radical reactions.[22] Thus, most workers are now recommending that patients be replete with ascorbic acid while discouraging its use in pharmacological doses. Nevertheless, a means of increasing the size of the chelatable pool in a safe manner would be a useful adjunct to chelation therapy.

<u>2,3-Dihydroxybenzoic Acid</u> - 2,3-Dihydroxybenzoic acid (2,3-DHB) has been shown to be a potentially useful orally effective iron-chelating agent.[9] Many naturally-occurring iron chelators are conjugates of 2,3-DHB.[23-25] In

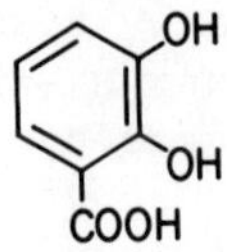

2,3-DHB

the case of these conjugates, both vicinal hydroxyls participate in iron binding while in that of 2,3-DHB itself, mixed complexes may form at physiological pH involving both hydroxyls or the carboxyl group and the adjacent hydroxyl.[26] The oral administration of 2,3-DHB to iron-overloaded rats promotes the excretion of urinary iron in a dose dependent fashion.[9] Preliminary clinical trials in patients with beta-thalassemia showed that iron excretion ranged from 1.4 to 19 mg per day following oral administration of 2,3-DHB.[27] The cause of this variability is not known although there is evidence which suggests that it may reflect the ability of a given person to transform 2,3-DHB into a more active metabolite which has not as yet been identified.[8] Also of note is the fact that the route of iron excretion induced by 2,3-DHB differs in rat and man.[27] In the rat, iron excretion is via the urine whereas in man, only fecal excretion of iron is elevated. A species difference is also observed in the case of DF which promotes predominantly fecal excretion in rats and urinary excretion in man. The basis for such species differences is unknown.

Clinical studies to date suggest that oral administration of 2,3-DHB, like the i.m. administration of desferrioxamine, is not capable of keeping patients in negative iron balance but rather is useful in retarding the rate of iron accumulation.[26] At present, it appears that slow subcutaneous infusion of DF is the only practical way of achieving iron balance in these patients. Another property of 2,3-DHB is its ability to act as a free radical scavenger[29]. As noted above, the tissue degeneration observed in iron overload is believed to result from free radical mediated damage to cellular components. Evidence for this resides in the fact that lipofuscin, which arises via the polymerization of unsaturated lipids, is commonly observed in this disease.[30] However, although 2,3-DHB is quite effective in scavenging radicals _in vitro_,[31] it was not possible to demonstrate decreased radical damage in patients who received 2,3-DHB for a period of one year.[28] Nevertheless, the adjunctive use of free radical trapping agents should decrease the pathology associated with iron overload, thus efforts to find more effective agents seem warranted.

The fact that 2,3-DHB is orally absorbed makes it extremely attractive for use in those parts of the world where the cost of daily parenteral administration of a drug is prohibitive. Attempts to improve the efficacy of 2,3-DHB have not been successful. In a series of structural analogues, none was found to be more effective than the parent compound.[32,32] However, since most of these derivatives contained only a single 2,3-DHB moiety and hence a relatively low binding constant for iron,[26] a series of compounds containing multiple 2,3-DHB moieties is being prepared in the hope of increasing efficacy while maintaining oral effectiveness.

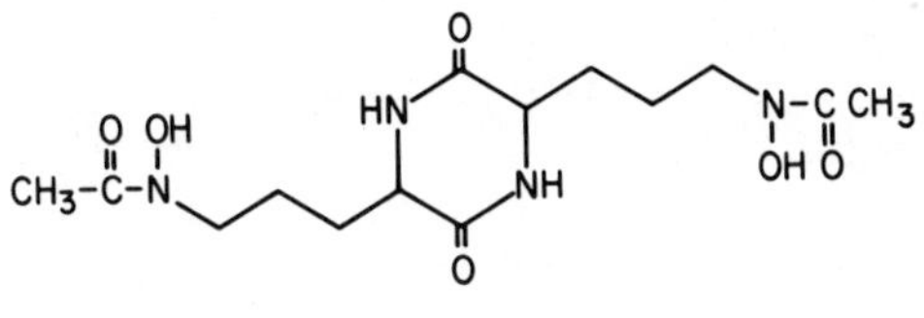

RA

Rhodotorulic Acid - Rhodotorulic acid (RA) is a quadridentate hydroxamic acid produced by the yeast *Rhodotorula pilimanae*. When this organism is grown in iron deficient medium, it produces in excess of 1 g of RA per liter.[34] This is more than 50 times the amount of DF produced by *Streptomyces pilosus*. Thus, if clinically useful, RA should be much more economical than DF. On a weight basis, it is more than 2 times as effective as desferrioxamine at inducing iron excretion in hypertransfused rats following i.p. administration.[35] Unfortunately, like DF, rhodotorulic acid is not orally absorbed, hence it must be given parenterally. It differs from the former compound, however, in that it is relatively insoluble in water. This property may prove advantageous. RA is a good candidate for administration as an intramuscular or subcutaneous depot. Administered in this fashion, the drug would be expected to dissolve at a rate more nearly matching that at which the chelatable iron pool is repleted. Pharmacokinetic studies in dogs have revealed the presence of RA in plasma up to 12 hours after an i.m. injection.[36] This contrasts sharply with the rapid loss of DF (half-life 76 minutes) following administration i.m.[13] In the absence of an effective oral chelator, the availability of a repository preparation would eliminate the necessity of portable infusion pumps as a means of delivering a sufficient amount of drug to place patients in iron balance. Clinical evaluation of rhodotorulic acid is currently underway.[36]

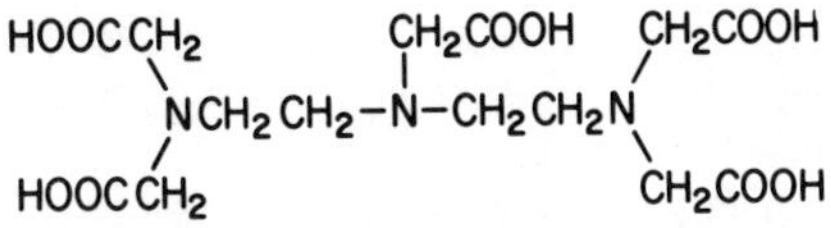

DTPA

Ethylenediamine Derivatives - The intravenous administration of diethylenetriaminepentaacetic acid (DPTA) was found to be more effective than desferrioxamine in promoting iron excretion by beta-thalassemics.[37] The drug is not specific for iron, however, causing significant excretion of magnesium. This, together with side effects including chills, fever, nausea, vomiting and localized pain at the injection site, has led to abandonment of its use.[38]

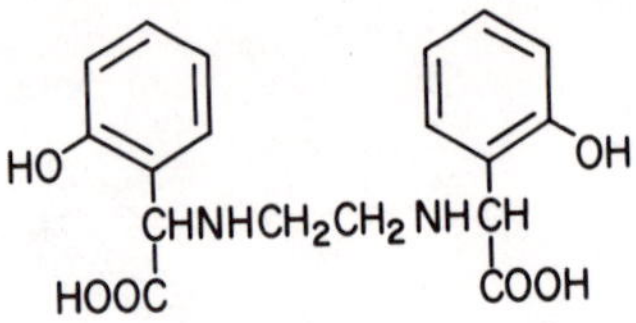

EHPG

Another analogue, ethylenediamine-N,N'-bis-(σ-hydroxyphenylglycine) (EHPG), is more selective and possesses a higher affinity for iron.[39] Nearly 20 years ago, this compound was administered to several iron-overloaded patients and found to promote iron excretion.[40] Unfortunately the work was not followed up until recently when EHPG was found to be the most effective iron chelator in a screen of potential drugs.[41] Of particular interest is the fact that this compound is orally absorbed. In fact, an oral dose of EHPG is more than 75% as effective as an equivalent intraperitoneal dose when administered to hypertransfused rats.[36] Further clinical studies are clearly warranted.

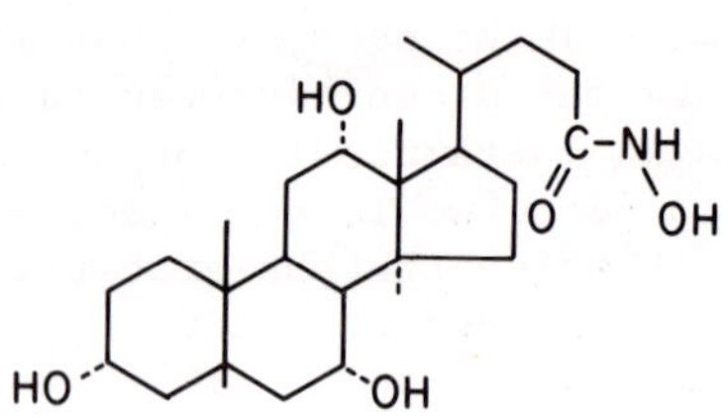

CHA

Cholylhydroxamic Acid - The hydroxamic acid moiety has an unusually high affinity for ferric ions. As noted above, neither DF nor RA is orally absorbed and hence they must be given parenterally. The evaluation of a number of natural and synthetic analogues has revealed that most such compounds are not absorbed from the gut.[32,33] The only orally effective compound found to date is cholylhydroxamic acid (CHA). When evaluated in iron-overloaded rats, cholylhydroxamic acid is as effective as an equivalent parenteral dose of desferrioxamine.[33] Presumably CHA acts as a bile acid and is transported to the liver via the enterohepatic circulation. The iron chelate would then be expected to exit via the bile. Ideally, a non-absorbable iron chelator in the diet, such as a tannin or a polymeric hydroxamic acid,[42] would then remove the iron from the chelate and allow the CHA to be recycled. Pharmacological studies of this compound are now in progress as well as a synthetic program aimed at developing cholic acid derivatives having more than one hydroxamate moiety.[36]

In conclusion, the development of drugs for the purpose of chelating iron is necessary if the sequelae of transfusion therapy are to be avoided. The rational design of such agents is now a challenge to medicinal chemists. Hopefully, in the years to come, an armamentarium of chelating agents will be available which will allow patients with iron overload to remain in iron balance, free of the complications which currently lead to their early demise.

References

1. M.M. Wintrobe in "Clinical Hematology," M.M. Wintrobe, Ed., Ten and Fiebeger, Philadelphia, 1974, p. 638.
2. B. Rotoli in"Iron Metabolism and Thalassemia," D. Bergsma, A. Cerami, C.M. Peterson and J.H. Graziano, Eds., Alan R. Liss, Inc., N.Y., 1976, p. 53.
3. M.J. Shahid, Brit. J. Hematol., 13, 713 (1967).
4. J.B. Neilands, Structure and Bonding, 1, 59 (1966).
5. H. Maehr, Pure and Appl. Chem., 28, 603, (1971).
6. G.W. Richter and M. Bessis, Blood, 25, 370 (1965).
7. J.T. Ellis, I. Schulman and C.H. Smith, Amer. J. Pathol., 30, 287 (1954).
8. G.P. White, A. Jacobs, R.W. Grady and A. Cerami, Brit. J. Hematol., 33, 487 (1976).
9. J.H. Graziano, R.W. Grady and A. Cerami, J. Pharmacol. Exp. Ther, 190, 570 (1974).
10. G.P. White, R. Bailey-Wood and A. Jacobs, Clin. Sci. Mol. Med., 50, 145 (1976).
11. M. Barry, D.M. Flynn, E.A. Letsky and R.A. Risdon, Brit. Med. J., 1, 16 (1974).
12. R.S. Smith, Ann. N.Y. Acad. Sci., 119, 776 (1964).
13. G. Peters, H. Keberle, K. Schmid and H. Brunner, Biochem. Pharmacol., 15, 93 (1966).
14. R.D. Propper, S.B. Shurin and D.G. Nathan, N. Engl. J. Med., 294, 1421 (1976).
15. M.A.M. Hussain, D.M. Flynn, N. Green, S. Hussein and A.V. Hoffbrand, Lancet, 2, 1278 (1976).
16. R.D. Propper, A. Rosenthal, B. Cooper, R.R. Rufo, H.F. Bunn, A.W. Nienhuis, W.F. Anderson and D. Nathan, N. Engl. J. Med., 297, 418 (1977).
17. T.H. Bothwell, B.A. Bradlow, P. Jacobs, K. Keeley, S. Kramer, H. Seftel and S. Zail, Brit. J. Hematol., 10, 50 (1964).
18. R.W. Charlton and T.H. Bothwell in "Iron Metabolism and Thalassemia," D. Bergsma, A. Cerami, C.M. Peterson and J.H. Graziano, Eds., Alan R. Liss, Inc., N.Y., 1976, p. 63.
19. R.T. O'Brien, Ann. N.Y. Acad. Sci., 232, 221 (1974).
20. A.W. Nienhuis, N. Engl. J. Med., 296, 114 (1976).
21. W.L. Henry and A.W. Nienhuis, Arch. Inter. Med., submitted (1977).
22. E.D. Wills, Biochim. Biophys. Acta, 98, 238 (1965).
23. T. Ito and J.B. Neilands, J. Amer. Chem. Soc., 80, 4645 (1958).
24. J.L. Corbin and W.A. Bulen, Biochemistry, 8, 757 (1969).
25. G.H. Tait, Biochem. J., 146, 191 (1975).
26. A. Andeef, S.R. Sofen, T.L. Bregante and K.N. Raymond, J. Amer. Chem. Soc., submitted (1977).

27. C.M. Peterson, J.H. Graziano, R.W. Grady, R.L. Jones, H.V. Vlassara, V.C. Canale, D.R. Miller and A. Cerami, Brit. J. Haematol., 33, 477 (1976).
28. C.M. Peterson, R.W. Grady, R.L. Jones, A. Cerami, J.H. Graziano, A.L. Markenson, V. Lavi, V.C. Canale, G.F. Gray and D.R. Miller, N. Engl. J. Med., 297, 1404 (1977).
29. J.H. Graziano in "Iron Metabolism and Thalassemia," D. Bergsma, A. Cerami, C.M. Peterson and J.H. Graziano, Eds., Alan R. Liss, Inc., 1976, p. 135.
30. C.B. Hyman, B. Landing, R. Alfin-Slater, L. Kozak, J. Weitzman and J.A. Ortega, Ann. N.Y. Acad. Sci., 232., 211 (1974).
31. J.H. Graziano, D.R. Miller, R.W. Grady and A. Cerami, Brit. J. Haematol., 32, 351 (1976).
32. R.W. Grady, J.H. Graziano, H.A. Akers and A. Cerami, J. Pharmacol. Exp. Ther., 196, 478 (1976).
33. R.W. Grady, J.H. Graziano, G.P. White, A. Jacobs and A. Cerami, J. Pharmacol. Exp. Ther., submitted (1977).
34. C.L. Atkin and J.B. Neilands, Biochemistry, 7, 2723 (1968).
35. R.W. Grady, J.H. Graziano, H.A. Akers and A. Cerami, Blood, 44, 911 (1974).
36. R.W. Grady, unpublished results.
37. M. Constantoulakis, J. Economidou, M. Karagiorga, A. Katsantoni and I. Gyftaki, Ann. N.Y. Acad. Sci., 232, 193 (1974).
38. J.L. Fahey, C.E. Rath, J.V. Princiotto, I.B. Brick and M. Rubin, J. Lab. Clin. Med., 57, 436 (1961).
39. A.E. Frost, H.H. Freedman, S.J. Westerback and A.E. Martell, J. Amer. Chem. Soc., 80, 530 (1957).
40. F. Cleton, A. Turnbull and C.A. Finch, J. Clin. Invest., 42, 327 (1963).
41. C.G. Pitt, unpublished observations.
42. A. Winston and G.R. McLaughlin, J. Polym. Sci., Polym. Chem. Ed., 14, 2155 (1976).

Chapter 24. Peptide Conformation and Biological Activity

Garland R. Marshall, Fredric A. Gorin and Michael L. Moore
Department of Physiology and Biophysics
Washington University School of Medicine
St. Louis, Missouri 63110

The primary event of a hormone-induced physiological response is that of recognition or binding. In order to adequately understand this process, one must know the conformation(s) of the hormone in physiological solution and the conformation(s) when bound to the receptor, presumably on the cell surface. Structure-activity studies of peptides have traditionally ignored conformational effects of chemical modification. Emphasis in this review will be to show how these may be used to distinguish between solution and receptor-bound conformations.

I. Solution Conformation - Nuclear magnetic resonance offers the ability to assign a resonance signal to each nucleus of the peptide molecule under study and interpret the chemical shift, relative intensity, and splitting patterns of these resonance signals in terms of angles and rotational freedom about bonds, and proximity of different groups[1]. Unfortunately, interpretation of results are often clouded by hidden assumptions and technical requirements which are not ideal. For example, exchange broadening of NH resonances at neutral or alkaline pH preclude measurement of J_{NC} coupling constants which yield information of the torsional angle ϕ. Interpretation of coupling constants is complicated by the degeneracy of the Karplus equation as well as by the time-scale of NMR, which renders distinguishing a unique conformer from a rapidly interconverting mixture difficult. These ambiguities may be resolved by measurement of multiple coupling constants especially in peptides enriched with either ^{13}C or ^{15}N, as exemplified with valinomycin[2]. Relaxation measurements offer insight into molecular dynamics but require high concentrations of peptide for natural abundance studies of ^{13}C NMR, leading to aggregation[3,4]. Interpretation of spin-lattice relaxation times in terms of overall rotational correlation times and segmental motions are model dependent[5] and inadequate determinations of correlation times have often been made. Measurements of nuclear Overhauser effects provide a valuable auxillary method for intermolecular distance constraints[6], but correlation times must be determined for rigorous interpretation. Other procedures which offer experimental advantages over NMR, due to lower concentration requirements, are laser Raman spectroscopy, e.g. valinomycin[7], and fluorescence energy transfer, e.g. enkephalin[8] and angiotensin[9] analogs.

Calculation of structures with potential energy minima ignore the observations that the conformation of most peptides is very dependent on solvent, which current computational techniques are inadequate to handle in detail. In addition, a dielectric function appears necessary[10] to adequately predict minima of charged molecules with the semi-empirical approach. Molecular orbital approximations of solvent-solute complexes may prove more realistic[11].

ISBN 0-12-040513-X

Considering the conformational lability of peptides in solution, one should not be surprised that interaction with an asymmetric receptor, which may include electrostatic, hydrogen-bonding, and hydrophobic interactions, affects the conformation of the peptide hormone. Evidence exists in studies[12,13] of the binding of S-peptide to S-protein to form ribonuclease-S' that binding of a peptide to a protein induces a conformational change from that observed in solution. Recent studies[14] on luliberin, the hypothalamic decapeptide which controls the release of gonadotropins from the pituitary, have led to the conclusion "that a predetermined solution conformation is not required for biological activity." A similar conclusion was reached[15] based on conformational studies on gramicidin S analogs with equivalent biological activity but with distinctly different conformations.

In summary, examination of the available information indicates that biologically active peptides in solution are flexible with time-averaged conformations which offer little insight into their biological activity.

II. Receptor-bound Conformation - While some workers have argued that the most highly populated conformer in solution will bind with the highest affinity to the receptor, there are excellent *a priori* reasons for believing that this will not be the general case[16], somewhat analogous to the observations that transition state analogs rather than the predominant conformers found in solution bind most tightly to enzymes. It is, therefore, necessary to develop approaches which allow one to deduce the receptor-bound conformation independent of solution observations. Systematic examination of semi-rigid analogs for their conformational effects and correlation with biological activity offers one rational approach. Marshall and Bosshard[17] first showed the dramatic effects of the α-methyl substitution in restricting the conformational flexibility at the substituted residue to a value near those for a right-handed (ϕ = -60, ψ = -50°) or a left-handed (ϕ = 60°, ψ = 50°) α-helix. These calculations have since been confirmed by two other groups[18,19] independently. Two crystal structures of fragments of alamethicin which contain a total of four residues of amino-isobutyric acid, i.e. α-methyl-alanine (Aib), have recently been solved[20,21]. Of the four Aib residues, three occupy the two predicted minima almost exactly (ϕ = -52°, ψ = -38°; ϕ = 48°, ψ = 42°; ϕ = -51°, ψ = -46°) while the fourth is well within the allowed area (ϕ = -72°, ψ = -11°), as shown in Fig. 1. These results confirm the calculations and indicate the strong constraints imposed by such residues when incorporated into peptide chains.

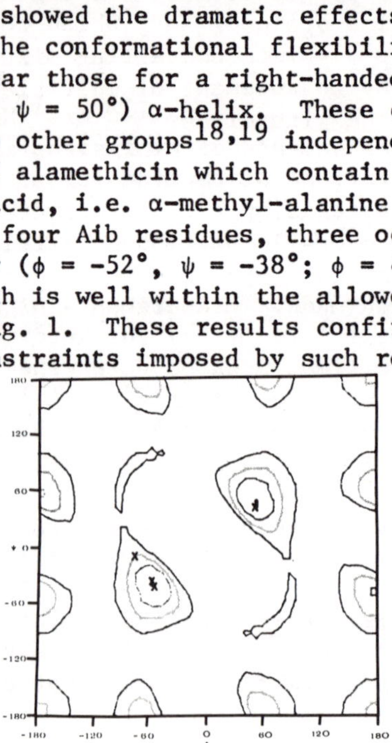

Fig. 1. Potential energy plot for N-acetyl-Aib-methylamide with experimental observations (X) of Aib residues.

The problem of interest is whether these calculated constraints apply to peptides when they bind to receptors. Agreement with the observed values from protein crystallography[22] argues in favor, as one would think that the range of potential distortions of the solution conformation which might occur on binding to the receptor had been adequately sampled in the folding of a large protein. A peptide would be expected to tolerate less distortion than a segment of a protein chain as the end residues can be moved without sacrificing a large number of energetically favorable interactions in order to relieve the local strain.

A basic assumption of a common backbone conformation which orients the essential functional group in the correct spatial positions for all active analogs underlies this approach. Intersection of the set of all possible conformations for each analog contains the biologically active conformer. Identification of essential functional groups by traditional structure-activity studies allows transformation of the problem from conformational space to orientation space where one examines possible pharmacophores, i.e. required groups and their orientation, and removes the objection of a possible analog with a different conformation having activity.

In order to illustrate these concepts, the current state of knowledge of conformation of three peptide hormones will be reviewed.

III. Thyroliberin - To the first level of approximation, six torsional angles are needed to describe the conformation of thyroliberin (TRH), the hypothalamic tripeptide which controls the release of thyroid stimulating hormone from the pituitary: ψ_1, ϕ_2, χ_1, χ_2, ψ_2, and ψ_3.

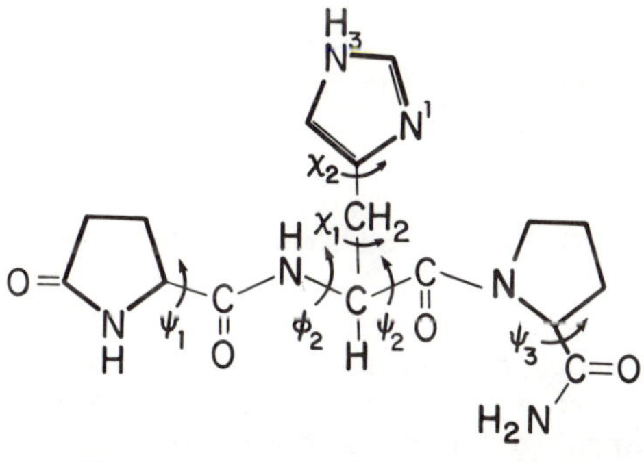

A. NMR Studies - A conformation for TRH in DMSO solution has been proposed[23] in which there is a hydrogen bond between the trans carboxamide hydrogen and the His-Pro carbonyl oxygen and another hydrogen bond between the imidazole N-1 and the Glp-His peptide bond hydrogen. This latter hydrogen bond is proposed because it stabilizes a structure with $\phi_2 = -150°$, compatible with the measured coupling constant. Double resonance techniques in which the $C_\beta H_a$-$C_\beta H_b$ coupling constants are measured lead to an interpretation that a value of $\chi_1 = +60°$ is slightly preferred, which agrees with the assigned hydrogen bond involving the imidazole ring.

Two groups[24,25] have re-evaluated the conformation of TRH in DMSO by pmr and find that $\chi_1 = +60°$ to have the lowest population. They identify the most highly populated rotamer as $\chi_1 = 180°$ because that is the one in which the imidazole is placed nearest the proline. They also measure the temperature dependence of the amide hydrogen chemical shifts and find no evidence for hydrogen bonds. They argue that the steric bulk of the histidine and proline force the peptide backbone into an extended conformation ($\phi_2 \simeq -150°$, $\psi_2 \simeq 150°$), which is consistent with the histidine J_{NC} of 7.2 Hz. The anisotropy of the proline δ and carboxamide hydrogens is due only to the proximity of the imidazole.

Donzel *et al.*[26] prepared the analog [MeHis^2]-TRH and reported its biological activity as 115%. This analog cannot possibly form a hydrogen bond involving the imidazole N1. They also studied its pmr spectrum in DMSO and concluded, from similar coupling constant analysis, that the histidine imidazole has no preferred orientation among the three staggered conformers. The rest of the spectrum is very similar to that of the parent compound.

Bellocq and Dubien[27] examined the pmr spectrum of [(3-methylimidazolyl)alanine^2]-TRH, an analog with 800% biological activity. Its spectrum in DMSO agrees very well with that of TRH. The temperature dependences of the chemical shifts for all the amide hydrogens were determined and found to be quite similar for all the hydrogens, implying that none are involved in hydrogen bonds. They suggest the anisotropy of the proline δ and carboxamide hydrogens to be due to the proximity of the imidazole ring. Bellocq *et al.*[28] also examined the pmr spectrum of [(2-thienyl)alanine^2]-TRH, an analog with 75% biological activity. Its spectrum in DMSO differs from that of TRH in that the non-equivalence of the proline δ hydrogens is abolished and that of the carboxamide hydrogens is reduced. Analysis of the rotamer population about χ_1 gives a distribution of 60% at $\chi_1 = -60°$. Thus, the data seem to indicate an extended conformation in DMSO, without intramolecular hydrogen bonds, determined mostly by the steric bulk of the histidine and proline residues. However, whatever the conformation of TRH in DMSO, it does not seem to be relevant to biological activity.

The pmr spectrum of TRH has been studied in water[25,29]. The overall model derived from these data is similar to the DMSO model. The molecule is in an extended conformation ($\phi_2 \simeq -150°$, $\psi_2 \simeq 155°$) unstabilized by hydrogen bonds and determined mainly by the steric bulk of the histidine and proline residues. There is less interaction between the imidazole and carboxamide groups compared to DMSO solution which may indicate more solvation of these groups in water or a change in the average value of ψ_3.

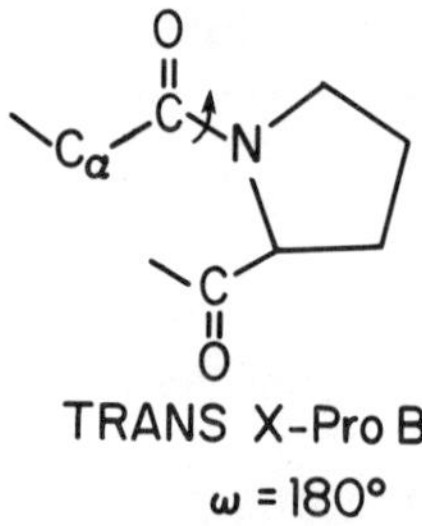

TRANS X-Pro Bond
$\omega = 180°$

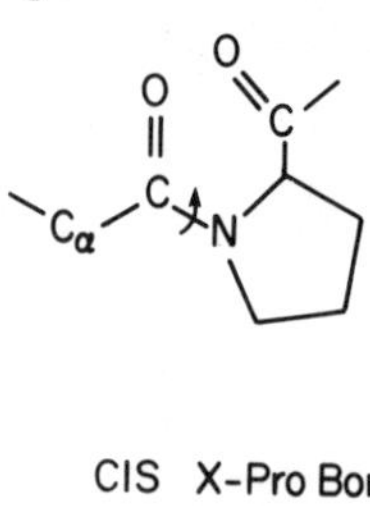

CIS X-Pro Bond
$\omega = 0°$

A number of ^{13}C studies[30,31] have demonstrated the presence of some cis isomer of Pro in TRH by the doubling of the pyrrolidine carbon resonances. The amount of cis isomer, estimated from relative peak heights, is uniformly reported as some 15-20%. This is in contrast to the behavior of N-acetyl-proline amide and other model X-Pro compounds, where the amount of cis isomer is some 25-40% in D_2O solution. This suggests some steric or conformational preference for a trans His-Pro bond in TRH. Deslauriers *et al.*[32] have examined the imidazole tautomer ratio in TRH by examining the pH dependence of the histidine carbon chemical shifts in D_2O solution. The behavior of thyroliberin is very similar to that of free histidine, which has been shown to be predominantly the N3-H tautomer. The spin-lattice relaxation times show no change for the imidazole carbons on going from pH 4.9 to pH 9.9, providing evidence against any conformer having a hydrogen bond involving the imidazole as a hydrogen bond acceptor[32,33]. The relaxation times of β, γ, and δ pyrrolidine carbons are appreciably higher than that of the alpha carbon, increasing in the order $\alpha < \beta \approx \delta < \gamma$. This suggests a rapid interconversion between endo and exo forms of the ring. Haar *et al.*[31] examined the ^{13}C vicinal coupling constants using [85% C-13 enriched proline^{3}]-TRH and propose the Cδ endo puckered conformer to predominate. It may be that there is a rapid conversion between exo and endo forms as suggested by the relaxation times. In general, the ^{13}C studies in D_2O give the overall impression of a relatively flexible molecule whose conformational mobility is similar to model dipeptides and acylamino acids. There is no evidence for hydrogen bonding.

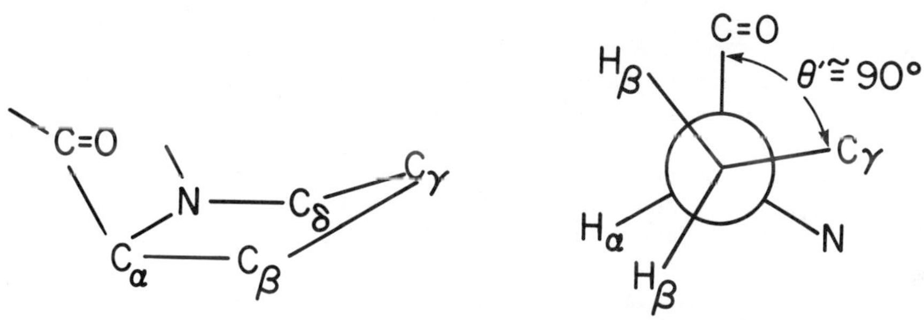

Cγ ENDO Proline

B. Theoretical Energy Calculations - There have been several attempts to calculate the minimum energy conformation of TRH. The calculated conformers all share one feature: they are stabilized by intramolecular hydrogen bonds. Blagdon *et al.*[34] find two minimum energy conformers. The global minimum features a "hairpin turn" with the histidine torsional angles ϕ_2 and ψ_2 approximately those of a right-handed alpha helix. There are hydrogen bonds between the imidazole N1 and Glp-His amide hydrogen and between the Glp-His amide carbonyl and the trans carboxamide hydrogen. The other low energy conformer features an extended conformation at the histidine residue. Burgess *et al.*[35] calculate a number of similar conformers, the lowest energy one being very near the extended conformer of Blagdon *et al.* There is one hydrogen bond, between the trans carboxamide hydrogen and the His-Pro amide carbonyl. Belle *et al.*[36] propose two hydrogen bonding schemes, one identical to that of Burgess *et al.* and, alternatively, one in which the imidazole is in the N1-H tautomer; there is a hydrogen bond between this N1-H and the His-Pro amide carbonyl. It is very difficult to assess the relevancy of energy calculations especially when the data indicates that TRH is well-solvated and lacks intramolecular hydrogen bonds.

C. Analog data - It is possible to probe the structural and conformational requirements for binding to the TRH receptor by evaluation of the biological activity of analogs of the hormone, in particular, those into which conformational constraints have been introduced. TRH is ideal for such a study because of the very close correlation between measured binding affinity and biological potency[39,40], suggesting that binding and activity are very closely coupled phenomena or at least have the same structural requirements. This is supported by the observation that the few inhibitory compounds known are only active at 10^4 higher concentrations than TRH[39].

There have been a number of reviews[40-43] of structure-activity relationships; the pertinent conclusions are summarized below.

1. The Glp residue: The lactam ring is necessary for good activity. Heteroatoms in the ring or short branches off the ring are compatible with activity. This implies that only the lactam structure is important and that the ring merely orients it. The fair amount of space available at the receptor at this point is emphasized if one considers the carbonyl of [N-formyl-Pro^1]-TRH, an analog with 10% activity, as equivalent to the lactam carbonyl.

2. The Pro amide residue: Proline monoalkyl amides and prolinol have good activity whereas the free acid is inactive, suggesting the necessity of a hydrogen bond donor in this position. Isosteric rings and MeAla which has conformational constraints similar to Pro, are active, as are the corresponding 4 and 6 membered ring amino acids. The purpose of Pro seems to be to hold the carboxamide in a certain orientation.

3. The His residue: The most active analogs contain a planar, five membered ring side chain with a nucleophile in the δ position. The activity of Phe, Leu, and cyclohexylalanine in this position, however, suggest that this is not an absolute requirement for binding and that only a branched amino acid is strictly required.

As has been noted, substitution of a methyl group for a backbone hydrogen in a peptide imposes severe conformational constraints. In particular, residues preceding an N-methyl residue are restricted to basically the extended conformation region ($-180° < \phi < -60°$, $+60° < \psi < +180°$), which puts limits on the angles ϕ_2 and ψ_2 of TRH. Similarily, since [MeHis^2]-TRH is an equipotent analog, it implies that ψ_1 is similarily constrained. [D,L-Glp(αMe)^1]-TRH is an analog with 50% activity[43]. Since [D-Glp^1]-TRH has only .02% activity, it is reasonable to assume that the L-α-methyl isomer is equipotent with TRH. When one considers the overlap in conformational space of the N-methyl and α-methyl analogs, one finds a small region of overlap, $+60° < \psi_1 < +120°$. This angle could be refined further by considering [Glp(αMe)^1, MeHis^2]-TRH. Its region of overlap with the two monosubstituted analogs is minute, $\psi_1 = +61°$. If the disubstituted analog is inactive, this implies that the methyl groups must be forced to occupy the same space when the molecule is bound to the receptor, which implies $\psi_1 \simeq +120°$. Using such conformationally restricted analogs, work is in progress to refine the receptor-bound conformation of

TRH.

IV. Enkephalin - An intense interest exists in the smallest of the opioid-like neuropeptides having the sequences Tyr-Gly-Gly-Phe-X, where X is either Leu (LENK) or Met (MENK). The existence of rigid opiates which interact with the same receptor offers a unique opportunity for deducing the pharmacophore and the receptor-bound conformation.

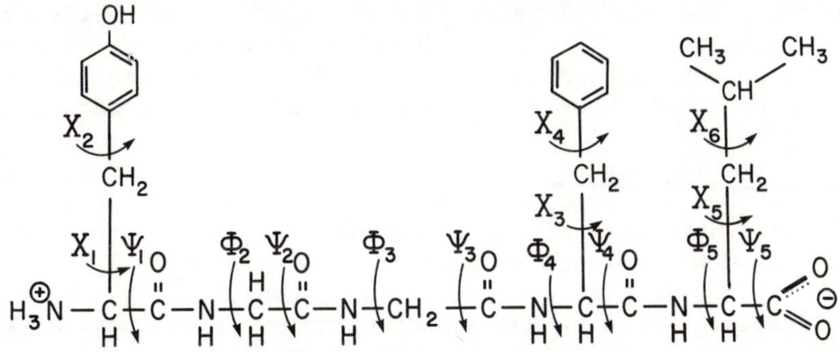

A. Crystal Structure - X-ray crystallographic structures have been reported for LENK[44] (Fig.6a) and the enkephalin fragments Tyr-Gly-Gly-Phe (TGGP)[45], Gly-Gly-Phe-Leu (GGPL)[45], and Tyr-Gly-Gly (TGG)[46]. The hydrogen bonding scheme and β-bend seen in the crystal of LENK is different from any proposed by theoretical calculations or solution NMR. Two points argue against the relevance of the crystal structure of LENK to biological activity. First, the tyrosine residue occurs in two conformers neither of which corresponds to the phenolic ring and nitrogen orientation seen in opiates. In addition, the backbone conformation has a hydrogen bond involving the amide hydrogen of Phe^4 and the carbonyl oxygen of Tyr^1, which would be incompatible with the exceptional activity of [D-Ala^2, N-Me-Phe^4]-LENK[47]. The crystal structure of the fragment TGGP has hydrogen bonding analogous to the pentapeptide but the orientation of the backbone and the side chains of Tyr^1 and Phe^4 are quite different. The other fragments of enkephalin have no intramolecular hydrogen bonding. For small, linear molecules with low internal barriers to rotation, intermolecular packing forces can dominate intramolecular forces[48], making correlation between solution or receptor conformation with solid state structures tenuous.

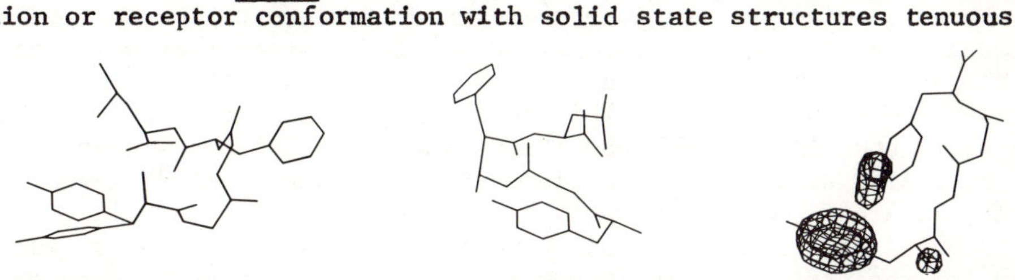

(a) Crystal structure of LENK[44]

(b) Theoretical Conformation of Isogai et al.[56]

(c) Receptor-bond conformer and morphine pharmacophore[72].

B. NMR Studies - Numerous proton studies[47,49-54] of MENK as well as ^{13}C NMR studies[50-53], have been reported; limited studies[50,54,4] on LENK indicate only minor differences. A number of discrepancies in the early studies have been resolved by noting that the zwitterionic form is compatible with a 2-5 βI turn in DMSO[50-51] while the cationic form exhibits a different conformation[51,54] not so well defined. These observations are complicated by the report[4] of association of enkephalin in a variety of solvents. The NT_1 values for the α-carbons of LENK in DMSO are very similar[50] which is compatible with an antiparallel β-dimer as proposed for the aggregated state[4]. In TGGP, the minimal fragment showing enkephalin activity, a 1-4 β-turn has been suggested[45]. [D-Ala^2]-MENK exhibits almost identical spectra as the parent compound and analysis of the C_α-C_β rotamer populations for both peptides shows significant populations for each rotamer[52].

C. <u>Other Physical Techniques</u> - Schiller and co-workers[8,55] have reported that [Trp^4]-MENK has the same affinity for the opiate receptor in rat brain as MENK. Examination of the intramolecular energy transfer between the Tyr^1 and the Trp^4 indicate an average separation of 9.3 Å either at pH 1.5 or pH 5.5. Since the concentration was only 3 x 10^{-5} M, one assumes the differences seen by NMR at these two pH values may reflect changes in aggregation. Furthermore, the observed phenol fluorescence in both aqueous solution and butanol rules out the proposed hydrogen bonded structures[4,56] which utilize the phenolic hydroxyl. The distance of 9.3 Å is supportive of a folded structure.

D. <u>Theoretical Energy Calculations</u> - Enkephalins have a minimum of seventeen variables, i.e. the rotatable bonds, if the amide unit is assumed planar and bond angles invariant. A 20° incremental systematic search would require analysis of about 10^{22} conformers. As a consequence, all reported semi-empirical energy calculations on enkephalin performed a limited exploration of conformational space[56-59]. Isogai <u>et al</u>.[56] found the most favorable conformer (Fig. 6b) to be a β-II' bend stabilized by a hydrogen bond between the phenolic hydroxyl of Tyr^1 and the carbonyl oxygen of Phe^4 which is not seen in aqueous solution[55]. The energetically most favored conformers are incompatible with the observation that [D-Ala^2]-MENK retains activity[60] while a large decrease in binding and activity accompanies the [L-Ala^2] analog[61] and thus the theoretically predicted structures must have little in common with the receptor-bound conformation. Momany[58] examined the lowest energy conformers of the charged and C-terminal amide forms of analogs of MENK. The conformation selected as being compatible with the active analogs examined has little structural correspondence with morphine. This conformation also conflicts with the observations that [Aib^2]-MENK and [L-Phe(αMe)^4]-LENK[62] are active and D-Ala^3 or L-Ala^3 analogs are inactive[63,64]. De Coen <u>et al</u>.[59] investigated the zwitterionic forms of MENK and LENK and three analogs: D-Ala^2, D-Ala^3, and D-Phe^4. A backbone conformation was selected which is not an energy minimum for the native enkephalins but is the minimum energy state for [D-Ala^2]-MENK and is not shared by the inactive [D-Ala^3] or [D-Phe^4] analogs. Strictly speaking, this conformer would contradict SAR data by predicting [Aib^2]-MENK and [L-Phe(αMe)^4]-LENK to be inactive. Because of the coarseness of the torsional scan, a ± 20° shift of predicted backbone angles could accommodate known structure-activity relationship (SAR) data. The side chain torsion angles of Tyr^1 proposed do not position the nitrogen and the phenolic ring in enkephalin in the same orientation as the tyramine moiety seen in most opiate compounds.

E. Receptor-Bound Conformation - Numerous analogs of enkephalin have been prepared[60-65] many of which contain substitutions with conformational information, e.g. D-amino acids. Beddell *et al.*[66] have examined the compatibility of active analogs containing such substitutions with particular conformations of the peptide backbone which are stabilized by intramolecular hydrogen bonds and previously characterized. Only 11 of the 26 possibilities considered were found to be consistent with the SAR data. Structures involving hydrogen bonding to the amide bond between residues 4 and 5 such as suggested by NMR can also be eliminated as essential due to the activity of analogs in which Phe^4 is replaced[67,68] with phenethylamine, eliminating the carboxamide group along with residue 5. Other highly active analogs with conformational constraints which must be considered are $[Phe(\alpha Me)^4]$-LENK[62] and $[D\text{-}Ala^2, MePhe^4]$-LENK[47].

An alternative approach has been to assume a pharmacophore for opiate activity and a correspondence between enkephalin and the essential groups of this pharmacophore. Correspondence between the tyramine moiety of morphine and Tyr^1 has been suggested[69-72]. Several investigations[70,71] have related the aromatic ring of Phe^4 with the 19-phenethyl substituent on 7-(1-phenyl-3-hydroxybutyl-3)-*endo*ethenotetrahydrothebaine (PET). Using 5-phenylbenzomorphan as a model, Gorin and Marshall[72] assumed a correspondence between the aromatic ring of Phe^4 and atoms C5 and C6 of morphine's non-aromatic C-ring. The activity of analogs in which Phe^4 has been replaced by cyclohexylalanine[68] or by carboranylalanine[73] indicates that aromaticity of Phe^4 is not essential. Assuming the correspondence of the conformation of Tyr^1 to that observed in morphine (χ_1 = 197°, χ_2 = -106°), conformational space was systematically explored at 31° torsional increments to determine those conformations in which the assumed correspondence between Phe^4 and the C-ring was possible. A single conformer (Fig. 6c) was found which appears consistent with the published SAR data[62,68].

V. Angiotensin - Of the eight amino acid residues, Asp-Arg-Val-Tyr-Ile-His-Pro-Phe, comprising angiotensin (AII), Val^3-Phe^8 is the minimal unit consistent with binding and activity. SAR studies[74,75] emphasize the importance of Tyr^4, His^6 and Phe^8. Single substitution of Tyr^4 and Phe^8 have led to partial agonists which have been used as competitive antagonists. The role of the C-terminal carboxylate has been reinvestigated[76] and may be essential to recognition, as analogs incapable of biotransformation to a free carboxyl in this position are devoid of activity. The other groups appear important for correct positioning of these functional groups and increased affinity.

A. Solution Studies - The combined results of the physical techniques used to study the solution conformation of $[Asn^1, Val^5]$-AII agree[22] that this linear octapeptide has a time-averaged preferred solution conformation. Proton NMR indicates two conformational changes, one with pKa of 5.5 and the other with pKa of 10.2. The first conformational change would appear associated with the titration of either the N-terminal amino group (pKa = 6.98), or the imidazole of His-6 (pKa = 6.26), or more likely both. The second is associated with ionization of the phenolic hydroxyl of Tyr-4. Measurement and assignment of the NH-CαH vicinal coupling constants limit the possible values for the torsional rotations about the amide to α-carbon bond. Exchange experiments indicate that Val-3, Val-5, and possibly Tyr-4 amide protons are either involved in intramolecular hydrogen bonds or sterically shielded from the solvent. Titration data[77] indicate that the N- and C-terminal ends of AII are in closer proximity then would be expected in a random coil. Carbon-13 spin-lattice relaxation studies[78] indicate that the α-carbons of the peptide backbone are approximately equally restricted in their motion. More recent investigation[3] of T_1's of AII as a function of field strength indicate overall motion (τ_R) of the molecule of approximately 6×10^{-9} sec which implies aggregation at pH 4.3 where these studies were done. This observation raises serious questions regarding the interpretation of data gathered previously on AII at this pH and concentration. The conformational change seen on going to alkaline pH as well as the presence[79] of cis-Pro at pH above 8 may simply imply a change in aggregation. Unfortunately, the question of aggregation will require re-examination of all the physical data obtained on angiotensin at higher concentration. The fluorescence energy transfer data gathered[9] at 10^{-5} M on [Trp^1, Val^5]-AII suggests close proximity (< 8 Å) of residue one and four and may be relevant to the monomeric state.

B. Receptor-Bound Conformation - By a variety of analogs with conformational constraints, the approximate values for the torsional rotations about the NH-CαH bond of residues 3, 4, and 5 when bound to the receptor have been deduced. In the case of position 3 and 5, the arguments were based on the high activity retained by substitution of the cyclic residue Pro at these positions. The constraint on position 4 is much better defined as [Phe(αMe)^4]-AII has the same activity at [Phe^4]-AII which implies that an α-methyl substitution at position 4 is fully compatible with biological activity[80]. Based on analysis of other analogs of AII which restrict conformational freedom, further constraints of the receptor-bound conformation have been proposed. While comparison of these values for ϕ with the values derived from examination of the NH-CH coupling constants has been made, two difficulties preclude a firm conclusion. First, the measurement of the coupling constants must be done at acid pH; and second, the state of aggregation of angiotensin under physiological conditions would appear different than that during most physical studies.

IV. Conclusion - The data currently available suggest strongly that the predominate solution conformation does not directly correspond to the biologically active conformer. Receptors either induce the conformation required for recognition and activation or select a minor conformer from the ensemble available in solution.

References

1. J. Feeney in "Drug Action at the Molecular Level", G.C.K. Roberts, ed., MacMillan Press, New York, N.Y., 1977, p. 55.
2. V.F. Bystrov, Y.D. Gavrilov, V.T. Ivanov and Y.A. Ovchinnikov, Eur J. Biochem., 78, 63 (1977).
3. J.A. Ferretti and G.R. Marshall, Biophys. J., 21, 79a (1978).
4. M.A. Khaled, M.M. Long, W.D. Thompson, R.J. Bradley, G.B. Brown and D.W. Urry, Biochem. Biophys. Res. Comm., 76, 224 (1977).
5. R. Deslauriers and R.L. Somorjai, J. Am. Chem. Soc., 98, 1931 (1976).
6. J.D. Glickson, S.L. Gordon, T.P. Pitner, D.G. Agresti and R. Walter, Biochem , 15, 5721 (1976).
7. K.J. Rothschild, I.M. Asher, H.E. Stanley and E. Anastassakis, J. Am. Chem. Soc., 99, 2032 (1977).
8. P.W. Schiller, C.F. Yam and M. Lis, Biochem., 16, 1831 (1977).
9. P.W. Schiller, Can. J. Biochem., 55, 75 (1977).
10. D.A. Greenberg, C.D. Barry and G.R. Marshall, J. Am. Chem. Soc. (in press).
11. E. Clementi, F. Cavallone and R. Scordamaglia, J. Am. Chem. Soc., 99, 5531 (1977).
12. I.M. Chaiken, M.H. Freedman, J.R. Lyerla, Jr. and J.S. Cohen, J. Biol Chem., 248, 884 (1973).
13. F.M. Finn and K. Hofman, Acc. Chem. Res., 6, 169 (1973).
14. S. Mabrey and I.M. Klotz, Biochem., 15, 234 (1976).
15. N.G. Kumar, N. Izumiya, M. Miyashi, H. Sugano and D.W. Urry, J. Am. Chem Soc., 97, 4105 (1975)
16. G.R. Marshall, in "Peptides: Chemistry and Biochemistry", B. Weinstein and S. Lande, eds., M. Dekker Inc., New York, N.Y., 1970, p. 151.
17. G.R. Marshall and H.E. Bosshard, Circulation Res., 31 (Suppl. 2), II-143 (1972).
18. A.W. Burgess and S.J. Leach, Biopolymers, 12, 2599 (1973).
19. V.Z. Pletney, E.P. Gromon and E.M. Popov, Khim. Prir. Soedin., 224 (1973).
20. G.D. Smith, W.L. Duax, E.W. Czerwinski, N.E. Kendrick, G.R. Marshall and F.S. Mathews, in "Peptides", M. Goodman and J. Meienhofer, eds., John Wiley and Sons, New York, N.Y., 1977, p. 277.
21. N. Shamala, R. Nagaraj and P. Balaram, Biochem. Biophys. Res. Comm., 79, 292 (1977).
22. G.R. Marshall, H.E. Bosshard, W.H. Vine, J.D. Glickson and P. Needleman, in "Recent Advances in Renal Physiology and Pharmacology", L.G. Wesson and G.M. Fanelli, University Park Press, Baltimore, Md, 1974, p. 215.
23. S. Fermandjian, P. Pradelles, P. Fromageot and J.J. Danand, FEBS Lett., 28, 156 (1972).
24. J. Feeney, G.R. Bedford and P.L. Wessels, FEBS Lett., 42, 347 (1974).
25. B. Donzel, J. Rivier, M. Goodman, Biopolymers, 13, 2631 (1974).
26. B. Donzel, M. Goodman, J. Rivier, M. Long and W. Vale, Nature, 256, 750 (1975).
27. A-M. Bellocq and M. Dubien, Biochem. Biophys. Acta, 420, 1 (1976).
28. A-M. Bellocq, S. Castensson and H. Sievertsson, Biochem. Biophys. Res. Comm., 74, 577 (1977).
29. M. Montagut, B. Lemanceau and A-M. Bellocq, Biopolymers, 13, 2615 (1974).
30. R. Deslauriers, R. Walter and I.C.P. Smith, Biochem. Biophys. Res. Comm., 53, 244 (1973).
31. W. Haar, S. Fermandjian, J. Vicar, K. Blaha and P. Fromageot, Proc. Nat. Acad Sci. USA, 72, 4948 (1975).
32. R. Deslauriers, W.H. McGregor, D. Sarantakis and I.C.P. Smith, Biochem , 13, 3443 (1974).
33. R. Deslauriers, I.C.P. Smith and R. Walter, J. Biol. Chem., 241, 7006 (1974).
34. D.E. Blagdon, J. Rivier and M. Goodman, Proc. Nat. Acad. Sci. USA, 70, 1166 (1973).
35. A.W. Burgess, F.A. Momany and H.E. Scheraga, Proc. Nat. Acad. Sci. USA, 70, 1456 (1973).
36. J. Belle, M. Montagut and A-M. Bellocq, C.R. Acad. Sci., Ser. C, 275, 471 (1972).
37. G. Grant, W. Vale and R. Guillemin, Endocrinology, 92, 1629 (1973).
38. P.M. Hinkle, E.L. Woroch and A.H. Tashjian, Jr., J. Biol. Chem. 249, 3085 (1974).
39. C.Y. Bowers, H. Sievertsson, J. Chang, J. Stewart, S. Castensson, S. Bjorkman, D. Chang and K. Folkers, Thyroid Research (1975), J. Robbins et al. (eds.), Excerpta Medica, Amsterdam, 1.
40. R. Guillemin, R. Burgess and W. Vale, Vitamins and Hormones, 29, 1 (1971).
41. C.Y. Bowers, A. Weil, J.K. Chang, H. Sievertsson, F. Enzmann and K. Folkers, Biochem. Biophys. Res. Comm., 40, 683 (1970).
42. W. Vale and C. Rivier, Handbook of Psychopharmacology, L.I. Iverson et al. (eds.), Plenum Press, New York, 5, 195 (1975).
43. H.J. Goren, L.G. Bauce and W. Vale, Molecular Pharmacol., 13, 606 (1977).
44. D.G. Smith and J.F. Griffin, Science, 199, 1214 (1978).
45. M.C. Fournic-Zaluski, T. Prange, C. Pascard and B.P. Roques, Biochem. Biophys. Res. Comm., 79, 1199 (1977).
46. M.L. Hachet and W.M. Carson, Abst. Am. Cryst. Assoc. Meeting, Michigan State Univ., 68 (1977).
47. D. Roemer, H.H. Buescher, R.C. Hill, J. Pless, W. Bauer, F. Cardinaux, A. Closse, D. Hauser and R. Huguenin, Nature, 268, 547 (1977).
48. J. Bernstein and A.T. Hagler, J. Am. Chem. Soc., 100, 673 (1978).
49. M. Anteunis, A.K. Lala, C. Garbay-Jaurequiberry and B.P. Roques, Biochem., 16, 1462 (1977).

50. C. Garbay-Jaurequiberry, B.P. Roques, R. Oberlin, M. Anteunis, S. Combrisson and J.Y. Lalleland, FEBS Letters, 276, 93 (1977).
51. C. Jones, V. Garsky and W. Gibbons, Biochem. Biophys. Res. Comm., 76, 619 (1977).
52. C.R. Jones, J.B. Alpers, M.-C. Kuo and W.A. Gibbons, in "Peptides", M. Goodman and J. Meinhofer, eds., John Wiley and Sons, New York, N.Y., 1977, p. 329.
53. H.E. Bleich, J.D. Cutnell, J.A. Glasel and J.F. McKelvey, Proc. Natl. Acad. Sci. USA, 73, 2589 (1976).
54. H.E. Bleich, A.R. Dry, R.J. Freer and J.A. Glasel, Biochem. Biophys. Res Comm., 74, 592 (1977).
55. P.W. Schiller, Biochem. Biophys. Res. Comm., 79, 493 (1977).
56. Y. Isogai, G. Nemethy and H.A. Scheraga, Proc. Natl. Acad. Sci. USA, 74, 414 (1977).
57. J.L. DeCoen, C. Humblet and M.H. Koch, FEBS Letters, 73, 414 (1977).
58. F.A. Momany, Biochem. Biophys. Res. Comm., 75, 1098 (1977).
59. C. Humblet and J.L. DeCoen, in "Peptides", M. Goodman and J. Meienhofer, eds., John Wiley and Sons, New York, N.Y., 1977, p. 88.
60. C.B. Pert, A. Pert, J.-K. Chang and B.T.W. Fong, Science, 194, 330 (1976).
61. L. Terenius, A. Wahlstrom, G. Lindeberg, S. Karlsson and U. Ragnarsson, Biochem. Biophys. Res. Comm., 71, 175 (1976).
62. G.R. Marshall and F.A. Gorin, in "Peptides", M. Goodman and J. Meienlhofer, eds., John Wiley and Sons, New York, N.Y., 1977, p. 84.
63. D.H. Coy, A.J. Kastin, A.V. Schally, O. Morin, N.G. Garon, F. Labrie, J.M. Walker, R. Fertel, G.G. Bernton and C.A. Sandmon, Biochem. Biophys. Res. Comm., 73, 632 (1976).
64. C.R. Beddell, R.B. Clark, G.W. Hardy, L.A. Lowe, F.B. Ubatuba, J.R. Vane, S. Wilkinson, K.J. Chang, P. Cuatrecasas and R.J. Miller, Proc. R. Soc. London B, 198, 249 (1977).
65. A.S. Dutta, J.J. Gormley, C.F. Hayward, J.S. Morley, J.S. Shaw, G.J. Stacey and M.T. Turnball, Life Sciences, 21, 559 (1977).
66. C.R. Beddell, R.B. Clark, L.A. Lowe, S. Wilkinson, K.-J. Chang, P. Cuatrecasas and R. Miller, Brit. J. Pharmacol., 61, 351 (1977).
67. B.A. Morgan, J.D. Bower, K.P. Guest, B.K. Handa, G. Metcalf and C.F.C. Smith, in "Peptides", M. Goodman and J. Meienhofer, eds., John Wiley and Sons, New York, N.Y., 1977, p. 111.
68. G.R. Marshall, T.M. Balasubramanian and F.A. Gorin, J. Supramol. Struc. (in press).
69. A.S. Horne, J.R. Rodgers, J. Pharm. Pharmacol., 29, 257 (1977).
70. A.F. Bradbury, D.G. Smythe and C.R. Snell, Nature, 260, 165 (1976).
71. A.P. Feinberg, I. Creese and S.H. Snyder, Proc. Natl. Acad. Sci. USA, 73, 4215 (1976).
72. F.A. Gorin and G.R. Marshall, Proc. Natl. Acad. Sci. USA, 74, 5179 (1977).
73. A. Eberle, O. Leukart, P. Schiller, J.-L. Fauchere and R. Schwyzer, FEBS Letters 82, 325 (1977).
74. F.M. Bumpus and M.C. Khosla, in "Hypertension", J. Genest, E. Koiw and O. Kuchel, eds., McGraw-Hill Book Co., New York, N.Y., 1977.
75. G.R. Marshall, Federation Proc., 35, 2494 (1976).
76. K.H. Hsieh, P. Needleman and G.R. Marshall, Abst. 172nd Natl. ACS Meeting, San Francisco, 1976.
77. L. Juliano and A.C.M. Paiva, Biochem., 13, 2445 (1974).
78. R. Deslauriers, A.C.M. Paiva, K. Schaumburg and I.C.P. Smith, Biochem , 14, 875 (1975).
79. R.E. Galardy, H.E. Bleich, P. Ziegler and L.C. Craig, Biochem , 15, 2303 (1976).
80. J. Turk, P. Needleman and G.R. Marshall, Mol. Pharmacol., 12, 217 (1976).

Chapter 25. Bacterial Resistance to β-Lactams: The β-Lactamases

Jed F. Fisher and Jeremy R. Knowles, Department of Chemistry, Harvard University, Cambridge, Massachusetts 02138

Bacteria can develop a number of ways of resisting the lethal consequences of exposure to β-lactam antibiotics, but one of the most effective is the production of an enzyme, the β-lactamase, that rapidly hydrolyzes the β-lactam to the β-amino acid derivative. These enzymes are extremely efficient catalysts, they may be constitutive or inducible, they can be coded for chromosomally or by readily transferable plasmids, and they may be largely intracellular, largely extracellular, or (for Gram-negative bacteria) predominantly periplasmic. While it is clear that the permeability of the cell's membrane to the antibiotic sharply affects β-lactam potency (for instance, it has been shown that a plasmid β-lactamase in E.coli protects the bacterium from penicillin G but not from cephaloridine, even though the enzyme hydrolyzes the latter 50% faster[1]), it appears that most commonly-encountered resistance to β-lactams derives from the presence of the β-lactamase.[2] Although the central role of the β-lactamases in resistance has been clear for some time, efforts to overcome this resistance by using β-lactamase inhibitors have not proved very fruitful because the specificity of β-lactamases is wide and broad-spectrum β-lactamase inhibitors were not available. This situation is changing however, and the tactical inclusion of β-lactamase-inhibitory function into an antibiotic, or the use of a β-lactamase inhibitor in synergy with a susceptible but effective antibiotic,[3] is becoming attractive. This short review is devoted to two topics: (a) properties of some of the better-studied β-lactamases; (b) the interaction with the E.coli RTEM β-lactamase of a number of recently-discovered β-lactams containing unusual structural features.

General - The β-lactamases (E.C. 3.5.2.6: penicillin amido-β-lactam hydrolase; E.C. 3.5.2.8: cephalosporin amido-β-lactam hydrolase) are monomeric enzymes typically of molecular weight around 30 000, that catalyze the hydrolysis of the β-lactam ring of a variety of penam (I) and cephem (II) derivatives. The enzymes are extremely efficient in catalyzing the hydrolysis of their more susceptible substrates showing k_{cat}/K_m values approaching that for a diffusion-limited reaction (e.g., 5×10^7 M^{-1} s^{-1} for the E.coli RTEM β-lactamase with benzylpenicillin). Pollock[4] has considered the evolutionary origins of the β-lactamases, bearing in mind that organisms known to have been dormant since before the clinical introduction of β-lactams have been shown to produce β-lactamase activity. He concluded that they are straightforward detoxification enzymes. β-Lactamases have been purified from a number of sources,[5] most of the detailed work having been done with the enzymes from Staphylococcus aureus, Bacillus cereus, Bacillus licheniformis, and Escherichia coli. Since it is not yet clear to what extent the characteristics of the enzyme from one source are applicable generally, we shall discuss the enzymes from these sources in turn.

ISBN 0-12-040513-X

β-Lactamases from Gram-Positive Bacteria

Staphlococcus aureus - The β-lactamase from S.aureus[6] may be inducible though most studies have used a penicillinase-constitutive strain[7] which produces large amounts of the enzyme, 60% of which is extracellular.[8] The sequence of the 257 amino acids of this enzyme is known,[9] and X-ray crystallographic studies have been started.[10] The catalytic activity of this enzyme is largely destroyed by iodine and by tetranitromethane, reaction with the latter leading to preferential nitration of tyrosine-82.[11] On treatment with guanidine hydrochloride, the enzyme is reversibly denatured via a definable partially unfolded state.[12] S.aureus β-lactamase is evidently a rather 'floppy' molecule. The S.aureus enzyme is a better penicillinase than cephalosporinase and the activity towards a number of

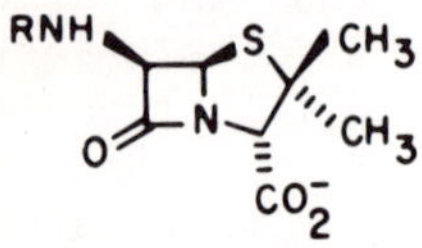

I

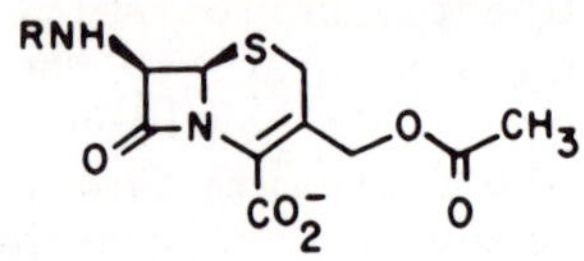

II

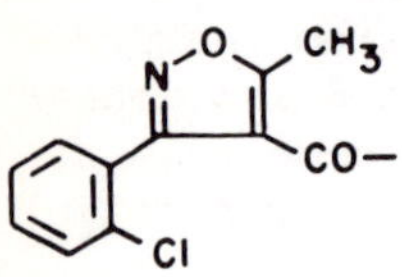

a

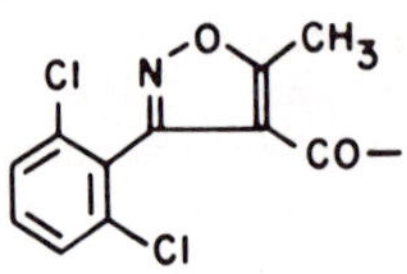

b

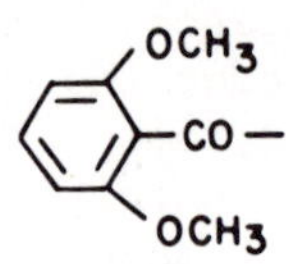

c

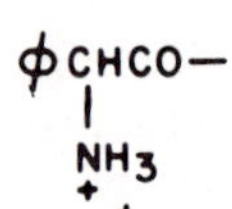

d

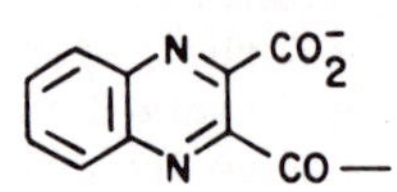

e

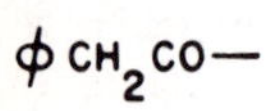

f

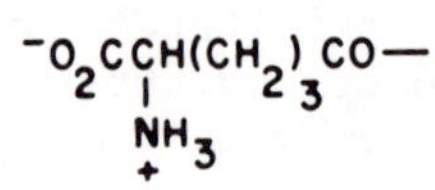

g

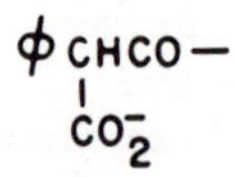

h

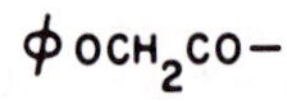

i

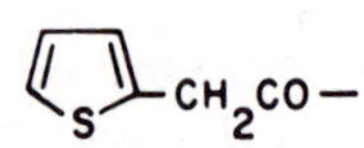

k

6-acylaminopenicillanic acids (I) depends unsurprisingly on the nature of the 6-acyl substituent. It has been suggested that the inhibition of the enzyme by resistant β-lactams such as dicloxacillin (I, R=b), cephaloglycin (II, R=d) and 7-aminocephalosporanic acid (II, R=H) is a function of the preincubation time of enzyme and inhibitor.[13,14]

Two detailed mechanistic studies have been made with the S.aureus β-lactamase. First, Halford (see ref. 10) has studied the hydrolysis of a chromogenic cephalosporin substrate by fast kinetic methods, and has concluded from the absence of a D_2O solvent kinetic isotope effect that the catalytic step (which involves proton release) may also include a rate-limiting enzyme conformational change that is insensitive to solvent isotope. In the second study, Virden, et al.[15] allowed the S.aureus enzyme to hydrolyze the poor substrate quinacillin (I, R=e), and quenched the reaction from the steady state using denaturants. They concluded that 0.3-0.7 moles of quinacillin become covalently linked to the enzyme in the steady-state. Although the kinetic competence of the complex was not established, the authors suggested that this was an acyl-enzyme intermediate in the normal catalytic cycle of this β-lactamase. One other intriguing observation on the S.aureus enzyme should be mentioned. Some preparations of this β-lactamase have been found to contain what appears to be two moles of non-covalently bound cell wall peptide. While this may be fortuitous, it is tempting to suggest that there may be some steric analogy between this peptide and penicillin, equivalent to the relationship between penicillin and the cell wall peptide originally suggested by Tipper and Strominger[16] and recently discussed by Boyd.[17]

Bacillus cereus - B.cereus produces two β-lactamases[18,19] which are coded for by separate genes and which do not cross-react immunologically. β-lactamase I is rather similar to the enzymes from other Gram-positive organisms, and its specificity is similar to the enzymes from S.aureus and B.licheniformis. β-Lactamase II is, in contrast, a zinc metalloenzyme[20] of 22 000 daltons, which shows a broader specificity including high activity towards cephalosporins. The B.cereus enzyme I has been largely sequenced[21] and it is homologous with the enzymes from B.licheniformis (60% homology) and S.aureus (40% homology). A small-scale purification using an affinity column has been reported.[22] Several attempts have been made to identify catalytically essential amino acids, using both amino acid-selective reagents (e.g., iodine, tetranitromethane, carbodiimide, triethyloxonium fluoroborate, N-bromosuccinimide, diethylpyrocarbonate) and enzyme specific reagents (e.g., the diazotization products of 6-aminopenicillanic acid (I, R=H) or of ampicillin (I, R=d).[23-27] Until the modified proteins from such studies have been properly characterized, only circumstantial statements can be made about the essentiality of particular amino acids.

In the presence of poor substrates that contain large aromatic 6-acyl side chains, B.cereus β-lactamase I becomes more susceptible to inactivation by such diverse treatments as heat, urea, or iodine.[5] This has led to the view that the β-lactamase is a 'floppy' enzyme, and the phenomenon has been studied by hydrogen-exchange.[28] For instance, the poor substrates methicillin (I, R=c) or cloxacillin (I, R=a) accelerate the rate of exchange of the enzyme's amide protons with those of the medium, which suggests that the protein conformation may be altered by the binding of these ligands. This conformational alteration apparently has kinetic consequences, too, and Samuni and Citri[29] have shown that while the hydrolysis rate of the 'natural' substrate benzylpenicillin (I, R=f) is linear from t=0, substrates such as methicillin (I, R=c) or cloxacillin (I, R=a) show biphasic "burst" kinetics. On the basis of this work it has been suggested that the enzyme conformation adjusts to accommodate the more sterically-hindered substrates giving a lower K_m value, and in doing so some catalytic capability is sacrificed by the enzyme.[30] The molecular details of these changes are unknown. Finally, some substrate-analogue competitive inhibitors have been investigated, and the pH-dependence of the steady-state parameters for benzylpenicillin (I, R=f) and for ampicillin (I, R=d) have been reported.[26,31]

Bacillus licheniformis - There are two β-lactamases from B.licheniformis, one of which is extracellular and the other a membrane-bound enzyme.[32] The extracellular enzyme has been sequenced.[33] The membrane-bound form has been shown to be a precursor of the extracellular enzyme and is a phospholipoprotein having an extra N-terminal peptide of 24 amino acids ending in phosphatidylserine.[34] While trypsin cleaves 25 amino acids from the N-terminus of the membrane enzyme (leaving an enzyme that differs only from the exo-enzyme in that it lacks N-terminal Lys), Aiyappa and Lampen[35] have isolated a 'penicillinase-releasing protease' that removes the 24 N-terminal amino acids. The B.licheniformis enzyme, like many other Gram-positive β-lactamases, has low activity against cephalosporin derivatives. This has been exploited in the use of Sepharose-bound cephalosporin C (II, R=g) as an affinity matrix for the purification of this enzyme.[36]

β-Lactamases from Gram-Negative Bacteria

β-Lactamases from Gram-negative organisms are generally constitutive, plasmid-coded, and are usually more effective in the hydrolysis of cephalosporins than are their Gram-positive counterparts.[37,38] Several papers dealing with β-lactamases in the Enterobacter,[39 40] Acinetobacter,[41] and Klebsiella groups[42] have appeared. The Pseudomonas are particularly opportunistic strains that are generally susceptible to carbenicillin (I, R=h), though P.aeruginosa strains containing the RTEM enzyme[43] or penicillinases that efficiently hydrolyze carbenicillin[44,45] are well-known. Labia and co-workers have suggested that the inhibition of a number of Gram-negative cephalosporinases by carbenicillin results from the formation of a rather stable non-covalent complex (K_i = 0.01 μM).[46]

Escherichia coli - Although some chromosomal enzymes are known from E.coli[47] most of the β-lactamases from Gram-negative organisms are encoded by plasmids. The enzyme from E.coli W3310 carrying the plasmid R6K (also called the TEM R-factor) has been purified,[48] and the almost complete amino acid sequence[49] has been favorably compared with the complete sequence of the structural gene from the plasmid pBR322.[50] There is some homology with the enzymes from Gram-positive species. The enzyme has been crystallized, and an X-ray map at 5.5 Å has been published.[51] Of the simple N-acyl penams benzylpenicillin (I, R=f) is the best substrate (relative V_{max} = 1.00; K_m = 0.02 mM) followed by ampicillin (I, R=d) (0.95; 0.02 mM), 6-aminopenicillanic acid (I, R=H) (0.79, 0.19 mM), phenoxymethylpenicillin (I, R=j) (0.50, 0.02 mM) and carbenicillin (I, R=h) (0.15, 0.05 mM). The cephalosporins suffer in terms of both V_{max} and K_m [cephaloglycin (II, R=d) (0.11, 0.46 mM), cephalothin (II, R=k) (0.06, 0.15 mM), and cephalosporin C (II, R=g)(0.014, 0.68 mM)]. In general, the RTEM enzyme is much better behaved kinetically than the B.cereus enzyme. The criterion used by Citri and co-workers[30] to identify kinetically anomalous penicillins (susceptibility relative to 6-aminopenicillanic acid) is not applicable to the RTEM β-lactamase, as all but two of the penams and cephems listed above are hydrolyzed more slowly than 6-aminopenicillanic acid,without any observable deviation from Michaelis-Menten kinetics. Experiments involving the sequential addition of different substrates indicate a greater conformational stability for the RTEM enzyme. Protein modification has been achieved using tetranitromethane, photooxidation, iodoacetic acid, and the C-3 isocyanate of benzylpenicillin.[52-54]

New Classes of β-Lactam and Their Interaction with the RTEM β-Lactamase

The recent discovery of a number of novel β-lactam-containing antibiotics[55] and the development of structures that both inhibit bacterial cell wall synthesis and inhibit β-lactamases, suggest that the interaction of these new structures with β-lactamases should be investigated at the molecular level. Interaction of these compounds with the RTEM β-lactamase is discussed below. The choice of the enzyme is dictated by the following: (a) By virtue of its plasmid origin, this is now the most widely distributed β-lactamase among the enteric Gram-negative bacteria. (b) The plasmid has the disturbing capability for transfer into previously susceptible species (e.g., N.gonorrhoeae and H.influenzae). (c) Infections derived from Gram-negative bacteria are becoming increasingly important clinically.

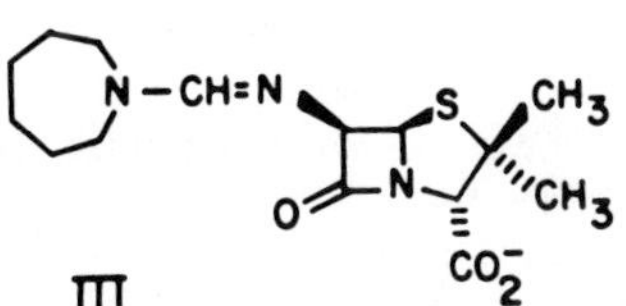

III

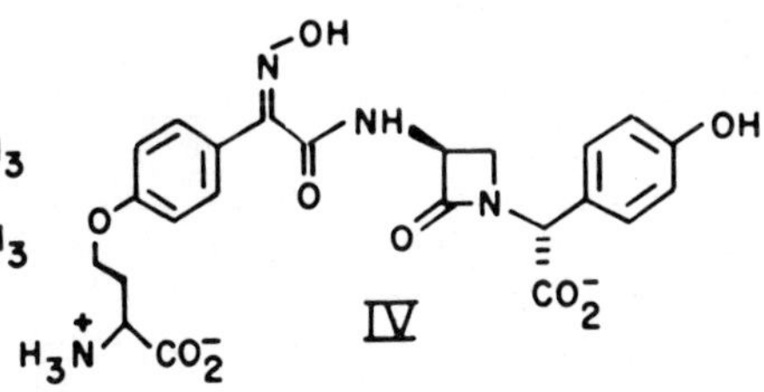

IV

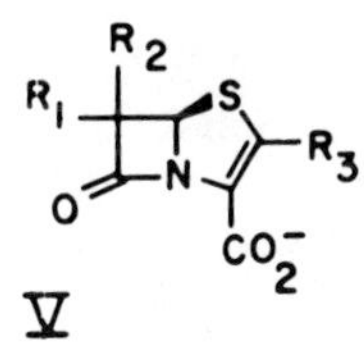

V

Mecillinam - The 6β-imidopenicillanic acids, exemplified by mecillinam (III), were the first class of β-lactams recognized to possess antibiotic activity in the absence of an N-acyl side chain.[56] The 6β-imidopenicillins are also unusual in terms of their bacteriocidal mechanism: they are lethal to certain Gram-negative bacteria (particularly E.coli) where the morphological change they elicit is the conversion of the cell rod to an ovoid.[57] Filamentation, which is the normal initial development in the expression of most other β-lactams, is not observed. Mecillinam binds specifically to a single penicillin binding protein (PBP2) of the inner membrane of E.coli,[58] and there is no significant binding to the other PBP species.[59,60] Mecillinam is 500 times more potent than ampicillin (I, R=d) against ampicillin-resistant (i.e., β-lactamase-producing) strains of E.coli, and has been shown to act synergistically with other β-lactam antibiotics.[61-63] Curiously, mecillinam is hydrolyzed very rapidly by β-lactamase, having the highest k_{cat} for any substrate yet discovered for this enzyme. The susceptibility of β-lactamase-producing strains of E.coli to this β-lactam must be dependent on factors other than the β-lactamase, and the killing locus (or loci) must scavenge the antibiotic very effectively before it is destroyed by the enzyme.

Nocardicin A - Nocardicin A (IV) is singular among β-lactam antibiotics in retaining antibiotic activity while having the relatively unreactive monocyclic β-lactam system. An account of its discovery, a summary of its antibiotic properties, and a total synthesis, has recently been presented by Kamiya.[64] This compound is particularly effective in vitro[65,66] and in vivo[67] (subcutaneous injection) against P.aeruginosa, the Proteus (with the exception of P.morganii) and the Neisseria groups, in comparison with carbenicillin (I, R=h). The in vitro inhibition behavior generally underestimates the efficacy of nocardicin A in vivo, and this is believed to be a consequence of the ability of nocardicin A to modify the cell surface structure and facilitate recognition and ingestion of the bacteria by polymorphonuclear leukocytes. From the antibacterial potency of a number of nocardicin derivatives it appears that the oxime in a syn relationship to the acylamino group, and the 3-amino-3-carboxypropoxy side chain are both necessary for optimal activity.[68,69]

The β-lactam ring of nocardicin A is rather resistant to β-lactamases, and only the chromosomal cephalosporinase from P.vulgaris and the E.coli RTEM β-lactamase show appreciable activity towards it.[65] As a substrate for the RTEM enzyme, nocardicin A has a V_{max} of 0.02 relative to benzylpenicillin. The product from the enzymatic action has not been fully characterized, although its properties are consistent with a normal hydrolytic cleavage of the β-lactam.

Penems - The total synthesis of a number of penems substituted at C-2 and C-6 (V) has been accomplished by Ernest, et al.[70] The rationale for their synthesis was to incorporate the Δ^3 double bond of the cephalosporins into the penicillin nucleus. These penems exhibit antibacterial activity. The observation that penems fragment in dilute acid to the ketene and the thiazole,[71] rather than suffer the normal β-lactam hydrolysis, suggested them as possible enzyme inactivators. It appears however, that the parent penem (V, $R_1=R_2=R_3=H$) is a normal substrate for the RTEM β-lactamase. This β-lactam is hydrolyzed at a relative V_{max} of 0.36, with a K_m of 310 μM. No loss in β-lactamase activity is detectable, even after 50,000 turnovers. The products from the enzymatic reaction have not yet been identified.

Cefoxitin - The finding that the addition of a 7α-methoxyl substituent enhanced cephalosporin antibacterial activity (whereas 6α-methoxy-penam is less effective than the parent penam), culminated in the synthesis of cefoxitin (VI). This β-lactam possesses an unusually broad activity spectrum, partly due to its exceptional resistance to hydrolysis by the β-lactamases.[72-74] Introduction of the 7α-methoxyl group depresses the rate of enzymatic hydrolysis by a factor of 3×10^4 for cefoxitin (VI) relative to cephalothin (II, R=k). However, the effects of the methoxyl substituent extend beyond a simple reduction in V_{max}, and the characteristics of the hydrolytic pathway are changed. Compare cefoxitin and 7-aminodesacetoxy cephalosporanic acid (7-ADCA), which shows an almost identical k_{cat}. If a portion of enzyme solution catalyzing 7-ADCA hydrolysis is diluted into a solution containing phenoxymethylpenicillin (I, R=j), the new substrate is hydrolyzed with a linear time course, at the predicted rate. If, however, cefoxitin replaces 7-ADCA as the first enzyme substrate, the rate of phenoxymethylpenicillin hydrolysis becomes biphasic, and accelerates over about 15 minutes to a new limiting velocity. No irreversible inactivation of the enzyme is detectable. This kinetic behavior is reminiscent of the observations of Citri and co-workers[30] with the B.cereus β-lactamase, which have been interpreted in terms of a substrate-induced conformational change of the enzyme. An alternative explanation may be offered, however, that is consistent with the kinetic behavior of clavulanic acid (VII, $R_1=CH_2OH$, $R_2=H$). The biphasic kinetics induced in the hydrolysis of the better substrate (phenoxymethylpenicillin) by preincubation with cefoxitin may derive from the slow decomposition of a transiently-inhibited form of the enzyme (see below).

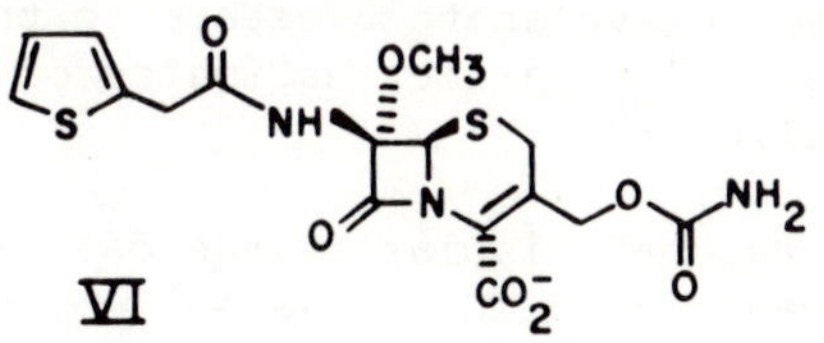
VI

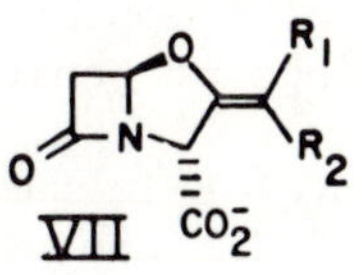
VII

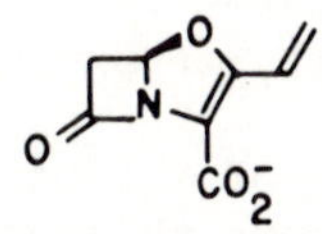
VIII

Clavulanic Acid - This unusual compound (VII, R_1=CH_2OH, R_2=H) was the first natural β-lactam shown to have specific, irreversible β-lactamase inhibitory activity.[75-79] A moderately active antibiotic itself, clavulanate acts synergistically at concentrations as low as 5 μg/mL to lower the MIC for a number of test organisms by as much as 10-fold (e.g., carbenicillin with P.aeruginosa Daglaish) to 10^3-fold (e.g., ampicillin with S.aureus Russel). There are three events that characterize the interaction of clavulanate with the RTEM β-lactamase. First, clavulanate is destroyed by the enzyme in what appears to be a normal hydrolytic reaction of the β-lactam. Secondly, two catalytically inactive forms are produced, one of which is an irreversibly inactivated species, and the other is only transiently inhibited and slowly decomposes to active enzyme. The transient complex is formed from the Michaelis complex at a rate which is some 3-fold faster than the rate of formation of the irreversibly inactivated complex. The transient complex is, therefore, the principle enzyme form present after short time periods. In the presence of excess clavulanate, however, all the enzyme accumulates into the irreversibly inactivated form. The number of clavulanate turnovers that occur before complete enzyme inactivation is 115. If the enzyme is totally irreversibly inactivated by incubation with a large (≥ 300-fold) molar excess of clavulanate, three different species of inactive enzyme are discerned on isoelectric focusing. Incubation of this mixture with hydroxylamine results in the recovery of about one-third of the catalytic activity, and one of the three bands on isoelectric focusing now runs as native enzyme. It seems clear that clavulanic acid is a 'suicide reagent' and that the enzyme generates from it, one or more acylating or alkylating agents that result in enzyme inactivation.[80,81]

Clavulanic Acid Derivatives - Although only a single naturally-occurring derivative of clavulanate (VII, R_1=CH_2OH, R_2=H) is known (VII, R_1=$CH_2OCOCH_2CH_2OH$, R_2=H),[82] a large number of derivatives have been prepared either by direct chemical functionalization of clavulanate or by total synthesis. The dihydro[83] and desoxy[84] (VII, R_1=CH_3, R_2=H) clavulanates have been prepared, as well as the sulfated[85] (VII, R_1=CH_2OSO_3H, R_2=H) and esterified (VII, R_1=CH_2OCOR, R_2=H) derivatives.[86] The allylic oxygen has been replaced with nitrogen[87] and with sulfur.[88] The double bond of clavulanate has been both photoisomerized[89,90] and cleaved with ozone.[91] Oxidation provides either the conjugated aldehyde or the unstable hept-2-ene (VIII).[92] Additionally, a number of other 7-oxo-4-oxa-1-azabicyclo-[3.2.0]hept-2-ane and hept-2-ene derivatives (e.g., IX) have been synthesized by the Beecham group.[93-100] Virtually every derivative mentioned is claimed to be a β-lactamase inhibitor and to act synergistically with other β-lactam antibiotics. A quantitative assessment of their efficacy is awaited. A procedure to hydrolyze clavulanate 3-esters to the free carboxylates in 0.1 M base[101] appears to belie earlier estimates of the instability of oxygen analogs of penicillins.[102]

Thienamycin - Of all of the novel β-lactams recently isolated, the carbocyclic β-lactams thienamycin[103] (X) and olivanic acid (XI, R_1=R_2=H) emerge as the β-lactam structures most responsible for rescuing this field from the quiescent state it had lapsed into in the years following the discovery of the cephalosporins. Thienamycin is truly a broad spectrum antibiotic, active against both Gram-negative and Gram-positive bacteria at MIC values lower than carbenicillin, ampicillin or the aminoglycosides. Thienamycin possesses a high affinity for all the PBPs of the *E.coli* inner membrane, causing ovoid formation at low concentrations and cell lysis at 0.6 μg/mL and above.[78] The 6α-configuration of the *R*-hydroxyethyl side chain is curious, and the suggestion has been made that the backbone mimics the 7α-methoxyl of the cephamycins while positioning the hydroxyl in the site normally occupied by the 6β-amide.[104] While this interpretation is supported by the lack of bacteriocidal activity in *O*-methylated thienamycin and in the *N*-methylated penicillins, it can only be part of the answer. Both the *cis* and *trans* hydroxyethyl penicillins and cephalosporins have been synthesized: all are very weak antibiotics, though interestingly, the *cis* compounds are the more active.[105]

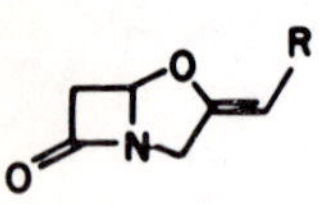

IX

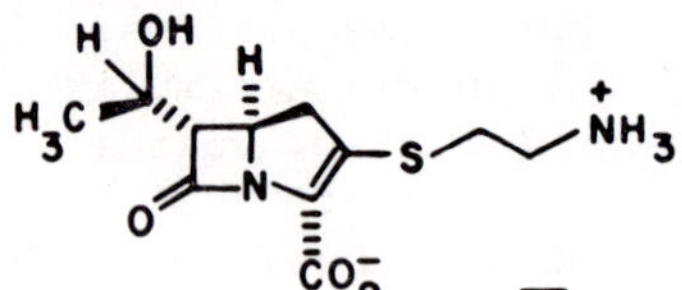

X

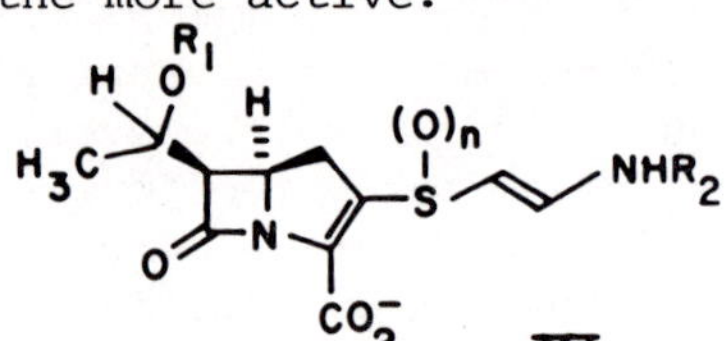

XI

Olivanic Acid - The structures of the β-lactam antibiotics and β-lactamase inhibitors MM13902 (XI, R_1=SO_3H, R_2=$COCH_3$, n=0) and MM4550 (XI, R_1=SO_3H, R_2=$COCH_3$, n=1) also known as MC696-SY2-A) have been simultaneously disclosed by two groups.[106,107] These antibiotics are present in several *Streptomyces* strains (but isolated from *S.olivaceus* and *S.fuloviridis*), and the trivial name olivanic acid has been suggested for the parent compound (XI, R_1=R_2=H, n=0). Their structural similarity to thienamycin is apparent, and a dihydroolivanate derivative (MM17880) has also been isolated.[108] The only structural difference of consequence between the two classes is the stereochemistry at C-6, with olivanic acid possessing the accustomed 6β-configuration. MM4550 and MM13902 are several-fold better than clavulanic acid as antibiotics for most test organisms (but still several-fold poorer than thienamycin). In synergy with ampicillin, MM4550 is equipotent with clavulanate towards *K.aerogenes A*, while clavulanate is marginally better than MM4550 in ampicillin synergy with *S.aureus* Russel.[109]

References

1 N. Curtis, J. Hughes, and G. Ross, Antimicrob. Agents. Chemother., 9, 208-213 (1976).
2 H. Ohmori, A. Azuma, Y. Suzuki, and Y. Hashimoto, J. Antibiot., 30, 267-269 (1977).
3 D. Greenwood and F. O'Grady, Chemotherapy (Basel), 21, 330-341 (1975).
4 M. Pollock, Proc. Roy. Soc. B, 179, 385-401 (1971).
5 N. Citri, in The Enzymes, Third Edition, Volume IV, pp. 23-46.
6 M. Richmond, Methods Enzymol., 43, 664-672 (1975).
7 R. Novick, J. Gen. Microbiol., 33, 121-136 (1963).
8 M. Richmond, Biochem. J., 88, 452-459 (1963).
9 R. Ambler, Biochem. J., 151, 197-218 (1975).
10 D. Thatcher, Nature, 225, 526 (1975).
11 A. Bristow and R. Virden, Biochem. J., 169, 381-396 (1978).
12 B. Robson and R. Pain, Biochem. J., 155, 325-330; 331-344 (1976).
13 J. Hou and J. Poole, Chemotherapy, 19, 129-147 (1973).
14 J. Hou and J. Poole, J. Pharm. Sci., 62, 783-788 (1973).
15 R. Virden, A. Bristow, and R. Pain, Biochem. J., 149, 397-401 (1975).
16 D. Tipper and J. Strominger, Proc. Natl. Acad. Sci. USA, 54, 1133-1141 (1965).
17 D. Boyd, Proc. Natl. Acad. Sci. USA, 74, 5239-5243 (1977).
18 S. Kuwabara and E. Abraham, Biochem. J., 103, 27c-30c (1967).
19 D. Thatcher, Methods Enzymol., 43, 640-652 (1975).
20 R. Davis and E. Abraham, Biochem. J., 143, 115-127 (1974).
21 D. Thatcher, Biochem. J., 147, 313-326 (1975).
22 R. Coombe and A. George, Anal. Biochem., 75, 652-655 (1976).
23 G. Patil and R. Day, Biochim. Biophys. Acta, 293, 490-496 (1973).
24 J. Durkin, G. Dmitrienko, and T. Viswanatha, Can. J. Biochem., 55, 453-457 (1977).
25 V. Csanyi, I. Ferencz, and I. Mile, Biochim. Biophys. Acta, 243, 484-488 (1971).
26 S. Waley, Biochem. J., 149, 547-551 (1975).
27 H. Ogawara and H. Umezawa, Biochim. Biophys. Acta, 391, 435-447 (1975).
28 P. Kiener and S. Waley, Biochem. J., 165, 279-285 (1977).
29 A. Samuni and N. Citri, Biochem. Biophys. Res. Commun., 62, 7-11 (1975).
30 N. Citri, A. Samuni, and N. Zyk, Proc. Natl. Acad. Sci. USA, 73, 1048-1052 (1976).
31 P. Kiener and S. Waley, Biochem. J., 169, 197-204 (1978).
32 D. Thatcher, Methods Enzymol., 43, 653-664 (1975).
33 R. Ambler and R. Meadway, Nature (London), 222, 24-26 (1969).
34 S. Yamamoto and J. Lampen, J. Biol. Chem., 251, 4095-4101; 4102-4110 (1976).
35 P. Aiyappa and J. Lampen, J. Bacteriol., 129, 191-197; J. Biol. Chem., 252, 1745-1747 (1977).
36 L. Crane, G. Bettinger, and J. Lampen, Biochem. Biophys. Res. Commun., 50, 220-227 (1973).
37 M. Richmond and R. Sykes, Advan. Microbial Physiol., 9, 31-88 (1973).
38 M. Richmond, J. Antimicrob. Chemother., 3 (Suppl. B), 29-39 (1977).
39 G. Ross, Methods Enzymol., 43, 678-687 (1975).
40 R. Letarte, M. Devaud-Felix, J. Pechere, and D. Allard-Leprohon, Antimicrob. Agents Chemother., 12, 201-205 (1977).
41 T. Morohoshi and T. Saito, J. Antibiot., 30, 969-973 (1977).
42 V. Petrocheilou, R. Sykes, and M. Richmond, Antimicrob. Agents Chemother., 12, 126-128 (1977).
43 R. Labia, A. Phillipon, F. LeGoffic, and J. Faye, Biochemie, 57, 139-143 (1975).
44 A. Furth, Biochim. Biophys. Acta, 377, 431-443 (1975).
45 R. Labia, M. Guionic, J. Masson, A. Phillipon, and M. Barthelemy, Antimicrob. Agents Chemother., 11, 785-790 (1977).
46 R. Labia and C. Fabre, Biochim. Biophys. Acta, 452, 209-218 (1976).
47 M. Richmond, Methods Enzymol., 43, 672-677 (1975).
48 J. Melling and G. Scott, Biochem. J., 130, 55-62 (1972).
49 R. Ambler and G. Scott, Nature (London), submitted (1978).
50 G. Sutcliffe, Nature (London), submitted (1978).
51 J. Knox, J. Kelly, P. Moews, and N. Murthy, J. Mol. Biol., 104, 865-875 (1976).
52 G. Scott, Biochem. Soc. Trans., 1, 159-162 (1973).
53 H. Ogawara and H. Umezawa, J. Antibiot., 27, 567-569 (1974).
54 H. Ogawara, Methods Enzymol., 46, 531-536 (1977).
55 Recent Advances in the Chemistry of the β-Lactam Antibiotics, J. Elks, Ed., Chemical Society Special Publication, 28, London (1977).
56 F. Lund, in ref. 55, pp. 25-45.
57 V. Lorian and B. Atkinson, Antimicrob. Agents Chemother., 11, 541-552 (1977).
58 B. Spratt, Antimicrob. Agents Chemother., 11, 161-166 (1977).
59 J. Park and L. Borman, Biochem. Biophys. Res. Commun., 51, 863-868 (1973).
60 S. Matsuhashi, T. Kamiryo, P. Blumberg, P. Linnett, E. Willoughby, and J. Strominger, J. Bacteriol., 117, 578-587 (1974).

61 H. Neu, Antimicrob. Agents Chemother., 9, 793-799 (1976); 10, 535-542 (1977).
62 S. Nagasawa, T. Nishino, N. Goto, K. Yonenaga, M. Yokete, S. Sugihara, and S. Yamada, Chemotherapy (Tokyo), 25, 28-45 (1977).
63 K. Okonogi, M. Kida, K. Tsuchiya, and M. Yoneda, Chemotherapy (Tokyo), 25, 94-99 (1977).
64 T. Kamiya, in ref. 55, pp. 281-294 (1977).
65 M. Nishida, Y. Mine, S. Nonoyama, K. Kojo, S. Goto, and S. Kuwahara, J. Antibiot., 30, 917-925 (1977).
66 H. Kojo, Y. Mine, M. Nishida, and T. Yokota, J. Antibiot., 30, 926-931 (1977).
67 Y. Mine, S. Nonoyama, H. Kojo, S. Fukada, M. Nishida, S. Goto, and S. Kuwahara, J. Antibiot., 30, 932-937; 938-944 (1977).
68 J. Hosada, T. Konomi, N. Tani, H. Aski, and H. Imanaka, Agr. Biol. Chem., 41, 2013-2020 (1977).
69 H. Hosada, N. Tani, T. Konomi, S. Ohsawa, H. Aski, and H. Imanaka, Agr. Biol. Chem., 41, 2007-2012 (1977).
70 I. Ernest, J. Gosteli, and R. Woodward, Ger. Offen. 2655298; Chem. Abstr., 87, 201516 (1977).
71 R. Woodward, in ref. 55, pp. 167-180 (1977).
72 H. Ohishi, D. Daost, S. Zimmerman, O. Hendlin, and E. Stapely, Antimicrob. Agents Chemother., 5, 38-48 (1974).
73 B. Christensen, K. Hoogsteen, F. Plavac, and R. Ratcliffe, in ref. 55, pp. 260-268 (1977).
74 G. Darland and J. Birnbaum, Antimicrob. Agents Chemother., 11, 725-734 (1977).
75 A. Brown, J. Goodacre, J. Harbridge, T. Howarth, R. Ponsford, I. Stirling, and T. King, in ref. 55, pp. 295-298.
76 P. Bentley, P. Berry, G. Brooks, M. Gilpin, E. Hunt, and I. Zomaya, Chem. Commun., 748-749 (1977).
77 C. Reading and M. Cole, Antimicrob. Agents Chemother., 11, 852-857 (1977).
78 B. Spratt, V. Jobanputra, and W. Zimmerman, Antimicrob. Agents Chemother., 12, 406-409 (1977).
79 J. Wust and T. Wilkins, Antimicrob. Agents Chemother., 13, 130-133 (1978).
80 J. Fisher, R. Charnas, and J.R. Knowles, Biochemistry, 17, in press (1978).
81 R. Charnas, J. Fisher, and J.R. Knowles, Biochemistry, 17, in press (1978).
82 C. Reading, Ger. Offen. 2708047; Chem. Abstr., 88, 4767v (1978).
83 A. Brown and T. Howarth, Ger. Offen. 2547698; Chem. Abstr., 85, 46641t (1976).
84 T. Howarth, J. Goodacre, and R. Ponsford, Ger. Offen. 2616088; Chem. Abstr., 86, 72625f (1977).
85 T. Howarth, Ger. Offen. 2616087; Chem. Abstr., 86, 89795j (1977).
86 T. Howarth, Ger. Offen. 2546243; Chem. Abstr., 85, 63051t (1976).
87 A. Brown, T. Howarth, I. Stirling, and T. King, Tetrahedron Lett., 4203-4204 (1976).
88 T. Howarth and I. Stirling, Ger. Offen. 2555626; Chem. Abstr., 85, 177397r (1976).
89 T. Howarth and I. Stirling, Ger. Offen. 2655675; Chem. Abstr., 87, 102313t (1977).
90 R. Ponsford, T. Howarth, and I. Stirling, Ger. Offen. 2646003; Chem. Abstr., 87, 84976 (1977).
91 R. Ponsford, Ger. Offen. 2702954; Chem. Abstr., 87, 152176 (1977).
92 D. Corbett, T. Howarth, and I. Stirling, Chem. Commun., 808 (1977); I. Stirling, Ger. Offen. 2655676; Chem. Abstr., 87, 135356 (1977).
93 A. Brown, D. Corbett, and T. Howarth, Chem. Commun., 359-361 (1977).
94 R. Alexander and R. Southgate, Chem. Commun., 405-407 (1977).
95 T. Howarth, A. Brown, D. Corbett, and R. Ponsford, Ger. Offen. 2623561; Chem. Abstr., 86, 189912p (1977).
96 P. Bentley, G. Brooks, M. Gilpin, and E. Hunt, Chem. Commun., 905-906 (1977).
97 A. Eglington, Chem. Commun., 720 (1977).
98 M. Cole, T. Howarth, and C. Reading, Ger. Offen. 2559410; Chem. Abstr., 86, 43960t (1977).
99 E. Hunt, Ger. Offen. 2702091; Chem. Abstr., 87, 168011, 168012 (1977).
100 E. Hunt, P. Bentley, G. Brooks, and M. Gilpin, Chem. Commun., 906-907 (1977).
101 J. Harbridge and T. Howarth, Ger. Offen. 2635477; Chem. Abstr., 87, 59445 (1977).
102 B. Christensen and R. Ratcliffe, Ann. Reports Med. Chem., 11, 271-280 (1976).
103 J. Kahan, F. Kahan, E. Stapely, R. Goegelman, and S. Hernandez, U.S. Patent 3950357 (1976).
104 D. Johnston, S. Schmitt, F. Bouffard, and B. Christensen, J. Am. Chem. Soc., 100, 313-315 (1978).
105 F. DiNinno, T. Beattie, and B. Christensen, J. Org. Chem., 42, 2960-2965 (1977).
106 A. Brown, D. Corbett, A. Eglington, and T. Howarth, Chem. Commun., 523-525 (1977).
107 K. Maeda, S. Takahashi, M. Sezaki, K. Iinuma, H. Nakanawa, S. Kondo, M. Ohno, and H. Umezawa, J. Antibiot., 30, 770-773 (1977).
108 D. Corbett, A. Eglington, and T. Howarth, Chem. Commun., 953-954 (1977).
109 D. Butterworth, M. Cole, and J. Hood, Brit. Patent 1467413 (1977).

Chapter 26. Selective Enzyme Inhibitors in Medicinal Chemistry

Michel J. Jung, Centre de Recherche Merrell International
16, rue d'Ankara 67084-Strasbourg Cedex, France

Introduction - Many old drugs have inhibitory properties on one or another enzyme, but only a few were conceived with that goal in mind. The knowledge of the structure and mechanism of action of enzymes has progressed tremendously over the past two decades so that the search of specific enzyme inhibitors as potential new drugs became more attractive and promising. In theory, if the primary and tertiary structure of an enzyme is known, for instance by X-ray crystallography, it should be possible to design compounds having optimal binding properties. This however is only rarely the case so that one has to rely on empirical methods to find structural requirements for a good binding, and this method has yielded some good competitive inhibitors.[1] This type of inhibitors is not always satisfactory because they are short-acting and high doses are often needed. The specificity of competitive inhibitors depends only on the recognition by an enzyme, so that different enzymes performing different reactions on the same substrate might be inhibited by such a compound. Additional selectivity can be gained if one takes into account what happens to the substrate after binding, and this has led to two classes of more potent and selective inhibitors: the transition state analogs[2] and the enzyme activated irreversible inhibitors, also called k_{cat} or catalytic inhibitors[3] or suicide enzyme inactivators.[4] The first example of an enzyme activated irreversible inhibitor was provided by K. Bloch's discovery of the interaction of β-hydroxydecanoylthioester dehydrase with the β,γ-unsaturated substrate analog CH_3-$(CH_2)_5$-C≡C-CH_2-CO-SCoA.[5] Nature has often developed potent and specific enzyme inhibitors and the systematic screening of extracts from mammalian tissue, bacterial or fungus culture has yielded enzyme inhibitors of various types of action.[6,7] Selective examples of the different kinds of enzyme inhibitors which have led or are likely to lead to biological applications, are presented. The review is divided into sections dealing with classes of enzymes metabolically linked or performing similar functions.

Enzymes Involved in Amino Acid Metabolism

Ornithine decarboxylase: α-Methylornithine,[8] α-hydrazino δ-amino valeric acid,[9] β,γ-dehydro-ornithine,[10] are potent competitive inhibitors of ornithine decarboxylase, the rate-limiting enzyme of polyamine biosynthesis. These compounds have been found to inhibit the proliferation or differentation of several cell lines in cultures[9,10,11]. The inhibition has been attributed to the depletion of spermidine. The competitive inhibitors have the disadvantage of increasing the amount of ornithine decarboxylase, probably by slowing down its degradation, which results in an increased ability to produce polyamines after the inhibitor has disappeared. Two irreversible inhibitors, α-difluoromethylornithine(1) and 5-hexyne 1,4-diamine (2), have been described.[12] Compound (1) blocks the proliferation of rat hepatoma tumor cells and mouse leukemia cells in culture.[13] The respective mechanisms of action are described in Scheme 1.

ISBN 0-12-040513-X

Scheme 1

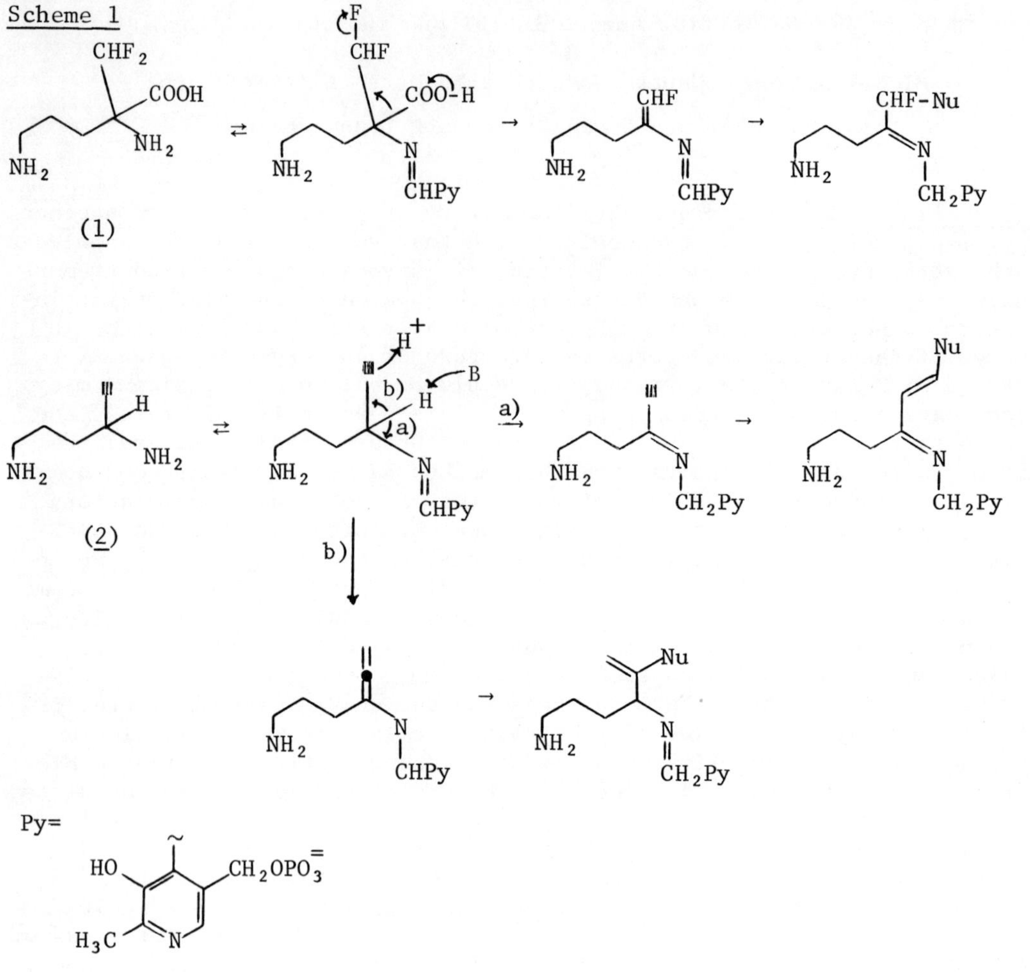

Nu= nucleophile

Histidine decarboxylase: Both hydrazinohistidine and tetrahydroisoquinolylhydrazino butyric acid are inhibitors of rat stomach histidine decarboxylase. They lower the histamine levels in stomach and reduce gastric secretion.[14] Structurally unrelated to histidine, lecanoric acid (3), a natural product isolated from a fungus broth, is an excellent reversible inhibitor of fetal rat histidine decarboxylase *in vitro*.[15] *In vivo*, the compound inhibits the development of rat paw edema induced by carrageenin, it remains, however, to be proved that these two actions are related. The synthetic amide analog (4) is more stable and is a stronger inhibitor of the enzyme and of edema formation.[15]

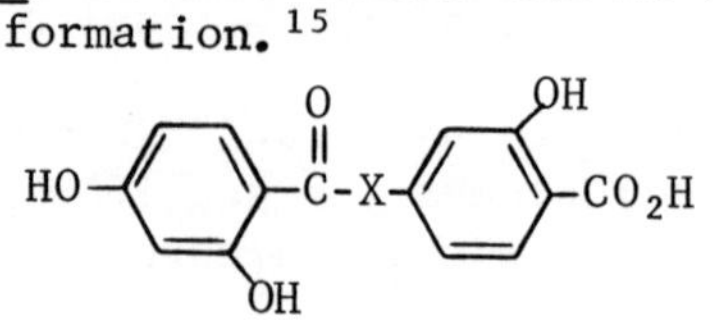

(3) X = O
(4) X = NH

4-Aminobutyric acid aminotransferase: The concentration of 4-aminobutyric acid (GABA), an inhibitory neurotransmitter in mammalian brain, can be elevated by inhibiting GABA-aminotransferase, the enzyme responsible for its degradation. As a result there is protection against electroshock, audiogenic and certain chemically induced seizures in animals. Until recently, inhibitors available were pyridoxal scavengers like aminooxyacetic acid,[16] hydrazino-propionic acid,[17] γ-glutamylhydrazone.[18] In recent years, four enzyme activated irreversible inhibitors have been described for this enzyme: ethanolamine-O-sulfate[19] (5), 4-aminohex 5-ynoic acid[20] (6), 4-aminohex 5-enoic acid[21] (7) and 5-amino-1,3-cyclohexadienyl carboxylic acid[22] (8). All of these compounds produce marked elevations of brain GABA levels and possess anticonvulsant action.[23-26] Their respective mechanisms of action are described in Scheme 2.

Scheme 2

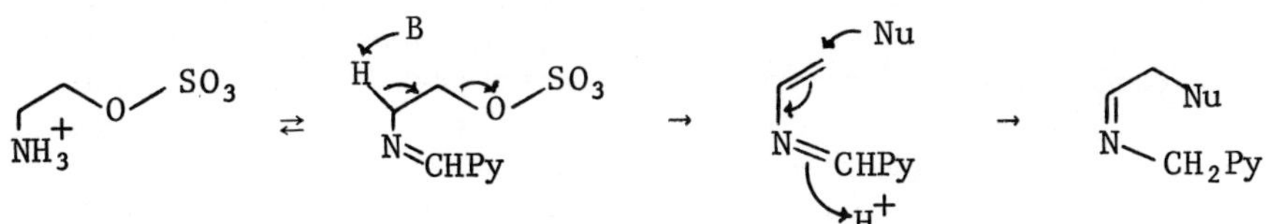

(5)

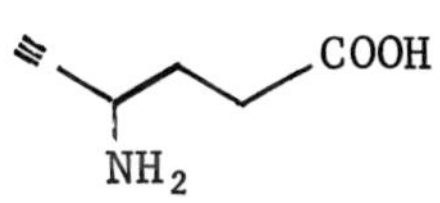

(6)

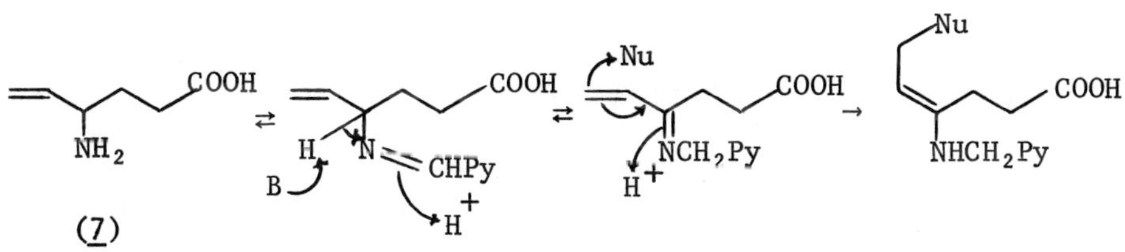

(7)

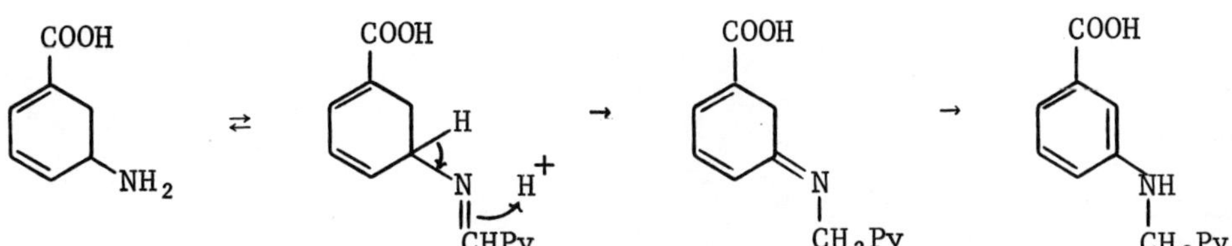

(8)

In addition, (6) inhibits irreversibly bacterial and mammalian glutamate decarboxylase,[27] probably by a mechanism similar to the one described for the inhibition of ornithine decarboxylase by (2) in Scheme 1.

Other pyridoxal-dependent enzymes: Much has been written during recent years about the irreversible inhibition of different pyridoxal-phosphate-dependent enzymes by mono or poly haloalanines[28,29] and propargyl,[30] allyl,[31] or vinyl[32] glycine. The mechanisms implied involve in all cases abstraction of the α-hydrogen from the pyridoxal-Schiff base by the enzyme, followed by elimination of a halide atom in the case of halo-alanines, tautomerisation of the conjugated Schiff base in the case of vinyl glycine, yielding reactive Michael-acceptors in the enzyme active site. The irreversible inhibition by propargyl and allyl glycine is more complex as it involves a second hydrogen abstraction to yield a conjugated Schiff base. This Michael acceptor can alkylate the enzyme which results in either a fully inhibited enzyme or an enzyme having modified properties. It can also be hydrolysed in either chemically reactive or unreactive species.[33] These compounds, although of limited utility in animal studies due to their lack of selectivity, helped to promote the search for more specific enzyme activated irreversible inhibitors of pyridoxal-dependent enzymes. Two compounds deserve a special mention, these are 3-fluoro-D-alanine and its 2-deutero analog.[34,35] Both compounds are irreversible inhibitors of alanine racemase and possess a broad spectral antibiotic activity. Animal toxicity is low with the protio compound and even lower with the deuterated compound. The anti-bacterial activity of D-carbamylserine and D-cycloserine, two natural antibiotics, is also due to the enzyme activated irreversible inhibition of alanine racemase.[36]

Enzymes involved in the synthesis or degradation of biogenic amines

Tyrosine hydroxylase: α-Methyl-p-tyrosine is a strong competitive inhibitor of tyrosine hydroxylase,[37] the key enzyme of catecholamine biosynthesis, and lowers dramatically the concentrations of brain, heart and adrenal catecholamines in animals, without any significant effect on serotonin levels.[38] Although this compound was promising in the treatment of pheochromocytoma,[39] it was not developed beyond the clinical phase because there was marked drug crystalluria[40] in experimental subjects. Benzimidazole alanine[41] (9) and its α-methyl analog[42] (10) are also good competitive inhibitors of tyrosine hydroxylase and block the synthesis of catecholamines in reserpinized animals.[43] Oudenone (11), a microbial product, inhibits tyrosine hydroxylase by competing with the pteridine cofactor,[44] and reduces catecholamine levels in mammalian brain and adrenal glands; the compound has hypotensive activity[45] in spontaneous hypertensive rats.

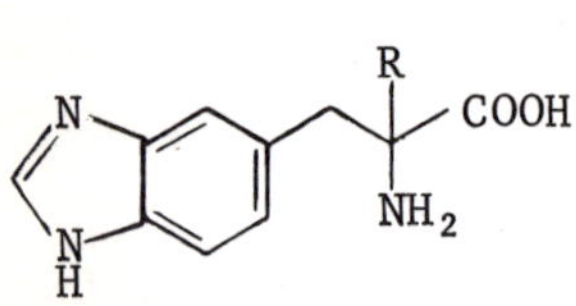

(9) R = H
(10) R = CH_3

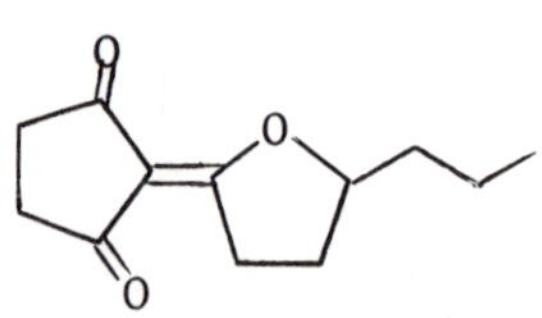

(11)

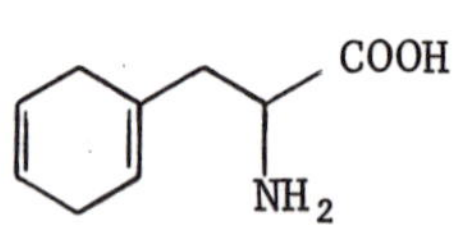

(12)

Tryptophan hydroxylase: p-Chlorophenylalanine, a competitive inhibitor of tryptophan hydroxylase *in vitro*, depletes serotonin levels *in vivo* by a more complex mechanism.[46] The serotonin depleting activity of α-methyl-tryptophan *in vivo* is probably due to its conversion to α-methyl serotonin rather than to tryptophan hydroxylase inhibition.[47] The Umezawa group has reported recently that 2,5-dihydrophenylalanine (12), a natural product isolated from a streptomyces strain, is a competitive inhibitor of tryptophan hydroxylase *in vitro*.[48]

Aromatic amino acid decarboxylase: Benserazide and Carbidopa are very potent inhibitors of peripheral decarboxylase, probably by forming hydrazones with the enzyme-bound pyridoxal-phosphate, and both compounds increase the amount of dopamine formed in brain after peripheral administration of Dopa to an animal.[49] The combinations of Dopa and Carbidopa or Dopa and Benzerazide are used clinically for the treatment of Parkinsonism.[50] Recently, the synthesis of α-vinyl Dopa (13) and α-ethynyl Dopa (14), two potential suicide inactivators of Dopa-decarboxylase, has been described by two independent groups.[51a,b]

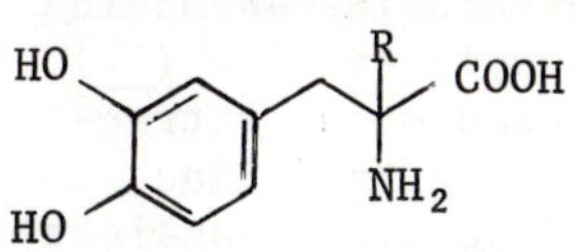

(13) R = /=
(14) R = -≡

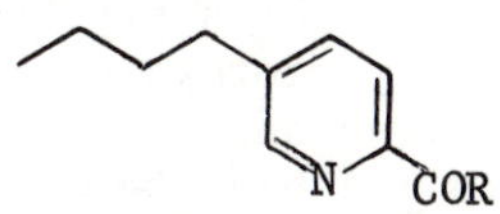

(15) R = OH
(16) R = NH_2

It was claimed without experimental details that (14) is a very potent inhibitor of this enzyme.[51a]

Dopamine-β-hydroxylase: This copper enzyme is inhibited by copper chelator. However, the only inhibitors, useful *in vivo*, are picolinic acids substituted in position 5 by aliphatic groups. The first member of this series is fusaric acid[52] (15), obtained from filtrates of microbial cultures; synthetic analogs have modified side chains,[53] or other functions in position 2[54] (16). All of these compounds have blood-pressure lowering effects.

Monoamine-oxidase inhibitors: The design of monoamine oxidase inhibitors is probably one of the fields in which medicinal chemists have been most active in the last decades. Some of the compounds are still in use to treat severe depression and hypertension. Mechanistically the most interesting are the propargylamine derivatives, like pargyline, clorgyline and deprenyl, which inhibit the flavin dependent enzyme irreversibly.[55] Very thorough investigations, including the characterization of the flavin adduct, have allowed Abeles and coworkers to propose the following reaction mechanism for the inhibition of mitochondrial MAO by a tertiary propargylamine[56] (Scheme 3).

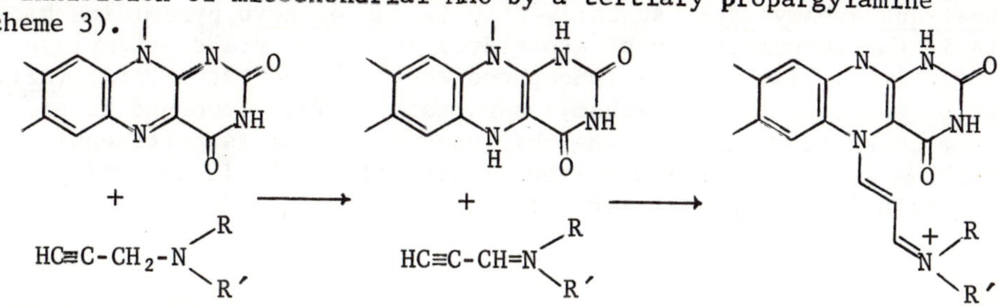

Plasma monoamine oxidase, a pyridoxal phosphate-dependent enzyme is inhibited irreversibly by aminoacetonitrile[57] and some esters of glycine.[58] The mechanisms implied, involve the formation of a keteneimine and a ketene by enzyme catalysis, followed by the alkylation of the enzyme by these reactive species.

Other flavin-dependent enzymes

Other flavin-dependent enzymes are also inhibited irreversibly by substrate analogs, suitably substituted by vinyl or acetylenic groups. The inhibition of sarcosine oxidase and dimethyl glycine oxidase, in vitro and in vivo by N-allyl or N-propargylglycine[59,60] may be of relevance with the long-known, prolonged pharmacological activity of N-allyl amines. Flavin dependent α-hydroxy acid and α-amino acid dehydrogenases are inhibited by H-C≡C-CH(OH)-COOH and propargylglycine, respectively.[33,61,62]

Enzymes involved in purine and pyrimidine synthesis or degradation

Adenosine deaminase: The anti-tumor activity of arabino-furanosyl adenine in animals can be increased by coadministration of tight-binding adenosine deaminase inhibitors[63] such as erythro-9-(2-hydroxy-3-nonyl) adenine (17) ($K_I = 10^{-9}M$)[64] and deoxycoformycin (18) which can be looked at as a transition state analog of adenosine during deamination.[65] Along this line, compounds (19, 20 and 21) have been synthesized and will be tested against the corresponding deaminases.[66]

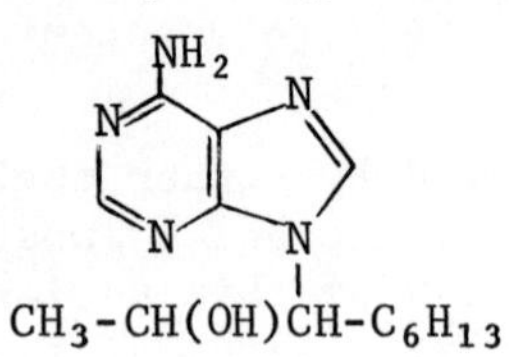

(17)

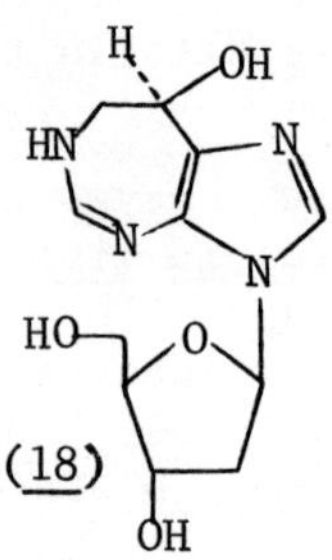

(18)

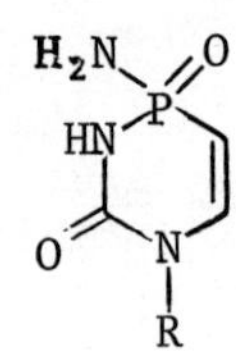

(19)

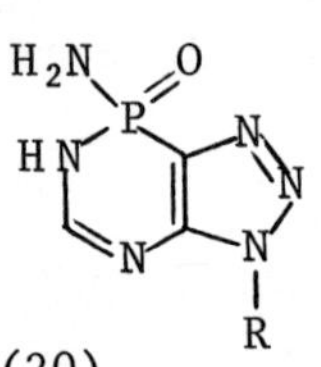

(20)

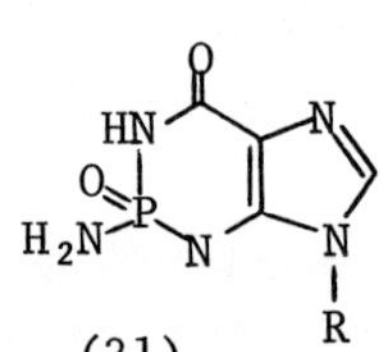

(21)

Aspartate-transcarbamylase: An early step in the de novo pyrimidine biosynthesis is the carbamylation of aspartate. Aspartate transcarbamylase can be effectively blocked by N-(phosphono-acetyl) aspartate (PALA) (22), a transition state analog of carbamyl aspartate.[67] This compound is effective in the mg/kg range in blocking this enzyme and the isoproterenol stimulated DNA synthesis in mouse submaxillary glands.[68] It is active against certain experimental tumors.[69]

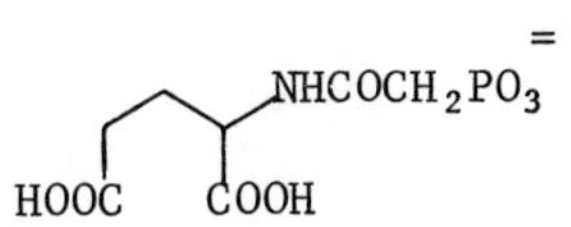

(22)

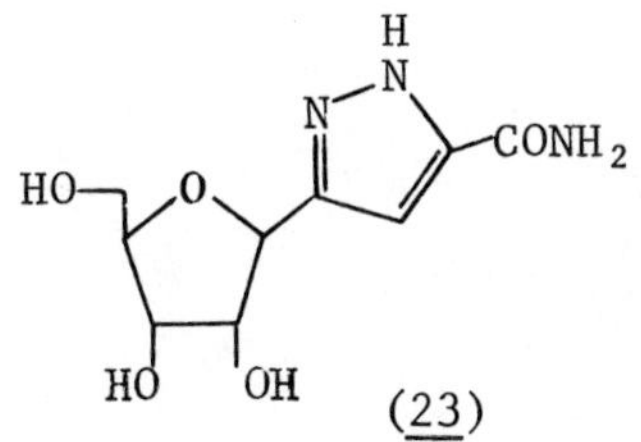

(23)

Orotate decarboxylase: Pyrazofurin (23), a natural antibiotic, is a very effective inhibitor of pyrimidine biosynthesis by blocking orotate decarboxylase. In combination with arabinosylcytosine, it increases greatly the cell toxicity of the latter compound.[70]

Thymidylate synthetase: Another key enzyme for DNA synthesis is thymidylate synthetase. This enzyme is irreversibly inhibited by fluorodeoxyuridine monophosphate formed in vivo from 2-fluorouracil, which had been used for about 20 years in cancer chemotherapy. The reader is referred to Ref. 71 for an excellent discussion on its mechanism of action. 5-Trifluoromethyl 2'-deoxyuridylic acid (24), formed from trifluoromethyl-uracil in vivo, is also an irreversible inhibitor of thymidylate synthetase.[72] The mechanism suggested by Santi and Sakai[73] is described in Scheme 4.

Scheme 4

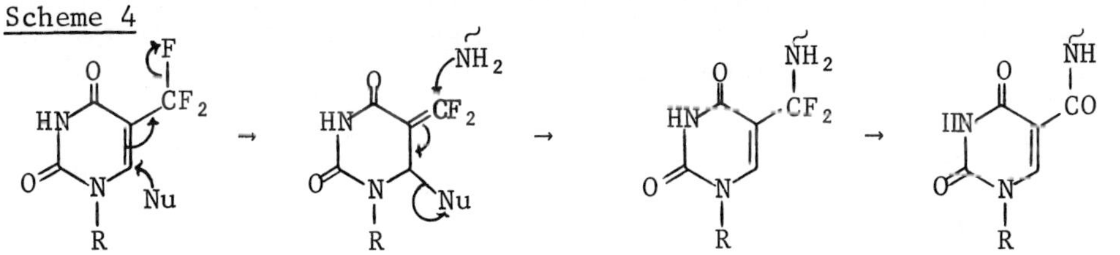

(24)

Ribonucleotide reductase: Since it has been shown that ribonucleotide reductase activity is increased dramatically in rapidly growing tissues and viral infection, much work has been done in understanding the mechanism[74] and designing inhibitors of this enzyme.[75] The antitumor action of hydroxyurea, a radical scavenger has been attributed to inhibition of this enzyme, and analogs of hydroxyurea have been found to increase life span of leukemic mice.[76] The dialdehyde derivatives of purine nucleosides (25) are inhibitors of ribonucleotide reductase, they inhibit DNA synthesis in cell cultures.[77]

2'-Deoxy-2'-azido (or 2'-chloro) ribonucleotide diphosphates (26, 27) are irreversible inhibitors of ribonucleotide reductase from E. Coli and (26) also inactivates the calf thymus enzyme.[78] In addition, azidocytidine inhibits cell growth in vitro,[79] however the inhibition was not related to a depletion of the deoxynucleotide pool and may be due to an interaction at the initiation stage of DNA synthesis.

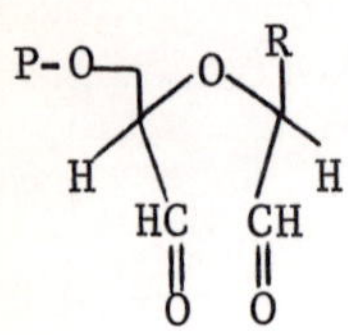

(25)

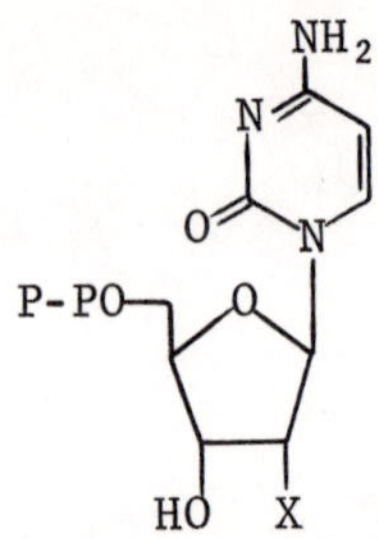

$X = N_3$ (26)

$X = Cl$ (27)

Inhibitors of steroid biosynthesis: The cytotoxic effects of several hydroxylated sterols against rat hepatoma cells in culture seem to be at least partly due to inhibition of 3-hydroxy-3-methyl-glutaryl CoA reductase[80] which catalyses an early step in cholesterol biosynthesis. These sterols are extracted from drugs used in chinese folk medicine for the treatment of cancer. The hypocholesterolemic action of clofibrate was attributed to the inhibition of mevalonic acid synthesis at an unspecified step[81] while citrinin, another hypocholesteremic agent, inhibits hydroxymethyl-glutaryl CoA reductase in a time-dependent irreversible manner.[82]
There are a number of competitive type inhibitors of steroid hormone biosynthesis. Recently enzyme activated irreversible inhibitors of bacterial Δ^5-3-ketosteroid isomerase and of Δ^4-3-ketosteroid reductase, namely β,γ-acetylenic 3-oxo-5,10-secosteroids (28) and allenic 3-oxo-5,10-secosteroids (29) have been described.[83,84] These compounds act also selectively on the mammalian enzymes from rat epididymis.[85] Their mechanism of action is described in Scheme 5.

Scheme 5

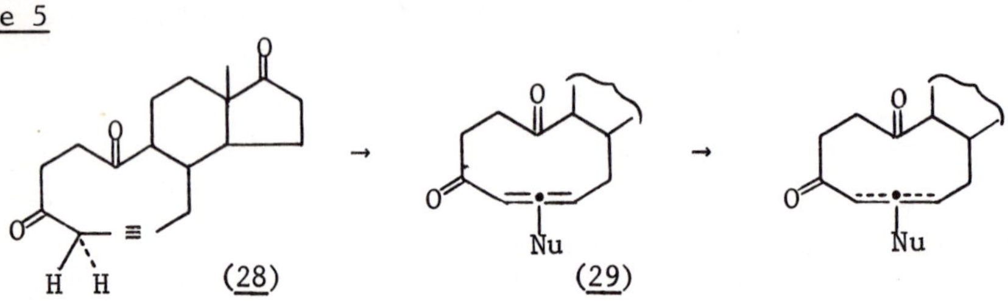

(28) (29)

Inhibitors of hydrolytic enzymes: There is no space to name the numerous proteolytic enzyme inhibitors found either in animals and plants[6] or in fungi and bacterial cultures.[7] Some of them have been tested clinically, such as pepstatine for the treatment of stomach ulcers, or leupeptin as an anti-coagulant. Leupeptin and antipain have terminal aldehyde functions which probably form hemi-acetals with a serine residue in the enzyme active site. It has been proposed that the unusual terminal amino acid of pepstatine, 4-amino-3-hydroxy-6-methylheptanoic acid, is an analog of the transition state in amide bond hydrolysis catalysed by acid proteases.[86] Inhibitors of angiotensin converting enzyme have a great potential as antihypertensive agents in renal hypertension. Active site mapping of such enzymes has lead to the design of a very powerful inhibitor, 3-mercapto-2-D-methylpropanoyl-L-proline (30) ($K_I = 1.7 \times 10^{-9}$M).[87] This compound is orally active and prevents angiotensin-induced hypertension in normotensive humans

with little side effects.[88]
α-Chymotrypsin and other acid proteases are inhibited in a time-dependent manner by halomethylated derivatives of dihydrocoumarins (31).[89] The mechanism suggested is described in Scheme 6.[90]

Scheme 6

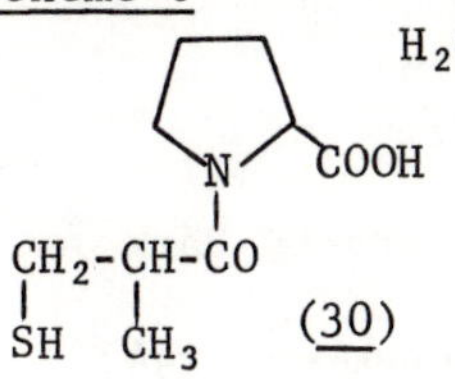

(30)

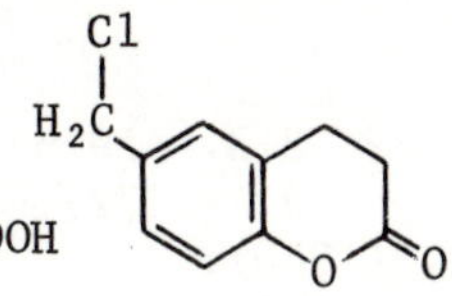

(31)

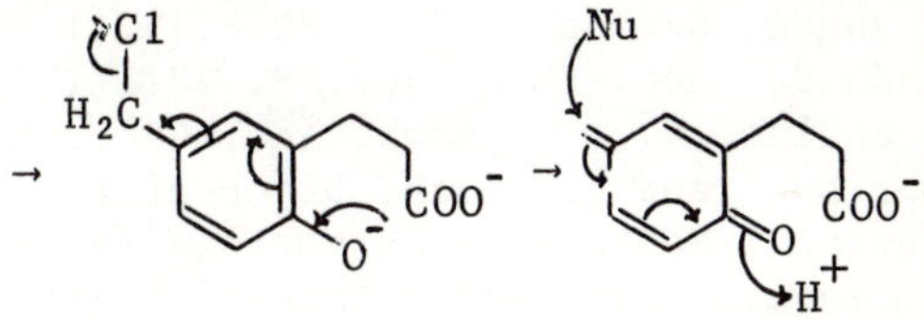

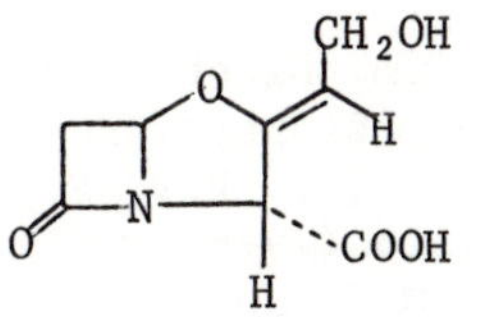

(32)

Penicillin G. inhibits cell wall biosynthesis in bacteria by several mechanisms one of which is irreversible acylation of D Ala-D Ala transpeptidase,[91] so that penicillin could be considered as a suicide enzyme inactivator.[3] Bacteria develop resistance to penicillin by developing specific β-lactamases. Medicinal chemists in turn, have tried to inhibit these β-lactamases. Over 1000 semi-synthetic penicillins have been screened for that purpose. Let us just mention clavulanic acid (32), a compound isolated from a streptomyces strain, which inhibits β-lactamases from both gram + and gram - bacteria in a time-dependent irreversible manner.[92]

Conclusion - Different possibilities to find selective enzyme inhibitors have been evaluated: The classical antimetabolic approach (like α-methyl analogs of amino acids), the systematic screening for active compounds (applied to microbial cultures) followed by chemical modifications to make stable and more potent products, (fusaric acid, lecanoric acid, etc.···), the active site mapping of enzymes (angiotensin converting enzyme), and when the enzymatic mechanism is known the design of transition analogs (PALA, adenosine deaminase inhibitors) or of enzyme activated irreversible inhibitors (GABA-transaminase inhibitors, seco-steroids). It often happens that the molecular mechanism of action is not understood until long after the compound is known (acetylenic monoamine oxidase inhibitors, penicillins, clavulanic acid).
It can be expected that with the advent of the potent, selective, long-lasting enzyme inhibitors like the enzyme activated irreversible inhibitors or transition state analogs, the usefulness of enzyme inhibitors in therapy will increase.

References

1. W. Shive and C.G. Skinner in Metabolic Inhibitors, Hochster and Quastel Eds, Acad. Press, New-York-London, Vol. 1, 2, (1963).
2. R. Wolfenden, Acc. Chem. Res., 5, 10, (1972).
3. R.R. Rando, Science, 185, 320, (1974).
   R.R. Rando, Acc. Chem. Res., 8, 281, (1975).
4. R.H. Abeles, A.L. Maycock, Acc. Chem. Res., 9, 313, (1976).
5. M. Morisaki and K. Bloch, Biochemistry, 11, 309, (1972).
6. B. Kassell, Methods in Enzymology, 19, 839, (1970).
7. H. Umezawa, Enzyme inhibitors of bacterial origin, University Park Press, Baltimore, 15, (1972).
8. M.M. Abdel-Monem, N.E. Newton and C.E. Weeks, J. Med. Chem., 17, 447, (1974).
9. S.I. Harik and S.H. Snyder, Biochim. Biophys. Acta, 327, 501,(1973).
10. N. Relyea and R.R. Rando, Biochem. Biophys. Res. Commun., 67, 392, (1975).
11. P.S. Mamont, P. Böhlen, P.P. McCann, P. Bey, F. Schuber and C. Tardif Proc. Natl. Acad. Sci. USA, 73, 1626, (1976).
12. B.W. Metcalf, P. Bey, C. Danzin, M.J. Jung, P. Casara and J.P. Vevert, J. Am. Chem. Soc. (in press).
13. P.S. Mamont, M.G. Duchesne, J. Grove and P. Bey, Biochem. Biophys. Res. Commun. (in press).
14. A. Castelluci and P. Megazzini, Arzneim. Forsch., 26, 62, (1976).
15. H. Umezawa, N. Shibamoto, H. Naganawa, S. Ayukawa, M. Matzusaki and T. Takeuchi, J. Antibiot., 27, 587, (1974).
16. D.P. Wallach, Biochem. Pharmacol., 5, 323, (1961).
17. N.M. Van Gelder, J. Neurochem., 15, 747, (1968).
18. R. Tapia, H. Pasantes, B.G. Ortega and C.H. Massieu, Biochem. Pharmacol. 15, 1831, (1966).
19. L.J. Fowler and R.A. John, Biochem. J., 130, 569, (1972).
    L.J. Fowler, J. Neurochem., 21, 437, (1973).
20. B.W. Metcalf, P. Casara, Tetrahedron Lett., 3337, (1975).
    M.J. Jung, B. Lippert, B.W. Metcalf, P.J. Schechter, P. Böhlen and A. Sjoerdsma, J. Neurochem., 28, 717, (1977).
21. B. Lippert, B.W. Metcalf, M.J. Jung and P. Casara, Eur. J. Biochem., 74, 441, (1977).
    M.J. Jung, B. Lippert, B.W. Metcalf, P. Böhlen and P.J. Schechter, J. Neurochem., 29, 797, (1977).
22. K. Kobayashi, S. Miyazawa, A. Terahara, H. Mishima and H. Kurihara, Tetrahedron Lett., 537, (1976).
    R.R. Rando and F.W. Bangerter, J. Am. Chem. Soc., 98, 6762, (1976).
23. G. Anlezark, R.W. Horton, B.S. Meldrum and M-C.B. Sawaya, Biochem. Pharmacol., 25, 413, (1976).
24. P.J. Schechter, Y. Tranier, M.J. Jung and A. Sjoerdsma, J. Pharmacol. Exp. Ther., 201, 606, (1977).
25. P.J. Schechter, Y. Tranier, M.J. Jung and P. Böhlen, Eur. J. Pharmacol. 45, 319, (1977).
26. Y. Matsui and T. Deguchi, Life Sci., 20, 1291, (1977).
27. B.W. Metcalf, M.J. Jung, B. Lippert, P. Casara and C. Danzin, 173rd Am. Chem. Soc. Meeting, New Orleans, Medi 26, (1977).

28. R.B. Silverman and R.H. Abeles, Biochemistry, 15, 4718, (1976).
29. S.S. Tate, N. Relyea and A. Meister, Biochemistry, 8, 5016, (1969).
30. R.H. Abeles and C. Walsh, J. Am. Chem. Soc., 95, 6124, (1973).
31. M. Orlowski, D.F. Reingold, M.E. Stanley, J. Neurochem., 28, 349, (1977).
32. R.R. Rando, Biochemistry, 13, 3859, (1974).
33. P. Marcotte and C. Walsh, Biochemistry, 15, 3070, (1976).
34. J. Kollonitsch, L. Barash, F.M. Kahan, H. Knopp, Nature, 243, 346, (1973).
35. J. Kollonitsch and L. Barash, J. Am. Chem. Soc. 98, 5591, (1976).
36. E. Wang, and C. Walsh, Biochemistry, 17, 1313 (1978).
37. T. Nagatsu, M. Levitt and S. Udenfriend, J. Biol. Chem., 239, 2910, (1964).
38. S. Spector, Pharmacol. Rev. 18, 599, (1966).
39. K. Engelman, D. Horwitz, E. Jequier and A. Sjoerdsma, J. Clin., Invest., 47, 577, (1968).
40. K. Engelman and A. Sjoerdsma, Circ. Res., 18, 1, (1966).
41. E.M. Johnson Jr., N. Zenker and J. Wright, Biochem. Pharmacol., 21, 1777, (1972).
42. N. Zenker, V.H. Morgenroth III and J. Wright, J. Med. Chem., 17, 1223, (1974)
43. N. Zenker, V.H. Morgenroth III, J. Wright, J.W. King and C.D. Arnett, Biochem. Pharmacol., 25, 585, (1976).
44. H. Umezawa, T. Takeuchi, H. Inuma, K. Suzuki, M. Ito, M. Matzuzaki, T. Nagatsu and O. Tanabe, J. Antibiot., 23, 514, (1970).
45. T. Nagatsu, I. Nagatsu, H. Umezawa, T. Takeuchi, Biochem. Pharmacol., 20, 2505, (1971).
46. S. Knapp and A.J. Mandell, Life Sci., 11, 761, (1972).
47. E.M. Gal and P.A. Cristiensen, J. Neurochem., 24, 89, (1975).
48. K. Okabayashi, H. Morishima, M. Hamada, T. Takeuchi and H. Umezawa, J. Antibiot., 30, 675, (1977).
49. G. Bartholini and A. Pletscher, Pharmacol. Ther., 1, (3), 407, (1975).
50. C.D. Marsden, J.D. Parkes and J.E. Rees, Lancet, 7844, (1973).
R.M. Pinder, R.N. Brogden, P.R. Sawyer, T.M. Speight and G.S. Avery, Drugs, 11, 329, (1976).
51. D. Taub and A.A. Patchett, Tetrahedron Lett., 2745, (1977).
B.W. Metcalf and K. Jund, Tetrahedron Lett., 3689, (1977).
52. H. Suda, T. Takeuchi, T. Nagatsu, M. Matzusaki, I. Matsumoto and H. Umezawa, Chem. Pharm. Bull., 17, 2377, (1969).
53. H. Umezawa, T. Takeuchi, K. Miyano, T. Koshigoe, H. Hamano, J. Antibiot 26, 189, (1973).
54. C.A. Kordura, J. Veals, A. Wohl, S. Symchowicz and I.I.A. Tabachnick, J. Pharmacol. Exp. Ther., 184, 671 (1973).
55. L. Hellerman and E.V. Erwin, J. Biol. Chem. 243, 5234 (1968).
56. A.L. Maycock, R.H. Abeles, J.I. Salach and T.P. Singer, Biochemistry 15, 115, (1976).
57. L.J. Riceberg, M. Simon, H. Van Vunakis and R.H. Abeles, Biochem. Pharmacol., 24, 119, (1975).
58. A.L. Maycock, R.H. Suva, R.H. Abeles, J. Am. Chem. Soc., 97, 5614, (1975).
59. J.L. Kraus, B. Belleau, Can. J. Chem., 20, 3141, (1975).
60. J.L. Kraus, and J.J. Yaouanc, Mol. Pharmacol., 13, 378, (1977).
61. T. Cromartie, J. Fisher, G. Kaczorowski, R. Laura, P. Marcotte and C. Walsh, J. Chem. Soc. Chem. Commun., 597, (1974).

62. K. Horiike, Y. Nashina, Y. Miyake and T. Yamano, J. Biochem., (Tokyo), 78, 57, (1975).
63. L. Lapi and S.S. Cohen, Biochem. Pharmacol., 26, 71, (1977).
64. H.J. Schaeffer and D.F. Schwender, J. Med. Chem., 17, 16, (1974).
65. S. Cha, R.P. Agawal, R.E. Parks Jr, Biochem. Pharmacol., 24, 2187, (1975).
66. P.A. Bartlett, J.L. Adams, J.T. Hunt, Abst. Papers Am. Chem. Soc. 174 Meet. Orgn 7, (1977).
67. K.D. Collins and G.R. Stark, J. Biol. Chem., 246, 6599, (1971).
68. T. Yoshida, G.R. Stark and N.J. Hoogenrad, J. Biol. Chem., 249, 6951, (1974).
69. R.K. Johnson, T. Inouye, A. Goldin and G.R. Stark, Cancer Res., 36, 2720, (1976).
70. M.J. Sweeney, F.A. Davis, G.E. Gutowski, R.L. Hamill, D.H. Hoffman and C.A. Poore, Cancer Res., 33, 2619, (1973).
71. P.V. Danenberg, Biochim. Biophys. Acta, 473, 73, (1977).
72. P. Reyes and C. Heidelberger, Mol. Pharmacol., 1, 14, (1965).
73. D.V. Santi and T.T. Sakai, Biochemistry, 10, 3598, (1971).
74. H. Follman, Angew Chem. (Int. Ed.), 13, 569, (1974).
75. C.H. Chang and Y.C. Cheng, The Pharmacologist, 18, 118, (1976).
76. H. Elford, Proc. Amer. Ass. Cancer Res. 18, 68 Meeting, 177, (1977).
77. C.B. George and J.G. Gory, Biochem. Pharmacol., 26, 1197, (1977).
78. L. Thelander and B. Larsson, J. Biol. Chem., 251, 1398, (1976).
79. L. Skoog, G. Bjursell, L. Thelander, T. Hagerström, J. Hobbs and F. Eckstein, Eur. J. Biochem., 72, 371, (1977).
80. M. Zander, P. Koch, Luu Bang, G. Ourisson and J.P. Beck, J. Chem. Res., (M) 2572, (1977).
81. K.V. Krishnaïah and T. Ramasarma, Biochem. J., 116, 321, (1970).
82. K. Tanzawa, M. Kuroda, A. Endo, Biochim. Biophys. Acta, 488, 97, (1977).
83. F.H. Batzold and C.H. Robinson, J. Am. Chem. Soc., 97, 2576, (1975).
84. D.F. Covey and C.H. Robinson, J. Am. Chem. Soc., 98, 5038, (1976).
85. B. Robaire, D.F. Covey, C.H. Robinson and L.L. Ewing, J. Steroid. Biochem., 8, 307, (1977).
86. J. Marciniszyn Jr., J.A. Hartsuck and J. Tang, J. Biol. Chem., 251, 7088, (1976).
87. M.A. Ondetti, D.W. Cushman, B. Rubin and E.F. Sabo, Proc. 173rd Am. Chem. Soc. Meeting New Orleans, Medi 24, (1977).
88. R.K. Ferguson, H.R. Brunner, G.A. Turini, H. Gavras and D.N. McKinstry, Lancet, 775, (1977).
89. J.J. Bechet, A. Dupaix, I. Blagoeva, Biochimie, 59, 231, (1977).
90. M. Wakselman, J.F. Hamon, M. Vilkas, Tetrahedron, 30, 4069, (1974).
91. D.J. Tipper and J.L. Strominger, Proc. Natl. Acad. Sci. USA, 54, 1113, (1965).
92. T.T. Hawarth, A.G. Brown and T.J. King, J. Chem. Soc. Chem. Commun., 266, (1976).

Chapter 27. The Inhibition of Proteolytic Enzymes

William B. Lawson, New York State Department of Health, Albany, NY 12201

This review will cover critically but not exhaustively the principal methods for efficient inhibition of proteolytic enzymes. Although the main emphasis is on serine proteases,[1-4] other proteases and other types of enzymes will be discussed to illustrate specific points. Much of the work over the years on enzyme inhibition has been purely theoretical, but the use of organophosphorus compounds (anticholinesterases) in insect control is well known, and the potential for specific enzyme inhibitors in medicine is becoming increasingly apparent.[5,6]

Concepts of Specific Enzyme Inhibition - An enzyme is specifically inhibited when its active site is blocked physically and/or chemically without significant alteration of the rest of the molecule. For the most part the kinetic complexities of inhibition[7,8] will not be dealt with. The emphasis is on various types of molecular interactions with active sites. Inhibitors may be categorized by the way they interact with active sites, but such categories may overlap and may not be assignable without considerable investigation. A broad division may be made between inhibitors that react chemically and those that interact only physically with an active site. Both groups include inhibitors that are for practical purposes either reversible or irreversible. It is a major thesis of this review that the efficiency of inhibition is directly related to the degree and correctness of binding for both reversible and irreversible inhibitors. As in the past, new types and examples of inhibitors will doubtless be discovered by accident, but as chemists learn more about the stereochemistry and reactivity of active site constituents, they will be increasingly successful in designing potent and selective inhibitors. It is really a question of exploiting the organic and physical chemistry of enzymes. The position has recently been taken that transition state inhibitors "are not likely to succeed in clinical utility" because they would "bind to the active site of the enzyme, i.e., where the enzymes from different cellular species show the greatest similarity or even identity."[9] Clinical utility is a very complex matter, but as will be seen, considerable selectivity in the inhibition of similar enzymes has already been achieved, and more can be expected from basic knowledge of the stereochemistry and mechanisms of action of active sites.

Substrates and Reversible Inhibitors - In order to design efficient and specific inhibitors of any type, it is necessary to know as much as possible about the mechanism of action and specificity of the enzyme and about the secondary binding sites, if any, near its active site. A classical method involves testing various substances as substrates, exemplified by the work of Bergmann's school on the specificity of proteolytic enzymes using small peptide substrates.[10] In a refinement of this method, oligopeptide substrates, sometimes containing D-amino acids, have been used to map the specificity and subsites of papain,[11,12] carboxypeptidase A,[13] and elastase.[14,15] Differences in the binding sites of

ISBN 0-12-040513-X

chymotrypsin, subtilisin Novo, and subtilisin Carlsberg were delineated by use of oligopeptide inhibitors.[16] Recently some oligopeptide inhibitors were developed for elastase in a search for medicinally useful compounds.[6] One of the most effective inhibitors was acetyl-Ala-Ala-Pro-Mec-Lac-$NHCH_3$ (Mec = 2-methylcarbazic acid; Lac = lactic acid), which has a K_i of 0.65 μM with pancreatic elastase.[6]

Much work has been done using simple molecules as reversible inhibitors to characterize binding sites of proteases. Some outstanding examples are the binding of amidines and guanidines to trypsin[17] and the inhibition (K_i's in the micromolar range) of trypsin, thrombin, and plasmin by aromatic amidines with ether functions[18] and by bis-amidines,[19] and tris-amidines for trypsinlike enzymes.[20] In the latter study, α,α',α''-tris(4-amidino-2-bromophenoxy)mesitylene (1) was found to inhibit pancreatic kallikrein with a K_i of 0.0243 μM, while α,α',α''-tris(3-amidinophenoxy)mesitylene was the best thrombin inhibitor with a K_i of 0.651 μM, and was a strong anticoagulant. Derivatives of dansylarginine are very good reversible thrombin inhibitors. One of the best is N^{α}-dansyl-L-arginine-4-ethylpiperidide (2; OM 205), which inhibits thrombin with an I_{50} of 0.03 μM but has little effect on plasmin (I_{50} 1 mM).[21] A well known reversible inhibitor that behaves almost irreversibly is methotrexate, which has a K_i of about 10^{-11} M in the inhibition of dihydrofolate reductase.[22]

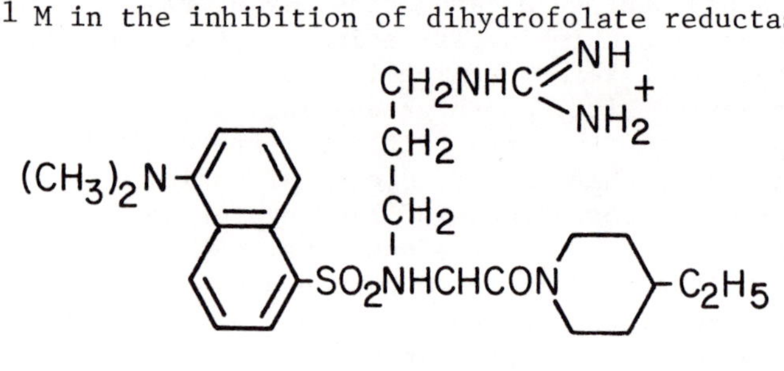

2 (OM 205)

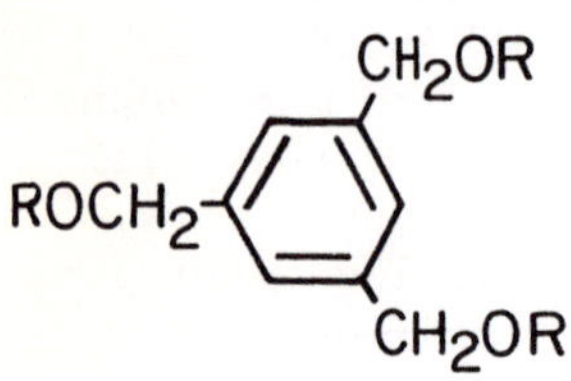

1: R = 4-amidino-2-bromophenyl

X-ray crystallographic studies of proteases have yielded fascinating results on the mode of binding of polypeptides, substrates, and inhibitors to the active site regions of chymotrypsin, trypsin, elastase, and subtilisin.[1-4,23-25] Since it is now relatively easy to construct a useful model (compatible with the widely used CPK models) of the active site of chymotrypsin,[26] and since models of the active sites of any enzymes for which x-ray data are available can be similarly constructed, the interactions of substrates and inhibitors with enzymes can be readily visualized. Study of these models should stimulate ideas for the design of effective inhibitors.

Affinity Labeling - In 1961 the idea of affinity labeling arose independently in four laboratories, where it was applied to glutamic dehydrogenase,[27] a hapten-antibody system,[28] and chymotrypsin.[29,30] This concept has proved very useful, and a vast literature on it has evolved.[31-36] The basic principle is that with knowledge of the specificity of the active site of an enzyme (or any other biological binding site) it is possible to design reagents which have both a group that binds specifically to the active site and a group that can react chemically with a constituent of (or group near) this site. Such reagents have been used frequently to identify groups in or near active sites and can be used to inactivate specifically one enzyme in a mixture.[37] In the design of affinity labeling agents a knowledge of techniques for chemical modification of proteins is essential.[38-40]

There are other reagents, besides affinity labeling agents, that react very specifically with an active site constituent on the basis of chemical reactivity. With the latter the reaction rate is often greatly accelerated by the concentration effect of the binding step, which may be evaluated by a Kitz-Wilson plot[41] from which a maximum rate constant (k_{max}) and a binding constant (K_m) can be obtained. Thus methanesulfonyl fluoride (3) irreversibly inactivates acetylcholinesterase without binding physically to the enzyme, while (3-hydroxyphenyl)trimethylammonium iodide methanesulfonate (4) binds to the site before chemically reacting with it because of its quaternary ammonium group.[41] Compound 4

CH_3SO_2F

3

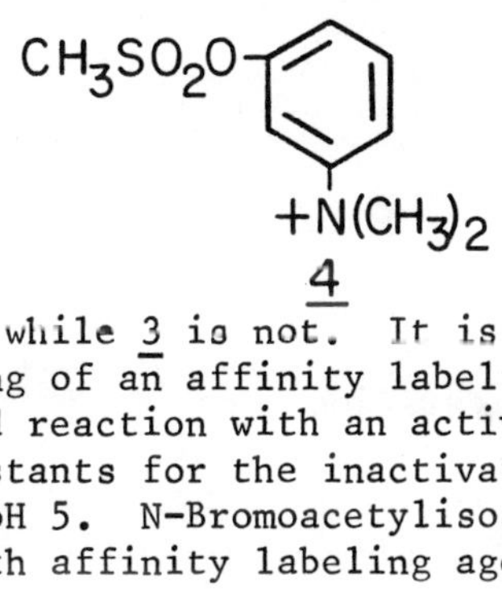

4

is therefore an affinity labeling agent while 3 is not. It is not commonly appreciated that correct binding of an affinity labeling agent may be of paramount importance for rapid reaction with an active site constituent. Table 1 shows kinetic constants for the inactivation of chymotrypsin by three α-bromoamides at pH 5. N-Bromoacetylisoindoline (5) and N-bromoacetylbenzylamine (6) are both affinity labeling agents that

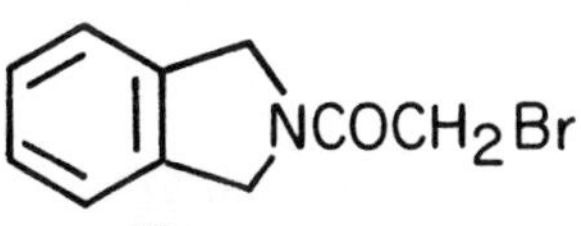

5

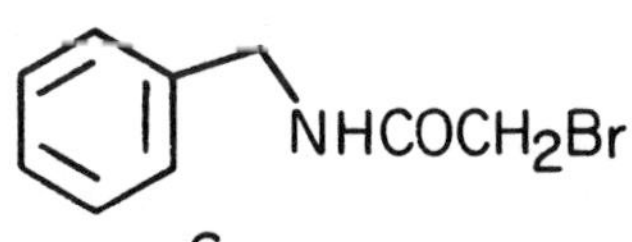

6

Table 1

Compound	$10^4\ k_{max}$	$10^3\ K_m$	$10^4\ k_2$	$V_{½}/V_2$
5	5880	4.0	-	13×10^3
6	12.5	6.7	-	15
7	-	-	57.5	-

alkylate Met 192 near the active site but at vastly different rates, which depend upon neither the reactivity of the bromine nor the binding constant (K_m). In the last column of the table, their half-maximal reaction rates are very roughly compared with the second order rate of inactivation by α-bromoacetamide (7), which does not show binding behavior. The difference in rate between 5 and 6 is due to the fact that the amide group is coplanar with the ring system in 5 and not in 6. Such conformational differences in these and other[42] site-specific α-bromoamides have been correlated[43] with the stereochemistry of the active site of chymotrypsin by use of the model mentioned above.[26] With the benzene ring of the coplanar α-bromoamide 5 in the binding site, the sulfur atom of Met 192 is in the right position for an attack on the back side of the CH_2Br group. Compound 6 does not fit correctly for an easy attack by Met 192.

Although α-haloamides[44,45] and α-haloketones[32] are very useful for studying active site constituents in vitro, they would probably not be of much use in vivo because they react rapidly with sulfhydryl groups. But the sulfonyl fluorides may be promising in vivo,[46,47] and they are much less toxic than organophosphates. For example, the oral LD_{50} in mice of the irreversible thrombin inhibitor, 4-aminomethylbenzenesulfonyl fluoride (8), is 1070 mg/kg, while that of diethyl 4-nitrophenyl phosphate is 8.0 mg/kg.[47] Diazomethyl ketones have recently been reinvestigated with cathepsin B_1 as affinity labeling agents that do not react

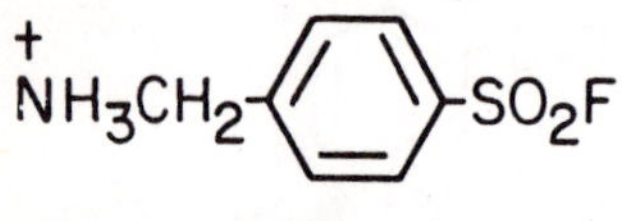

8

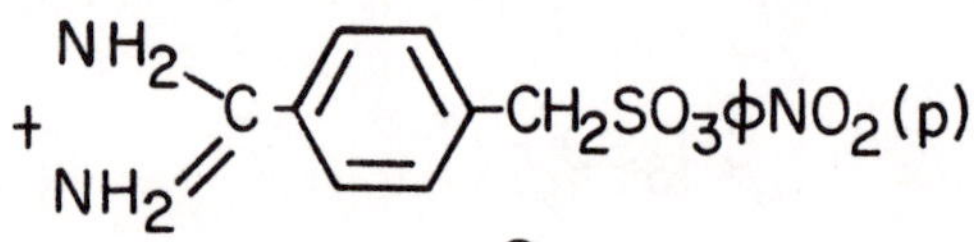

9

with sulfhydryl groups.[48] Although p-nitrophenyl esters might also not be desirable in vivo, p-nitrophenyl p'-amidinophenylmethanesulfonate (9) is worth consideration because of its high selectivity. It binds well to thrombin, trypsin, plasmin, chymotrypsin, and plasma kallikrein, but of these it irreversibly inactivates only thrombin.[49] The meta amidino analog is only a competitive inhibitor of these enzymes.[49] Further, the ortho and meta nitro analogs of 9 show much less selectivity: they irreversibly inactivate trypsin and kallikrein in addition to thrombin but do not affect plasmin.[50]

Occasionally there are reports that an enzyme is not inactivated by an inhibitor that might be expected to be effective. In such cases it is best to vary the reaction conditions and try other inhibitors of the same type. Urokinase is inhibited by DFP but not by tosyl-L-lysine chloromethyl ketone (TLCK),[51] which would be unexpected for a trypsin-like serine protease. The authors wisely did not, as some might, ascribe the lack of reactivity of urokinase toward TLCK to lack of a histidine residue at its active site. Rather they pointed to a difference between the active site of urokinase and that of other trypsinlike enzymes. It was later found that the peptide chloromethyl ketones acetyl-Gly-Lys-CH_2Cl and norleucyl-Gly-Lys-CH_2Cl inactivate urokinase by labeling a histidine residue at the active site.[52] In another case it was erroneously concluded that thrombin has no essential histidine at its active site from the fact that it was not activated by tosyl-L-phenylalanine chloromethyl ketone (TPCK) and from the belief that TPCK is a reagent for histidine residues.[53] Actually TPCK is not specific for histidine, but it is specific for chymotrypsinlike enzymes. The same group later found that TLCK inhibits bovine thrombin,[54] a result consistent with the known specificity of thrombin.

Suicide Inhibitors - A fascinating new group of irreversible enzyme inhibitors developed in recent years are called k_{cat} or suicide inhibitors.[35,55,56] Such an inhibitor is basically an affinity labeling agent with a masked active group that can be activated by the target enzyme's active site mechanism. There is considerable promise in this type of inhibitor because the potentially reactive group may be rather innocuous in a mixture of enzymes or in vivo until the inhibitor reaches and is activated by the target enzyme.

Practically all of the work done with suicide inhibitors has been on nonproteolytic enzymes, especially pyridoxal- and flavin-dependent enzymes, and much of the recent work is reviewed in the preceding chapter of this volume by Jung. While it has been suggested that a bromolactone of the general type 10 could be a suicide inhibitor of chymotrypsin because the acyl enzyme would rearrange to an α-bromoketone,[55] no experimental work on this has appeared. Chymotrypsin has been irreversibly inactivated by the nitrosoamide 11. The acyl enzyme from 11 would be expected to convert to the carbonium ion 12, which can alkylate one or more groups in or around the active site, but the place(s) of attack has not been established.[57]

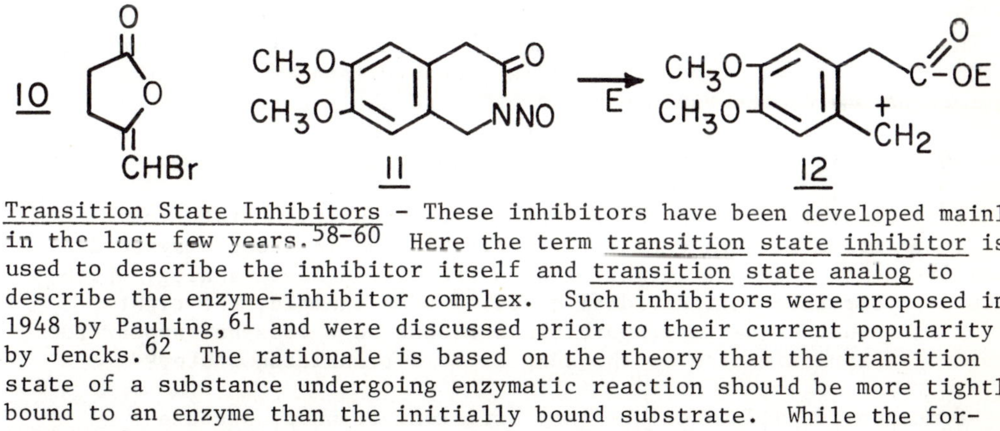

Transition State Inhibitors - These inhibitors have been developed mainly in the last few years.[58-60] Here the term transition state inhibitor is used to describe the inhibitor itself and transition state analog to describe the enzyme-inhibitor complex. Such inhibitors were proposed in 1948 by Pauling,[61] and were discussed prior to their current popularity by Jencks.[62] The rationale is based on the theory that the transition state of a substance undergoing enzymatic reaction should be more tightly bound to an enzyme than the initially bound substrate. While the formation of a normal transition state accelerates an enzymic reaction, the formation of an abnormal one should lead to inhibition. The following scheme applies,[58] where the upper line shows the nonenzymatic route and

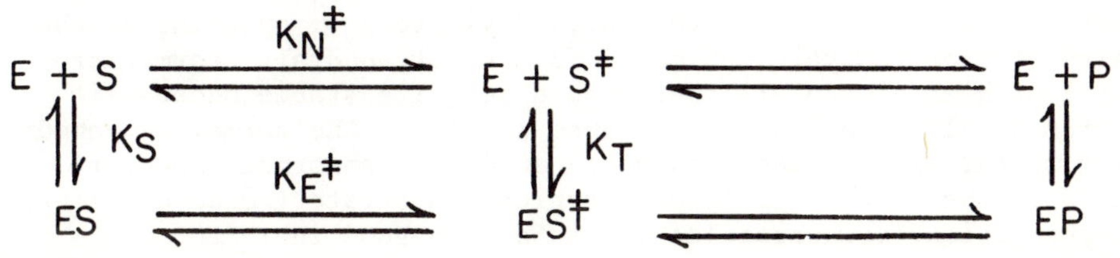

the lower line the enzymatic route. The binding constants for these inhibitors can theoretically be much better than 10^{-10} M.[60] It has been stated that "it appears meaningless to distinguish between 'binding sites' and 'catalytic sites' since catalysis requires an enhanced degree of binding,"[59] but examples will be given to show that the primary and secondary specificity of binding (K_s) is related to the final degree of binding (K_T). Sometimes this selectivity shows up in the reactivity (k_{cat}) of a substrate rather than in K_s,[60] but whatever the exact kinetic situation, high specificity is necessary for the design of good inhibitors for particular enzymes. The lack of emphasis on K_s sometimes seen in the literature may be due to misinterpretation of the importance of increased binding in the transition state ($K_E\ddagger$). The strain that is induced in a substrate in going from the Michaelis complex ES to the transition state ES$\ddagger$ reduces the activation energy of the ensuing reaction but also results in an observed K_s less favorable than would be possible for an optimum fit.[62] In no way do these considerations reduce the importance of primary binding. In the above scheme K_s represents the initial binding of substrate that is enhanced in the second step ($K_E\ddagger$); K_T represents the idealized binding of the substrate's transition state to a complementary conformation of the enzyme's active site, and it should be a much better binding constant than K_s. To the extent that a transition state analog approaches the true transition state, the binding constant should approach K_T.

The enhancement in binding of some transition state inhibitors has been less than predicted by theory, and this has been attributed to the imperfect nature of the inhibitors.[63,64] Changes in entropy have also been invoked to account for such binding.[64] It seems likely, however, that the less-than-expected binding "is probably largely due to the imperfect nature of the analogs rather than to the incorrectness of the theory."[63] This view not only seems reasonable but also provides a stimulus to design more nearly perfect inhibitors.

Very tight binding is characteristic of transition state inhibitors and must be measured with care.[8] But such binding in itself may be due to factors other than the formation of a transition state analog, which has to be determined in individual cases.[60] For example, the tight binding of methotrexate to dihydrofolate reductase[22] does not appear to be caused by approximation of the complex to a transition state.[65]

Some peptide aldehydes are very efficient transition state inhibitors of proteolytic enzymes. The rationale is that an aldehyde exists in hydroxylic media largely in a tetrahedral state as either a hydrate or an acetal. The aldehyde group should be able to react with the hydroxyl group of serine or the sulfhydryl group of cysteine at the active site of a proteolytic enzyme to form a tetrahedral intermediate (hemiacetal or hemithioacetal) that should be quite stable because it derives from an aldehyde and also because it mimics the normal tetrahedral transition state. This transition state analog is abnormal, however, since it lacks the leaving group of a typical substrate (amide or ester). Acetyl-L-phenylalanylaminoacetaldehyde is a very good inhibitor

(K_i 0.046 μM) of papain.[66] The importance of the detailed structure of this inhibitor and therefore of primary binding is borne out by the facts that benzoylaminoacetaldehyde had a K_i of 25 μM and propionaldehyde of about 1 M.[66] Recently, physical evidence was obtained to support the view that aldehydes form a hemithioacetal with the reactive sulfhydryl group of papain.[67,68] The serine protease elastase has been inhibited by synthetic peptide aldehydes, the most potent of which was acetyl-Pro-Ala-Pro-alaninal (K_i 0.8 μM). The corresponding alcohol was a much poorer inhibitor (K_i 600 μM), and the primary structure of the aldehyde was quite important: acetyl-Ala-Pro-alaninal had a K_i of 62 μM.[69]

Peptide aldehydes of microbial origin had been discovered to be efficient inhibitors of proteolytic enzymes before the recent interest in transition state analogs, and much of this work has been reviewed.[70-72] Leupeptins, which terminate in argininal, inhibit trypsinlike enzymes[73] while synthetic analogs ending in aromatic amino acid aldehydes inhibit chymotrypsin.[74] Elastinal, an unusual tetrapeptide terminating in -Gln-alaninal,[75] is a good inhibitor of elastase but a very poor one for a number of other proteolytic enzymes.[76]

Boronic acids have been investigated as transition state inhibitors of proteases, but the best of these do not have outstanding binding constants. More potent inhibitors of this type might be obtained by synthesizing compounds analogous in structure to the better aldehyde inhibitors. There is, however, good evidence that boronic acids can form tetrahedral intermediates at the active sites of proteases.[77]

The much better inhibition of chymotrypsin by phenylethaneboronic acid (K_i 0.05 mM) and styreneboronic acid (K_i 0.026 mM) than by hydrocinnamaldehyde (K_i 0.38 mM) and cinnamaldehyde (K_i 2.6 mM) was attributed to transition state binding.[78,79] Phenylethaneboronic acid (K_i 2.6 mM) and benzeneboronic acid (K_i 0.8 mM) are far better inhibitors of subtilisin Carlsberg than methaneboronic acid (K_i 250 mM).[80] The most convincing evidence for a tetrahedral complex in these inhibitions was obtained by x-ray diffraction with adducts of benzene- and phenylethaneboronic acids with subtilisin BPN' (Novo): The boron atom was found to be coordinated tetrahedrally, with one of the two additional boronic acid oxygen atoms lying in the "oxyanion hole" and the other at the leaving group site. Moreover, the structure of the tetrahedral intermediate for substrate hydrolysis is isosteric with these boronic acid adducts. Thus the adducts can be considered good models for the transition state complex.[77]

Stable acyl enzymes can be formed by reaction with low molecular weight compounds, mostly active esters, which may be called titrants, because several have been used to titrate the concentration of proteolytic enzyme solutions.[81-83] In the case of crystalline indoleacryloylchymotrypsin, a correct transition state is difficult to achieve as the carbonyl group attached to Ser 195 is not properly oriented for deacylation.[24] Some natural protease inhibitors form stable acyl enzymes. The chemistry[84] and structure[85] of the complex between soybean trypsin inhibitor and trypsin have been especially well investigated.

A number of cyclic esters inhibit chymotrypsin.[83] For example, 13 and 14 react with it to form relatively stable acyl enzymes, but the products behave differently. While the acyl enzyme from 14 hydrolyzes

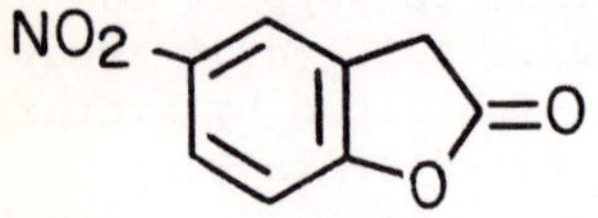

13

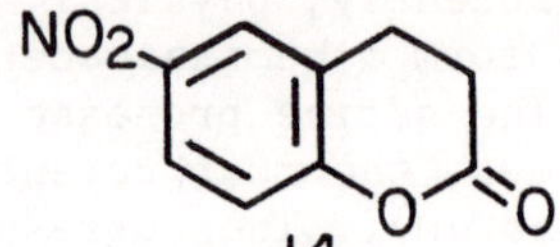

14

to give the free acid, that from 13 releases 13 itself. There is an equilibrium between free chymotrypsin, the acyl enzyme, and 13, which slowly hydrolyzes nonenzymatically to the corresponding acid.[86] To the extent that cyclic titrants can be regenerated readily, their effect is the same as that of reversible inhibitors, though the mechanism is different.

Most titrants studied are acyclic ones that lose the acyl substituent upon reaction with an enzyme. The majority of these are p-nitrophenyl (NP) esters, which are convenient for measuring reaction rates. Other esters can be used for enzyme inhibition,[87] and the particular ester chosen can affect specificity.[50] Perhaps the best known of titrants is p-nitrophenyl-p'-guanidinobenzoate (NPGB), which is used to determine the concentration of various trypsinlike enzymes. The acyl enzyme from trypsin itself is particularly stable.[81,87] In a study of deacylation rates of para-substituted benzoyl trypsins and chymotrypsins, compound 15 was found useful for titrating chymotrypsin in the presence of trypsin.[88]

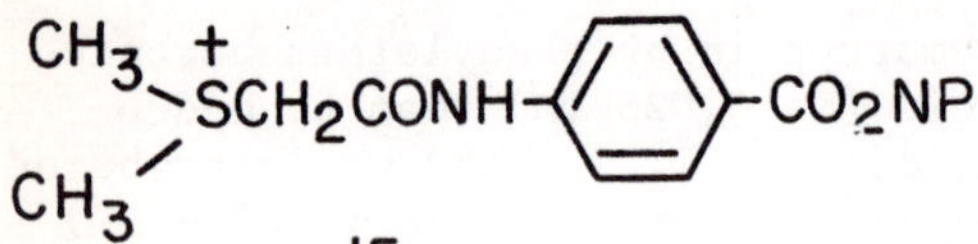

15

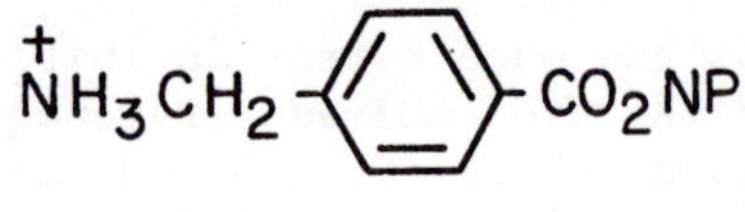

16

With compound 16 it is possible to titrate plasmin contaminated by thrombin (up to about 50%). The kinetics of the reactions of NPGB and 16 with trypsin, thrombin, and plasmin were compared and considered to support strongly the idea that acylation is the most significant parameter for specificity in these enzymes.[89] This is probably true, but specificity in acylation is intimately connected with specificity in binding. Further, the specificity of deacylation determines the efficiency of a titrant as an inhibitor. Although the principle of microscopic reversibility dictates that deacylation is the reverse of acylation,[90] it cannot be applied strictly to an acyclic titrant, since the latter loses its acyl substituent to the medium upon acylation. Because of this there is considerable scope in the design of titrants as inhibitors.

By-Product Analogs - This new type of inhibitor is so constructed that it resembles the collected substrates for the reverse of an enzymatic reaction all combined in one molecule. Consequently such an inhibitor binds with an affinity resembling the combined affinity of the products of the reaction. In the first good example of this sort of inhibitor, L-benzylsuccinate (17), which may be considered as part of the combined

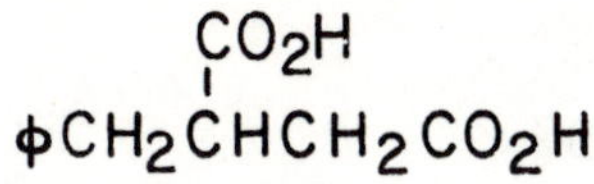

17

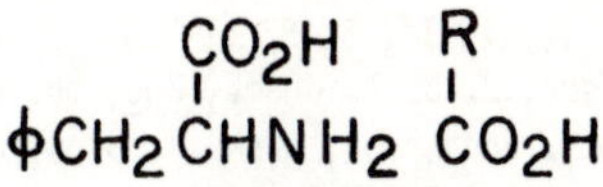

18

structures (18; R = ϕCONHCH$_2$-) of hippuric acid and L-phenylalanine, had a K_i of 0.45 μM in the inhibition of carboxypeptidase A.[91] Recently S-(guanidinoethyl)mercaptosuccinic acid was found to be the most effective (K_i 4 μM) of a series of by-product analogs of carboxypeptidase B.[92] Perhaps the most fascinating example of this type of inhibitor is D-3-mercapto-2-methylpropanoyl-L-proline (SQ 14,225), which inhibits angiotensin converting enzyme with a K_i of 0.0017 μM[5] (cf Chapter 9 of this volume). In this case the second carboxyl group of the previously reported inhibitors of this class is replaced by a sulfhydryl group that can coordinate with the zinc atom at the active site of the enzyme. Several principles discussed and illustrated in this review were applied in the evolution of SQ 14,225: 1) The concept of inhibition was based upon the probable mechanism of action of the target enzyme. 2) The binding specificity of the enzyme was very important, and in this case had to be worked out in detail by testing a large number of compounds. 3) Chemical ingenuity led to the selection of an excellent substituent (sulfhydryl group) for the design of the best inhibitor.

References

1. H. Fritz, H. Tschesche, L.J. Greene, and E. Truscheit, Eds., "Protease Inhibitors," Springer Verlag, New York, 1974.
2. D.M. Blow, Accts. Chem. Res. 9, 145 (1976).
3. J. Kraut, Ann. Rev. Biochem., 46, 331 (1977).
4. D.A. Matthews, R.A. Alden, J.J. Birktoft, S.T. Freer, and J. Kraut, J. Biol. Chem., 252, 8875 (1977).
5. D.W. Cushman, H.S. Cheung, E.F. Sabo, and M.A. Ondetti, Biochemistry, 16, 5484 (1977).
6. C.P. Dorn, M. Zimmerman, S.S. Yang, E.C. Yurewicz, B.M. Ashe, R. Frankshun, and H. Jones, J. Med. Chem., 20, 1464 (1977).
7. I.H. Segel, "Enzyme Kinetics,"Wiley-Interscience, New York, 1975.
8. S. Cha, Biochem. Pharmacol., 24, 2177 (1975).
9. A. Burger, J. Med. Chem., 21, 1 (1978).
10. M. Bergmann and J.S. Fruton, Adv. Enzymol., 1, 63 (1941).
11. I. Schechter and A. Berger, Biochem. Biophys. Res. Commun., 27, 157 (1967).
12. A. Berger and I. Schechter, Phil. Trans. Roy. Soc. Lond., B257, 249 (1970).
13. N. Abramowitz, I. Schechter, and A. Berger, Biochem. Biophys. Res. Commun., 29, 862 (1967).
14. E. Harper and A. Berger, ibid, 46, 1956 (1972).
15. R.C. Thompson and E.R. Blout, Biochemistry, 12, 66 (1973).
16. H.R. Bosshard and A. Berger, ibid, 13, 266 (1974).
17. M. Mares-Guia and E. Shaw, J. Biol. Chem., 240, 1579 (1965).
18. P. Walsmann, H. Horn, H. Landmann, F. Markwardt, J. Stürzebecher, and G. Wagner, Pharmazie, 30, 386, (1975).
19. P. Walsmann, H. Horn, F. Markwardt, P. Richter, J. Stürzebecher, H. Vieweg, and G. Wagner, Acta Biol. Med. Germ., 35, Kl (1976).
20. R.R. Tidwell, L.L. Fox, and J.D. Geratz, Biochim. Biophys. Acta, 445, 729 (1976).

21. A. Hijikata, S. Okamoto, E. Mori, K. Kinjo, R. Kikumoto, S. Tonomura, Y. Tamao, and H. Hara, Thromb. Res. Suppl. II, 8, 83 (1976)
22. W.C. Werkheiser, J. Biol. Chem., 236, 888 (1961).
23. T.A. Steitz, R. Henderson, and D.M. Blow, J. Mol. Biol., 46, 337 (1969).
24. R. Henderson, ibid, 54, 341 (1970).
25. R. Huber and W. Bode, Accts. Chem. Res., 11, 114 (1978).
26. F.H. Clarke, J. Chem. Ed., 54, 230 (1977).
27. B.R. Baker, W.W. Lee, E. Tong, and L.O. Ross, J. Am. Chem. Soc., 83, 3713 (1961).
28. L. Wofsy, H. Metzger, and S.J. Singer, Biochemistry, 1, 1031 (1962).
29. G. Schoellmann and E. Shaw, Biochem. Biophys. Res. Commun., 7, 36 (1962).
30. W.B. Lawson and H.J. Schramm, J. Am. Chem. Soc., 84, 2017 (1962).
31. B.R. Baker, "Design of Active-Site-Directed Irreversible Enzyme Inhibitors," Wiley, New York, 1967.
32. E. Shaw, Physiol. Rev., 50, 244 (1970); The Enzymes, 3rd Ed., 1, 91 (1970).
33. T.F. Spande, B. Witkop, Y. Degani, and A. Pachornik, Adv. Protein Chem., 24, 97 (1970).
34. D.S. Sigman and G. Mooser, Ann. Rev. Biochem., 44, 889 (1975).
35. W.B. Jakoby and M. Wilchek, Eds., Methods in Enzymology, 46 (1977).
36. F. Wold, in ref. 35, p. 3.
37. V. Kostka and F.H. Carpenter, J. Biol. Chem., 239, 1799 (1964).
38. L.A. Cohen, The Enzymes, 3rd Ed., 1 147 (1970).
39. G.E. Means and R.E. Feeney, "Chemical Modification of Proteins," Holden Day, San Francisco, 1971.
40. C.H.W. Hirs and S.N. Timasheff, Eds., Methods in Enzymology, 25B (1972).
41. R. Kitz and I.B. Wilson, J. Biol. Chem., 237, 3245 (1962).
42. H.J. Schramm and W.B. Lawson, Z. Physiol. Chem., 332, 97 (1963).
43. W.B. Lawson and G.J.S. Rao, Biochemistry, in press.
44. W.B. Lawson and H.J. Schramm, Biochemistry, 4, 377 (1965).
45. W.B. Lawson, M.D. Leafer, A. Tewes, and G.J.S. Rao, Z. Physiol. Chem., 349, 251 (1968).
46. B.R. Baker and G.J. Lourens, J. Med. Chem., 10, 1113 (1967).
47. F. Markwardt, P. Walsmann, M. Richter, H.-P. Klöcking, J. Drawert, and H. Landmann, Pharmazie, 26, 401 (1971).
48. R. Leary and E. Shaw, Biochem. Biophys. Res. Commun., 79, 926 (1977).
49. S.-C. Wong and E. Shaw, Arch. Biochem. Biophys., 161, 536 (1974).
50. S.-C. Wong and E. Shaw, ibid, 176, 113 (1976).
51. H. Landmann and F. Markwardt, Experientia, 26, 145 (1970).
52. E.B. Ong, A.J. Johnson, and G. Schoellmann, Biochim. Biophys. Acta, 429, 252 (1976).
53. W.H. Seegers, D. Heene, E. Marciniak, N. Ivanovic, and M.J. Caldwell, Life Sci., 4, 425 (1965).
54. W.H. Seegers and T.J. Andary, Thromb. Res., 4, 869 (1974).
55. R.R. Rando, Science, 185, 320 (1974); Accts. Chem. Res., 8, 281 (1975).
56. R.H. Abeles and A.L. Maycock, Accts. Chem. Res., 9, 313 (1976).
57. E.H. White, D.F. Roswell, I.R. Politzer, and B.R. Branchini, in ref. 35, p. 216.
58. G.E. Lienhard, Ann. Rep. Med. Chem., 7, 249 (1972).
59. R. Wolfenden, Accts. Chem. Res., 5, 10 (1972).
60. R. Wolfenden, in ref. 35, p. 15.
61. L. Pauling, American Scientist, 36, 51 (1948); Nature, 161, 707 (1948).
62. W.P. Jencks, "Catalysis in Chemistry and Enzymology," McGraw-Hill, New York, 1969, pp. 282-320.
63. G.E. Lienhard, Science, 180, 149 (1973).
64. K. Schray and J.P. Klinman, Biochem. Biophys. Res. Commun., 57, 641 (1974).
65. D.A. Matthews, R.A. Alden, J.T. Bolin, S.T. Freer, R. Hamlin, N. Xuong, J. Kraut, M. Poe, M. Williams, and K. Hoogsteen, Science, 197, 452 (1977).
66. J.O'C. Westerik and R. Wolfenden, J. Biol. Chem., 247, 8195 (1972).
67. M.R. Bendall, I.L. Cartwright, P.I. Clark, G. Lowe, and D. Nurse, Eur. J. Biochem., 79, 201 (1977).
68. C.A. Lewis, Jr. and R. Wolfenden, Biochemistry, 17, 4890 (1977).

69. R.C. Thompson, ibid, 12, 47 (1973).
70. H. Umezawa, "Enzyme Inhibitors of Microbial Origin," University Park Press, Baltimore, 1972.
71. W. Wigender, in ref. 1, p. 548.
72. T. Aoyagi and H. Umezawa, "Proteases and Biological Control," E. Reich, D.B. Rifkin, and E. Shaw, Eds., Cold Spring Harbor Laboratory, 1975, p. 429.
73. T. Aoyagi, S. Miyata, M. Nanbo, F. Kojima, M. Matsuzaki, M. Ishizuka, T. Takeuchi, and H. Umezawa, J. Antibiotics (Tokyo), 22, 558 (1969).
74. A. Ito, K. Tokawa, and B. Shimizu, Biochem. Biophys. Res. Commun., 49, 343 (1972).
75. A. Okura, H. Morishima, T. Takita, T. Aoyagi, T. Takeuchi, and H. Umezawa, J. Antibiotics (Tokyo), 28, 337 (1975).
76. H. Umezawa, T. Aoyagi, A. Okura, H. Morishima, T. Takeuchi, and Y. Okami, ibid, 26, 787 (1973).
77. D.A. Matthews, R.A. Alden, J.J. Birktoft, S.T. Freer, and J. Kraut, J. Biol. Chem., 250, 7120 (1975).
78. K.A. Koehler and G.E. Lienhard, Biochemistry, 10, 2477 (1971).
79. J.D. Rawn and G.E. Lienhard, ibid, 13, 3124 (1974).
80. R.N. Lindquist and C. Terry, Arch. Biochem. Biophys., 160, 135 (1974).
81. T. Chase, Jr. and E. Shaw, Methods in Enzymology, 19, 20 (1970).
82. F.J. Kézdy and E.T. Kaiser, ibid, 19, 3 (1970).
83. E.T. Kaiser, in ref. 1, p. 523.
84. D. Kowalski, T.R. Leary, R.E. McKee, R.W. Sealock, D. Wang, and M. Laskowski, Jr., in ref. 1, p. 311.
85. R.M. Sweet, H.T. Wright, J. Janin, C.H. Chothia, and D.M. Blow, Biochemistry, 13, 4212 (1974).
86. P. Tobias, J.H. Heidema, K.W. Lo, E.T. Kaiser, and F.J. Kézdy, J. Am. Chem. Soc., 91, 202 (1969).
87. M. Mares-Guia and E. Shaw, J. Biol. Chem., 242, 5782 (1967).
88. C.-C. Wang and E. Shaw, Arch. Biochem. Biophys., 150, 259 (1972).
89. T.J. Ryan, J.W. Fenton, T. Chang, and R.D. Feinman, Biochemistry, 15, 1337 (1976).
90. M.L. Bender and F.J. Kézdy, Ann. Rev. Biochem., 34, 49 (1965).
91. L.D. Byers and R. Wolfenden, Biochemistry, 12, 2070 (1973).
92. T.J. McKay and T.H. Plummer, Jr., ibid, 17, 401 (1978).

Section VI - Topics in Chemistry

Editor: H.B. Renfroe, CIBA-GEIGY Corporation, Ardsley, N.Y. 10502

Chapter 28. Reactions of Interest in Medicinal Chemistry

David M. Spatz, American Cyanamid Company, Princeton, N.J.

Useful reference books published in 1977 include: Compendium of Organic Synthetic Methods, Volume 3, by L. S. Hegedus and L. G. Wade, Jr; Reagents for Organic Synthesis, Volume 6, by M. Fieser and L. M. Fieser; Synthetic Methods of Organic Chemistry, Volume 31, edited by W. Theilheimer; Organic Synthesis, Volumes 56 and 57, edited by G. H. Büchi and C. R. Johnson, respectively; Organic Reactions, Volume 25, edited by W. G. Dauben; Advances in Heterocyclic Chemistry, Volumes 20, 21, 22, edited by A. R. Katritzky and A. J. Boulton; Annual Reports in Organic Synthesis - 1976, by R. B. Miller and L. G. Wade, Jr.

Reviews - Dimetalated heterosubstituted organic molecules,[1] cyclometalation,[2] Claisen rearrangements,[3] ketene equivalents,[4] phase transfer catalysis,[5] O-silylated enolates,[6] titanium tetrachloride in synthesis,[7] and umpolung through sulfur compounds[8] have been reviewed. A useful table for selective oxidations and reductions has been published.[9]

C-C Bond Formations - Several improvements in the aldol reaction have been noted. Coupling of an α-bromocarbonyl compound with another carbonyl compound via dialkylaluminum chloride-zinc produces the aldol regiospecifically in high yield.[10] Fluoride ion catalyzed reaction of enol silyl ethers and carbonyl compounds prepares aldol products regiospecifically.[11] Aldol-type products are stereoselectively synthesized by Claisen rearrangement of silylketene acetals.[12]

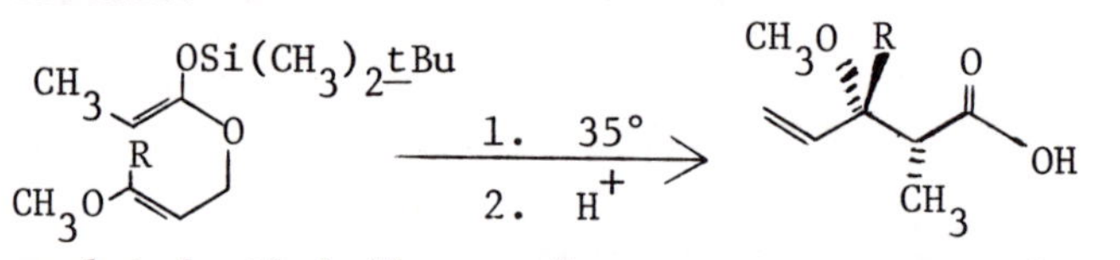

1-Ethoxy-1-trimethylsiloxycyclopropane acts as a homoenolate anion precursor with $TiCl_4$.[13]

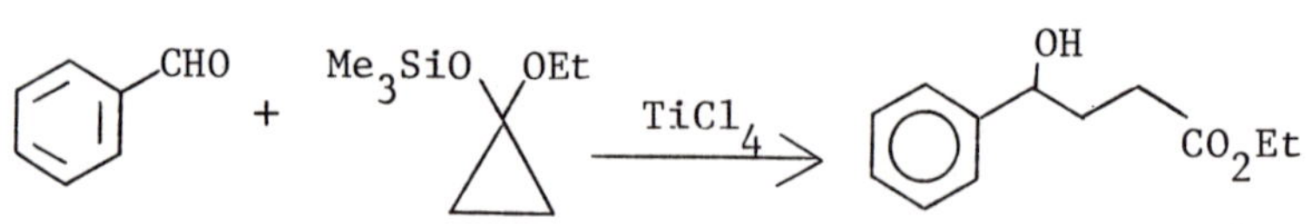

Nucleophiles readily add to 2-chloro-1,3-dithiane, a formyl cation equivalent.[14,15]

An alkyl copper-boron trifluoride complex gives complete γ-alkylation of γ-substituted allylic halides.[16]

$$\text{Ph-CH=CH-CH}_2\text{Cl} \xrightarrow{\text{BuCu}\bullet\text{BF}_3} \text{Ph-}\underset{}{\overset{\text{Bu}}{\text{CH}}}\text{-CH=CH}_2$$

ISBN 0-12-040513-X

Tosylmethyl isocyanide (TosMIC) can be used to prepare both symmetrical and unsymmetrical α-diketones and ketones.[17,18]

An acyl anion-type Michael addition can be achieved via an organotetracarbonylferrate.[19]

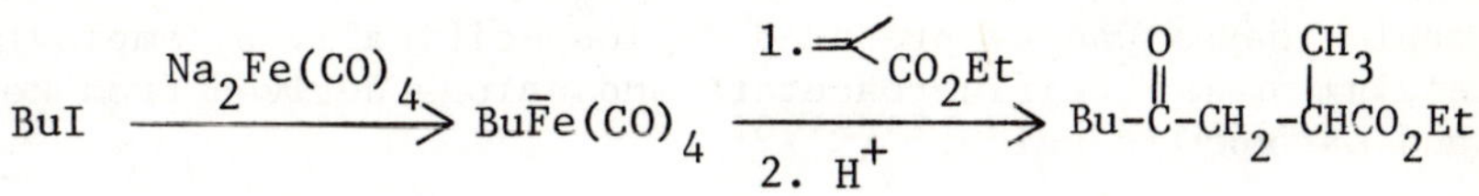

Chloromethyl ketones are prepared by addition of lithio chloromethyl phenyl sulfoxide to aldehydes.[20]

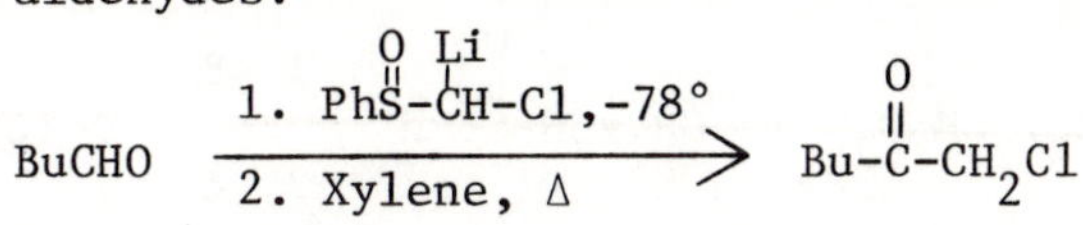

Addition of α-chloro-α-trimethylsilyl carbanion to carbonyl compounds, however, generates α,β-epoxysilanes which are convertible to the homologated carbonyl or alkene compounds.[21,22]

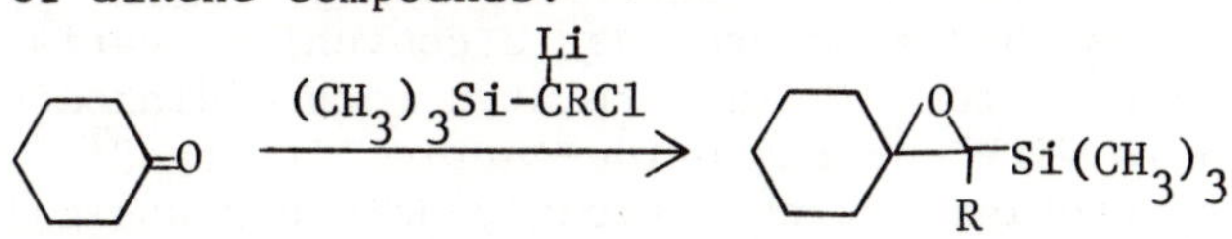

Organotin compounds offer an attractive route to dialkylative enone transposition.[23] Trialkylstannyllithium adds exclusively 1,4. Alkylation of the resultant enolate, methyllithium addition and oxidation afford the transposed enone.

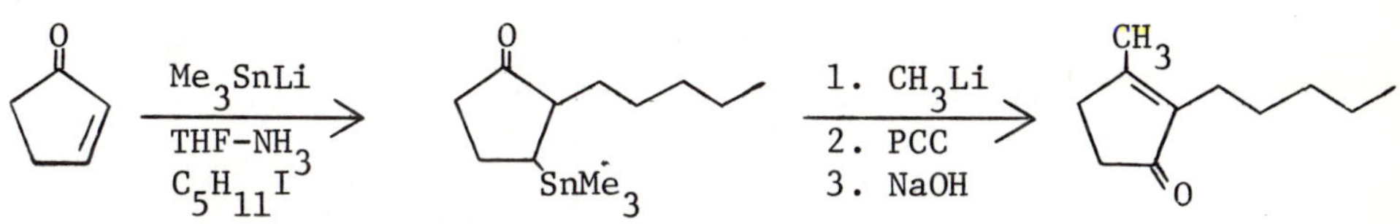

Stabilized carbanions add to simple olefins and allyl amines and sulfides through the intermediacy of palladium complexes.[24,25] Addition occurs predominately at the more substituted position. The resulting palladocycle may be reduced to the hydrocarbon or transformed further by an oxidative addition-reductive elimination sequence.[42]

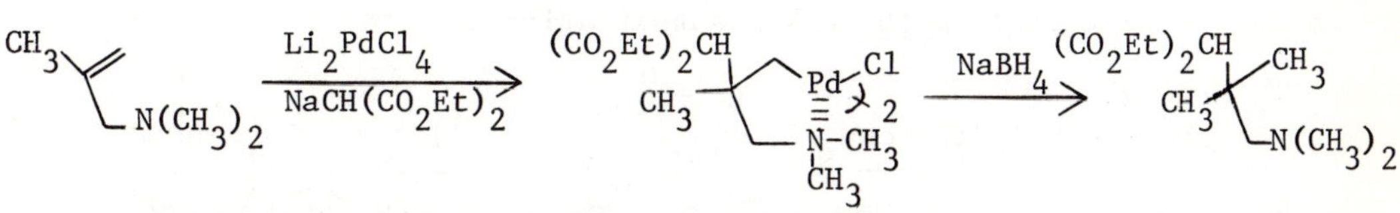

Zirconium alkenyls, available by hydrozirconation of acetylenes, add to α,β-unsaturated ketones with catalytic nickel (II).[26] Zirconium alkenyls also couple with arylhalides under nickel catalysis.[27] More difficultly prepared aluminum alkenyls and copper (I) alkenyls are available by transmetalation of zirconium compounds.[28,29]

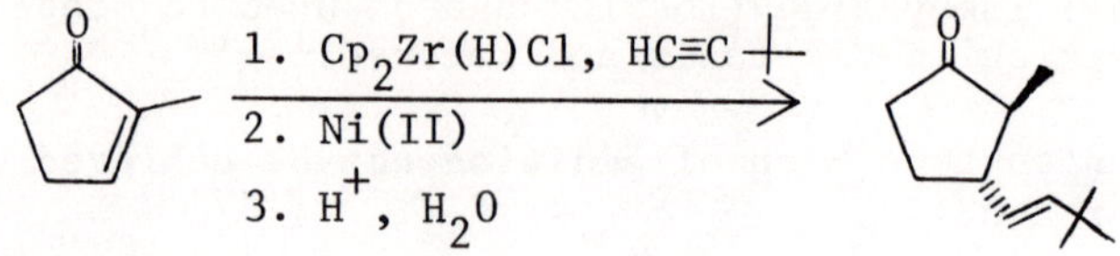

Mannich bases can be prepared regiospecifically by employing dimethyl (methylene)ammonium trifluoroacetate and anions derived from ketones, esters and carboxylic acids.[30,31,32]

Interesting olefins can be prepared by Michael addition to aryl vinyl sulfoxides followed by sulfoxide elimination.[33]

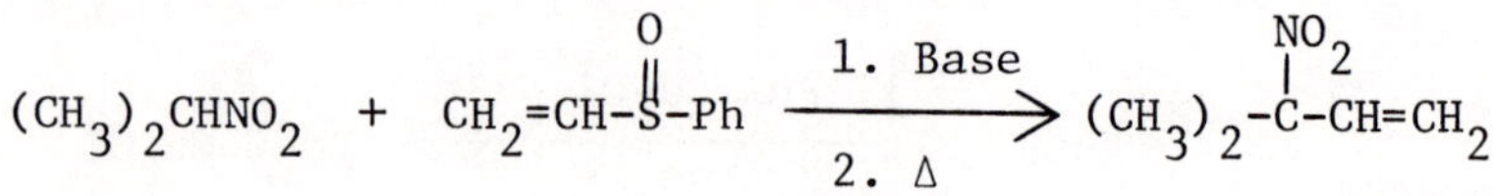

Aromatic Substitution - Arylamines are directly converted to aromatic hydrocarbons by alkyl nitrites in DMF.[34] Alternatively an aryl halide is produced when cupric halides are added in acetonitrile.[35] The alkyl-nitrite deamination method also provides a convenient variant of the Meerwein arylation reaction.[36] In a related method diazonium ions are converted to phenols with cuprous oxide-cupric nitrate.[37] This radical process avoids the problems of the strongly acidic classical transformation.

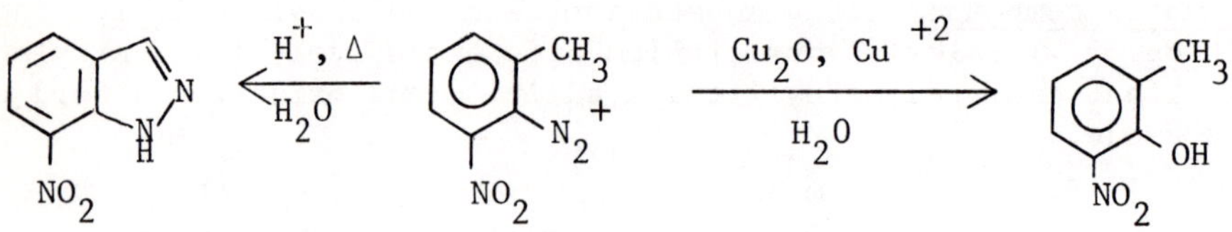

Phenols may also be converted to anilines via a Smiles rearrangement that is greatly accelerated by HMPA solvent.[38]

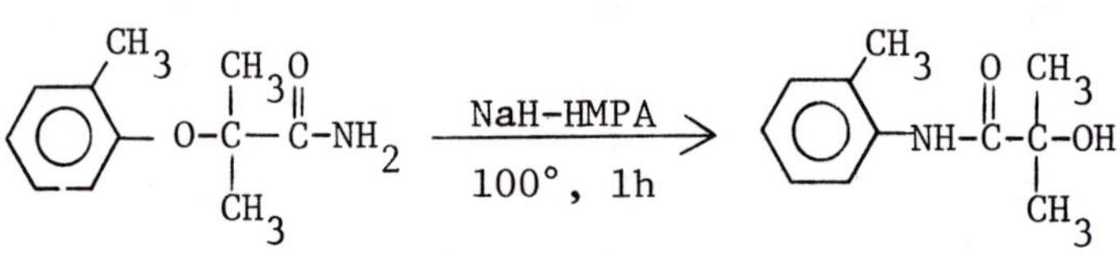

N-Acyl-N-arylhydroxylamines are converted into the ortho-alkylated benzamides via a two step procedure.[39] Variations generate ketone, ester or amide functionalized ortho-alkyl substitutions.

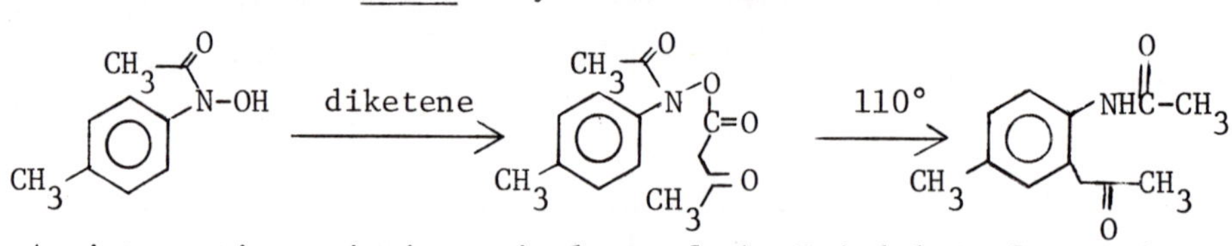

An interesting anionic equivalent of the Friedel-Crafts cycloacylation has been demonstrated.[40]

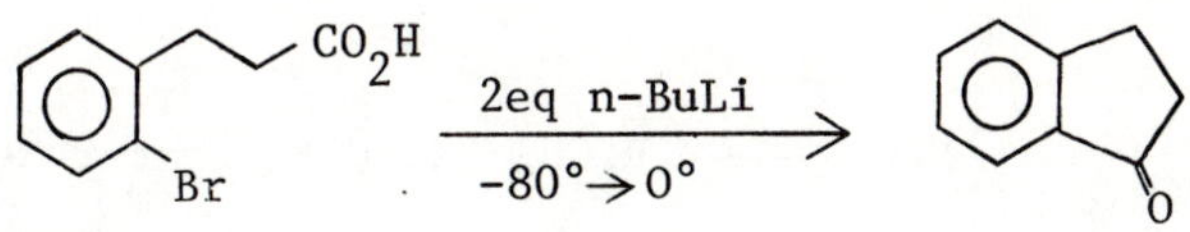

o-(Aminoaryl)oxazolines are prepared by a facile methoxy displace-ent with lithium amides.[41]

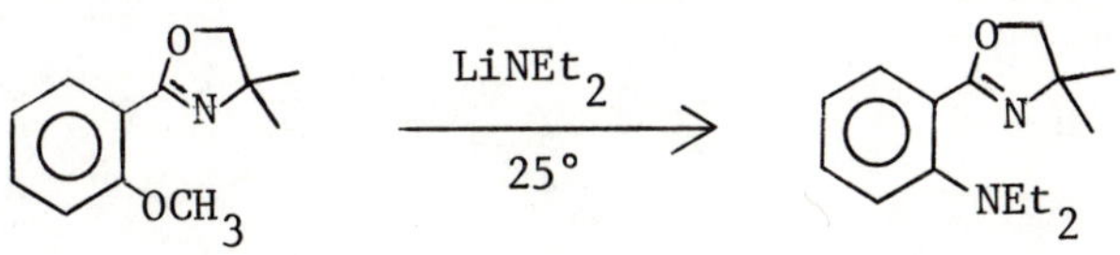

Transition metal catalyzed aromatic substitution continues to be a fruitful area. Aromatic palladium complexes of benzylamines and benzoic acids add enones to generate vinyl substituted aryl derivatives.[42,43,44]

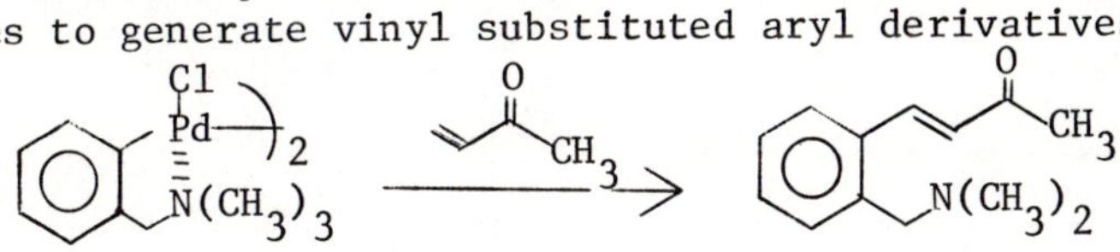

Direct arylation and vinylation of lithium ester enolates is catalyzed by nickel.[45]

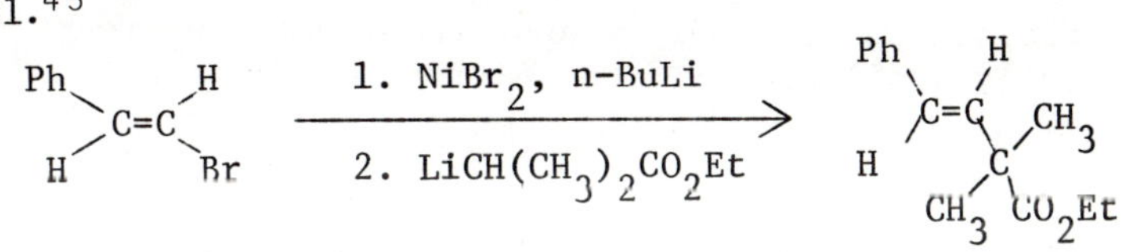

Heterocycles - Two new direct preparations of cyanated indoles and pyrroles utilize either triphenylphosphine-thiocyanogen or anodic electrochemical substitution with methanolic cyanide solution.[46,47]

Indoles are efficiently prepared from o-tolyl isocyanide.[48]

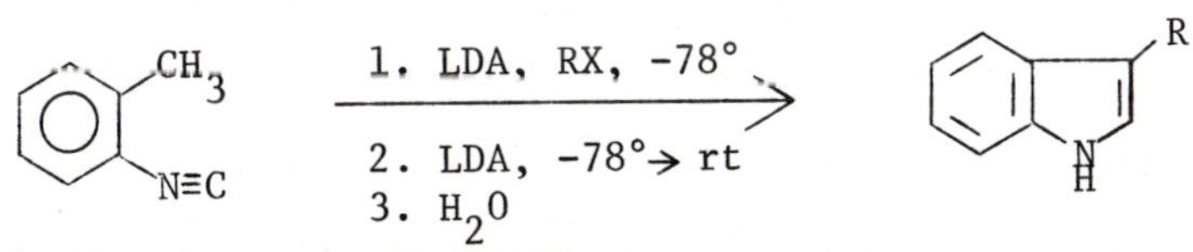

Gassman and coworkers have extended their [2,3] sigmatropic rearrangement of N-aryl-azasulphonium ylides to the synthesis of isatins,[49] and N-methyl-2-quinolones.[50]

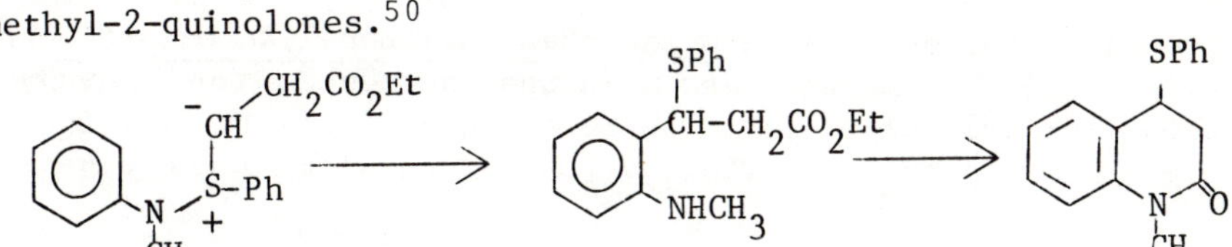

Substituted 2-pyridones are formed by base catalyzed condensation of secondary propargylic alcohols and 1-cyanopyrrolidine.[51]

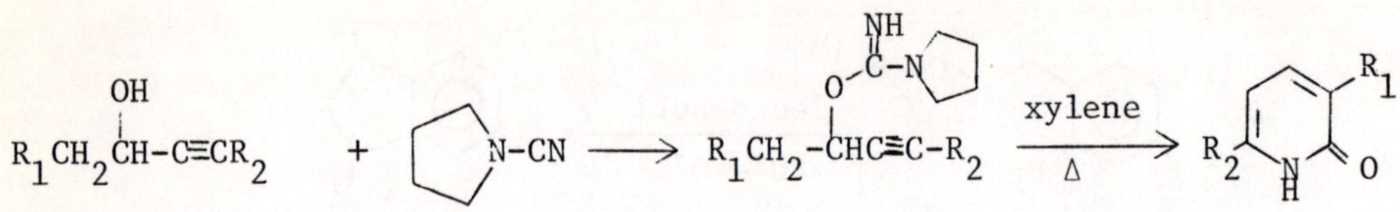

A general route to five-membered mesoionic compounds uses α-bromoacyl chlorides and monoprotonic 1,3-binucleophiles such as N-monosubstituted thioamides.[52] The 1,3-dithiolium and 1,3-oxathiolium systems were also prepared.

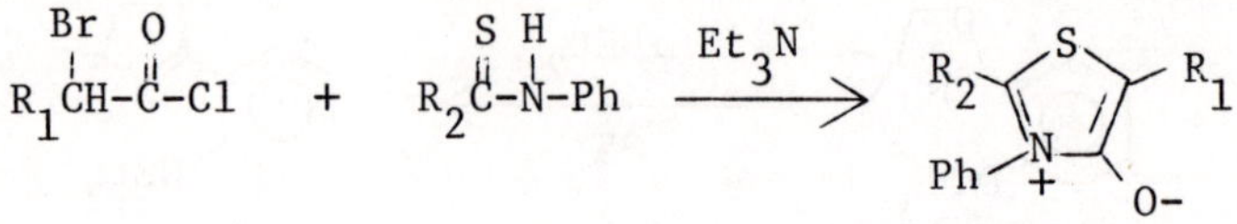

The Darzens condensation has been extended to the synthesis of 1,3-diphenylaziridines.[53]

Halogenations - Primary, secondary and tertiary alcohols can be converted to the iodides with trimethylsilyl iodide.[54]

Primary amines can be converted into iodides with 2,4,6-triphenylpyrylium iodide.[55]

Aliphatic trifluoromethyl groups are prepared by reaction of amines with commercially available trifluoronitroso methane followed by photolysis.[56]

$$\text{n-octyl-NH}_2 \xrightarrow{CF_3NO} \text{n-octyl-N=N-CF}_3 \xrightarrow[\underline{t}\text{-BuOH}]{h\nu} \text{n-octyl-CF}_3$$

α-Iodoketones are conveniently synthesized with silver chromate-iodine.[57]

$$\text{Ph-CH=CHCH}_2\text{OAc} \xrightarrow{AgCrO_3\text{-I}} \text{Ph-}\overset{O}{\overset{\|}{C}}\text{-}\overset{I}{\overset{|}{C}}\text{H-CH}_2\text{OAc}$$

Carboxylic Acids and Derivatives - Esters are mildly converted to amides or t-butylthioesters by trimethyl aluminum and the primary or secondary amine or t-butyl thiol.[58,59]

Thiol and selenol esters are prepared from the corresponding thiol or selenol and the carboxylic acid-imidazolides.[60]

Procedures for phenylseleno and phenylsulphenyllactonization have appeared.[61,62,63] The methods are mild and introduce, for instance, the useful phenylselenyl moiety into the molecule. Similarly cyclic ethers can be prepared from an appropriately positioned alcohol and alkene.[64]

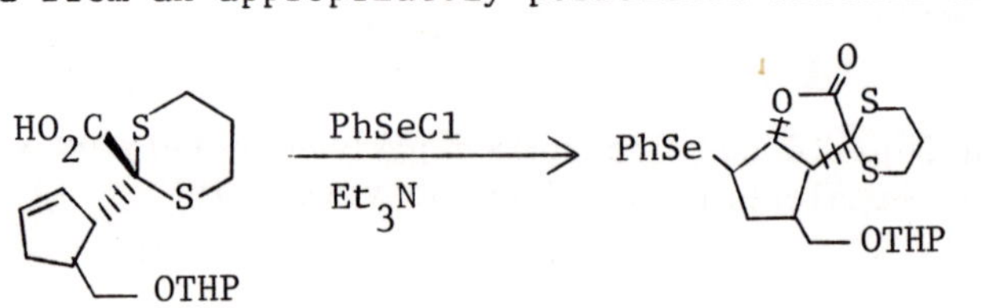

Lactones are cleaved by sodium phenyl selenolate to the ω-phenylselenyl carboxylic acids. Esterification, oxidation and elimination generates ω-olefinic esters.[65,66]

Nitriles can be prepared directly from primary nitro compounds using phosphorus trichloride.[67] β-Acetoxy nitromethanes yield cyanohydrin acetates.

Catalytic dimsylsodium induces a very mild O-alkylimidate to N-alkyllactam conversion.[68] The reaction appears to be both mild and gentle.

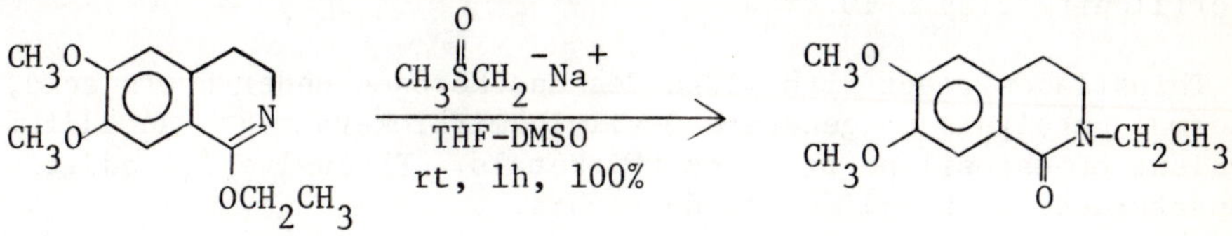

N-Alkylamides are formed by alkylaluminum reduction of the methylol.[69]

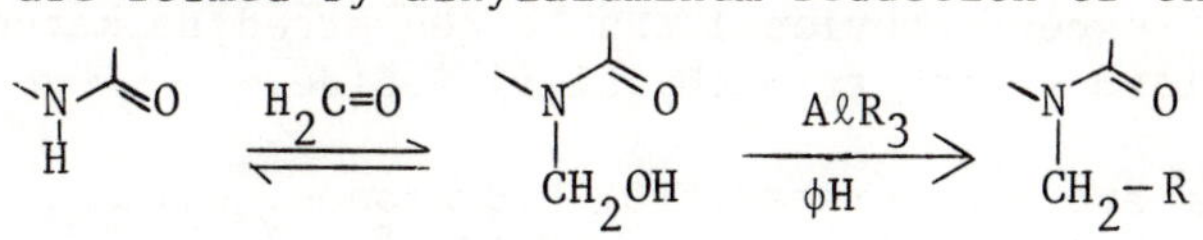

Oxidations - The use of oxidants absorbed on alumina or silica has blossomed. These reagents are generally milder and more selective and provide for convenient reaction workup. Oxidations of cyclobutanol to cyclobutanone and β-hydroxysulfides and selenides to the β-keto compounds are accomplished by trichloroacetaldehyde on alumina.[70,71] Basic dry silica gel converts nitro groups into carbonyls[72] and chromyl chloride on silica-alumina oxidizes alcohols.[73]

Pyridinium chlorochromate (PCC) will directly oxidize cyclic and acyclic enol ethers to lactones and esters.[74]

PCC oxidizes tertiary allylic alcohols to the transposed 3-alkyl α,β-unsaturated ketones.[75]

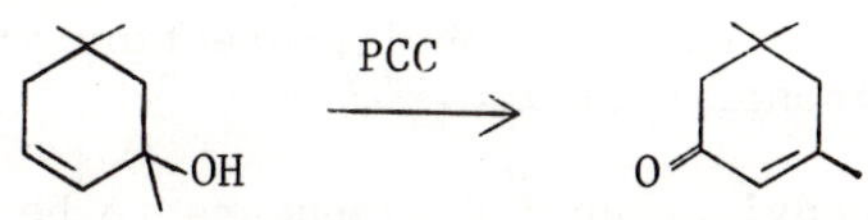

α-Keto sulfides, prepared by sulfenylation of enolates with diphenyl disulfide, are acetoxylated by lead tetraacetate to afford mono-protected 1,2-dicarbonyl compounds.[76]

Reductions - The experimental details and scope of alumina as a medium for carbonyl reductions have been published.[77]

Aldehydes are selectively reduced in the presence of ketones and other functional groups by either 9-borabicyclo [3.3.1] nonane-pyridine or sodium borohydride modified by thiols.[78,79]

Lithium triethylborohydride causes a number of useful reductions. Tertiary amides are cleaved by carbon-nitrogen fission to alcohols[80] and alkyl methanesulfonate esters are reduced to hydrocarbons.[81] Additionally, $LiEt_3BH$ adds to substituted styrenes in a Markownikoff manner.[82]

$$\text{Ph-CH=CH-CH}_3 \xrightarrow[\text{THF, }\Delta]{\text{LiEt}_3\text{BH}} \text{Ph-}\underset{\text{BEt}_2}{\text{CH}}\text{CH}_2\text{CH}_3$$

Protecting Groups - Acetals are formed rapidly in high yields at room temperature using trimethylorthoformate absorbed on commercially available montmorillonite clay K-10.[83]

Thiosilanes react with aldehydes and ketones under Lewis acid, anion or thermal catalysis to generate O-silylhemithioketals.[84] An additional equivalent of thiosilane produces thioketals. Exclusive 1,4-addition to α,β-unsaturated carbonyl compounds occurs.

Ketals (except ethylene) can be converted to ketones under non-aqueous conditions with trimethylsilyl iodide.[85]

Ketones are regenerated from hydrazones, oximes, semicarbazones and thioketals by benzeneseleninic anhydride.[86,87]

Acylation of sterically hindered hydroxyl groups is facile with an anhydride and fluoride ion.[88] Additionally a silyl group may be directly replaced by an acyl group using the anhydride and tetrabutylammonium fluoride. This transformation permits the in situ exchange of an alkali resistant for an alkali sensitive protecting group.

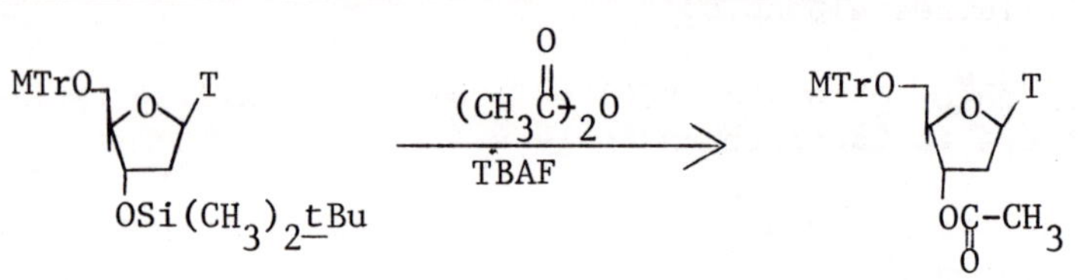

Crotonyl esters are useful alcohol protecting groups removable with dilute hydrazine in methanol-pyridine.[89]

The vinyloxy carbonyl group (VOC) appears to be very useful for alcohol and amine protection and an extremely mild reagent for amine dealkylation.[90,91,92] For example, one equivalent of vinyl chloroformate produces the VOC ester (R_1=VOC, R_2=CH_3). An additional equivalent of VOC-Cl in methylene chloride at 25° produces the N-demethylated compound (R_1=R_2=VOC). The ester can be cleaved in the presence of the urethane with dilute base while the urethane can be cleaved in the presence of the ester by one equivalent of HBr in methanol. Refluxing 5% methanolic-HCl cleaves both protecting groups.

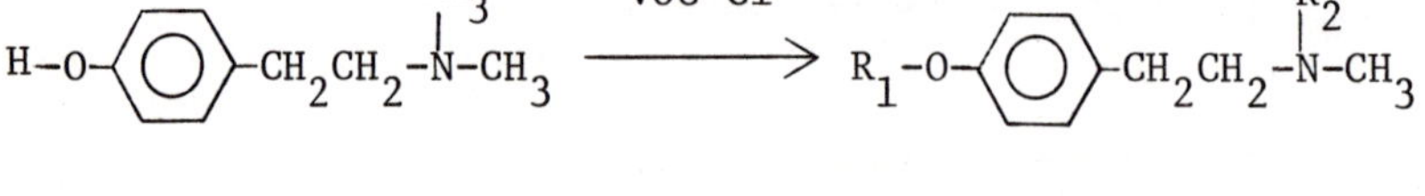

Esters and ethers can be cleaved with trimethylsilyl iodide.[93,94]

Miscellaneous - Azides are converted to amines in a non-reductive aza transfer reaction to acetylacetone.[95]

Thioethers are formed when an alcohol, sulfenamide and tri-n-butylphosphine react.[96]

Nitrile oxides are converted into isocyanates by catalytic sulfur dioxide in refluxing benzene.[97]

Primary amines are transformed into acetates or benzoates via a two step procedure by reaction with triphenylpyrylium tetrafluoroborate and subsequent pyrolysis of the pyridinium salt in the presence of acetate or benzoate.[98]

Alumina and silica have been used as catalysts for opening arene oxides and vinyl epoxides using weak oxygen and amine nucleophiles[99] and dry ozonization of amines to nitro compounds.[100]

Triphase catalysis allows conversion of alkyl halides to nitriles and alkyl bromides to chlorides.[101]

Vinyl bromides, enol acetates, enol ethers and enamides can be prepared stereospecifically from α,β-epoxysilanes.[102]

References

1. E. M. Kaiser, J. D. Petty and P. L. A. Knutson, Synthesis, 509 (1977).
2. M. I. Bruce, Angew. Chem. Int. Ed. Engl., 16, 73 (1977).
3. G. B. Bennett, Synthesis, 589 (1977).
4. S. Ranganathan, D. Ranganathan and A. K. Mehrotra, ibid., 289, (1977).
5. E. V. Dehmlow, Angew. Chem. Int. Ed. Engl., 16, 493 (1977).
6. J. K. Rasmussen, Synthesis, 91 (1977).
7. T. Mukaiyama, Angew. Chem. Int. Ed. Engl., 16, 817 (1977).
8. B.-T. Gröbel and D. Seebach, Synthesis, 357 (1977).
9. M. Hudlicky, J. Chem. Educ., 54, 100 (1977).
10. K. Maruoka, S. Hashimoto, Y. Kitagawa, H. Yamamoto and H. Nozaki, J. Amer. Chem. Soc., 99, 7705 (1977).
11. R. Noyori, K. Yokoyama, J. Sakata, I. Kuwajima, E. Nakamura and M. Shimizu, ibid., 99, 1265 (1977).
12. R. E. Ireland and C. S. Wilcox, Tetrahedron Lett., 2839, (1977).
13. E. Nakamura and I. Kuwajima, J. Amer. Chem. Soc., 99, 7360 (1977).
14. E. C. Taylor and J. L. LaMattina, Tetrahedron Lett., 2077 (1977).
15. C. G. Kruse, N. L. J. M. Broekhof, A. Wijsman and A. van der Gen, ibid., 885 (1977).
16. K. Maruyama and Y. Yamamoto, J. Amer. Chem. Soc., 99, 8068 (1977).
17. D. van Leusen and A. M. van Leusen, Tetrahedron Lett., 4233 (1977).
18. O. Possel and A. M. van Leusen, ibid., 4229 (1977).
19. M. P. Cooke, Jr. and R. M. Parlman, J. Amer. Chem. Soc., 99, 5222 (1977).
20. V. Reutrakul and W. Kanghae, Tetrahedron Lett., 1225 (1977).

21. C. Burford, F. Cooke, E. Ehlinger and P. Magnus, J. Amer. Chem. Soc., 99, 4536 (1977).
22. F. Cooke and P. Magnus, Chem. Commun., 513 (1977).
23. W. C. Still, J. Amer. Chem. Soc., 99, 4836 (1977).
24. J. Hayashi and L. S. Hegedus, ibid., 99, 7093 (1977).
25. R. A. Holton and R. A. Kjonaas, ibid., 99, 4177 (1977).
26. M. J. Loots and J. Schwartz, ibid., 99, 8045 (1977).
27. E.-i. Negishi and D. E. Van Horn, ibid., 99, 3168 (1977).
28. D. B. Carr and J. Schwartz, ibid., 99, 638 (1977).
29. M. Yoshifuji, M. J. Loots, and J. Schwartz, Tetrahedron Lett., 1303 (1977).
30. J. L. Roberts, P. S. Borromeo and C. D. Poulter, ibid., 1621 (1977).
31. J. L. Roberts, P. S. Borromeo and C. D. Poulter, ibid., 1299 (1977).
32. N. L. Holy and Y. F. Wang, J. Amer. Chem. Soc., 99, 944 (1977).
33. R. Tanikaga, H. Sugihara, K. Tanaka and A. Kaji, Synthesis, 299 (1977).
34. M. P. Doyle, J. F. Dellaria, Jr., B. Siegfried and S. W. Bishop, J. Org. Chem., 42, 3494 (1977).
35. M. P. Doyle, B. Siegfried and J. F. Dellaria, Jr., ibid., 42, 2426 (1977).
36. M. P. Doyle, B. Siegfried, R. C. Elliott and J. F. Dellaria, Jr., ibid., 42, 2431 (1977).
37. T. Cohen, A. G. Dietz, Jr., and J. R. Miser, ibid., 42, 2053 (1977).
38. R. Bayles, M. C. Johnson, R. F. Maisey and R. W. Turner, Synthesis, 33 (1977).
39. R. M. Coates and I. Md. Said, J. Amer. Chem. Soc., 99, 2355 (1977).
40. R. J. Boatman, B. J. Whitlock, H. W. Whitlock, Jr., ibid., 99, 4822 (1977).
41. A. I. Meyers and R. Gabel, J. Org. Chem., 42, 2653 (1977).
42. R. A. Holton, Tetrahedron Lett., 355 (1977).
43. B. A. Patel, C. B. Ziegler, N. A. Cortese, J. E. Plevyak, T. C. Zebovitz, M. Terpko and R. F. Heck J. Org. Chem., 42, 3903 (1977).
44. R. A. Holton and R. G. Davis, J. Amer. Chem. Soc., 99, 4175 (1977).
45. A. A. Millard and M. W. Rathke, ibid., 99, 4833 (1977).
46. Y. Tamura, T. Kawasaki,M. Adachi, M. Tanio and Y. Kita, Tetrahedron Lett., 4417 (1977).
47. K. Yoshida, J. Amer. Chem. Soc., 99, 6111 (1977).
48. Y. Ito, K. Kobayaski and T. Saegusa, ibid., 99, 3532 (1977).
49. P. G. Gassman, B. W. Cue, Jr., and T.-Y. Luh, J. Org. Chem., 42, 1344 (1977).
50. P. G. Gassman and R. L. Parton, Chem. Commun., 694 (1977).
51. L. E. Overman and S. Tsuboi, J. Amer. Chem. Soc., 99, 2813 (1977).
52. K. T. Potts, S. J. Chen, J. Kane and J. L. Marshall, J. Org. Chem., 42, 1633 (1977).
53. L. Wartski, Chem. Commun., 602 (1977).
54. M. E. Jung and P. L. Ornstein, Tetrahedron Lett., 2659 (1977).
55. N. F. Eweiss, A. R. Katritzky, P.-L. Nie and C. A. Ramsden, Synthesis, 634 (1977).
56. P. Gölitz and A. de Meijere, Angew. Chem. Int. Ed. Eng., 16, 854 (1977).
57. G. Cardillo and M. Shimizu, J. Org. Chem., 42, 4268 (1977).
58. A. Basha, M. Lipton and S. M. Weinreb, Tetrahedron Lett., 4171 (1977).
59. R. P. Hatch and S. M. Weinreb, J. Org. Chem., 42, 3960 (1977).

60. H.-J. Gais, Angew. Chem. Int. Ed. Engl., 16, 244 (1977).
61. K. C. Nicolaou and Z. Lysenko, J. Amer. Chem. Soc., 99, 3185 (1977).
62. D. L. J. Clive and G. Chittattu, Chem. Commun., 484 (1977).
63. K. C. Nicolaou and Z. Lysenko, ibid., 293 (1977).
64. K. C. Nicolaou and Z. Lysenko, Tetrahedron Lett., 1257 (1977).
65. R. M. Scarborough, Jr. and A. B. Smith, III, ibid., 4361 (1977).
66. D. Liotta and H. Santiesteban, ibid., 4369 (1977).
67. P. A. Wehrli and B. Schaer, J. Org. Chem., 42, 3956 (1977).
68. S. Kano, T. Yokomatsu, S. Hibino, K. Imamura and S. Shibuya, Heterocycles, 6, 1319 (1977).
69. A. Basha and S. M. Weinreb, Tetrahedron Lett., 1465 (1977).
70. G. H. Posner and M. J. Chapdelaine, Synthesis, 555 (1977).
71. G. H. Posner and M. J. Chapdelaine, Tetrahedron Lett., 3227 (1977).
72. E. Kienan and Y. Mazur, J. Amer. Chem. Soc., 99, 3861 (1977).
73. J. San Filippo, Jr. and C.-I. Chern, J. Org. Chem., 42, 2182 (1977).
74. G. Piancatelli, A. Scettri and M. D'Auria, Tetrahedron Lett., 3483 (1977).
75. W. B. Dauben and D. M. Michno, J. Org. Chem., 42, 682 (1977).
76. B. M. Trost and G. S. Massiot, J. Amer. Chem. Soc., 99, 4405 (1977).
77. G. H. Posner, A. W. Runquist and M. J. Chapdelaine, J. Org. Chem., 42, 1202 (1977).
78. H. C. Brown and S. U. Kulkarni, ibid., 42, 4169 (1977).
79. Y. Maki and K. Kikuchi, Tetrahedron Lett., 263 (1977).
80. H. C. Brown and S. C. Kim, Synthesis 635 (1977).
81. R. W. Holder and M. G. Matturro, J. Org. Chem., 42, 2166 (1977).
82. H. C. Brown and S. C. Kim, ibid., 42, 1482 (1977).
83. E. C. Taylor and C.-S. Chiang, Synthesis, 467 (1977).
84. D. A. Evans, L. K. Truesdale, K. G. Grimm and S. L. Nesbitt, J. Amer. Chem. Soc., 99, 5009 (1977).
85. M. E. Jung. W. A. Andrus and P. L. Ornstein, Tetrahedron Lett., 4175 (1977).
86. D. H. R. Barton, D. J. Lester and S. V. Ley, Chem. Commun., 445 (1977).
87. D. H. R. Barton, N. J. Cussans and S. V. Ley, ibid., 751 (1977).
88. S. L. Beaucage and K. K. Ogilvie, Tetrahedron Lett., 1691 (1977).
89. R. Arentzen and C. B. Reese, Chem. Commun., 270 (1977).
90. R. A. Olofson and R. C. Schnur, Tetrahedron Lett., 1571 (1977).
91. R. A. Olofson, R. C. Schnur, L. Bunes and J. P. Pepe, ibid., 1567 (1977).
92. R. A. Olofson, Y, S. Yamamoto and D. J. Wancowicz, ibid., 1563 (1977).
93. T.-L. Ho and G. A. Olah, Angew. Chem. Ind. Ed. Engl., 15, 774 (1976).
94. M. E. Jung and M. A. Lyster, J. Org. Chem., 42, 3761 (1977).
95. B. Stanovnik, M. Tisler, S. Polanc and J. Zitnik, Synthesis,491 (1977).
96. K. A. M. Walker, Tetrahedron Lett., 4475 (1977).
97. G. Trickes and H. Meier, Angew. Chem. Int. Ed. Engl., 16, 555 (1977).
98. U. Gruntz, A. R. Katritsky, D. H. Kenny, M. C. Rezende and H. Sheikh, Chem. Commun., 701 (1977).
99. G. H. Posner and D. Z. Rogers, J. Amer. Chem. Soc., 99, 8214 (1977).
100. E. Keinan and Y. Mazur, J. Org. Chem. Soc., 42, 844 (1977).
101. S. L. Regen, ibid., 42, 875 (1977).
102. P. F. Hudrlik, A. M. Hudrlik, R. J. Rona, R. N. Misra and G. P. Withers J. Amer. Chem. Soc., 99, 1993 (1977).

Chapter 29. Asymmetric Synthesis

Donald Valentine Jr. and John W. Scott
Chemical Research Department, Hoffmann-La Roche Inc.,
Nutley, New Jersey, U.S.A. 07110

In an asymmetric synthesis an achiral substrate is transformed by a chiral reagent to produce an excess of one enantiomer of the chiral product. Asymmetric synthesis is a lively field whose early promise is being realized in development of several useful processes. Effective use of asymmetric synthesis to obtain a chiral substance requires that a suitable substrate be found which can be transformed to a synthetically useful (typically > 50%) enantiomeric excess (e.e.) of a chiral product which can be fractionated to give pure enantiomer. This article briefly summarizes the best results currently obtainable by asymmetric synthesis using chemical reagents. More detailed treatments are available.[1-4]

Asymmetric transamination (1→2) is a useful route to α-amino acids. Catalytic reduction of imine 1 (R^2 and/or R^3 chiral) to the corresponding amine and hydrogenolysis (R^2 is usually benzylic) gives the amino acid 2. Usually R^2 and R^3 can be chosen so that 2 is obtained in high e.e.[5,6] Typical is synthesis of (S)-alanine 7 in 63% e.e. (4→7).[7] A similar synthesis of amines,[8-14] well suited to preparation of amphetamine derivatives, is available, i.e. 8→10.[14] Replacing amine by hydrazine,[15-18] the best being 11,[17] allows transamination to be achieved without losing the original chiral center, e.g. 11+12→14+15.[17]

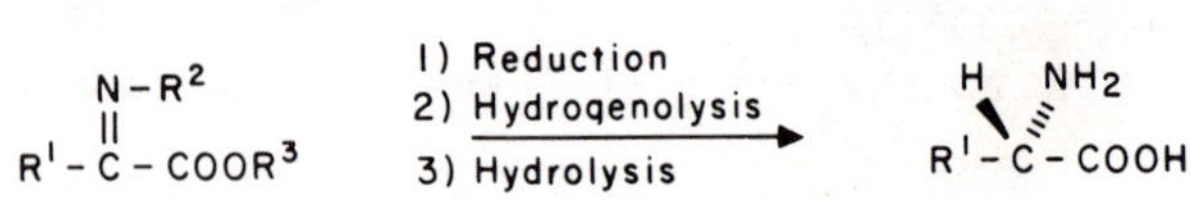

1 2

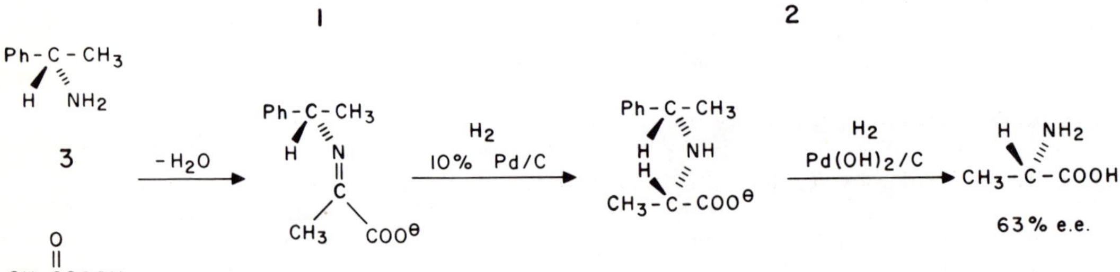

4 5 6 7

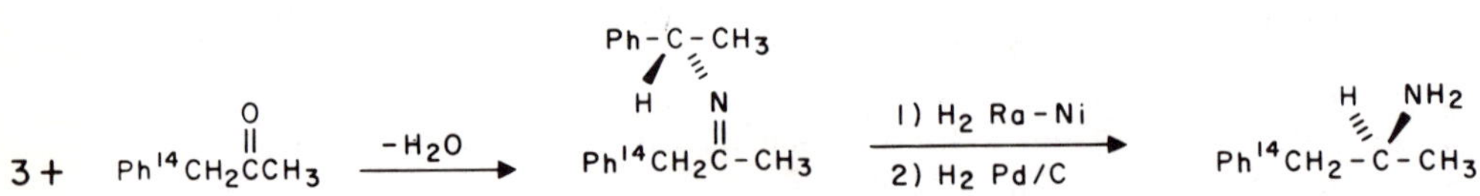

8 9 10

ISBN 0-12-040513-X

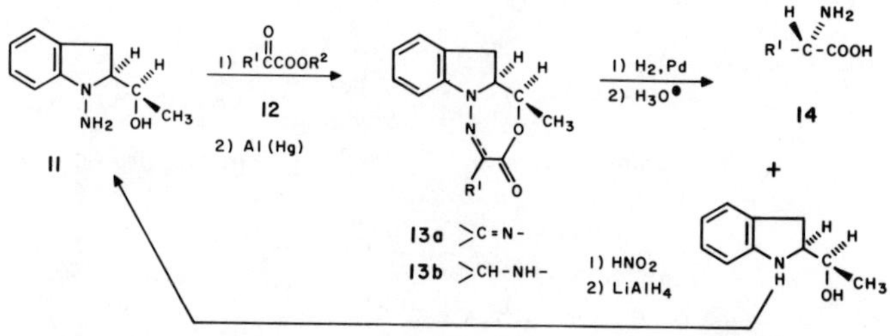

Chiral amines and amino acids have been made via additions of nucleophiles to amines, e.g. asymmetric Strecker synthesis wherein cyanide adds to 16 giving selectively one diastereomeric form of 17. Nitrile hydrolysis and reductive benzyl cleavage complete the synthesis.[19] The amino acids 18 can typically be obtained in only 20-60% e.e. unless it is possible to purify the aminonitrile intermediate by crystallization. Numerous modifications of the basic procedure have been tried without much success[20-23] although improved (61-75%) e.e. of 18 results from Lewis acid catalyzed condensation of imine 16 with trimethylsilylcyanide to give 19 whose acid hydrolysis under mild conditions yields (S,S)-17. Enantioselectivity in conversion of 16 to 19 depends on the catalyst. Zinc chloride is preferred.[24] Use of ephedrine[25] and (S,S)-5-amino-2,2-dimethyl-4-phenyl-1,3-dioxane[26] as amines for Strecker-type amino acid syntheses have been reported, the former being restricted to preparations of aromatic N-methylamino acids and the latter to preparations of α-methylamino acids. An asymmetric Strecker synthesis is used in commercial synthesis of the antihypertensive agent α-methyl DOPA.[27]

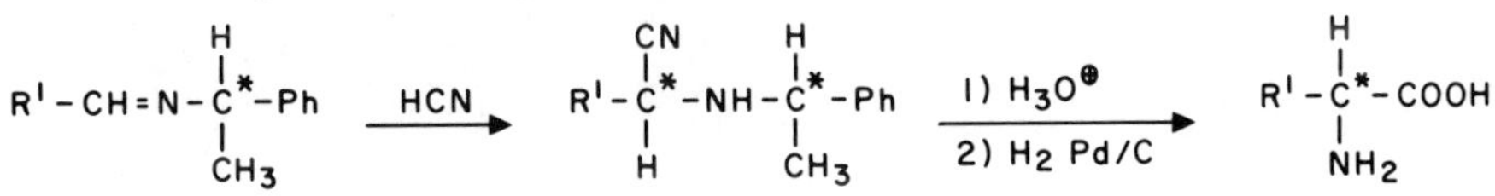

16 17 18

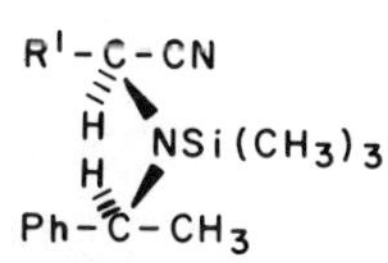

19

The iminium cation intermediate in Pictet-Spengler ring closures is implicated in a 1,3-asymmetric transfer process which gives chiral alkaloids.[28] Condensation of (S)-DOPA methyl ester hydrochloride, (S)-20, with glycidate 21 (3,4-dimethoxybenzaldehyde precursor) gives isoquinoline 22 in 76% e.e. Methylation and 3 step removal of the carbomethoxy group (and thus of the original center of asymmetry) gives (S)-laudanosine (S)-23.[29] The method was used also to prepare (R)-laudanosine,[30] (S)-reticuline[31] and, in modified form, to prepare (+)-maritidine.[32] In a related process, borohydride reduction of 25 followed by hydrogenolysis gives (S)-salsolidine, (S)-26, in 36-44% e.e.[33]

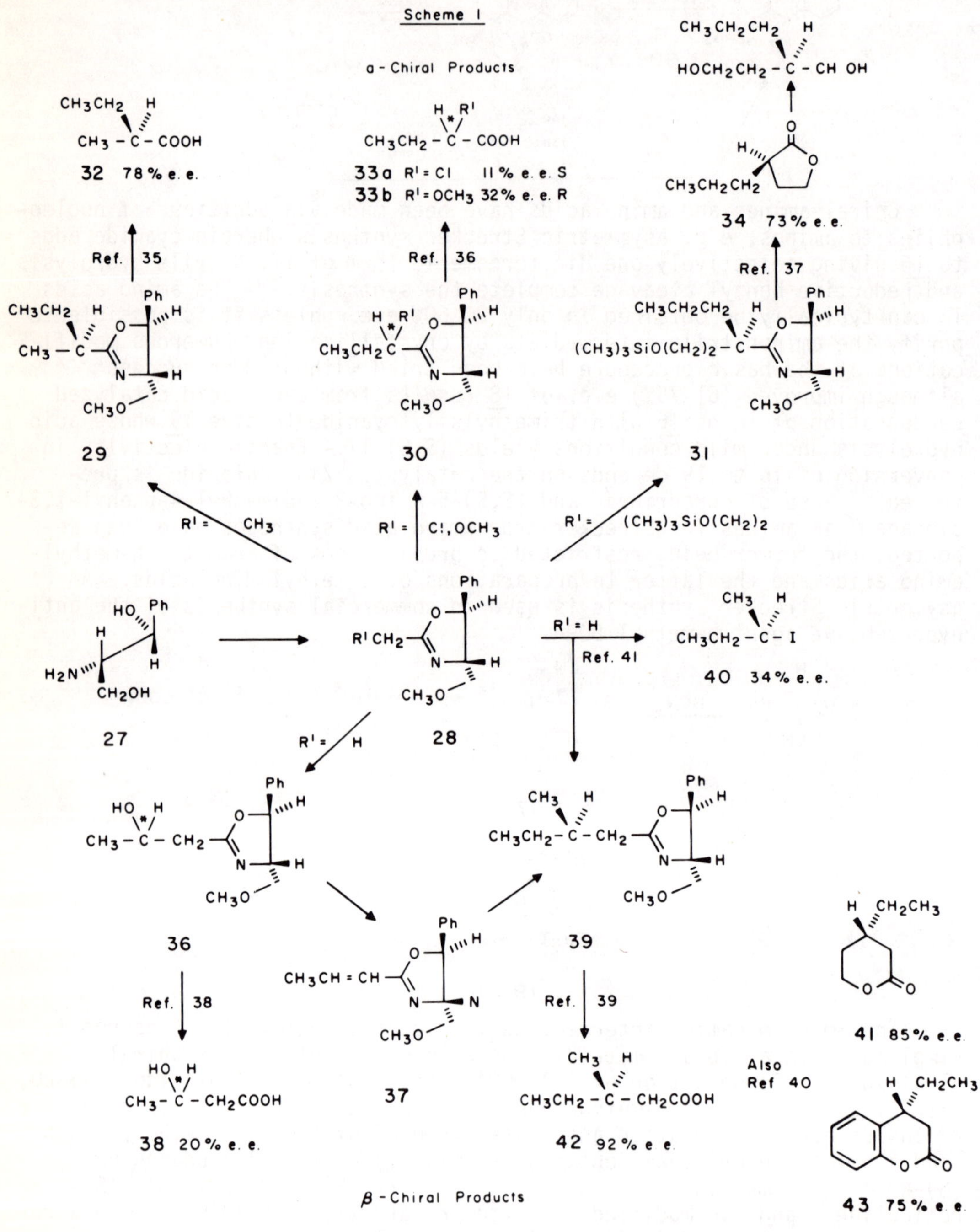
Scheme I
a-Chiral Products
CH3CH2 H
CH3 - C - COOH
32 78% e.e.
H R'
CH3CH2 - C - COOH
33a R' = Cl 11% e.e. S
33b R' = OCH3 32% e.e. R
CH3CH2CH2 H
HOCH2CH2 - C - CH OH
CH3CH2CH2
34 73% e.e.
Ref. 35
Ref. 36
Ref. 37
29
30
31
R' = CH3
R' = Cl, OCH3
R' = (CH3)3SiO(CH2)2
(CH3)3SiO(CH2)2 - C
R' = H
Ref. 41
CH3CH2 - C - I
40 34% e.e.
27
28
R'CH2
H2N
CH2OH
CH3O
Ph
36
37
39
CH3CH = CH
Ref. 38
Ref. 39
HO H
CH3 - C - CH2COOH
38 20% e.e.
CH3 H
CH3CH2 - C - CH2COOH
42 92% e.e.
Also
Ref 40
H CH2CH3
41 85% e.e.
43 75% e.e.
β-Chiral Products

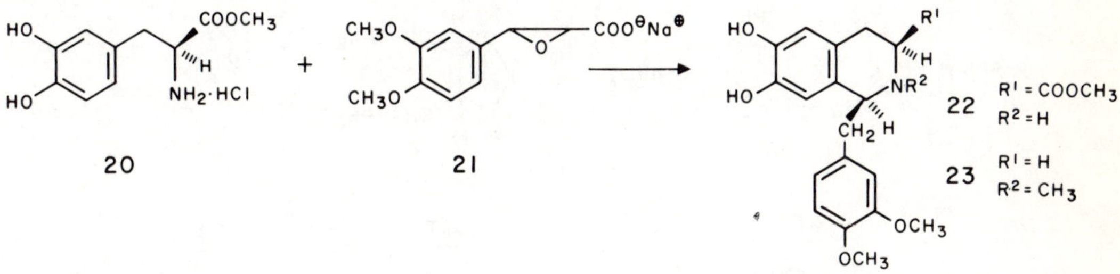

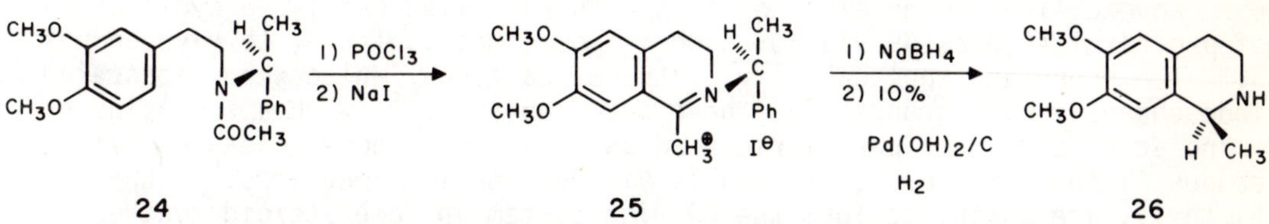

Very useful asymmetric transformations of imine anions, especially anions of oxazoline 28, have been reported.[34] These are practical synthetic procedures which often afford high e.e. products. Some examples of the α- and β-chiral carboxylic acids prepared by this method[34-43] are given in Scheme 1.

A catalytic asymmetric hydrogenation (reviews: ref. 4,44) of (Z)-44 gives (S)-45 in ca. 95% e.e. when Rh-46[45] catalyst is used. This reaction is the basis for a commercial L-DOPA synthesis.[46] Similar catalysts with phosphine enantiomers ligated to rhodium have been used to transform other enamides, certain prochiral C=C, C=O and C=N chromophores into chiral hydrogenation and hydrosilylation products. Many other useful phosphine ligands have been discovered - the most widely used is DIOP, 47,[44] which often affords good enantioselectivity and has the virtue of being commercially available. It is useful to recognize that substrates which can be hydrogenated with high enantioselectivity at reasonable rates by these catalysts are primarily those which are at least formally able to coordinate to Rh in a bidentate fashion, e.g. 48, (X=O,CHR,NR;Y-O,N,CH_2, etc.).

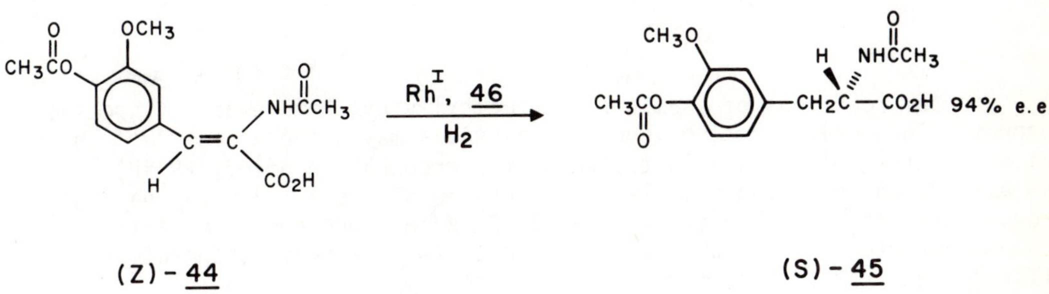

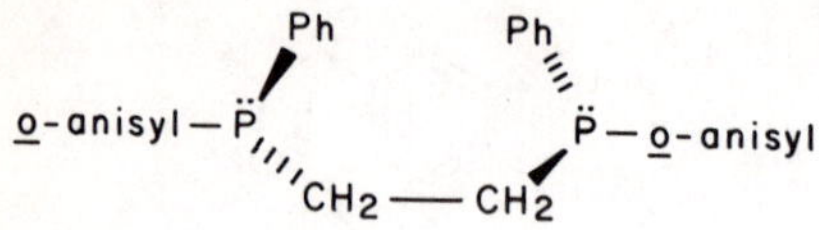

46

(DIPAMP)

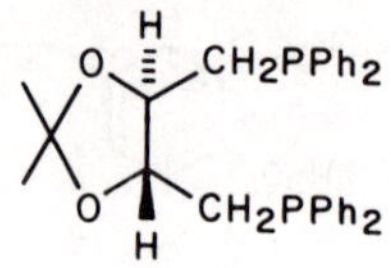

47

(-)-DIOP

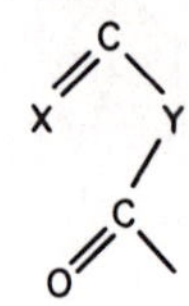

48

An exciting new development is the chiral amine catalyzed cyclization of prochiral triones 49 via 50 which is sometimes isolable, to give enones 51. The scope and applicability of these reactions, which were discovered independently by 2 groups, [47-48] have been reviewed.[49] With amino acids or amino acids and added perchloric acid as catalysts, these reactions afford enones 51 in 60-97% e.e., presumably via enamine intermediates.[49] Enones 51 (n=1), are useful to form the CD ring system in some steroid syntheses while 51 (n=2, R^1=R^2=H) is the chiral Wieland-Miescher ketone[50] which is a steroid AB ring synthon[49] and a valuable starting material for terpene syntheses.

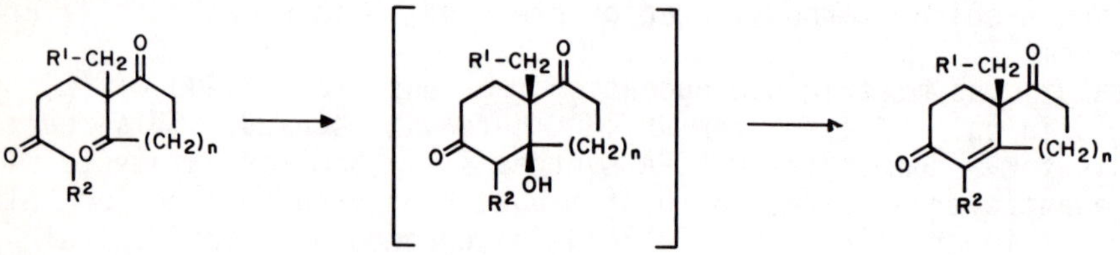

49 n=1,2 50 51

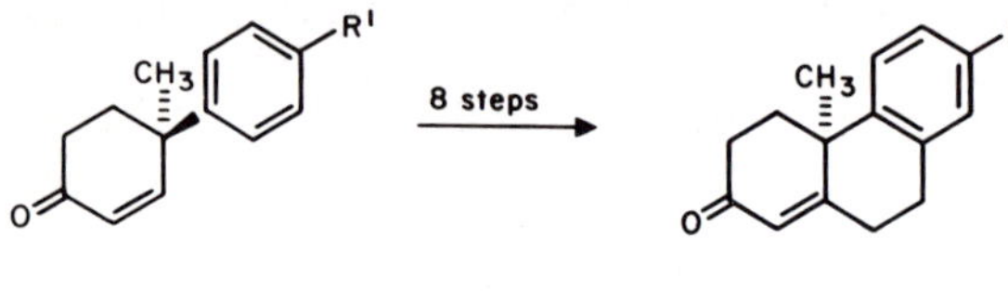

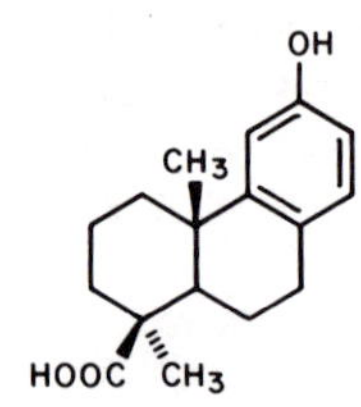

52 53 54 Podocarpic Acid

Michael reactions of enamines with methyl vinyl ketone are of special interest since chiral cyclohexenone derivatives may be obtained.[51,52] The utility of the method is illustrated by the preparation of 52, (R^1=H) in 44% e.e.,[53] which is convertible in 8 steps to 53, useful in many natural product syntheses.[54] The enantiomer of 53 (R^1=H), prepared similarly can be converted to natural podocarpic acid.[55] An analogous preparation affords unnatural (+)-mesembrine.[56] The same type of reaction yields (R)- or (S)-$\Delta^{1,9}$-2-octalone.[57] Also, acid catalyzed cyclization of enamine 55 gives (R)-α-cyclocitral, 56, (converted to trans-α-damascone 57) in 33% e.e.[58]

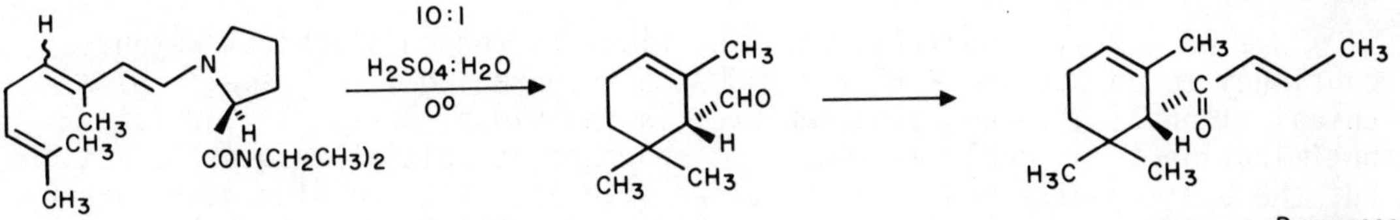

trans-α-Damascone

55 56 57

A catalytic asymmetric process with evident potential is decomposition of diazo esters by enantiomeric copper chelates in the presence of olefins, e.g. to prepare optically active chrysanthemates 58 and 59 in about 60% e.e.[59]

Another promising method which affords chiral centers not otherwise easy to obtain in enantiomeric form is catalytic displacement on allylic acetates, e.g. 60, under the influence of enantiomeric palladium (0) complexes, to give optically active chiral sulfone derivatives 61 in moderate e.e. This reaction proceeds via Pd π-allyl complexes and may also be run stoichiometrically on preformed complex.[60-69]

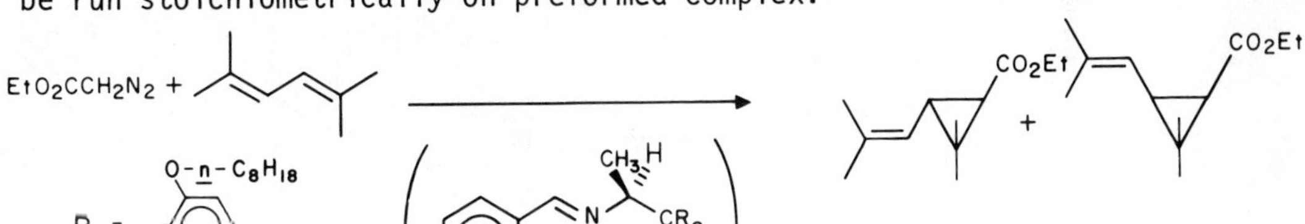

(1S,3S)-58 (1S,3R)-59

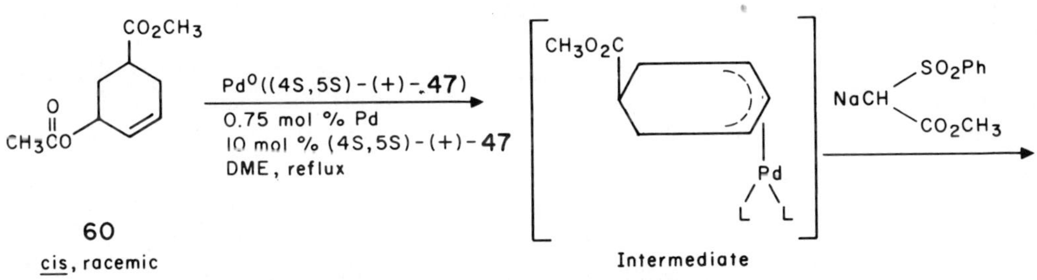

60

cis, racemic

Intermediate

Achiral if L achiral

Chiral if L chiral

2L = (4S,5S)-(+)-47

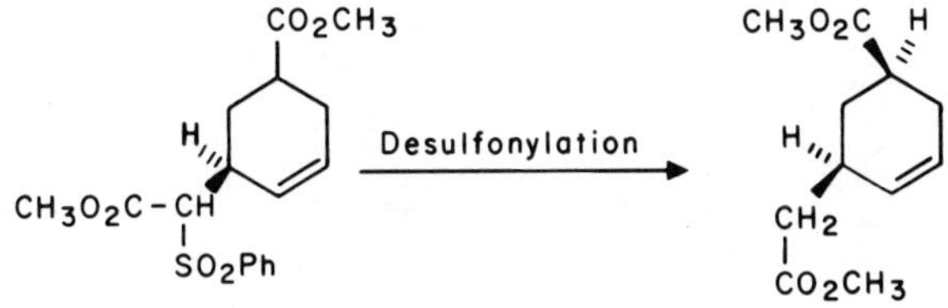

61 (R,R)-62

Use of chirally modified metal hydrides to reduce prochiral ketones continues to be studied actively and some encouragingly high e.e.'s of chiral alcohols have now been reported in individual cases.[70] Careful optimization is probably at least as important as initial reagent selection but the best results have been obtained with an $LiAlH_4$ complex with Darvon alcohol. Reduction of rac.-63 using $LiAlH_4$-(2R,3S) Darvon alcohol gives a 38% yield of 1S,2R,3S-64 (64% e.e.) and 21% yield of 1R,2R,3R-65 (at least 77% e.e.)[71-72] The $LiAlH_4$-Darvon alcohol reagent affords highly enantio-selective reductions of prochiral acetylenic ketones. Reduction of 66 gives 67 (84% e.e.).[73] This alcohol is a precursor to 11α-hydroxyprogesterone, and, ultimately, cortisone.[74]

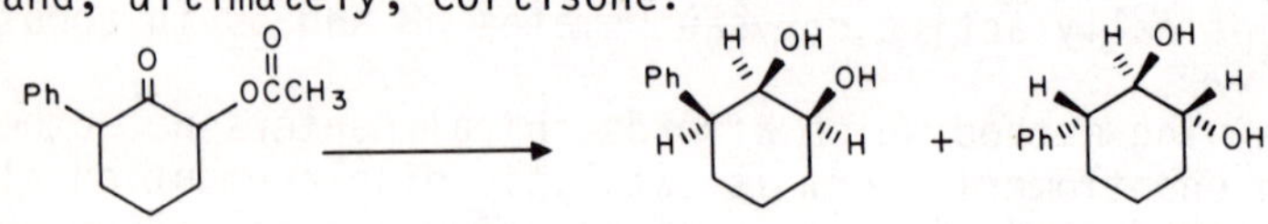

63 64 65

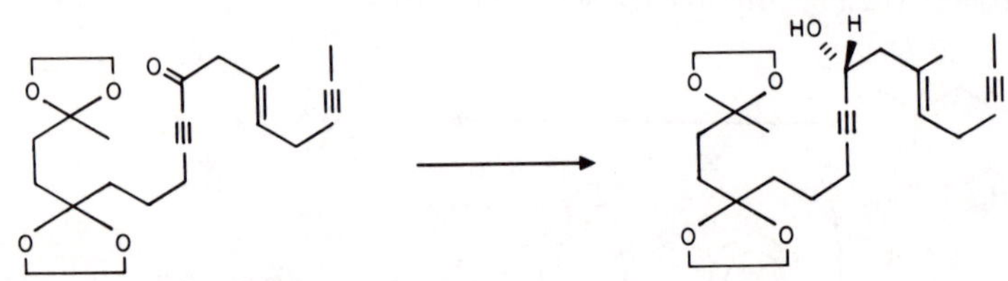

66 67

Intramolecular rearrangements, usually proceeding via doubly suprafacial [2,3] or [3,3] sigmatropic pathways, may sometimes be used to transfer asymmetry creating a new asymmetric center while sacrificing one which is easier to obtain. The most useful of these reactions involve Claisen[75] or modified Claisen[76] rearrangements. Both cyclic[77-80] and acyclic systems[81-85] give good results, for instance, the following examples:[86]

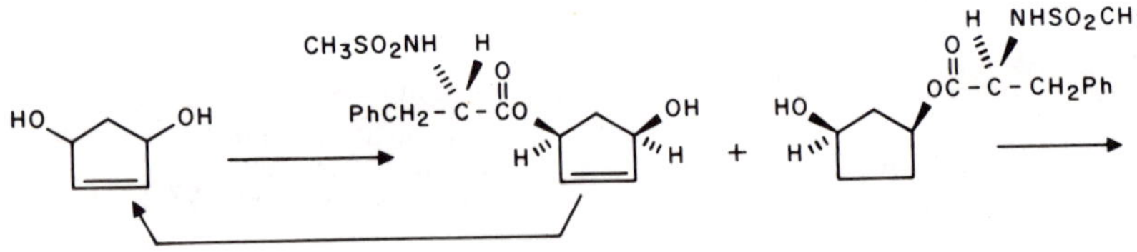

68 70 71

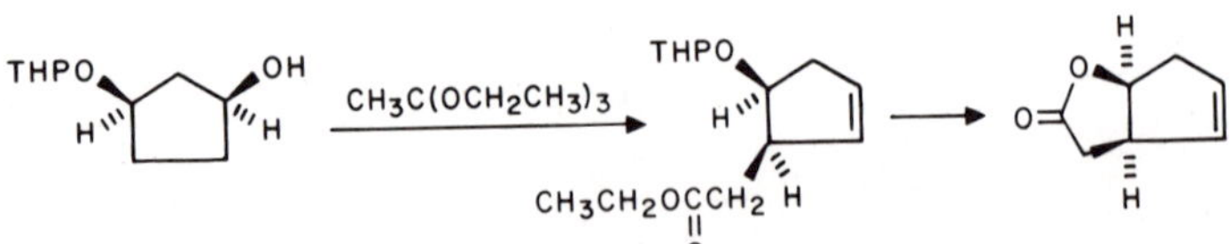

72 73 74

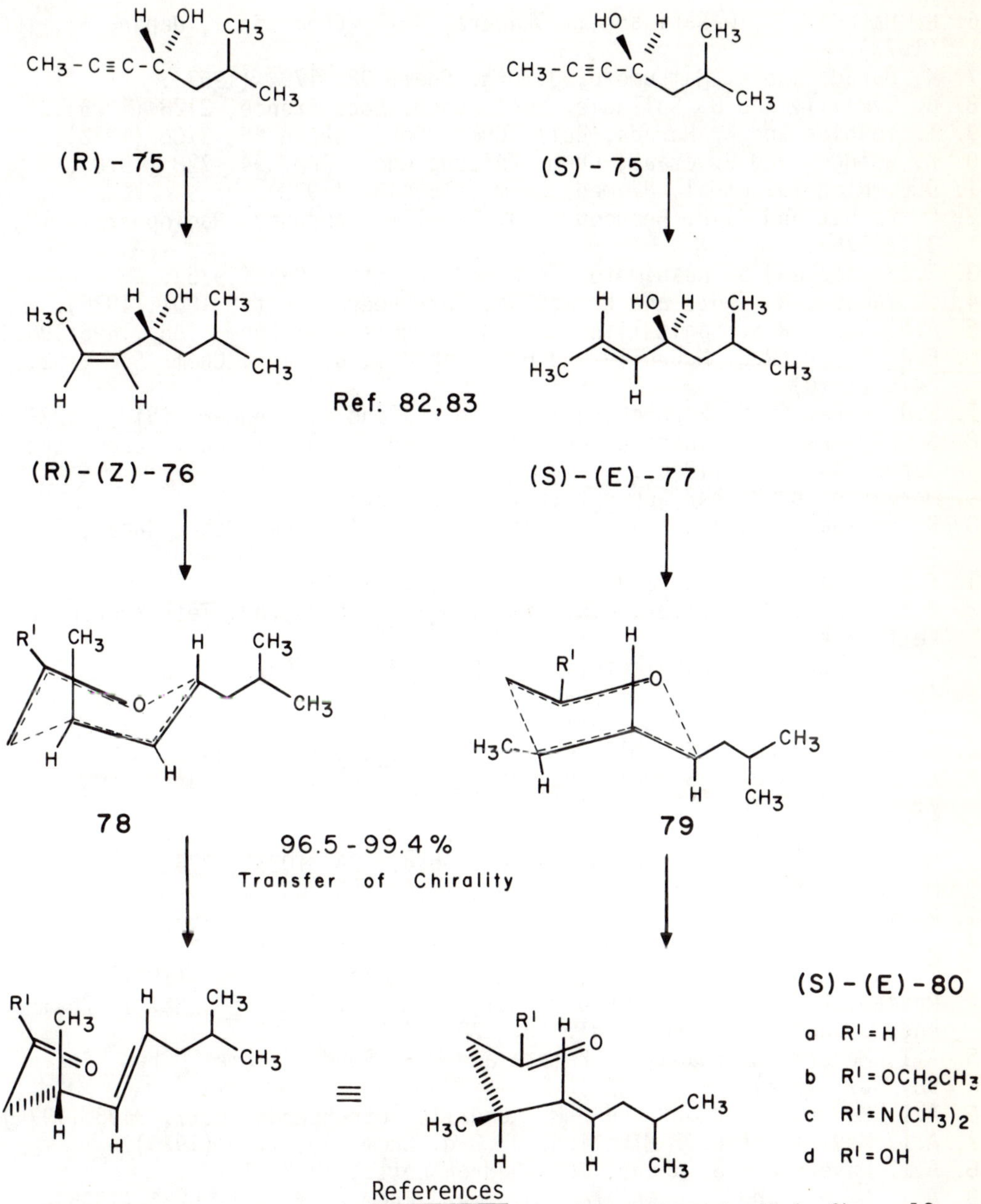

References

1. C.J. Sih, E. Abushanab and J.B. Jones, Annu. Reports Med. Chem. 12, 298 (1977).
2. J.D. Morrison and H.S. Mosher, Asymmetric Organic Reactions, Prentice Hall, 1971.
3. J.W. Scott and D. Valentine Jr., Science 184, 943 (1974).
4. D. Valentine Jr. and J.W. Scott, Synthesis, in press.
5. R.G. Hiskey and R.C. Northrop, J. Amer. Chem. Soc., 87, 1753 (1965).

6. K. Harada, T. Iwasaki and T. Okawara, Bull. Chem. Soc., Japan, 46, 1901 (1973).
7. K. Harada and K. Matsumoto, J. Org. Chem. 32, 1794 (1967).
8. G. Demailly and G. Solladie, Bull. Chem. Soc. France, 2128 (1975).
9. T. Yoshida and K. Harada, Bull. Chem. Soc., Japan 45, 3706 (1972).
10. K. Weinges and G. Graab, Chem. Zeitung Chem. App. 94, 728 (1970).
11. D.E. Nichols, et al. J. Med. Chem., 16, 480 (1973).
12. L. Pichat and J.-P. Beaucourt, J. Labelled Compounds Radiopharm., 12, 31 (1976).
13. S. Yamada and S. Hashimoto, Tetrahedron Lett., 997 (1976).
14. S. Yamada, N. Ikota and K. Achiwa, Tetrahedron Lett., 1001 (1976).
15. A.N. Kost, R.S. Sagitullin and M.A. Yurgovskaja, Chem. Ind.,1496(1966).
16. E.J. Corey, R.C. McCaully and H.S. Sachdev, J. Amer. Chem. Soc., 92, 2476 (1970).
17. E.J. Corey, H.S. Sachdev, J.Z. Gougoutas and W. Saenger, ibid., 4288.
18. S. Kiyooka, K. Takeshima, H. Yamamoto and K. Suzuki, Bull. Chem. Soc., Japan, 49, 1897 (1976).
19. Morrison and Mosher, op cit (ref. 2) p. 327.
20. K. Harada, T. Okawara and K. Matsumoto, Bull. Chem. Soc., Japan, 46, 1865 (1973).
21. K. Harada and T. Okawara, ibid., 46, 191 (1973).
22. U.E. Diner, M. Worsley, J.W. Lown and J.-A. Forsythe, Tetrahedron Lett. 3145 (1972).
23. S. Yamada and S. Hashimoto, Chem. Lett. 921 (1976).
24. I. Ojima, S. Inaba and Y. Nagai., ibid., 737 (1975).
25. L. Neelakantan, J. Org. Chem. 36, 2253 (1971).
26. K. Weinges and B. Stemmle, Chem. Ber., 106, 2291 (1973).
27. K. Weinges and B. Stemmle, Recent Develop. Chem. Nat. Carbon Cmpds., 7, 89-115 (1976). See p. 106.
28. H. Akimoto, et al. Chem. Pharm. Bull. 22, 2614 (1974).
29. M. Konda, T. Shioiri and S. Yamada, ibid., 23, 1025 (1975).
30. M. Konda, T. Oh-ishi and S. Yamada, ibid., 25, 69 (1977).
31. M. Konda, T. Shioiri and S. Yamada, ibid, 23, 1063 (1975).
32. S. Yamada, K. Tomioka and K. Koga, Tetrahedron Lett., 57 (1976).
33. T. Kametani and T. Okawara, J. Chem. Soc. Perkin I, 599 (1977).
34. Review: A.I. Meyers and E.D. Mihelich, Angew. Chem. 88, 321 (1976); Angew. Chem. Intl. Ed. Engl. 15, 270 (1976).
35. A.I. Meyers, G. Knaus, K. Kamata and M.E. Ford, J. Amer. Chem. Soc. 98, 567 (1976).
36. A.I. Meyers, G. Knaus and P.M. Kendall, Tetrahedron Lett., 3495 (1974).
37. A.I. Meyers and E.D. Mihelich, J. Org. Chem. 40, 1186 (1975).
38. A.I. Meyers and G. Knaus, Tetrahedron Lett., 1333 (1974).
39. A.I. Meyers and C.E. Whitten, J. Amer. Chem. Soc., 97, 6266 (1975).
40. A.I. Meyers and C.E. Whitten, Tetrahedron Lett. 1947 (1976).
41. A.I. Meyers and K. Kamata, J. Amer. Chem. Soc., 98, 2290 (1976).
42. J.F. Hanson and C.S. Cooper, J. Org. Chem. 41, 3219 (1976).
43. A.I. Meyers and C.E. Whitten, Heterocycles 4, 1687 (1976).
44. H.B. Kagan, Pure App. Chem. 43, 401 (1975).
45. B.D. Vineyard, W.S. Knowles, M.J. Sabacky, G.L. Bachman and D.J. Weinkauff, J. Amer. Chem. Soc., 99, 5946 (1977).
46. J. Solodar, Paper presented at the 173rd A.C.S. Meeting, New Orleans,

March 20-25, 1977.
47. Z.G. Hajos and D.R. Parrish, J. Org. Chem., 39, 1615 (1974).
48. U. Eder, G. Sauer and R. Wiechert, Angew. Chem. 83, 492 (1971); Angew Chem. Int'l. Ed. Engl. 10, 496 (1971).
49. N. Cohen, Accounts Chem. Res. 9, 412 (1976).
50. W. Acklin, V. Prelog and A. Pietro, Helv. Chim. Acta 41, 1416 (1968).
51. G. Otani and S. Yamada, Chem. Pharm. Bull. 21, 2125 (1973).
52. T. Sone, K. Hiroi and S. Yamada, ibid., 2331.
53. T. Sone, S. Terashima and S. Yamada, ibid., 24, 1273 (1976).
54. Ref. 53, footnote 9.
55. T. Sone, S. Terashima and S. Yamada, Chem. Pharm. Bull. 24, 1288(1976).
56. G. Otani and S. Yamada, ibid., 21, 2130 (1973).
57. T. Igarishi, J. Oda and Y. Inouye, Bull, Inst. Chem. Res., Kyoto Univ. 50, 222 (1972); Chem. Abstracts 77, 164105 (1972).
58. M. Shibasaki, S. Terashima and S. Yamada, Chem. Pharm. Bull, 23, 279 (1975).
59. T. Aratani, Y. Yoneyoshi and T. Nagase, Tetrahedron Lett., 1707 (1975).
60. B.M. Trost and P.E. Strege, J. Amer. Chem. Soc., 99, 1649 (1977).
61. B.M. Trost and T.J. Dietsche, J. Amer. Chem. Soc. 95, 8200 (1973).
62. B.M. Trost and P.E. Strege, Tetrahedron Lett., 2603 (1974).
63. B.M. Trost and L. Weber, J. Org. Chem. 40, 3617 (1975).
64. B.M. Trost and T.J. Fullerton, J. Amer. Chem. Soc. 95, 292 (1973).
65. B.M. Trost, T.J. Dietsche and T.J. Fullerton, J. Org. Chem. 39, 737 (1974).
66. B.M. Trost and L. Weber, J. Amer. Chem. Soc., 97, 1612 (1975).
67. B.M. Trost and P.E. Strege, J. Amer. Chem. Soc. 97, 2534 (1975).
68. B.M. Trost and T.R. Verhoeven, J. Org. Chem. 41, 3215 (1976).
69. B.M. Trost and T.R. Verhoeven, J. Amer. Chem. Soc., 98, 630 (1976).
70. Review: ref. 4.
71. K. Kabuto and H. Ziffer, J. Org. Chem. 40, 3467 (1975).
72. K. Kabuto, H. Shindo and H. Ziffer, ibid., 42, 1742 (1977).
73. W.S. Johnson, R.S. Brinkmeyer, V. Kapoor and T.M. Yarnell, in press
74. W.S. Johnson, S. Escher and B.W. Metcalf, J. Amer. Chem. Soc., 98, 1039 (1976).
75. W.H. Watanabe and L.E. Conlon, J. Amer. Chem. Soc., 79, 2828 (1957).
76. W.S. Johnson, et al., ibid., 92, 741 (1970).
77. R.K. Hill and A.G. Edwards, Tetrahedron Lett., 3239 (1964).
78. R.K. Hill and M.E. Synerholm, J. Org. Chem., 33, 925 (1968).
79. R.J. Ferrier and N. Vethivayasar, J. Chem. Soc. Perkin Trans. I, 1791 (1973).
80. S. Terashima and S. Yamada, Tetrahedron Lett. 1001 (1977).
81. E.J. Corey, M. Shibasaki and J. Knolle, ibid., 1625.
82. R.K. Hill, R. Soman and S. Sawada, J. Org. Chem. 37, 3737 (1972).
83. K.K. Chan, et al., J. Org. Chem. 41, 3497 (1976).
84. N. Cohen, et al., ibid, 41, 3512 (1976).
85. K.K. Chan and G. Saucy, J. Org. Chem., 42, 3828 (1977).
86. K. Hermann, Nachrichten Chem. Tech., 25, 87 (1977).

Chapter 30. Quantitative Structure-Activity Relationships in Drug Design

John G. Topliss and James Y. Fukunaga
Schering-Plough Research Division, Bloomfield, N. J. 07003

Introduction - This review covers new developments concerning the methodological aspects of quantitative structure-activity relationships (QSAR), the physicochemical/structural parameters employed, applications of QSAR approaches to various problems and the significance of the results in drug design. Particular emphasis has been placed on uses of QSAR approaches. Expansion of activity in this field has continued since the last Annual Reports review two years ago. The proceedings of two symposia have been published[1,2] and the second Gordon Conference on QSAR was held in 1977. The most widely used approach continues to be the linear-free energy related model.[3]

Methods - Several newer methods for correlating biological activities such as cluster analysis,[4] pattern recognition[5,6] and Fibonacci numbers[7] have been discussed. The DARC-PELCO[8] and the sequential simplex[9] procedures have been advanced as possible means of more rapidly approaching the most active drug congener. Molecular orbital (MO) indices[10] and calculations of lowest energy conformations have continued to draw interest.[11]

A set of molecular connectivity parameters was derived and used in correlating various molecular and physical properties. Biological data were also correlated and parabolic relationships between molecular connectivity parameters and biological activities were formulated. The method has the advantage that experimentally measured physico-chemical constants are not required.[12] To date, however, only one study has dealt with testing the correlations.[13]

The Free-Wilson (F-W) model and the modified version of Fujita and Ban has been carefully analyzed. The method has been extended to include combinations of continuous parameters (e.g. π, π^2, etc.) and F-W parameters, a concept that is equivalent to Hansch's idea of using indicator variables.[14] The F-W model has been limited by its inability to predict activities of congeners having substituents not present in the matrix. This limitation was due to the usually imprecise correlation of "de novo" constants with experimentally measured constants. Kubinyi has shown that a multiparameter correlation can be used to extend the applicability of the F-W model.[15]

ISBN 0-12-040513-X

The theory of linear equations has been reviewed and difficulties in application to QSAR examined.[16] A method has been proposed for incorporating drug ionization in QSAR equations.[17] A bilinear model was formulated whereby lower activity congeners were related by a linear equation and the higher activity congeners by an asymptotic rather than a parabolic equation.[18,19] A method for applying the Hansch approach without the use of a computer was described. The procedure involves comparison of the potency order of a small initial set of compounds with that calculated for various parameter dependencies.[20] One limitation of the Hansch approach has been its inability to deal with different activities of stereoisomers. However, a means of incorporating stereoisomers into one equation has been devised whereby the physico-chemical constants of the groups on the chiral center are treated as independent variables.[21,22] Progress has also been made in reply to the criticism that the validity of regression equations are not evaluated by the synthesis and testing of new compounds.[23-25]

Parameters - Hansch and coworkers have updated their 1973 compilation of substituent parameters by adding 48 new substituents.[26] σ^0 values for 190 substituents have been determined from infrared spectroscopy.[27] Steric constants for 161 groups have been compiled.[28] Molar refraction (MR) and its use has been reviewed.[29] Some newer parameters were proposed as alternatives to log P in correlating biological data (e.g. solubility,[30] distribution,[31] and chromatographic R[32]). A hydrogen-bonding parameter was discussed.[33] Photoionization potential was used as an index for correlating the brain levels of psychotropic drugs.[34]

Log P continued as the important parameter. The most recent Pomona College output has over 10,000 measured log P's. Chromatographic techniques[35,36] and a solvent extraction method[37] for determining log P's were described. Methods for estimating log P were developed. The SCAP model predicted octanol-water log P with an average absolute deviation of 9%.[38] The hydrophobic fragmental constant, f, its derivation and additive nature was described.[39,40] Deviations between calculated and experimental values were attributed to conformational differences[41] or dimer formation.[42] The relationship of log P to surface area,[43] molecular volumes[44] and van der Waals volume[45] was discussed.

Applications of QSAR Approaches - Hansch and coworkers correlated the inhibition of dihydrofolate reductase (DHFR) from different organisms with physicochemical parameters in three compound series. These studies represented attempts to discern variations in enzyme characteristics. An indicator variable merged parallel sets of DHFR inhibition by dihydrotriazines from two distinct tumor cells.[46] Two equations were necessary for correlating the inhibitory activities of pyrimidines, possibly because of species variations and because two separate sets of pyrimidines were investigated.[47,48] Two quinazoline QSAR equations differ significantly from each other in that the bacterial DHFR equation shows no dependence on substituent properties at position 6. These two quinazoline equations can be quantitatively compared since common congeners were used in the two enzyme studies.[48,49] Based on these results, a map of the active site of DHFR was constructed and specific areas of the map were described as hydrophobic, polar and sterically sensitive. The X-ray structure of methotrexate-bound DHFR was determined[50] and its characteristics differ from the map proposed by Hansch.

As with DHFR, interest in chymotrypsin centered on characterizing the active site environment. A single equation correlated the binding constants of stereoisomeric D- and L-amides acting as inhibitors and substrates, respectively, with MR terms.[22] The presence of the MR terms allowed the identification of three "pockets" as polar and not lipophilic areas. Further support for these descriptions was elaborated in an extensive study where sets of esters and amides were related to MR and not π.[51]

Studies on the binding of two sets of ligands to papain, another hydrolytic enzyme, demonstrated the importance of MR.[52] The X-ray structure, however, showed a bank of lipophilic amino acids near the cleft in papain. A separate set of substrates were designed to specifically explore this area, care being taken to ensure orthogonality between π and MR. The QSAR for this new set of substrates was related to lipophilicity and not MR. The three equations, taken together, clearly define a lipophilic and a polar pocket for papain.[53]

Tumor cells exhibit abnormal levels of certain enzymes. The enzymes are involved in DNA synthesis, proteolysis or cellular oxidations. QSAR summarized in a consistent way, the bulk of the data gathered by Baker and his group. Inhibitory potencies of the various compound series were related to MR and/or π. Indicator variables were used to parameterize major structural variations.[47,54] QSAR studies on malate dehydrogenase,[55] thymidylate synthetase[56] and ribonucleotide diphosphate reductase[57] were reported. Electronic and hydrophobic factors were involved in the inhibition of cholinesterase by carbamates[58] and displacement of vinblastine from tubulin by Vinca alkaloids.[59] Size (E_s) and hydrophilicity ($-\pi$) of substituents were important in the uncoupling of mitochondrial oxidative phosphorylations by dicoumarol derivatives.[60]

Applications of QSAR approaches have been quite numerous

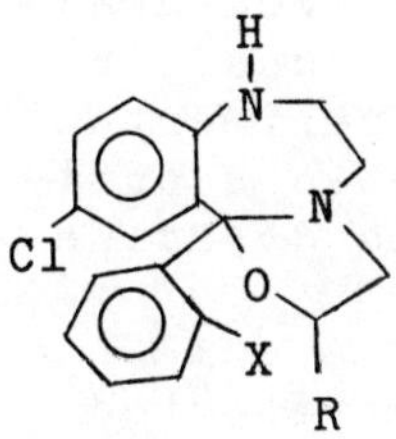

1

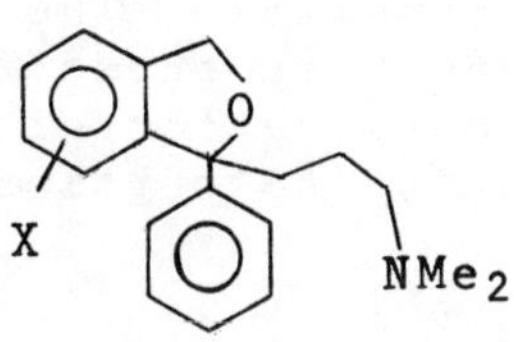

2

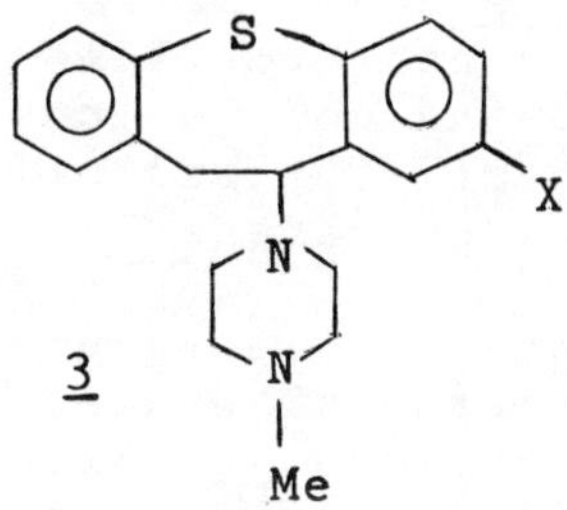

3

in the CNS field. Electronic indices seemed to be a major factor in a number of studies. Correlations were observed between various CNS activities of benzodiazepines (minor tranquilizers) and calculated total molecular dipole moment.[61] QSAR for benzodiazepinooxazoles 1, also of interest as minor tranquilizers, demonstrated the significance of the field effect, as measured by F, for nine biological test systems. These equations did not identify factors for selectivity of action.[62] Hansch and F-W analyses for a series of 1-aryl-1-[3-(di- and monoalkylamino)propyl] phthalans 2 possessing potent selective 5-HT uptake inhibiting properties appeared to demonstrate an impact of F of the aromatic substituents on drug-receptor interaction.[63] The monoamine oxidase inhibitory potencies of N-isopropylaryl hydrazides related to the antidepressant drug iproniazide were found to correlate with the electron withdrawing capacity of the aryl ring substituents.[69] This result along with previously published data on other classes of MAO inhibitors[65] led to a proposal of a general model for the inhibitor pharmacophore. A relationship was established between log P, steric bulk in the para position and the ability to stimulate serotonin receptors in an in-vitro sheep umbilical artery preparation for a series of psychotomimetic phenylethylamine derivatives. The log P and steric bulk terms for the para substituents were interpreted as indicating directional hydrophobicity. The relative activity in man of a group of four compounds was successfully predicted using this model.[66] An equation correlating potency with three connectivity terms and permitting an interpretation of SAR was found. The equation gave reasonable predictions of potencies for amphetamines not in the list as well as mescalines and tryptamines.[13] Electronic (σ) and molar volume terms were used to correlate the ataxic activities of 10-piperazinodibenzo[b,f]thiepins 3.[67] The role of hydrophobic and electronic factors in the binding of eleven tricyclic tranquilizers and antidepressants to human serum albumin was studied. The results indicated that the major factor influencing binding is the ability of the drugs to form a strong charge transfer complex with the tryptophan residue of HSA, with hydrophobicity playing only a minor role.[68] Conformations of the tricyclic and butyrophenone type neuroleptics have been compared to the *trans* conformation of dopamine. The need to consider neuroleptic conformations other than those found experimentally, in drawing conclusions about the correlation between antipsychotic activity and similarity to portions of the dopamine structure, was stressed.[11]

In the cardiovascular field QSAR studies were reported for antihypertensive agents and β-blockers. In a series of clonidine analogs 4, differing in the aromatic ring substitution, a QSAR analysis showed the critical dependence of the α-mimetic activity in the pithed rat on a steric effect in the

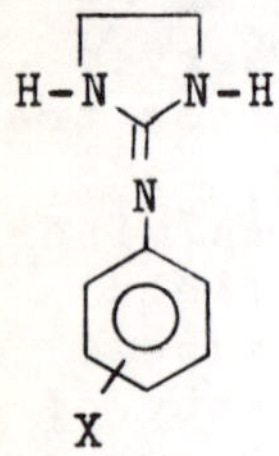

4

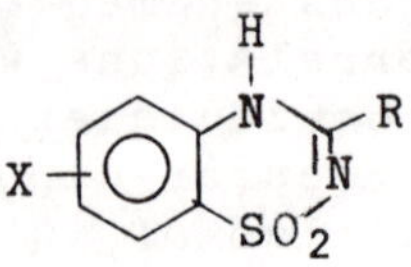

5

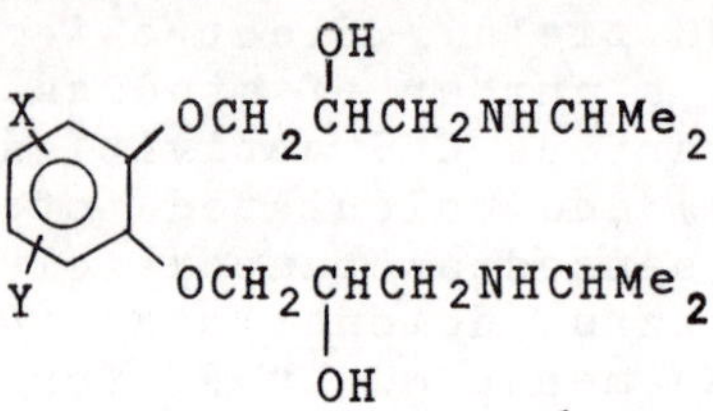

6

ortho positions. The resulting equation allowed the accurate prediction of the activities of three subsequently synthesized highly active compounds. However, no significant correlation between physicochemical parameters and central hypotensive activity, for the seven analogs having such activity, was found.[69] Another study of 26 clonidine analogs successfully correlated hypotensive activity with steric, electronic and lipophilic factors. An ingenious approach was developed in which "kinetic" aspects of the compounds were separated out allowing drug activity at the central α-adrenoreceptor level to be related to molecular structural characteristics of the compounds. The results were used to construct an interesting speculative working model for drug-receptor interactions in this series.[70] The activities of a series of antihypertensive substituted benzothiadiazine derivatives 5 has been correlated with their binding energies to a receptor model calculated using the monopole bond polarizability method.[71] This compound series had been previously analyzed using MO, Hansch and F-W methods.[72] A parabolic relationship between hydrophobicity, measured by octanol-water partition coefficients, and the non-specific antiarrhythmic and cardiodepressant actions of a series of β-adrenergic blocking drugs, determined in the isolated frog heart, guinea pig and cat models was established. Thus, the hydrophobicity of β-adrenergic blocking drugs should be a useful predictor of their non-specific activities.[73] A similar parabolic dependence of the non-specific activities of a small series of alkyl substituted 1,1'-(*o*-phenylenedioxy)bis(3-isopropylamino-2-propanols) 6 on hydrophobicity was noted. Tracheal β-adrenergic blocking activity correlated with the steric parameter E_s whereas affinity to right atrial β-adrenoreceptors was dependent on both E_s and π.[74]

A compelling example of activity enhancement using the Hansch approach for a series of substituted 8-azapurines 7 having anti-allergic properties was reported. Through a series of stages in which predictive use of the Hansch technique played a major role, the activity of the original lead compound was enhanced over 10^5 times.[75] Also in the allergy field a quantitative linear relationship was obtained between the activity of a series of substituted oxalinic acids 8 in preventing the release of mediators of immediate hypersensitivity from the rat mast cell and the energy of a low-lying anti-bonding π orbital localized in the phenyl ring. A theoretical basis for the correlation involving a charge-transfer interaction in which the drug acts as an electron acceptor was proposed.[76]

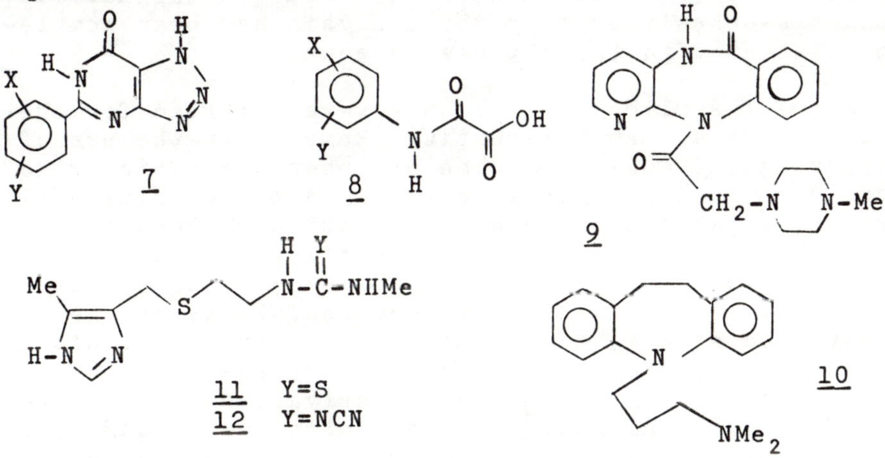

That partitioning characteristics can have a profound effect on the pharmacological activity of a compound is illustrated by pirenzepine 9, a new type of anti-ulcer drug. Despite structural similarities with psychotropic tricyclic compounds, pirenzepine is devoid of any central activity. In rats it does not penetrate the blood brain barrier and produces no CNS effects after intracerebral administration. The inability of the compound to pass the blood brain barrier and to activate the psychotropic receptors was attributed to thermodynamic factors relating to its low partition coefficient, log P 0.10 compared to 4.80 for imipramine 10.[77] The pharmacological equivalence of the thiourea and cyanoguanidine groupings in the antiulcer H_2 receptor antagonists metiamide 11 and cimetidine 12 respectively, was linked to the close correspondence in the physicochemical properties of these groupings with regard to acidity, hydrophobicity, dipole moment and geometry. Thiourea and cyanoguanidine are therefore established as bioisosteres and the development of cimetidine from metiamide is an excellent example of the use of the concept of bioisosterism in drug design.[78]

Conformational analysis of antiinflammatory arylacetic acids was used to hypothesize a detailed model for the active site of the fatty acid dioxygenase unit of the PG synthetase enzyme and the mechanism of PGG formation was interpreted in terms of this model. The model rationalizes observed structure-activity relationships among enzyme substrates and inhibitors, including several nonsteroidal antiinflammatory drugs and is of potential utility in designing novel specifically acting antiinflammatory drugs.[79] The antiinflammatory effects of a series of 4-benzyloxyarylacetic acids substituted in the 3-position showed a parabolic dependence on the lipophilicity of the variable substituents and a positive relationship with the electron withdrawing effect of substituents in the meta position with respect to the acetic acid chain. The activity of a compound synthesized after the analysis had been completed was consistent with the regression equation.[80]

A number of applications of QSAR were reported for chemotherapeutic agents. An interesting example was the use of QSAR in studying the mode of action of tuberculostatic drugs of the isonicotinic acid hydrazide type. Antibacterial activity and rate constants for the quaternization of 2-substituted pyridines with methyl iodide showed a similar dependence on the steric and electronic effects of the substituents. These correlations provided evidence that the reactivity of the pyridine nitrogen atom is essential for the biological activity of 2-substituted isonicotinic acid hydrazides and support the hypothesis that isonicotinic acid derivatives are incorporated into an NAD analogue.[81] In a similar vein QSAR studies of antifungal 1-alkylsulfonyl-2-arylacetylenes 13 supported a mechanism of action based on a reaction of the compounds with nucleophiles present in the fungal cells which was confirmed by kinetic studies with a model nucleophile. A compound designed for high activity based on the regression equation was synthesized but was far less active than predicted.[82] A high inverse correlation was found between antibacterial activity against a dental plaque forming organism and the size of the substituents as measured by MR, in the 5-position of a series of 5-substituted 8-hydroxyquinolines.[83] A QSAR analysis, based on the Hansch model, of the antibacterial properties of a series of long chain aliphatic monoamines related activity principally to the surface active parameter, critical micelle concentration.[84] The in-vitro antibacterial activity of a series of 1-phenyl-4,6-diamino-1,2-dihydro-2,2-dimethyl-s-triazines 14 showed a parabolic dependence on partition with no significant contribution from electronic or steric terms. That no in-vivo activity was observed was attributed to strong non-specific binding in view of the high value of the optimum partition for the series.[85]

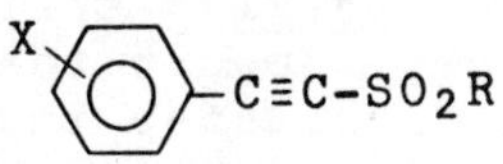

13

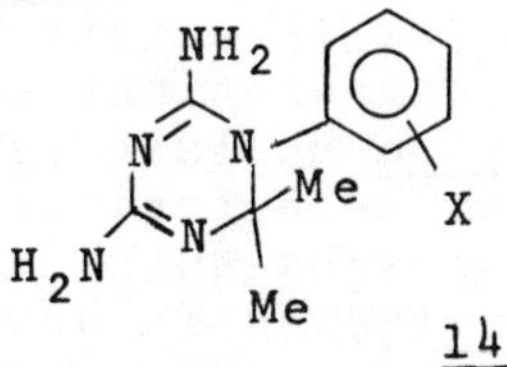

14

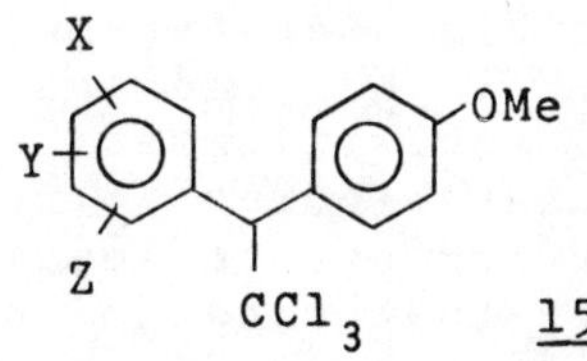

15

In a well designed test of the practical worth of the method of physicochemical-activity relationships, a series of substituted 2-aryl-2-(p-methoxyphenyl)-1,1,1-trichloroethanes 15 were selected to obtain well-spread sets of minimally correlated physicochemical parameter values. The compounds were then synthesized and tested for toxicity towards houseflies. A statistically significant regression equation was obtained indicating that toxicity increases with lipophilic character and donation of electrons to the benzene ring by resonance, and decreases by the introduction of bulky substituents in the benzene ring particularly at the ortho positions. The regression equation obtained forecast the activity of eight further members of the series sufficiently well so that by a statistical test the hypothesis that the same function applies to all members of the series could not be rejected.[86]

The method of discriminant analysis was used to analyze structure-activity relationships in a series of antitumor 1-phenyl-3-benzyl-3-methyltriazenes. The analysis classified 11 of 13 compounds correctly.[87] Antileukemic activity (L-1210) for three series of homologous dialkanesulfonic esters was correlated with a binomial expression in lipophilic-hydrophilic balance. Since the sulfonyloxy function is strongly hydrophilic considerable latitude is available for the introduction of various lipophilic moieties in alkylating agents with sulfonate esters as leaving groups.[88] In a study on the delivery of a variety of antitumor agents to the central nervous system brain level measurements indicated that most drugs, even those with very low log P values, have some accessibility to the CNS. In addition to the well known considerations of lipid solubility, degree of ionization and protein binding, molecular size plays an important role in determining penetration of the blood brain barrier.[89] Absorption of antitumor rhodium II carboxylates by cells is governed primarily by the compound's hydrophobic character. Optimum activity was obtained in the pentanoate.[90]

In the hormone field a detailed QSAR study of androst-4-en-3-one derivatives and their affinity for putative progesterone receptors led to the derivation of a six variable regression equation which satisfactorily predicted the affinities of other literature compounds. A novel feature of the analysis was the use of a surface area parameter for non-hydroxyl substituents as a measure of hydrophobic bonding of relatively nonpolar groups.[91] In a comprehensive QSAR study of thyroid hormone analogs correlations between in-vivo anti-goiter activities and in-vitro nuclear receptors support the idea that binding to nuclear receptors is the first step in initiating events leading to subsequent hormonal effects. Factors that need to be considered in designing new analogues were identified.[92]

Finally an impressive case of the use of molecular models in conjunction with knowledge of the structure of the receptor site to design compounds which should bind to and stabilize the deoxy conformation of human haemoglobin has been described. The compounds so designed were not closely related to the natural starting substance but had the expected property of promoting oxygen liberation and their relative potencies were in the predicted sequence. This example illustrates the potential of drug design when the receptor site is understood in sufficient detail and may well be a portent of a future era in quantitative drug design.[93]

References

1. M. Tichy, Ed., "Quantitative Structure Activity Relationships," Birkhauser, Basel and Stuttgart 1976.
2. J.A.K. Buisman, Ed., "Biological Activity and Chemical Structure," Elsevier, Amsterdam 1977.
3. C. Hansch, J.Med.Chem., 19, 1 (1976).
4. W.J. Dunn, III, M.J. Greenberg and S.S. Callejas, J.Med. Chem., 19, 1299 (1976).
5. A. Cammarata and G.K. Menon, J.Med.Chem., 19, 739 (1976).
6. G.K. Menon and A. Cammarata, J.Pharm.Sci., 66, 304 (1977).
7. S.N. Deming, J.Med.Chem., 19, 977 (1976).
8. J.-E. Dubois, D. Laurent, P. Bost, S. Chamband and C. Mercier, Eur.J.Med.Chem., 11, 225 (1976).
9. R.D. Gilliom, W.P. Purcell and T.R. Bosin, Eur.J.Med.Chem., 12, 187 (1977).
10. R. Carbo, M. Martin and V. Pons, Afinidad, 34, 348 (1977).
11. J.P. Tollenaere, H. Moereels and M.H.J. Koch, Eur.J.Med. Chem., 12, 199 (1977).
12. L.B. Kier and L.H. Hall, "Molecular Connectivity in Chemistry and Drug Research," Academic Press, New York, 1976.
13. L.B. Kier and L.H. Hall, J.Med.Chem., 20, 1631 (1977).
14. H. Kubinyi, J.Med.Chem., 19, 587 (1976).
15. H. Kubinyi and O.-H. Kehrhahn, J.Med.Chem., 19, 1040 (1976).
16. L.J. Schaad and B.A. Hess, Jr., J.Med.Chem., 20, 619 (1977).
17. Y.C. Martin and J.J. Hackbarth, J.Med.Chem., 19, 1033 (1976).
18. H. Kubinyi, Arzneim.-Forsch., 26, 1991 (1976).

19. H. Kubinyi, J.Med.Chem., 20, 625 (1977).
20. J.G. Topliss, J.Med.Chem., 20, 463 (1977).
21. E.J. Lien, J.F. Rodrigues de Miranda and E.J. Ariens, Mol. Pharmacol., 12, 598 (1976).
22. M. Yoshimoto and C. Hansch, J.Org.Chem., 41, 2269 (1976).
23. C. Hansch and J.Y. Fukunaga, Chem.Tech., 7, 20 (1977).
24. C. Hansch, M. Yoshimoto and M.H. Doll, J.Med.Chem., 19, 1089 (1976).
25. C. Grieco, C. Silipo, A. Vittorio and C. Hansch, J.Med. Chem., 20, 586 (1977).
26. C. Hansch, S.D. Rockwell, P.Y.C. Jow, A. Leo and E.E. Steller, J.Med.Chem., 20, 304 (1977).
27. A.R. Katritzky and R.D. Topsom, Chem.Rev., 77, 639 (1977).
28. S.H. Unger and C. Hansch, Prog.Phys.Org.Chem., 12, 91 (1977).
29. W.J. Dunn, III, Eur.J.Med.Chem., 12, 109 (1977).
30. S.A. Khalil, M.A. Moustafa, O.Y. Abdallah, Can.J.Pharm. Sci., 11, 121 (1976).
31. R.A. Scherrer and S.M. Howard, J.Med.Chem., 20, 53 (1977).
32. D. Henry, J.H. Block, J.L. Anderson and G.R. Carlson, J. Med.Chem., 19, 619 (1976).
33. T. Fujita, T. Nishioka and M. Nakajima, J.Med.Chem., 20, 1071 (1977).
34. L.N. Domelsmith, L.L. Munchausen and K.N. Houk, J.Amer. Chem.Soc., 99, 4311 (1977).
35. M.S. Mirrlees, S.J. Moulton, C.T. Murphy and P.J. Taylor, 19, 615 (1977).
36. D. Maysinger, W. Wolf, J. Casanova and M. Tarle, Croatica Chemica Acta, 49, 549 (1977).
37. S.S. Davis, G. Elson, E. Tomlinson, G. Harrison and J.C. Dearden, Chem.Ind., 677 (1976).
38. A.J. Hopfinger and R.D. Battershell, J.Med.Chem., 19, 569 (1976).
39. R.F. Rekker, "The Hydrophobic Fragmental Constant," Elsevier, New York, 1977.
40. A. Leo, P.Y.C. Jow, C. Silipo and C. Hansch, J.Med.Chem., 18, 865 (1975).
41. G.R. Parker, T.L. Lemke and E.C. Moore, J.Med.Chem., 20, 1221 (1977).
42. M. van Damme, M. Hanocq, J. Topart and L. Molle, Eur.J. Med.Chem., 11, 209 (1976).
43. S.H. Yalkowsky and S.C. Valvani, J.Med.Chem., 19, 727 (1976).
44. A. Leo, C. Hansch and P.Y.C. Jow, J.Med.Chem., 19, 611 (1976).
45. I. Moriguchi, Y. Kanada and K. Komatsu, Chem.Pharm.Bull., 24, 1799 (1976).
46. C. Silipo and C. Hansch, J.Amer.Chem.Soc., 97, 6849 (1975).
47. M. Yoshimoto and C. Hansch, J.Med.Chem., 19, 71 (1976).
48. J.Y. Fukunaga, C. Hansch and E.E. Steller, J.Med.Chem.,

19, 605 (1976).
49. C. Hansch, J.Y. Fukunaga, P.Y.C. Jow and J.B. Hynes, J. Med. Chem., 20, 96 (1977).
50. D.A. Matthews, R.A. Alden, J.T. Bolin, S.T. Freer, R. Hamlin, N. Xuong, J. Kraut, M. Poe, M. Williams and K. Hoogsteen, Science, 197, 452 (1977).
51. C. Hansch, C. Grieco, C. Silipo and A. Vittoria, J.Med. Chem., 20, 1420 (1977).
52. C. Hansch and D. Calef, J.Org.Chem., 41, 1240 (1976).
53. C. Hansch, R.N. Smith, A. Rockoff, D. Calef, P.Y.C. Jow and J.Y. Fukunaga, Arch.Bioch.Bioph., 183, 383 (1977).
54. C. Silipo and C. Hansch, J.Med.Chem., 19, 62 (1976).
55. K.J. Shah and E.A. Coats, J.Med.Chem., 20, 1001 (1977).
56. Y. Wataya, D.V. Santi and C. Hansch, J.Med.Chem., 20, 1469 (1977).
57. W.J. Dunn, III and E.M. Hodnett, Eur.J.Med.Chem., 12, 113 (1977).
58. Y.A.I. Abdel-Aal, Bioch.Pharmacol., 26, 2187 (1977).
59. R.J. Owellen, D.W. Donigian, C.A. Hartke and F.O. Hains, Bioch.Pharmacol., 26, 1213 (1977).
60. J.-J. Godfroid, C. Deville and C. Laruelle, Eur.J.Med. Chem., 12, 213 (1977).
61. T. Blair and G.A. Webb, J.Med.Chem., 20, 1206 (1977).
62. M. Yoshimoto, T. Kamioka, T. Miyadera, S. Kobayashi, H. Takagi and R. Tachikawa, Chem.Pharm.Bull., 25, 1378 (1977).
63. A.J. Bigler, K.P. Bøgesø, A. Toft and V. Hansen, Eur.J. Med.Chem., 12, 289 (1977).
64. C.L. Johnson, J.Med.Chem., 19, 600 (1976).
65. T. Fujita, J.Med.Chem., 16, 923 (1973).
66. D.E. Nichols, A.T. Shulgin and D.C. Dyer, Life Sciences, 21, 569 (1977).
67. J.P. Tollenaere, H. Moereels and M. Protiva, Eur.J.Med. Chem., 11, 293 (1976).
68. D. Sharples, J.Pharm.Pharmac., 28, 100 (1976).
69. B. Rouot, G. Leclerc, C.-G. Wermuth, F. Miesch and J. Schwartz, J.Med.Chem., 19, 1049 (1976).
70. P.B.M.W.M. Timmermans and P.A. van Zwieten, J.Med.Chem., 20, 1636 (1977).
71. H.-D. Höltje, Arch.Pharm., 309, 480 (1976).
72. W.J. Dunn, Ann.Rep.Med.Chem., 8, 313 (1973).
73. D. Hellenbrecht and L. Gortner, Pol.J.Pharmacol.Pharm., 28, 625 (1976).
74. J. Zaagsma and W.Th. Nauta, J.Med.Chem., 20, 527 (1977).
75. K.R.H. Wooldridge, Proc. 5th Int. Symp. Med. Chem., Paris, July 19-22, 1976, J. Mathieu (Ed.), p 427.
76. B.V. Cheney, J.B. Wright, C.M. Hall and H.G. Johnson, Abstracts 15th Nat. Med. Chem. Symp., Salt Lake City, Utah, 1976.
77. W. Eberlein, G. Schmidt, A. Reuter and E. Kutter, Arzneim.-Forsch., 27, 356 (1977).
78. G.J. Durant, J.C. Emmett, C.R. Ganellin, P.D. Miles, M.E.

Parsons, H.D. Prain and G.R. White, J.Med.Chem., 20, 901 (1977).
79. P. Gund and T.Y. Shen, J.Med.Chem., 20, 1146 (1977).
80. M. Kuchar, B. Brunova, V. Rejholec, J. Grimova and O. Nemecek, Coll.Czech.Comm., 42, 1723 (1977).
81. J.K. Seydel, K.-J. Schaper, E. Wempe and H.P. Cordes, J. Med.Chem., 19, 483 (1976).
82. H.A. Selling and A. Tempel, Pestic.Sci., 7, 19 (1976).
83. V.D. Warner, J.D. Musto, J.N. Sane, K.H. Kim and G.L. Grunewald, J.Med.Chem., 20, 92 (1977).
84. G.E. Bass, L.J. Powers and E.O. Dillingham, J.Pharm.Sci., 65, 1525 (1976).
85. R.J.A. Walsh, K.R.H. Wooldridge, D. Jackson and J. Gilmour, Eur.J.Med.Chem., 12, 495 (1977).
86. P.J. Goodford, A.T. Hudson, G.C. Sheppey, R. Wootton, M.H. Black, G.J. Sutherland and J.C. Wickham, J.Med.Chem., 19, 1239 (1976).
87. W.J. Dunn, III and M.J. Greenberg, J.Pharm.Sci., 66, 1416 (1977).
88. B.F. Cain and W.A. Denny, J.Med.Chem., 20, 515 (1977).
89. L.B. Mellet, Cancer Treatment Rep., 61, 527 (1977).
90. R.A. Howard, E. Sherwood, A. Erck, A.P. Kimball and J.L. Bear, J.Med.Chem., 20, 943 (1977).
91. D.L. Lee, P.A. Kollman, F.J. Marsh and M.E. Wolff, J.Med. Chem., 20, 1139 (1977).
92. S.W. Dietrich, M.B. Bolger, P.A. Kollman and E.C. Jorgensen, J.Med.Chem., 20, 863 (1977).
93. C.R. Beddell, P.J. Goodford, F.E. Norrington, S. Wilkinson and R. Wootton, Br.J.Pharmac., 57, 201 (1976).

Chapter 31. Enantioselectivity in Drug Metabolism

Lawrence K. Low and Neal Castagnoli, Jr., Dept. of Pharmaceutical Chemistry, University of California, San Francisco, California 94143

Introduction - The inherent asymmetry of biological systems leads to diastereomeric interactions between small chiral molecules and the binding sites of biomacromolecules. These interactions contribute to the stereochemical differences in pharmacological activity observed for a variety of asymmetric drugs.[1-3] Such diastereomeric interactions may occur with membrane components involved in transport,[2,4,5] with receptors,[6,7] and with enzymes responsible for the stereoselective biotransformation of drugs and other xenobiotics. As pointed out in a previous review by Jenner and Testa,[8] stereoselective biotransformations often are difficult to delineate *in vivo* since absorption, distribution and excretion may contribute to the overall disposition of chiral molecules. Therefore, in reports where enrichment of one enantiomer is seen in plasma, urine or tissue, caution must be exercised in assessing the contribution of metabolism.

Three stereochemical metabolic events have been defined:[8,9] (1) Substrate stereoselectivity in which the two enantiomers of a chiral molecule are differentially metabolized; (2) Substrate-product stereoselectivity in which a prochiral center of a chiral molecule is metabolized preferentially to one of the two possible diastereomers; and (3) Product stereoselectivity in which a prochiral center of a symmetric molecule is metabolized preferentially to one of the two possible enantiomers. The present chapter is primarily concerned with recent reports (1974-1977) on substrate dependent enantioselective metabolism of chiral CNS agents, autonomic and cardiovascular agents, and miscellaneous drugs and xenobiotics.

CNS Agents

Narcotic Analgesics - The greater analgesic potency of R(-)-methadone (1) compared to its S(+)-enantiomer is reported to result from stereochemical differences in affinity for the opiate receptor rather than from stereoselective differences in disposition or metabolism.[10,11] This conclusion conflicts with several studies which report the enantioselective metabolism of either S(+)-1 [8] or R(-)-1 .[12] Differences in the biotransformation of the enantiomers of both isomethadone (2) and α-acetylmethadol (3) have been reviewed.[8]

In rats, the pharmacologically active 2S,3R(+)-propoxyphene (4) undergoes slower N-demethylation and binds to liver microsomes less tightly than does (-)-propoxyphene.[13] Higher plasma levels, slightly longer half-life, and slower tissue uptake have been observed for the (+)-enantiomer after oral adminstration of racemic propoxyphene in dogs.[14] Enantiomeric interactions[15,16] have been suggested to be responsible for the enhanced analgesic activity and higher plasma and brain levels of (+)-propoxyphene when racemic propoxyphene is adminstered compared to the corresponding values obtained with (+)-propoxyphene alone.[16]

ISBN 0-12-040513-X

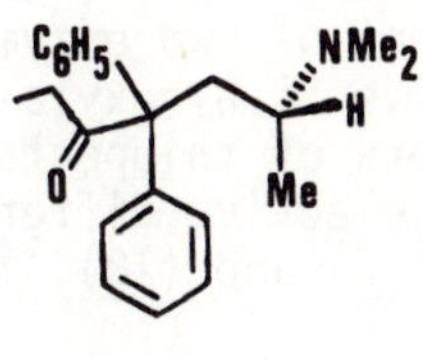

R(-)- 1

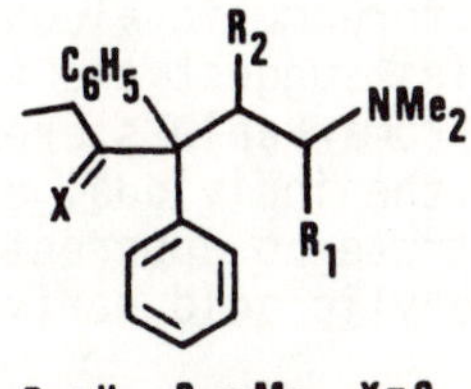

2 R_1=H, R_2=Me, X=O

3 R_1=Me, R_2=H, X= (O-acetyl, H)

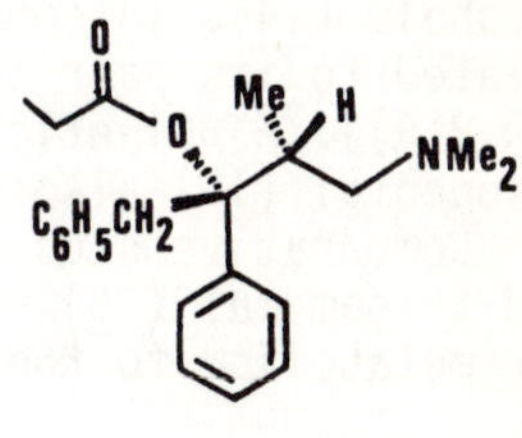

2S,3R(+)-4

Conflicting results concerning the enantioselectivity of the N-,O- and N,O-dealkylation pathways of opiates have been discussed.[8] Recent studies investigating the reduction of the 6-keto function in various dihydromorphinones and dihydrocodeinones indicate marked species variations in the stereoselective formation of the two possible diastereomeric 6α- and 6β-hydroxy metabolites.[17-19] For example, naloxone (5) and naltrexone (6) are metabolized in the chicken to 6α-naloxol and 6α-naltrexol, respectively, whereas in the rabbit, they are metabolized to the corresponding epimeric 6β-metabolites. In man, naltrexone is primarily reduced to 6β-naltrexol.[19] Different soluble hepatic reductases appear to be responsible for the observed product stereoselectivity.[17,18] Other substrates undergoing 6-keto reduction such as oxymorphone (7), hydromorphone (8), oxycodone (9), and hydrocodone (10) also demonstrate species dependency.[17]

	R_1	R_2	R_3
5	allyl	OH	H
6	CH_2-cyclopropyl	OH	H
7	Me	OH	H
8	Me	H	H
9	Me	OH	Me
10	Me	H	Me

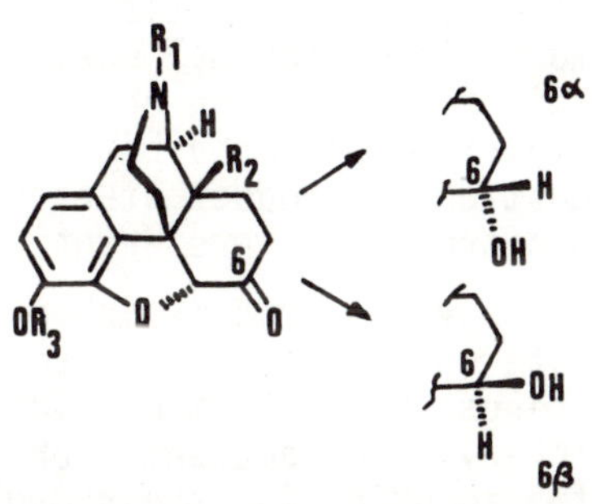

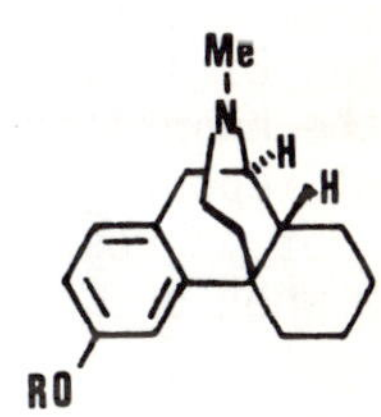

[-]-11 R=H

[-]-12 R=Me

N-Methylmorphinan derivatives also show differences in the metabolism of their enantiomers. The analgesically active (-)-3-hydroxy-N-methylmorphinan or levorphanol (11) is N-demethylated to a greater extent than its (+)-isomer, dextrorphan but undergoes less extensive glucuronidation or excretion compared to the (+)-enantiomer.[21] The O-methylated derivative of (-)-11, levomethorphan (12), also undergoes more rapid N-demethylation than its inactive (+)-isomer, dextromethorphan.[13] Enantiomeric interactions have been reported whereby dextromethorphan enhances and prolongs the analgesic activity of its enantiomer, levomethorphan.[15]

Barbiturates and Related Compounds - The more active S(-)-pentobarbital (13) undergoes stereoselective hydroxylation at the prochiral C-3' atom giving a 5:1 ratio of the two possible diastereomeric (1'S,3'R) and (1'S, 3'S) alcohols (14). In contrast, the R(+)-enantiomer is less selectively hydroxylated to its pair of diastereomeric alcohols {1:1 ratio (1'R,3'S) and (1'R,3'R)}.[22] Kinetic studies suggest the involvement of two enzymes.[23] S(-)-Thiopental (15) also shows remarkable stereoselective 3'-hyroxylation.[24] Comparative studies of the individual enantiomers of thiopental (15) and thioamylal (16) demonstrate no apparent stereoselective difference in their metabolism to the carboxylic acid derivatives (17) and (18).[24]

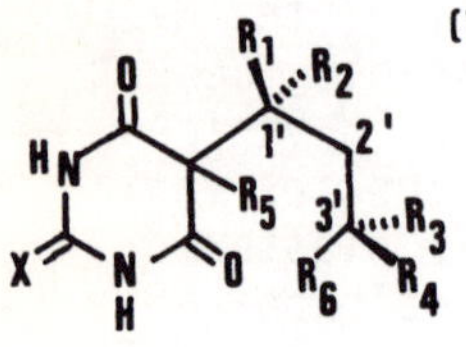

	R1	R2	R3	R4	R5	R6	X
S(-)-13	Me	H	H	H	Et	Me	O
(1'S,3'R)-14	Me	H	OH	H	Et	Me	O
15	Me,H		H	H	Et	Me	S
16	Me,H		H	H	allyl	Me	S
17	Me,H		H	H	Et	COOH	S
18	Me,H		H	H	allyl	COOH	S

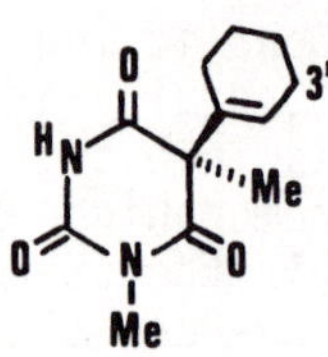

R(-)-19

Preferential metabolism (primarily 3'-hydroxylation and 3'-keto formation) of the enantiomers of hexobarbital (19) has been reviewed.[8,25] In man[26] and mouse[27] the less active R(-)-isomer is metabolized more rapidly whereas the opposite is true in the rat.[27,28] Kinetic and binding spectral studies suggest that the preferential binding of S(+)-19 in the rat and R(-)-19 in the mouse to microsomal enzymes might be responsible for the enantioselective biotransformation observed in each species.[27,29] Recent reports on N-hydroxylation of amobarbital[29a] and pentobarbital[29b] have not addressed the question of product stereoselectivity which might arise when one of the two nitrogens is preferentially hydroxylated.

Biotransformation of phenytoin or 5,5-diphenylhydantoin (20) in man and dog reveals striking stereoselectivity in aromatic hydroxylation of the two prochiral phenyl rings.[30,31] In man, highly preferential 4-hydroxylation of the pro-S phenyl ring accounts for the 10:1 ratio of S(-)-21 to R(+)-21 excreted in urine (as their β-glucuronide conjugates). In contrast, dogs stereoselectively carry out 3-hydroxylation of the pro-R phenyl ring to yield R(+)-22 although some 4-hydroxylation is observed. The overall ratio of R(+)-22/S(-)-21/R(+)-21 found in dogs is 18:2:1.[31]

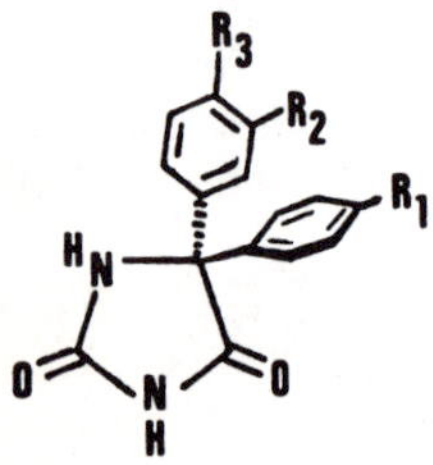

	R1	R2	R3
20	H	H	H
S(-)-21	OH	H	H
R(+)-21	H	H	OH
R(+)-22	H	OH	H

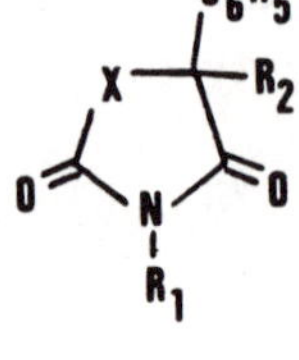

	R1	R2	X
23	Me	Et	NH
24	Et	H	NH
25	H	H	NH
26	Me	H	CH_2
27	Me	Me	CH_2

The enantioselective biotransformations (N-dealkylation or hydrolysis) of chiral hydantoins, mesantoin (23), ethotoin (24), 5-phenylhydantoin (25) and the chiral succinimide, phensuximide (26) have been discussed in detail previously.[8,9,32] More recent studies report enantiomeric differences in the N-demethylation of methsuximide (27).[33] The metabolism of racemic 5-phenylhydantoin (25) to only R(-)-2-phenylhydantoic acid (28) has been shown to be a consequence of stereospecific hydrolysis by a dihydropyrimidinase enzyme and spontaneous *in vivo* racemization of S(+)-25.[34,35]

Amphetamine and Related Compounds - The stereoselective metabolism of amphetamine (29) and related compounds remains complex and controversial.[8,36] The species variation in stereoselective biotransformation of amphetamine must be appreciated.[8] Recent studies reveal that rabbit liver microsomes metabolize R(-)-29 more rapidly {to N-hydroxyamphetamine (30) and 1-phenyl-2-propanol (31)} than its active S(+)-enantiomer in separate incubations.[37,38] However, racemic amphetamine is metabolized at the same rate as S(+)-29 and shows enrichment of metabolites 30 and 31 derived

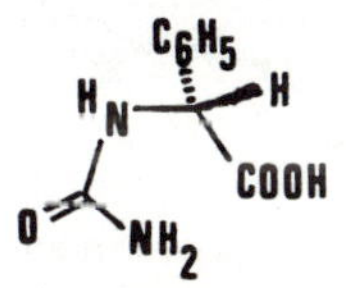

R(-)-28

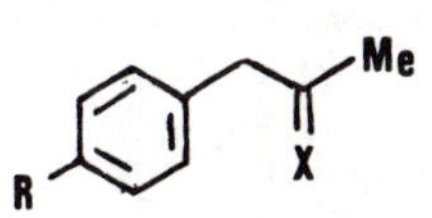

	R	X
29	H	NH_2, H
30	H	NHOH, H
31	H	OH, H
32	OH	NH_2, H
33	H	N-OH

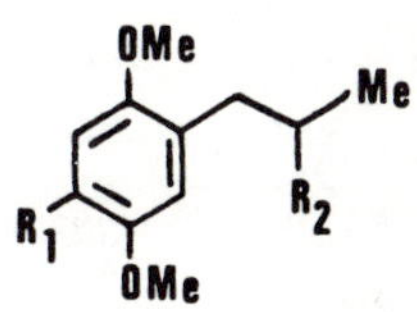

	R_1	R_2
34	Me	NH_2
35	COOH	NH_2
36	Me	NHOH

from S(+)-29. This reversal in stereoselectivity indicates that S(+)-amphetamine or one of its metabolites is inhibiting the metabolism of R(-)-amphetamine. Similar enantiomeric interactions may be occurring in the biotransformation of R(-)- and S(+)-29 to their corresponding p-hydroxylated metabolites 32 in rats.[39,40] Pharmacokinetic studies indicate that S(+)-amphetamine ($t_{1/2}$ 13-15 hrs) is cleared faster from the plasma than its R(-)-enantiomer ($t_{1/2}$ 24-30 hrs) in man after oral administration of individual isomers or racemate.[41] Enantioselective metabolism of R(-)-N-hydroxyamphetamine (30) to the propanol 31 and oxime 33 has also been reported.[38] Thermodynamic aspects of enantioselective metabolism of N-alkylamphetamine derivatives have been reported.[42]

Stereochemical studies on the metabolism of the psychotomimetic amine (±)-1-(2,5-dimethoxy-4-methylphenyl)-2-aminopropane (34) show that the pharmacologically less active S(+)-34 is metabolized more extensively (aromatic C-4 methyl oxidation to 35, O-demethylation and oxidative deamination) than R(+)-34 in rabbits.[43-47] An exception involves N-hydroxylation to 36 which is enantioselective for the R(-)-isomer.[44] In contrast to the enantioselectivity observed with racemic 34, recent studies (no product analysis) show that the individual enantiomers are metabolized at the same rate.[48] These results have been interpreted in terms of an enantiomeric interaction in which the S(+)-isomer or its derived metabolite(s) is inhibiting the metabolism of the R(-)-antipode. Rats dosed with racemic 34 excrete more of the R(-)-enantiomer in the urine.[49]

Miscellaneous CNS Agents - N-Oxidation of the two enantiomers of nicotine show no substrate stereoselectivity but does exhibit marked product stereoselectivity.[8,50] Naturally occurring S(-)-nicotine (37) and its R(+)-enantiomer 38 are oxidized preferentially to the 1'R - N-oxides 39 and 40, respectively.

Although enantioselective metabolism and disposition are unlikely to explain the thirteen-fold greater pyschotomimetic activity of naturally occurring (-)-Δ^1-tetrahydrocannabinol (41) over (+)-41, they may account for the 1.8-fold higher brain levels (in mice) of the 7-hydroxylated metabolite 42 derived from (+)-41.[51]

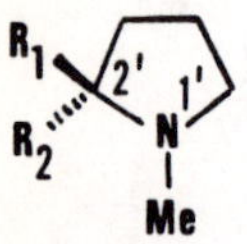

	R_1	R_2
S(-)-37	H	3-pyridyl
R(+)-38	3-pyridyl	H

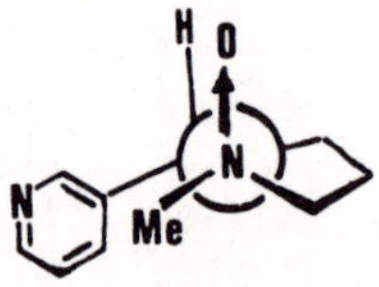

39 (1'R,2'S)

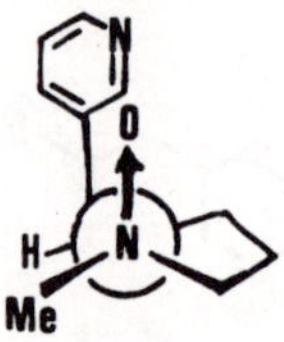

40 (1'R,2'R)

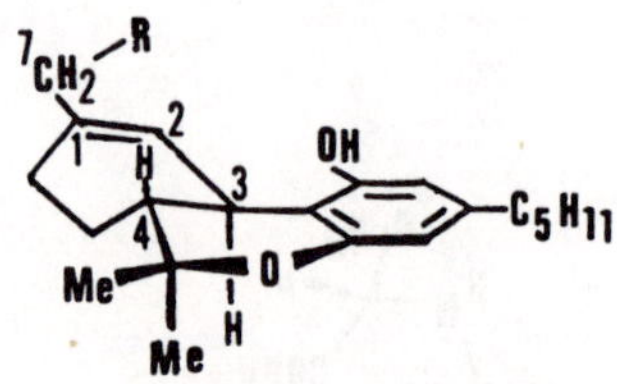

3R,4R (-)-41 R = H

42 R = OH

Microsomal hydroxylations of diazepam (43) and desmethyldiazepam (44) proceed stereoselectively at the prochiral C-3 carbon atom to yield optically active (S)-N-methyloxazepam (45) and S(+)-oxazepam (46), respectively.[52] Since the 3-hydroxylated metabolites are pharmacologically active,[53] the stereochemistry about C-3 may be important in the CNS activity of benzodiazepine enantiomers. The enhanced stereoselectivity observed for the hydrolysis of S(+)-oxazepam hemisuccinate (47) compared to its R(-)-enantiomer may account for the greater CNS activity of the (+)-iso-

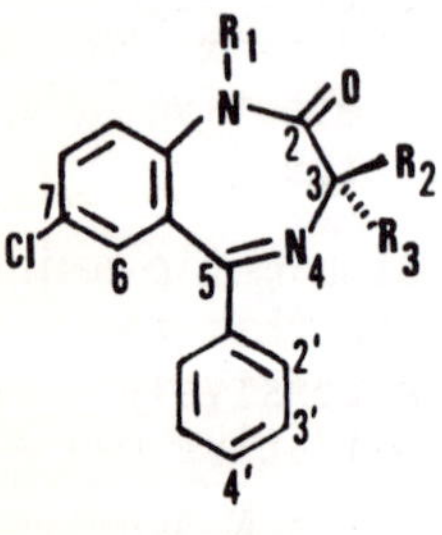

	R_1	R_2	R_3
43	Me	H	H
44	H	H	H
45	Me	H	OH
46	H	H	H
47	H	H	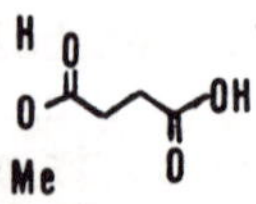
48	Me	H	Me
49	H	H	Me

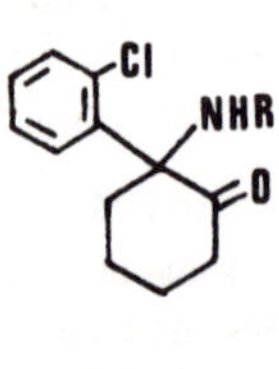

50 R = Me

51 R = H

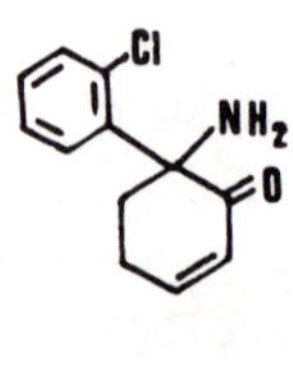

52

mer.[54,55] In a series of optically active 3-substituted 1,4-benzodiazepin-2-ones, the enantiomers with the (3S)-configuration (e.g. 48 and 49) appear to possess greater pharmacological activity than the essentially inactive (3R)-enantiomers.[56] Preferential aromatic hydroxylations (at C-3' and C-4') are observed for S(+)-48 and S(+)-49.[57] Other metabolic pathways for 48 and 49 (e.g. N-demethylation and C-3 hydroxylation) display no enantioselective differences.[56,57] Recent reports indicate that the (+)-enantiomers of some benzodiazepines have 100 to 200-fold greater affinity for a "CNS benzodiazepine receptor" than do their (-)-enantiomers.[7]

Stereoselective differences in the metabolism of the two enantiomers of the dissociative anesthetic agent ketamine (50) have been observed in rats[58] and mice.[59] Plasma pharmacokinetic studies indicate enantioselective N-demethylation of (+)-ketamine to the corresponding norketamine (51) and stereoselective conversion of (-)-ketamine to the cyclohexenone metabolite 52.[59]

Differential disposition of the enantiomers of the non-steroidal anti-inflammatory agents, ibuprofen (53) and cicloprofen (54) is complicated by observations that the (-)-enantiomers of both 53 and 54 can undergo metabolic inversion of configuration to the corresponding (+)-enantiomers. This novel unidirectional bioinversion may account for the predominance of (+)-53 in urine and plasma after adminstration of racemic or (-)-ibuprofen.[60,61] Similar isomerizations have been reported for (±)- and (-)-cicloprofen leading to accumulation of the (+)-enantiomer.[62,63] Preferential elimination of the (-)-isomer is not responsible for these effects.[64] Instead, (+)-cicloprofen appears to be metabolized and excreted more rapidly than its (-)-antipode.

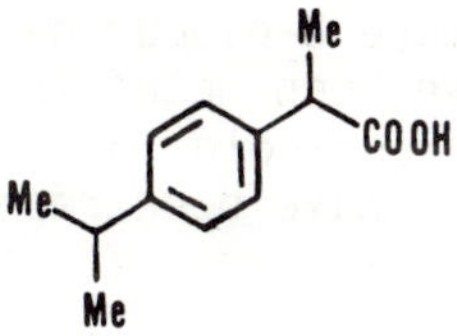

53

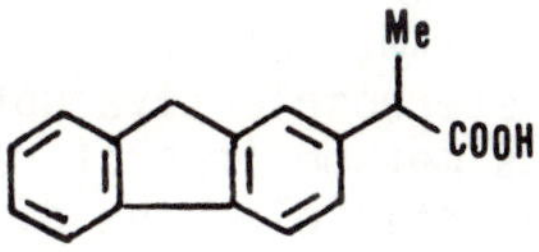

54

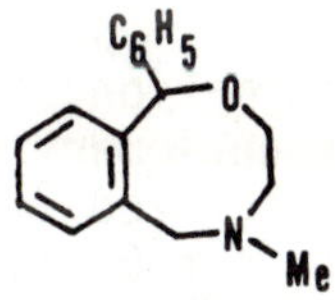

55

Stereoselective microsomal oxidation of the two enantiomers of nefopam (55) (an antidepressant and muscle relaxant) has been examined and indicate that the (+)-isomer is more rapidly N-demethylated.[65] Kinetic studies demonstrate that one enzyme is demethylating both enantiomers and indicate inhibition of metabolism at high substrate concentrations.

Autonomic and Cardiovascular Agents

Enantioselective transport, uptake and metabolism of endogenous catecholamines and adrenergic drugs have been reviewed.[2] Studies with the antihypertensive drug, α-methyldopa, have demonstrated enantioselective transport of the active S(-)-isomer 56 into rat brain and its metabolic conversion to the false neurotransmitters S(+)-α-methyldopamine (57)[4] and 1R,2S(-)-α-methylnorepinephrine (58).[2] Previous reviews[2,8] have emphasized the importance of stereospecific transport and decarboxylase activity in contributing to the observed differences in absorption and metabolism of S(-)-dopa (59) and its enantiomer.

Stereoselective differences in the biotransformation and excretion of the enantiomers of ephedrine have been reported in rabbits.[66] The more active 1R,2S(-)-60 is more rapidly oxidized but more slowly excreted than the (+)-enantiomer. The 1S,2S(+)-isomer, pseudoephedrine (61) is N-demethylated more rapidly that its (-)-antipode.[8] In rats, (-)-ephedrine is ring hydroxylated but (+)-ephedrine is not.

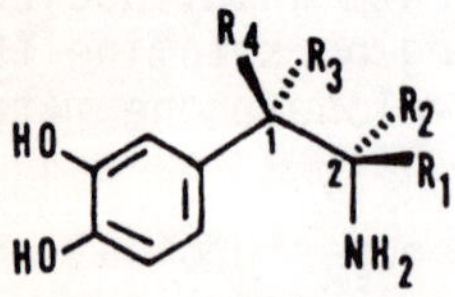

	R_1	R_2	R_3	R_4
S(-)-56	COOH	Me	H	H
S(+)-57	H	Me	H	H
1R,2S(-)-58	H	Me	H	OH
S(-)-59	COOH	H	H	H

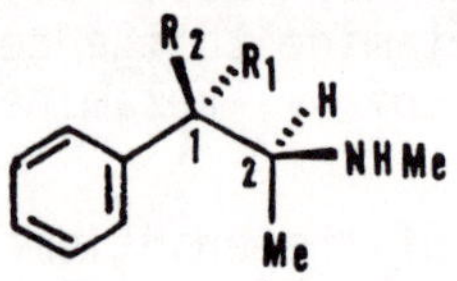

	R_1	R_2
1R,2S (-)-60	H	OH
1S,2S(+)-61	OH	H

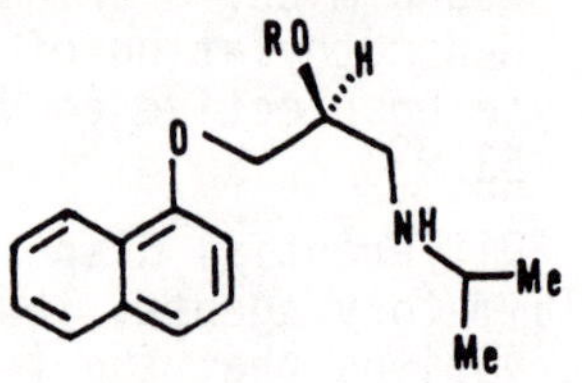

S(-)-62 R = H

63 R = glucuronyl

Differences in the disposition of the active S(-)-62 enantiomer of the adrenergic β-blocker, propranolol, and its R(+)-enantiomer have been reported.[67-69] Slower metabolism, longer half-life, more O-glucuronide (63) formation, and more stereoselective uptake have been noted for the S(-)-enantiomer. Numerous metabolites of racemic propranolol have been characterized[70,71] but enantioselective differences have been reported only for the O-glucuronides.[69]

Enantioselective metabolism of the antiarrhythmic agent, drobuline (64) has been reported.[72] Three-fold higher plasma levels of the (-)-isomer than the (+)-isomer are observed when dogs are dosed with the racemate or with the individual enantiomers. More rapid metabolism of the (+)-isomer appears to account for the difference in plasma levels of the two enantiomers.

Chiral local anesthetic agents also demonstrate enantioselective disposition.[73] The less active R(-)-enantiomer of prilocaine (65) is prefer-

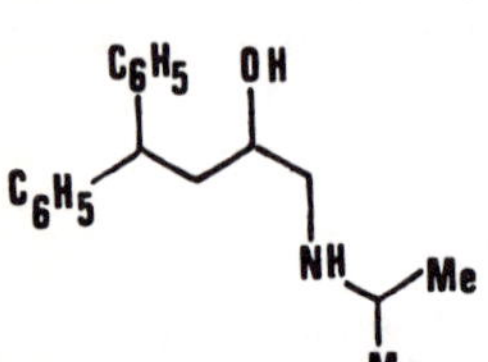

64

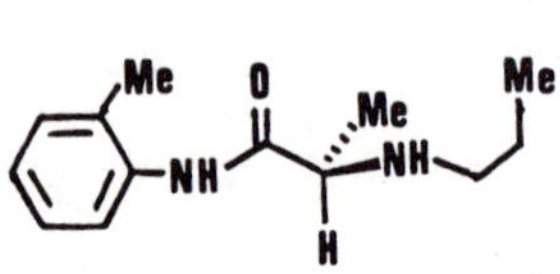

R(-)-65

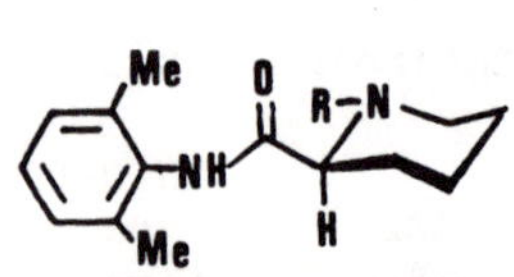

S(+)-66 R = Me

S(+)-67 R = n-C_4H_9

entially hydrolyzed and may be responsible for its greater methemoglobinemic toxicity. Absorption of the active S(+)-enantiomers of both mepivacaine (66) and bupivacaine (67) is more rapid that that observed for the more toxic R(-)-antipodes.

Intriguing species differences have been observed in the disposition of the oral anticoagulant, warfarin. In man,[74,75] the more active S(-)-warfarin (68A) is eliminated more rapidly than the R(+)-enantiomer 68B but the converse is true in the rat.[76] In humans, S(-)-warfarin is primarily 7-hydroxylated while the R(+)-isomer is reduced to the (R,S)-alcohol 69.[77,78] However, in rats, the S(-)-enantiomer is primarily 4-hydroxylated while the R(+)-isomer is 7-hydroxylated.[79-81] Kinetic[79-81] and spectral binding[82] studies with normal, phenobarbital, and 3-methylcholanthrene induced rat liver microsomes indicate that the observed differences in the oxidative metabolism of S(-)- and R(+)-warfarin are due to interactions with different forms of cytochrome P-450. Another oral anti-

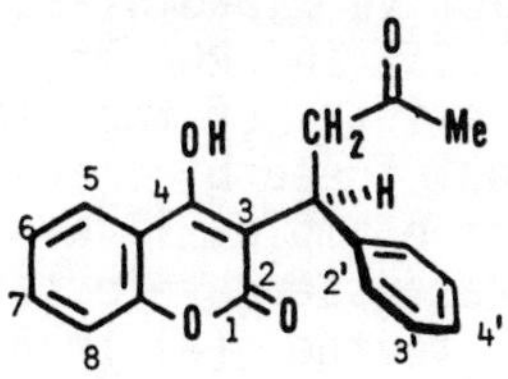

S(-)-68A

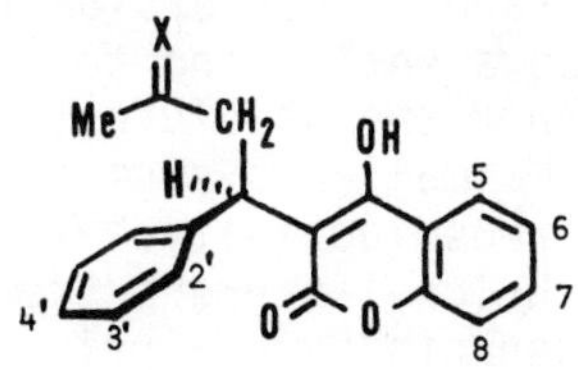

R(+)-68B X = O

(R,S)-69 X = H OH

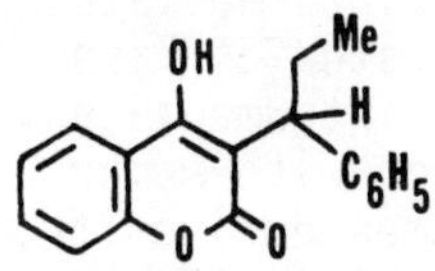

70

coagulant, phenprocoumon (70), also shows species variations in disposition of its enantiomers. The more potent S(-)-70 is less rapidly cleared from plasma than R(+)-70 in man[83] while the reverse holds in the rat.[84] These differences are related to enantioselective protein binding and tissue distribution.

Miscellaneous Drugs and Xenobiotics

The two enantiomers of norgestrel follow different metabolic pathways. The biologically active (+)-enantiomer (71) has a longer half-life and yields metabolites resulting from enantioselective reduction (to 3α,5β-tetrahydronorgestrel) and 2α-hydroxylation. In contrast, the (-)-isomer undergoes preferential 16β-hydroxylation, A-ring aromatization to phenolic metabolites, oxidative rearrangement of the ethynyl group to the novel D-homoannulated metabolite 72 and other minor stereoselective biotrans-

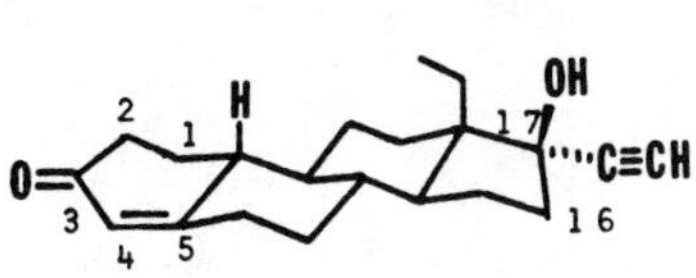

(+)-71

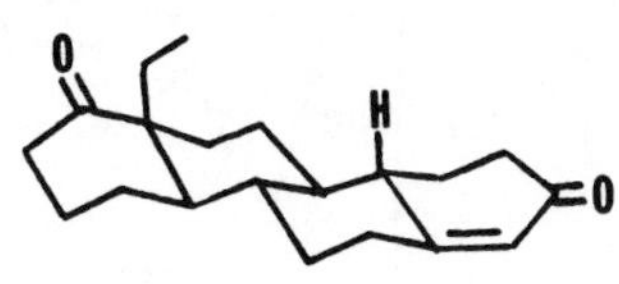

72

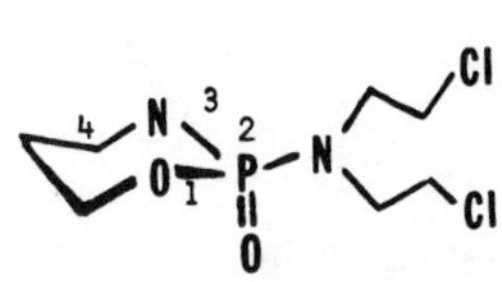

S(-)-73

formations.[85,86]

The chiral phosphorous atom in the antitumor agent, cyclophosphamide (73), gives rise to two enantiomers whose absolute configurations have been assigned recently.[87,88] The S(-)-enantiomer appears to be the more potent antitumor agent.[89] The preferential excretion of S(-)-73 in patients dosed with racemic drug suggests enantioselective metabolism of the R(+)-isomer.[89,90] It has been postulated that the improved antitumor activity of the (-)-isomer could reflect its less efficient detoxification by tumor tissues.[91,92] In mice, markedly more 4-ketocyclophosphamide and slightly less carboxyphosphamide are formed from R(+)-73 than from S(-)-73. The minor amount of unchanged cyclophosphamide detected is not enriched in either enantiomer.[91] In comparison, the individual stereoisomers of (±)-cis- and (±)-trans-4-methylcyclophosphamide reportedly display no marked differences in metabolism.[93]

The toxicity of the environmental carcinogen, benzo(a)pyrene (74) is believed to be mediated by metabolic conversion to reactive 7,8-diol-9,10-epoxide intermediates which covalently bind to crucial DNA and RNA.[94-97] Elegant studies have established the absolute stereochemistry of the diol epoxide intermediates.[98,99] Mammalian systems carry out these biotransformation with remarkable stereoselectivity.[99,100] For example, liver microsomes derived from 3-methylcholanthrene treated rats stereoselectively metabolize the prochiral benzo(a)pyrene principally to the (-)-trans-diol 75A which in turn undergoes stereoselective epoxidation to give a 9:1 ratio of the diastereomeric diol epoxides, (+)-76A and (-)-77A. On the other hand, the enantiomeric (+)-trans-diol 75B is epoxidized with even greater stereoselectivity to a 22:1 ratio of (+)-77B to (-)-76B. Results with normal or phenobarbital treated microsomes show qualitatively similar but less dramatic stereoselectivity in the epoxidation step.[99] This enantioselective difference in epoxidation is especially revelant in terms of the mutagenic and carcinogenic potential of the resulting diol

	Absolute configuration (as shown)
75A	7R,8R
75B	7S,8S
76A	7R,8S,9R,10R
76B	7S,8R,9S,10S
77A	7R,8S,9S,10S
77B	7S,8R,9R,10R

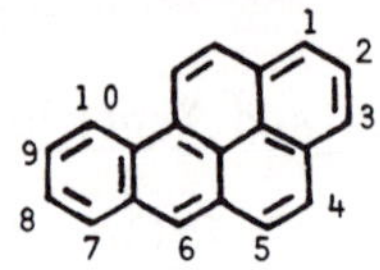

74

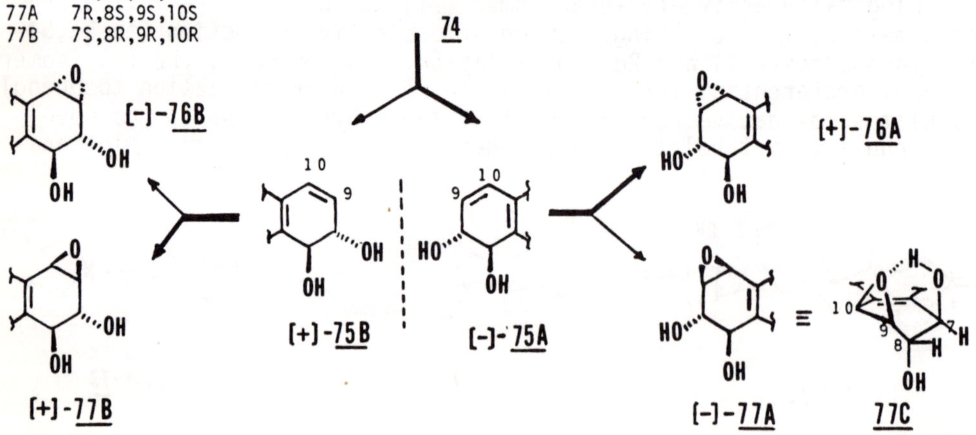

epoxides[101,102] (especially 77A and 77B in which the 9,10-epoxide may be more reactive towards nucleophilic attack as a result of anchimeric assistance by the neighboring cis C-7 hydroxyl group, see 77C [102]). Diol epoxide products formed from the (+)-75B diol are twice as mutagenic as those formed from (-)-75A.[99]

Other environmental pollutants such as insecticides also demonstrate enantiomeric differences in their metabolism. The (+)-enantiomer of O-methyl S-methyl 1-naphthyl phosphorothiolate is more rapidly O-demethylated than its (-)-isomer.[103] The prochiral O,O-dimethyl 1-naphthyl phosphorothionate shows remarkable stereoselective product formation yielding 90% of (-)-O-methyl 1-naphthyl phosphorothionate on O-demethylation.[103] Enantioselective hydration of chlordane-related cyclodiene epoxides to trans-diols[104,105] and enantioselective oxidation of (±)-cis- and (±)-trans-resmethrin[106] have been reported.

Differential disposition of R(+)- and S(-)-1-phenylethanol (formed from the metabolism of ethylbenzene) continues to be of interest.[8,107,108] The mechanism for the stereoselective conversion of ethylbenzene to S(-)-mandelic acid has also been reported.[108]

References

1. A.F. Casy in "Medicinal Chemistry", 3rd Ed., A. Burger, Ed., Wiley-Interscience, N.Y. 1970, p. 81.
2. P.N. Patil, D.D. Miller and U. Trendelenburg, Pharmacol. Rev., 26, 323 (1975).
3. B.V. Rama Sastry, Ann. Rev. Pharmacol., 13, 253 (1973).
4. M.M. Ames, K.L. Melmon and N. Castagnoli, Jr., Biochem. Pharmacol, 26, 1757 (1977).
5. J.A. Gray, H. Lüllmann, F. Mitchelson and G.-H. Reil, Br. J. Pharmacol., 56, 485 (1976).
6. Y.F. Jacquet, W.A. Klee, K.C. Rice, I. Iijima and J. Minamikawa, Science, 198, 842 (1977).
7. H. Möhler and T. Okada, Science, 198, 849 (1977).
8. P. Jenner and B. Testa, Drug Metab. Rev., 2, 117 (1973).
9. B. Testa and P. Jenner, "Drug Metabolism: Chemical and Biochemical Aspects", Marcel Dekker, Inc., N.Y., 1976, p. 237.
10. H.R. Sullivan, S.L. Due and R.E. McMahon, J. Pharm. Pharmacol., 27, 728 (1975).
11. N. Gerber, R.M. Leger, P. Gordon, R.G. Smith, J. Bauer and R.K. Lynn, J. Pharmacol. Exp. Ther., 200, 487 (1977).
12. A.L. Misra and S.J. Mulé, Nature (London), 241, 281 (1973).
13. M.W. Anders, M.J. Cooper and A.E. Takemori, Drug Metab. Disposition, 1, 642 (1973).
14. R.E. McMahon and H.R. Sullivan, Res. Comm. Chem. Path. Pharmacol., 14, 631 (1976).
15. M.J. Cooper and M.W. Anders, Life Sci., 15, 1665 (1975).
16. P.J. Murphy, R.C. Nickander, G.M. Bellamy and W.L. Kurtz, J. Pharmacol. Exp. Ther., 199, 415 (1976).
17. S.H. Pollock and K. Blum in "Alcohol and Opiates", K. Blum, D.L. Bard and M.G. Hamilton, Eds., Academic Press, N.Y., 1977, p. 359.
18. S. Roerig, J.M. Fujimoto, R.I.H. Wang and D. Lange, Drug Metab. Disposition, 4, 53 (1976).
19. H. Dayton and C.E. Inturrisi, Drug Metab. Disposition, 4, 474 (1976).
20. A.L. Misra, R. Bloch, J. Vardy, S.J. Mulé and K. Verebely, Drug Metab. Disposition, 4, 276 (1976).
21. A.L. Misra, N.L. Vadlamani, R. Bloch and S.J. Mulé, Res. Comm. Chem. Path. Pharmacol., 7, 1 (1974).
22. K.H. Palmer, M.S. Fowler and M.E. Wall, J. Pharmacol. Exp. Ther., 175, 38 (1970).
23. J.L. Holtzman and J.A. Thompson, Drug Metab. Disposition, 3, 113 (1975).
24. F.I. Carroll, D. Smith, L.C. Mark, L. Brand, and J.M. Perel, Drug Metab. Disposition, 5, 343 (1977).
25. M.T. Bush and W.L. Weller, Drug Metab. Rev., 1, 249 (1972).
26. D.D. Breimer and J.M. VanRossum, J. Pharm. Pharmacol., 25, 762 (1973).
27. J. Noordhoek, A.P. VandenBerg, E.M. Savenije-Chapel and E. Koppman-Kool, in "Microsomes and Drug Oxidations", V. Ullrich, I. Roots, A. Hildebrandt, R.W. Estabrook, and A.H. Conney, Eds., Pergamon Press, Oxford, England, 1977, p. 534.

28. D.D. Breimer and J.M. VanRossum, Eur. J. Pharmacol, 26, 321 (1974).
29. D.R. Feller and W.C. Lubawy, Pharmacology, 9, 129 (1973).
29a. B.K. Tang, T. Inaba and W. Kalow, Biomed. Mass Spectrom., 4, 73 (1977).
29b. B.K. Tang, T. Inaba, and W. Kalow, Drug Metab. Disposition, 5, 71 (1977).
30. T.C. Butler, K.H. Dudley, D. Johnson and S.B. Roberts, J. Pharmacol. Exp. Ther., 199, 82 (1976).
31. J.H. Poupaert, R. Cavalier, M.H. Claesen and P.A. Dumont, J. Med. Chem., 18, 1268 (1975).
32. J.D. Alvin and M.T. Bush, in "Anticonvulsants", J.A. Vida, Ed., Academic Press, N.Y., 1977, p. 113.
33. M.G. Horning, C.M. Butler, and A.J. Glasko, Pharmacologist, 18, 155 (1976).
34. K.H. Dudley, T.C. Butler and D.L. Bius, Drug Metab. Disposition, 2, 103 (1974).
35. K.H. Dudley and D.L. Bius, Drug Metab. Disposition, 4, 340 (1976).
36. N. Castagnoli, in "Handbook of Psychopharmacology", Vol. 11, L.L. Iverson, S.D. Iver and S.H. Snyder, Eds., Plenum Press, N.Y., 1978 (in press).
37. J. Gal, J. Wright and A.K. Cho, Res. Comm. Chem. Path. Pharmacol., 15, 525 (1976).
38. J. Wright, A.K. Cho and J. Gal, Xenobiotica, 7, 257 (1977).
39a. J.A. Jonsson, Biochem. Pharmacol., 23, 3191 (1974).
39b. A.K. Cho, B.J. Hodshon, B. Lindeke, and J. Jonsson, Xenobiotica, 5, 531 (1975).
40. J. Gal, Biomed. Mass Spectrom., 5, (1978), in press.
41. S.B. Matin, S.H. Wan and J.B. Knight, Biomed. Mass Spectrom., 4, 118 (1977).
42. P.T. Henderson, T.B. Vree, C.A.M. vanGinneken and J.M. vanRossum, Xenobiotica, 4, 121 (1974).
43. S.B. Matin, P.S. Callery, J.S. Zweig, A. O'Brien, R. Rapoport and N. Castagnoli, Jr., J. Med. Chem., 17, 877 (1974).
44. J. Gal, L.D. Gruenke and N. Castagnoli, Jr., J. Med. Chem., 18, 683 (1975).
45. R.J. Weinkam, J. Gal, P. Callery, N. Castagnoli, Jr., Anal. Chem., 48, 203 (1976).
46. J.S. Zweig and N. Castagnoli, Jr., J. Med. Chem., 20, 414 (1977).
47. J.S. Zweig and N. Castagnoli, Jr., Psychopharmacol. Commun., 1, 359 (1975).
48. N.P. McGraw, P.S. Callery and N. Castagnoli, Jr., J. Med. Chem., 20, 185 (1977).
49. J. Gal, J. Pharm. Sci., 66, 169 (1977).
50. B. Testa, P. Jenner, A.H. Beckett and J.W. Gorrod, Xenobiotica, 6, 553 (1976).
51. G. Jones, R.G. Pertwee, E.W. Gill, W.D.M. Patton, I.M. Nilsson, M. Widman and S. Agurell, Biochem. Pharmacol., 23, 439 (1974).
52. A. Corbella, P. Gariboldi, G. Jommi, A. Forgione, F. Marcucci, P. Martelli, E. Mussini and E. Mauri, J. Chem. Soc., Chem. Comm., 721 (1973).
53. S. Garattini, F. Marcucci and E. Mussini in "Psychotherapeutic Drugs", E. Usdin and I.S. Forrest, Eds., Marcel Dekker, N.Y., 1977, p. 1039.
54. M. Salmona, C. Saronio, R. Bianchi, F. Marcucci and E. Mussini, J. Pharm. Sci., 63, 222 (1974).
55. M. Lescovelli, A. Castellani and D. Perbellini, Arzneim-Forsch, 26, 1623 (1976).
56. S. Rendić, V. Šunjić, F. Kajfež, L. Klasing and P. Mildner, Chimia, 28, 232 (1974).
57. S. Rendić, V. Šunjić, F. Kajfež and N. Blažević, in "Microsomes and Drug Oxidations", V. Ullrich, I. Roots, A. Hildebrandt, R.W. Estabrook and A.H. Connery, Eds., Pergamon Press, Oxford, England, 1977, p. 622.
58. M.P. Marietta, W.L. Way, N. Castagnoli, Jr., and A.J. Trevor, J. Pharmacol. Exp. Ther., 202, 157 (1977).
59. S. Ryder, W.L. Way and A.J. Trevor, Eur. J. Pharmacol., 47, (1978) in press.
60. G.J. Vangiessen and D.G. Kaiser, J. Pharm. Sci., 64, 798 (1975).
61. R.F.N. Mills, S.S. Adams, E.E. Cliffe, W. Dickinson and J.S. Nicholson, Xenobiotica, 3, 589 (1973).
62. A.V. Dean, S.J. Lan, K.J. Kripalani, L.T. Difazio and E.C. Schreiber, Xenobiotica, 7, 549 (1977).
63. S.J. Lan, K.J. Kripalani, A.V. Dean, P. Egli, L.T. Difazio and E.C. Schreiber, Drug Metab. Disposition, 4, 330 (1976).
64. K.J. Kripalani, A. Zein El-Abdin, A.V. Dean and E.C. Schreiber, Xenobiotica, 6, 159 (1976).
65. A.G. Bolt, G. Graham and P. Wilson, Xenobiotica, 4, 355 (1974).
66. D.R. Feller and L. Malspeis, Drug Metab. Disposition, 5, 37 (1977).
67. K. Kawashima, A. Levy and S. Spector, J. Pharmacol. Exp. Ther., 196, 517 (1976).
68. C.F. George, T. Fenyvesi, M.E. Connolly, and C.T. Collery, Eur. J. Clin. Pharmacol., 4, 74 (1972).
69. H. Ehrsson, J. Pharm. Pharmacol., 27, 971 (1975).
70. T. Ishizaki, P.J. Privitera, T. Walle and T.E. Gaffney, J. Pharmacol. Exp. Ther., 189, 626 (1974).

71. T. Walle and T.E. Gaffney, J. Pharmacol. Exp. Ther., 183, 83 (1972).
72. P.J. Murphy, T.L. Williams, J.K. Smallwood, G. Bellamy and B.B. Molloy, Pacific Conference on Chemistry and Spectroscopy, Anaheim, CA, Oct. 12-14, 1977, Abstracts, p. 61.
73. R.H. deJong, "Local Anesthetics", 2nd Ed., Charles C. Thomas Publishers, Springfield, Ill., 1977, pp. 196, 240, 243.
74. R.A. O'Reilly, Clin. Pharmacol. Ther., 16, 348 (1976).
75. D.S. Hewick and J. McEwen, J. Pharm. Pharmacol., 25, 458 (1973).
76. A. Yacobi and G. Levy, J. Pharmacokin., Biopharm., 2, 239 (1974).
77. R.J. Lewis, W.F. Trager, K.K. Chan, A. Breckenridge, M. Orme, M. Roland and W. Schary, J. Clin. Investig., 53, 1607 (1974).
78. T.A. Moreland and D.S. Hewick, Biochem. Pharmacol., 24, 1953 (1975).
79. L.R. Pohl, S.D. Nelson, W.R. Porter and W.F. Trager, Biochem. Pharmacol., 25, 2153 (1976).
80. L.R. Pohl, R. Bales and W.F. Trager, Res. Comm. Chem. Pathol. Pharmacol., 15, 233 (1976).
81. W.F. Trager in "Drug Metabolism Concepts", D.M. Jerina, Ed., American Chemical Society, Washington, D.C., 1977, p. 81.
82. M.J. Fasco, L.J. Piper and L.S. Kaminsky, in "Microsomes and Drug Oxidations", V. Ullrich, I. Roots, A. Hildebrandt, R.W. Estabrook and A.H. Conney, Eds., Pergamon Press, Oxford, England, 1977, p. 136.
83. E. Jähnchen, T. Meinertz, H.-J. Gilfrich, Ulrich Groth and A. Martini, Clin. Pharmacol. Ther., 20, 342 (1976).
84. W. Schmidt and E. Jänchen, J. Pharm. Pharmacol., 29, 266 (1977).
85. S.F. Sisenwine, H.B. Kimmel, A.L. Liu and H.W. Ruelius, Drug Metab. Disposition, 3, 180 (1975).
86. S.F. Sisenwine, H.B. Kimmel, A.L. Liu and H.W. Ruelius, Drug Metab. Disposition, 2, 65 (1974).
87. D.A. Adamaik, R. Kinas, W. Saenger and W.J. Stec, Agnew. Chem., Internat. Ed., 16, 330 (1977).
88. I.L. Karle, J.M. Karle, W. Egan, G. Zon and J.A. Brandt, J. Am. Chem. Soc., 99, 4803 (1977).
89. P.J. Cox, P.B. Farmer, M. Jarman, M. Jones, W.J. Stec and R. Kinas, Biochem. Pharmacol., 25, 993 (1976).
90. P.J. Cox, P.B. Farmer, A.B. Foster, E.D. Gilby and M. Jarman, Cancer Treatment Rep., 60, 483 (1976).
91. P.J. Cox, P.B. Farmer, A.B. Foster, L.J. Griggs, M. Jarman, R. Kinas, K. Pankiewicz and W.J. Stec, Biomed. Mass Spectrom., 4, 371 (1977).
92. P.J. Cox, B.J. Phillips and P. Thomas, Cancer Treatment Rep., 60, 321 (1976).
93. P.B. Farmer, M. Jarman, T. Facchinetti, K. Pankiewicz and W.J. Stec, Chem.-Biol. Interactions, 18, 47 (1977).
94. P.D. Moore, M. Koreeda, P.G. Wislocki, W. Levin, A.H. Conney, H. Yagi and D.M. Jerina, in "Drug Metabolism Concepts", D.M. Jerina, Ed., American Chemical Society, Washington, D.C., 1977, p. 197.
95. I.B. Weinstein, A.M. Jeffrey, K.W. Jennette, S.H. Blobstein, R.G. Harvey, C. Harris, H. Autrup, H. Kasai and K. Nakanishi, Science, 193, 592 (1976).
96. A.M. Jeffrey, K.W. Jennette, S.H. Blobstein, I.B. Weinstein, F.A. Beland, R.G. Harvey, H. Kasai, I. Miura and K. Nakanishi, J. Am. Chem. Soc., 98, 5714 (1976).
97. K. Nakanishi, H. Kasai, H. Cho, R.G. Harvey, A.M. Jeffrey, K.W. Jennette and I.B. Weinstein, J. Am. Chem. Soc., 99, 258 (1977).
98. H. Yagi, H. Akagi, D.R. Thakker, H.D. Mah, M. Koreeda and D.M. Jerina, J. Am. Chem. Soc., 99, 2358 (1977).
99. D.R. Thakker, H. Yagi, H. Akagi, M. Koreeda, A.Y.H. Lu, W. Levin, A.W. Wood, A.H. Conney and D.M. Jerina, Chem.-Biol. Interaction, 16, 281 (1977).
100. S.K. Yans, D.W. McCourt, P.P. Roller and H.V. Gelboin, Proc. Natl. Acad. Sci., USA, 73, 2594 (1976).
101. A.W. Wood, P.G. Wislocki, R.L. Chang, W. Levin, A.Y.H. Lu, H. Yagi, O. Hernandez, D.M. Jerina and A.H. Conney, Cancer Res., 36, 3358 (1976).
102. H. Yagi, D.R. Thakker, O. Hernandez, M. Koreeda and D.M. Jerina, J. Am. Chem. Soc., 99, 1604 (1977).
103. D.H. Hutson, Chem.-Biol. Interactions, 16, 315 (1977).
104. W.D. Danterman, in "Insecticide Biochemistry and Physiology", C.F. Wilkinson, Ed., Plenum Press, N.Y., 1976, p. 169.
105. G.T. Brooks, A. Harrison and S.E. Lewis, Biochem. Pharmacol., 19, 255 (1970).
106. K. Ueda, L.C. Gaughan and J.E. Casida, Pesticide Biochem. Physiol., 5, 280 (1975).
107. G.A. Maylin, M.J. Coopers and M.W. Anders, J. Med. Chem., 16, 606 (1973).
108. H.R. Sullivan, W.M. Miller and R.E. McMahon, Xenobiotica, 6, 49 (1976).

Chapter 32. Stereochemistry of Drug-Nucleic Acid Interactions and its Biological Implications

Chun-che Tsai, Department of Chemistry, Kent State University, Kent, Ohio

Introduction - The nucleic acids DNA and RNA are undoubtedly among the best defined of all target molecules for the action of drugs, antibiotics, antineoplastic agents, antiparasitic agents, and antibacterial agents.[1,2] This has encouraged many workers over the years to define the molecular geometries of such drug-nucleic acid interactions and to understand the mechanisms of drug action for a wide spectrum of drugs and antibiotics known to bind to double-stranded nucleic acids, often with the hope of more effective and rational drug design.

A variety of techniques have been used to study the binding of drugs to nucleic acids and to provide information concerning the precise nature of drug-nucleic acid interactions,[3-24] Two main modes of binding drugs to nucleic acids have been suggested.[3-6] The primary and generally stronger mode of binding has been interpreted as intercalation where a planar part of the bound drug molecule slides between adjacent base-pairs in the DNA helix.[3,4] The second and generally weaker mode of binding is thought to be an electrostatic interaction between the phosphate groups in the double-stranded nucleic acids and the drug molecules.[5,6] This review focuses primarily on the stereochemical studies of the interaction of drugs with double-stranded nucleic acids.

It has been suggested that three classes of intercalative drugs or agents may be distinguished by their directional entrance into the DNA helix.[39] The first class intercalates exclusive from the minor groove. Drugs in this class may include actinomycin D and ethidium. The second class may intercalate exclusively from the major groove. Examples of drugs in this class may be daunomycin, proflavine, and acridine orange. Finally, there may be a third class of intercalative drugs that can intercalate from either the major or minor grooves. Drugs in this class may include 9-aminoacridine and ellipticine. It is possible that the biological activities of these drugs and the kinetics of their binding reactions to DNA reflect their directional entrance into DNA helix, as defined by these three classes.[39]

The stereochemistry of actinomycin D binding to DNA demonstrates a general principle that drugs and proteins may utilize in recognizing symmetrically arranged nucleotide sequences on the DNA helix, and suggests a rationale for the synthesis of new variants of the actinomycin molecule that may be used clinically in the chemotherapy for neoplastic disease and viral infection.[12,75]

Le Pecq et al.[74] have used the intercalating properties of ellipticine in a systematic attempt to obtain highly active anticancer drugs by consideration of various ellipticine molecular modifications, and have

ISBN 0-12-040513-X

demonstrated that 9-hydroxyellipticine had the highest DNA affinity and the strongest pharmacological activity. It seems plausible that the introduction of the hydroxy group has enhanced binding, by means of a hydrogen bond to a DNA phosphate.

Recently there have been encouraging signs that interpretation of the molecular model for the interaction of daunomycin with DNA proposed by Pigram et al.[56] may well lead to more active derivatives of daunomycin.[60] A detailed examination of the daunomycin-DNA model reveals that intercalation of the chromophore is only partial compared with simple intercalative agents such as proflavine; on the basis of the model it was proposed that removal of the bulky methoxy group on the chromophore ring would result in a molecule that could intercalate more effectively. Di Marco and his co-workers[61] have now synthesised, and exhaustively examined new daunomycin derivatives that lack just this methoxy group. The modified molecule does indeed bind to DNA somewhat better than its parent molecule. Significantly, in vivo testing of these 4-demethoxy derivatives in mouse cancer systems, both of the leukaemic and solid tumor type, show that it is as effective as daunomycin itself, but at dose levels four to eight times lower.

In a recent report,[23] Krugh and Young have shown that daunomycin and adriamycin facilitate strong binding of actinomycin D to poly(dA-dT).poly (dA-dT). This new observation suggests that combinations of intercalative drugs, such as daunomycin (or adriamycin) with actinomycin D, should be explored clinically.[23]

The concept of drug-DNA intercalation has stimulated the synthesis and study of a new compound, bis(methidium)spermine,[76] that binds DNA very tightly by polyintercalation as echinomycin[77,78] and bisacridine.[79] The compound is a dimer of a well-characterized DNA-binding compound, ethidium. The two ethidium molecules in the dimer are joined by spermine; the linker is long enough to permit the planar ethidium portions to fit between non-adjacent DNA base-pairs. The binding of bis(methidium)spermine not only is tight, but it has significant sequence specificity for p(dC-dG), a synthetic DNA polymer, over calf thymus DNA.[76]

Unifying Structural Concepts in Understanding Drug-Nucleic Acid Interactions and their Broader Implications in Understanding Protein-DNA Interactions - The structural information and stereochemical features afforded by the X-ray crystallographic studies of ethidium-dinucleoside monophosphate crystalline complexes have led Sobell, Tsai et al.[39,42] to generate a detailed molecular model for ethidium-DNA binding. The model predicts that at maximal drug-nucleic acid binding ratios, ethidium intercalates between every other base pair in DNA (i.e. a neighbor exclusion model for intercalative drug binding); this follows from the mixed sugar puckering pattern, C3'endo (3'-5') C2'endo, that is observed in the crystalline complexes. Base-pairs in the immediate region of intercalation are twisted by 10°; this gives rise to an angular unwinding of -26° at the immediate site of the drug intercalation. Base-pairs in the immediate region of intercalation are separated by about 6.7 Å; this distance reflects the presence of an ethidium molecule intercalated between base-pairs. The phenyl and ethyl groups of the ethidium molecule lie in the minor groove of DNA; this suggests that the direction of entrance by this drug is from the minor groove of the double helix. A weak pyrimidine-purine sequence binding preference is predicted from stacking considerations of ethidium on adjacent base pairs. The model explains a large mass of physical and biochemical data concerning the interaction of ethidium with DNA and contains the more general stereochemical postulate that drug intercalation gives rise to a helical screw axis dislocation in DNA, a variable whose magnitude determines the relative ring overlap between an intercalative drug molecule and adjacent base-pairs. The conformational changes in the sugar-phosphate backbone that accompany drug intercalation

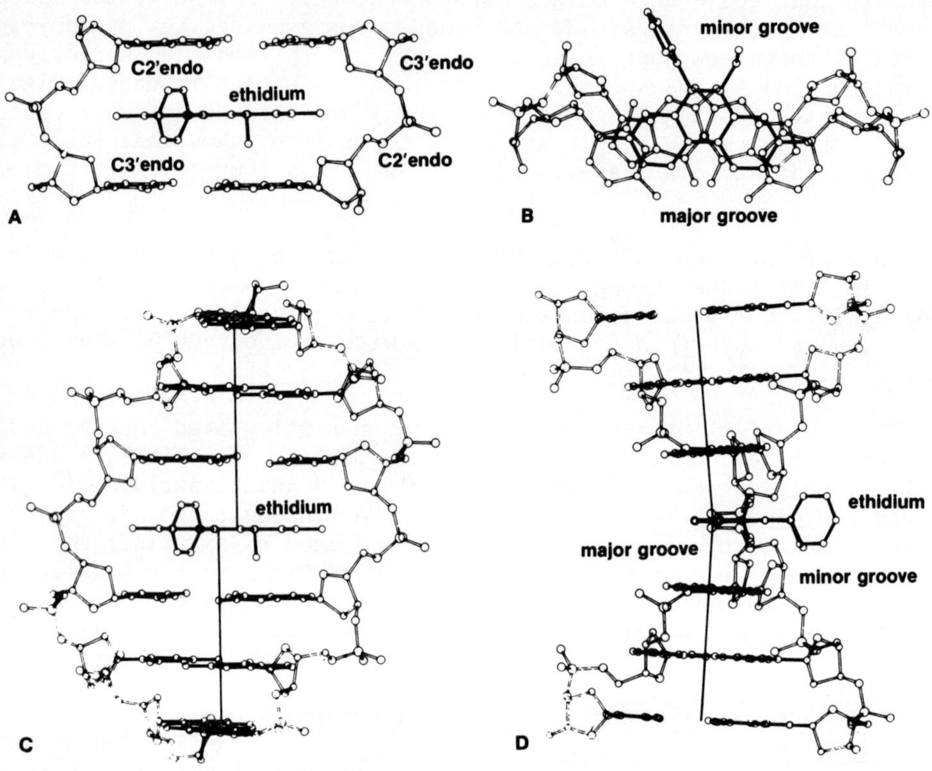

Fig. 1. Computer-graphic illustrations of the detailed stereochemistry for ethidium-DNA binding. (From Ref. 39 with permission of publisher.)
(A) Structure of ethidium-CpG intercalated complex, viewed down the dyad axis and parallel to the planes of ethidium and base-pair molecules.
(B) Structure of ethidium-CpG intercalated complex, viewed perpendicular to the planes of ethidium and base-pair molecules.
(C) Ethidium-DNA intercalation, shown down the dyad axis.
(D) Ethidium-DNA intercalation, side view. Long solid lines indicate helix axes for B-form DNA sections above and below ethidium intercalation structures. Notice that these helix axes are not colinear.

and a small residual "kink" of 8° at the intercalation site have led Sobell, Tsai et al.[39,42] to propose that DNA first bends or "kinks" to accept an intercalative drug or dye. This is made possible by altering the normal C2'endo deoxyribose sugar ring puckering in B-DNA to a mixed puckering pattern of the type: C3'endo (3'-5') C2'endo and partially unstacking base-pairs.

Utilizing the structural features of drug-DNA intercalation, Sobell, Tsai et al.[39,42] have proposed a detailed molecular model for the kinking of B-DNA. A variety of superhelical DNA structures can be formed by kinking B-DNA periodically varying numbers of base-pairs apart. Perhaps the most interesting of these is the one in which a kink occurs every ten base pairs. This gives rise to a left-handed superhelical structure that contains 1½ turns per 140 base pairs and has an axial length of 80 Å. These and other structural features make it an attractive model for the organization of DNA within the nucleosome in chromatin.[39,42]

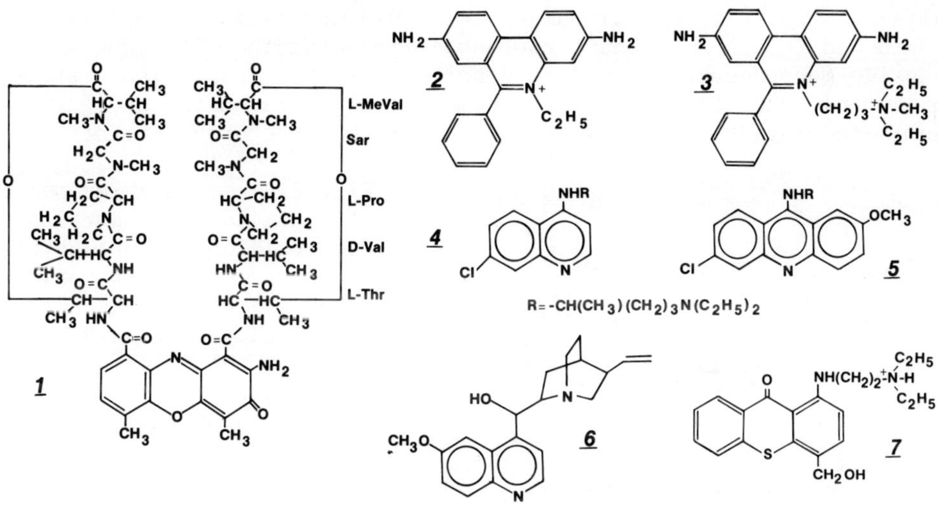

Drugs Intercalate from the Minor Groove of DNA - Actinomycin D (1) is a cyclic polypeptide-containing antibiotic which is a potent antitumor agent. The activity of the antibiotic stems from its ability to bind double-stranded DNA and inhibit RNA synthesis.[12] The interaction of actinomycin D with DNA has been studied by a variety of techniques.[13-28] When actinomycin D binds to DNA, there is a general, but not absolute, requirement for the presence of a guanine base at the interaction site. Sobell and coworkers have cocrystallized actinomycin D with its DNA substrate, deoxyguanosine, and have solved the three-dimensional structure of the complex by X-ray crystallography.[28-30] The structure of the cocrystalline complex provided an excellent basis for proposing a model for the actinomycin D-DNA binding.[30] The model involves intercalation of the phenoxazone ring system between base pairs in the DNA double helix and the utilization of specific hydrogen bonds, van der Waals forces, and hydrophobic interaction between pentapeptide chains on actinomycin D and chemical groups in the minor groove of the DNA helix. Important elements in the recognition of actinomycin D for DNA are the guanine specificity and the use of symmetry in the interaction. A mixed sugar puckering has been postulated to occur at the intercalation site of the type: C3'endo (3'-5') C2'endo.

Ethidium (2) and propidium (3) are phenanthridinium compounds which are useful as tools for binding studies of nucleic acids. Of the two, ethidium is a well-established drug in widespread use for the chemotherapy of trypanosomiasis. Propidium is not employed in chemotherapeutic practice; it has only recently become of interest for its value in closed circular DNA isolation studies.[32] The medicinal action of ethidium stems from its ability to bind to DNA and RNA and to inhibit nucleic acid function.[32] The precise nature of ethidium binding to nucleic acids has been elucidated.[31-41] It is generally believed that ethidium binds to DNA (and perhaps to RNA) through intercalation. Although a variety of physical techniques have been used to provide evidence concerning intercalative binding, direct information has been provided by the single-crystal X-ray analysis of ethidium-nucleic acid crystalline complexes. Tsai, Jain and Sobell [35-38] have cocrystallized ethidium with several dinucleoside monophosphates, and have solved the three-dimensional structure of two of these (ethidium:5-iodouridylyl(3'-5')adenosine and ethidium:5-iodocytidylyl(3'-5')guanosine). Both structures demonstrate

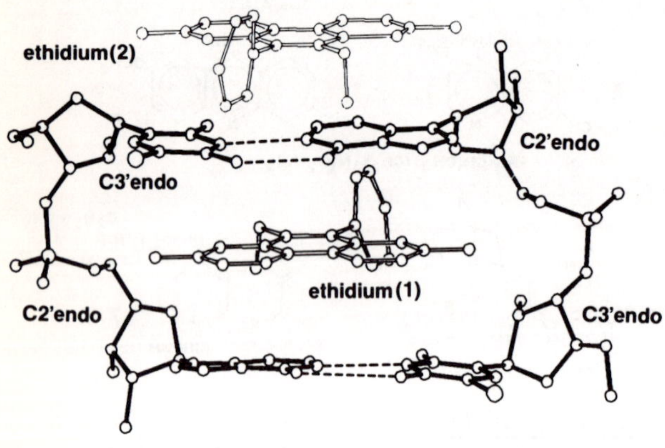

Fig. 2. A computer-graphic illustration of a portion of the ethidium:iodoUpA crystal structure viewed approximately parallel to the planes of the base-pairs and ethidium molecules. (Redrawn from Ref. 36 with permission of publisher.)

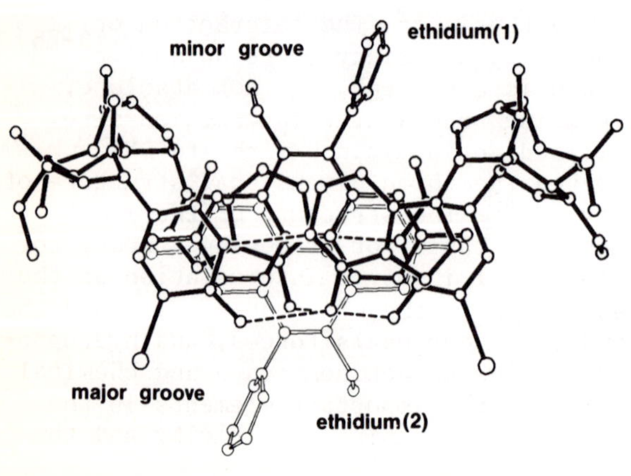

Fig. 3. A computer-graphic illustration of the ethidium: iodoUpA complex viewed perpendicular to the planes of the base-pairs and ethidium molecules. This figure illustrates the non-crystallographic 2-fold symmetry that is found in this model drug-nucleic acid interaction. (Redrawn from Ref. 36 with permission of publisher.)

drug intercalation into Watson-Crick-type double helices. In each structure, one ethidium molecule is intercalated between base pairs, while the second ethidium molecule is stacked above (and below) this intercalated base-paired dinucleoside monophosphate structure. The phenyl and ethyl substitutents of the intercalated ethidium molecule lie in the minor groove of the double helix. Non-crystallographic 2-fold symmetry is utilized in this model drug-nucleic acid interaction; this reflects the pseudo-2-fold symmetry of the phenanthridinium ring system in ethidium coinciding with the approximate 2-fold symmetry that relates the base-paired dinucleoside monophosphates. Adjacent base-pairs within the paired dinucleoside monophosphate structure are separated by about 6.7 Å; this separation results from the intercalative binding by one ethidium molecule between base pairs. A mixed sugar puckering of the type: C3'endo (3'-5') C2'endo is observed in both structures. This sugar-phosphate conformational change partly results in the 8° twist angle that is observed between base pairs. Base-pairs are not parallel to each other, but instead are tilted about 8° to form a V-type notch that opens into the minor groove of the miniature double helix (this is best seen in the stereo picture of the intercalated complex, shown in Fig. 4). On the basis of these two structures a detailed molecular model for ethidium-DNA binding, a nearest neighbor exclusion model for intercalative drug binding to DNA, and a detailed sequence of conformational changes leading to drug-DNA intercalation have been proposed and applied to a wide range of drug-DNA interactions.[39]

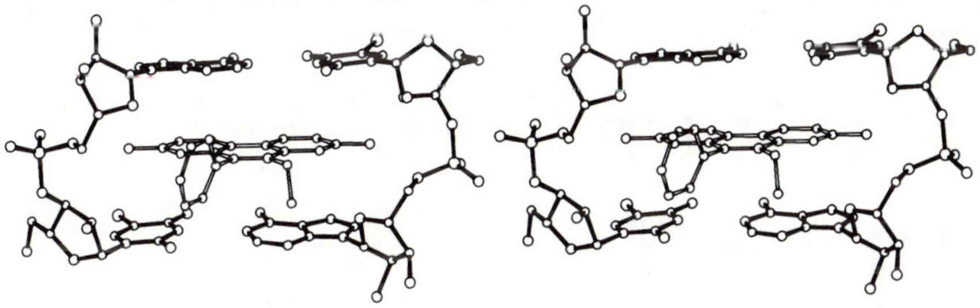

Fig. 4. Stereo pair of ethidium:iodoUpA intercalated complex, as visualized in the ethidium:iodoUpA crystal structure. (Redrawn from Ref. 37 with permission of publisher.)

The antimalarial drugs chloroquine (4), quinacrine (5), and quinine (6) have been shown to interact with DNA and to inhibit the ability of DNA to act as a template for DNA replication and for RNA synthesis.[43-45] These effects are thought to result from intercalation of the drugs with DNA and may account for part of their antimalarial activity. Hahn and coworkers[46] have shown that the probable mode of action for chloroquine involves formation of a complex with DNA through intercalation of the chloroquine aromatic ring system and interaction of the positively charged side chain with the negatively charged DNA phosphate groups. The evidence for this model, its simplicity, and the lack of a definite bioreceptor for alternative models have helped it gain widespread acceptance; chemists have used the model to design new antimalarial drugs.[44]

Hycanthone (7) has been used in the treatment of schistosomiasis.[47] The accumulated evidence suggests that hycanthone binds to DNA through intercalation in the same manner as actinomycin D and ethidium. The three-ring heterocyclic system in a planar configuration provides strong hydrophobic interaction with the DNA base pairs; the proximal nitrogen atom of the molecule has an intramolecular hydrogen bond; and the terminal nitrogen atom contributes to hycanthone activity by interacting with a phosphate group at the periphery of the DNA helix, thereby stabilizing the drug-DNA complex.[48,49]

Drugs Intercalate from the Major Groove of DNA - Daunomycin (8), adriamycin (9), and carminomycin (10) are anthracycline antibiotics that have been used in the treatment of a wide spectrum of cancer. Their biological activities have been related to their ability to interact with double-stranded DNA by intercalation.[50-55] Pigram, Fuller and Hamilton[56] have suggested a molecular model for the interaction of daunomycin with DNA, based on X-ray fiber diffraction data and molecular model-building study. They proposed that the aromatic chromophore of the drug intercalates into the DNA helix, and the sugar is hydrogen-bonded to the nucleic acid backbone through its amino group. Di Marco and his coworkers have done the majority of mechanistic studies on the anthracycline antibiotics,[57-61] and Di Marco and Arcamone[57] have recently reviewed this subject, and have suggested that DNA-adriamycin interaction involves three types of binding: hydrophobic interaction due to the intercalated aglycone, electrostatic attraction between the protonated 3'-amino group of the daunosamine and phosphate groups of the helix, and hydrogen bonds of unspecified character.

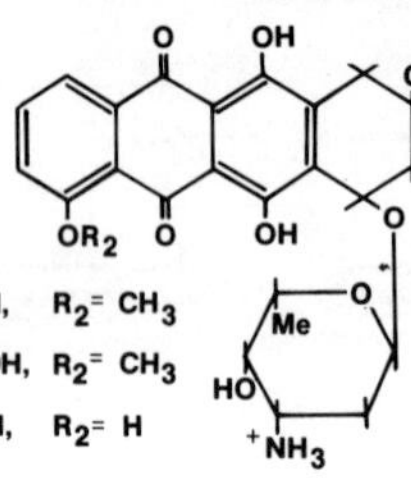

8 R_1= H, R_2= CH_3
9 R_1= OH, R_2= CH_3
10 R_1= H, R_2= H

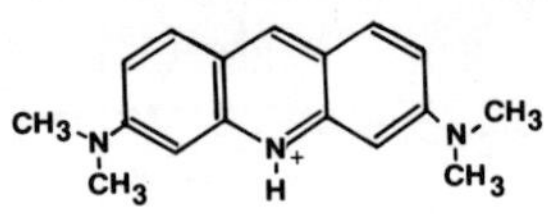

11

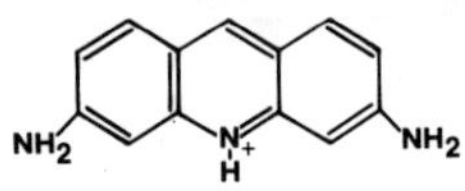

12

Acridine orange (11) and proflavine (12) are aminoacridine dyes that bind to DNA and possess mutagenic activity.[3,4] The precise nature of aminoacridine-DNA binding was proposed by Lerman[3,4] over a decade ago, who introduced the stereochemical concept of drug intercalation to explain his spectroscopic and hydrodynamic DNA-dye binding data. Recently several aminoacridine-dinucleoside monophosphate complexes have been cocrystallized and their structures have been determined by X-ray crystallographic analysis.[62-66]

The X-ray crystallographic study of acridine orange:5-iodocytidylyl-(3'-5')guanosine crystalline complex by Reddy et al.[66] demonstrates the intercalative binding by this drug to miniature Watson-Crick double-helical structure. The amino groups of the intercalated acridine lie in the major groove. A mixed sugar puckering conformation of the type: C3'endo (3'-5') C2'endo is observed in the structure.

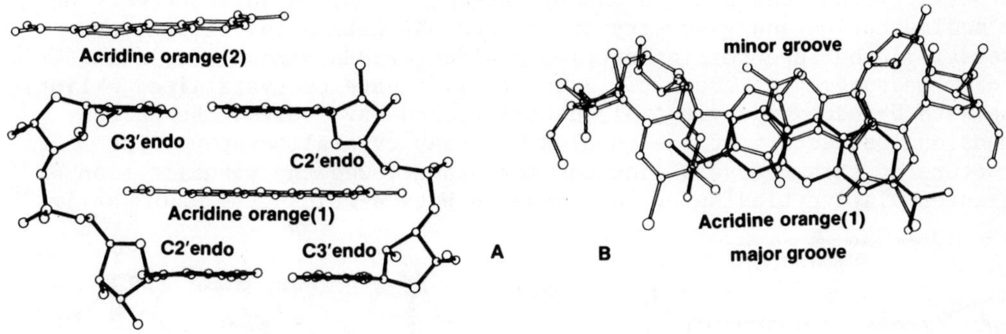

Fig. 5. Structure of acridine orange:iodoCpG complex.
(A) Viewed down the dyad axis and parallel to the planes of acridine and base-pair molecules.
(B) Viewed perpendicular to the planes of acridine and base-pair molecules.

The crystal structure of proflavine:5-iodocytidylyl(3'-5')guanosine complex (reported by Seshadri et al.[65]) and the crystal structure of proflavine:cytidylyl(3'-5')guanosine (reported by Neidle et al.[64]) both demonstrate the intercalative binding by this drug to miniature Watson-Crick double-helical structure. Some unexpected features are observed in these two structures: all the sugars are in C3'endo conformation; base-pairs in the immediate region of intercalation are twisted by about 33°.

Drugs Intercalate from either the Major or Minor Grooves of DNA - 9-Aminoacridine (13) has long been known to be a potent mutagen.[67] It is one in a general class of aminoacridine dyes that bind to DNA. The precise nature of 9-aminoacridine binding to nucleic acids has been elucidated.[3,4] The structure analysis of 9-aminoacridine:5-iodocytidylyl(3'-5')guanosine crystalline complex by Sakore et al.[62] demonstrates two distinct intercalative binding modes by this drug to miniature Watson-Crick double-helical structures. There are two 2:2 complexes in one crystal; each complex has an intercalated and a stacked acridine. In one complex, the intercalated 9-aminoacridine is oriented such that its amino group points toward the minor groove. For the other complex, the amino group of the intercalated acridine is oriented such that it points toward the major groove. The same C3'endo (3'-5') C2'endo mixed sugar puckering conformation is observed in both complexes.

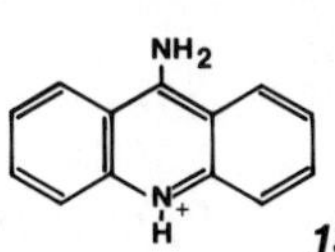

13

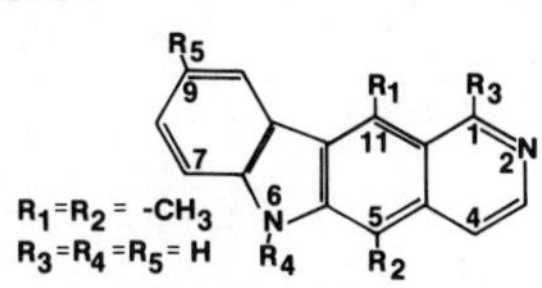

14

Ellipticine (14) is a plant alkaloid which has a planar ring structure capable of being inserted between base pairs in the DNA helix. Ellipticine has received widespread attention on account of its high anti-leukaemia activity, which is believed to be related to its ability to bind nucleic acids.[69-72] Kohn, Waring and their coworkers[73] have established that ellipticine does bind to DNA by intercalation, based on effects on the sedimentation and viscosity of sheared DNA fragments, removal and reversal of the supercoiling of closed circular DNA, and electric dichroism measurements. Recently Jain et al.[68] have cocrystallized ellipticine with 5-iodocytidylyl(3'-5')guanosine, and have solved the three-dimensional structure of the complex by X-ray crystallography. The structure of this cocrystalline complex has allowed the visualization of the intercalative binding by this drug to Watson-Crick-type double helix.[68]

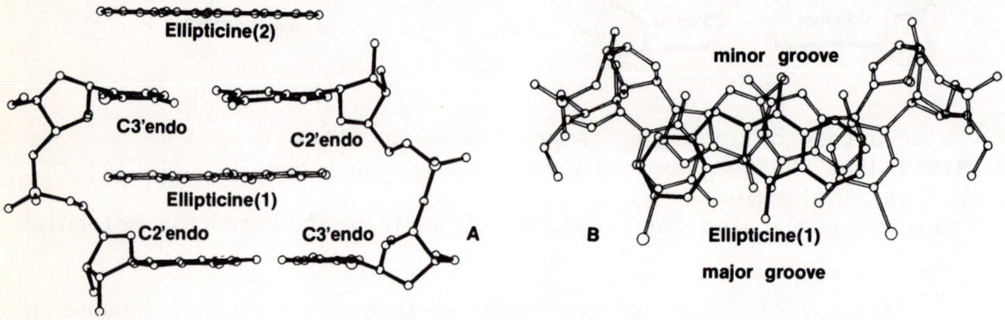

Fig. 6. Structure of ellipticine:iodoCpG complex. (A) Viewed down the dyad axis and parallel to the planes of ellipticine and base-pairs. (B) Viewed perpendicular to the planes of ellipticine and base-pairs.

References

1. I.H. Goldberg and P.A. Friedman, Ann. Rev. Biochem., 40, 775 (1971).
2. J.W. Corcoran and F.E. Hahn, Eds., "Antibiotics, Vol. III, Mechanism of Action of Antimicrobial and Antitumor Agents", Springer-Verlag, Berlin-Heidelberg-New York, 1974.
3. L.S. Lerman, J. Mol. Biol., 3, 18 (1961).
4. L.S. Lerman, Proc. Natl. Acad. Sci. USA, 49, 94 (1963).
5. A.R. Peacocke and J.N.H. Skerrett, Trans. Faraday Soc., 52, 261 (1956).
6. D.F. Bradley and M.K. Wolf, Proc. Natl. Acad. Sci. USA, 45, 944 (1959).
7. H.J. Li and D.M. Crothers, J. Mol. Biol., 39, 461 (1969).
8. J.L. Bresloff and D. M. Crothers, J. Mol. Biol., 95, 103 (1975).
9. W. Müller and D.M. Crothers, Eur. J. Biochem., 54, 267 (1975).
10. W. Müller, H. Bünemann and N. Dattagupta, Eur. J. Biochem., 54, 279 (1975).
11. D.J. Patel and L.L. Canuel, Proc. Natl. Acad. Sci. USA, 74, 2624 (1977).
12. H.M. Sobell, Prog. Nucleic Acid Res. & Mol. Biol., 13, 153 (1973).
13. M.J. Waring, J. Mol. Biol., 54, 247 (1970).
14. R.D. Wells and J.E. Larson, J. Mol. Biol., 49, 319 (1970).
15. W. Müller and D.M. Crothers, J. Mol. Biol., 35, 251 (1968).
16. T.R. Krugh, Proc. Natl. Acad. Sci. USA, 69, 1911 (1972).
17. T.R. Krugh and J.W. Neely, Biochemistry, 12, 1775 (1973).
18. T.R. Krugh and J.W. Neely, Biochemistry, 12, 4418 (1973).

19. T.R. Krugh and Y.-C. Chen, Biochemistry, 14, 4912 (1975).
20. T.R. Krugh, E.S. Mooberry and Y.-C. Chen Chiao, Biochemistry, 16, 740 (1977).
21. Y.-C. Chen Chiao and T.R. Krugh, Biochemistry, 16, 747 (1977).
22. C.G. Reinhardt and T.R. Krugh, Biochemistry, 16, 2890 (1977).
23. T. R. Krugh and M.A. Young, Nature, 269, 627 (1977).
24. D.J. Patel, Biochemistry, 13, 2396 (1974).
25. U. Hollstein, Chem. Rev., 74, 625 (1974).
26. J. Meienholer and E. Atherton, Adv. Appl. Microbiol., 16, 203 (1973).
27. J.C. Wang, Biochim. Biophys. Acta, 232, 246 (1971).
28. H.M. Sobell, S.C. Jain, T.D. Sakore and C.E. Nordman, Nature New Biol., 231, 200 (1971).
29. S.C. Jain and H.M. Sobell, J. Mol. Biol., 68, 1 (1972).
30. H.M. Sobell and S.C. Jain, J. Mol. Biol., 68, 21 (1972).
31. J.C. Wang, J. Mol. Biol., 89, 783 (1974).
32. M.J. Waring, in Ref. 2, p 141.
33. M.J. Waring, in "Topics in Infectious Diseases, Vol. 1", J. Drews and F.E. Hahn, Eds., Springer-Verlag, Wien-New York, 1974, p 77.
34. R.J. Douhart, J.P. Burnett, F.W. Beasley and B.H. Frank, Biochemistry, 12, 214 (1973).
35. C.-c. Tsai, S.C. Jain and H.M. Sobell, Phil. Trans. R. Soc. London, B 272, 137 (1975).
36. C.-c. Tsai, S.C. Jain and H.M. Sobell, Natl. Acad. Sci. USA, 72, 628 (1975).
37. C.-c. Tsai, S.C. Jain and H.M. Sobell, J. Mol. Biol., 114, 301 (1977).
38. S.C. Jain, C.-c. Tsai and H.M. Sobell, J. Mol. Biol., 114, 317 (1977).
39. H.M. Sobell, C.-c. Tsai, S.C. Jain and S.G. Gilbert, J. Mol. Biol., 114, 333 (1977).
40. T.R. Krugh, F.N. Wittlin and S.P. Cramer, Biopolymers, 14, 197 (1974).
41. T.R. Krugh and C.G. Reinhardt, J. Mol. Biol., 97, 133 (1975).
42. H.M. Sobell, C.-c. Tsai, S.G. Gilbert, S.C. Jain and T.D. Sakore, Proc. Natl. Acad. Sci. USA, 73, 3068 (1976).
43. E.J. Olmstead, J.W. Panter, D.W. Boykin, Jr. and W. D. Wilson, Biochemistry, 14, 521 (1975).
44. V.E. Mårguez, J.W. Cranston, R.W. Ruddon and J.H. Burckhalter, J. Med. Chem., 17, 856 (1974).
45. M.W. Davidson, B.G. Griggs, D.W. Boykin and W.D. Wilson, J. Med. Chem., 20, 1117 (1977).
46. F.E. Hahn, R.L. O'Brien, J. Ciak, J.L. Allison and J.G. Olenick, Mil. Med., 131, 1071 (1966).
47. D. Rosi, G. Peruzzotti, E.W. Dennis, D.A. Berberian, H. Freele, B.F. Tullar and S. Archer, J. Med. Chem., 10, 867 (1967).
48. I.B. Weinstein and E. Hirschberg, in "Progress in Molecular and Subcellular Biology", Vol. 2, F.E. Hahn, Ed., Springer-Verlag, Berlin, 1971, p 232.
49. E. Hirschberg, in Ref. 2, p 274.
50. D.W. Henry, in "Cancer Chemotherapy", A.C. Sartorelli, Ed., Am. Chem. Soc. Symp. Ser. 30, 1976, p 15.
51. A. Theologides, J.W. Yarbro and B.J. Kennedy, Cancer, 21, 16 (1968).
52. A. Rusconi and A. Di Marco, Cancer Res., 29, 1507 (1969).
53. W.D. Meriwether and N.R. Bachur, Cancer Res., 32, 1137 (1972).

54. K. Dano, S. Frederiksen and P. Hellung-Larsen, Cancer Res., 32, 1307 (1972).
55. G.F. Gauze, M.A. Sveshikova, R.S. Ukholina, G.V. Gavrilina, V.A. Filicheva and E.G. Gladkikh, Antibiotiki, 18, 675 (1973).
56. W.J. Pigram, W. Fuller and L.D. Hamilton, Nature New Biol., 235, 17 (1972).
57. A. Di Marco and F. Arcamone, Arzneimittel Forsch., 25, 368 (1975).
58. A. Di Marco, A.M. Casazza, R. Gambetta, R. Supino and F. Zunino, Cancer Res., 36, 1962 (1976).
59. F. Zunino, R. Gambetta, A. Di Marco, A. Velcich, A. Zaccara, F. Quadrifoglio and V. Crescenzi, Biochimica et Biophysica Acta, 476, 38 (1977).
60. F. Zunino, R. Cambetta, A. Di Marco, G. Luoni and A. Zaccara, Biochem. Biophy. Res. Comm., 69, 744 (1976).
61. F. Arcamone, L. Bernardi,P. Giardino, B. Patelli, A. Di Marco, A.M. Casazza, G. Pratesi and P. Reggiani, Cancer Treatment Repts., 60, 829 (1976).
62. T.D. Sakore, S.C. Jain, C.-c. Tsai and H.M. Sobell, Proc. Natl. Acad. Sci. USA, 74, 188 (1977).
63. N.C. Seeman, R.O. Day and A. Rich, Nature, 253, 324 (1975).
64. S Neidle, A. Achari, G.L. Taylor, H.M. Berman, H.L. Carrell, J.P. Glusker and W.C. Stallings, Nature, 269, 304 (1977).
65. T.P. Seshadri, T.D. Sakore, B.S. Reddy and H.M. Sobell, Amer. Cryst. Assoc. Winter Meeting, Norman, Oklahoma, Abstract F3 (1978).
66. B.S. Reddy, T.P. Seshadri, T.D. Sakore and H.M. Sobell, Amer. Cryst. Assoc. Winter Meeting, Norman, Oklahoma, Abstract F2 (1978).
67. F.H.C. Crick, L. Barnett, S. Brenner and R.J. Watts-Tobin, Nature, 192, 1227 (1961).
68. S.C. Jain, K.K. Bhandary and H.M. Sobell, Amer. Cryst. Assoc. Winter Meeting, Norman, Oklahoma, Abstract F1 (1978).
69. J. Hartwell and B. Abbott, Advan. Chemotherap. Pharmacol., 7, 117 (1969).
70. W. Kersten, H. Kersten and W. Szybalski, Biochemistry, 5, 236 (1966).
71. L.P.G. Wakelin and M.J. Waring, Mol. Pharmacol., 9, 544 (1974).
72. M.J. Waring, in "The Molecular Basis of Antibiotic Action", E. F. Gale, E. Cundiffe, P.E. Reynolds, M.H. Richmond and M.J. Waring, Eds., John Wiley and Sons, Inc., New York, 1972, p 173.
73. K.W. Kohn, M.J. Waring, D. Glaubiger and C.A. Friedman, Cancer Res., 35, 71 (1975).
74. J.B. Le Pecq, N.D. Xuong, C. Gosse and C. Paoletti, Proc. Natl. Acad. Sci. USA, 71, 5078 (1974).
75. H.M. Sobell, Cancer Chemother. Rep., 58, 101 (1974).
76. P.B. Dervan and M.M. Becker, Abstracts, The Amer. Chem. Soc. 175th National Meeting, Anaheim, California, March 12-17, 1978, Abstract ORGN 005; Chem. & Eng. News, 56, 22 (1978).
77. M.J. Waring and L.P.G. Wakelin, Nature, 252, 653 (1974).
78. L.P.G. Wakelin and M.J. Waring, Biochem. J., 157, 721 (1976).
79. J.B. Le Pecq, M. Le Bret, J. Barbet and B. Roques, Proc. Natl. Acad. Sci. USA, 72, 2915 (1975).

ISBN 0-12-040513-X

A B C 8 D 9 E 0 F 1 G 2 H 3